ILLUSTRATED PHARMACOLOGY
FOR NURSES

ILLUSTRATED PHARMACOLOGY
FOR NURSES

Terje Simonsen MD, Specialist in Clinical Pharmacology & Chief Physician, Department of Clinical Pharmacology, University Hospital of Tromsø, Norway

Jarle Aarbakke MD, Professor of Pharmacology, University of Tromsø, Specialist in Clinical Pharmacology, Department of Clinical Pharmacology, University Hospital of Tromsø, Norway

Ian Kay PhD, Department of Biological Sciences, Manchester Metropolitan University, Manchester, UK

Paul Sinnott RGN, BSc (Hons), Division of Medicine (Acute Medicine), Manchester Royal Infirmary, Manchester, UK

Iain Coleman PhD, Biomedical Sciences Division, School of Applied Sciences, University of Wolverhampton, Wolverhampton, UK

Illustrated by **Roy Lysaa** Dr (Scient), Post. Doc. Pharmacology, Institute of Pharmacy, University of Tromsø, Norway

Hodder Arnold

A MEMBER OF THE HODDER HEADLINE GROUP

First published in two volumes in Norway in 1997 by
Fagbokforlaget Vigmostad & Bjørke AS
Published in two volumes in Denmark in 1999 by Glydendalske Boghandel,
Nordisk Forlag A/S
Published in two volumes in Sweden in 2001 by
Bokforlaget Natur och Kultur
This edition published in 2006 by
Hodder Arnold, an imprint of Hodder Education and a member of the
Hodder Headline Group,
338 Euston Road, London NW1 3BH

http://www.hoddereducation.com

Distributed in the United States of America by
Oxford University Press Inc.,
198 Madison Avenue, New York, NY10016
Oxford is a registered trademark of Oxford University Press

© 2006 Terje Simonsen, Jarle Aarbakke, Roy Lysaa, Ian Kay, Paul Sinnott, Iain Coleman

Whilst the advice and information in this book are believed to be true and
accurate at the date of going to press, neither the author[s] nor the publisher
can accept any legal responsibility or liability for any errors or omissions
that may be made. In particular (but without limiting the generality of the
preceding disclaimer) every effort has been made to check drug dosages;
however it is still possible that errors have been missed. Furthermore,
dosage schedules are constantly being revised and new side-effects
recognized. For these reasons the reader is strongly urged to consult the
drug companies' printed instructions before administering any of the drugs
recommended in this book.

British Library Cataloguing in Publication Data
A catalogue record for this book is available from the British Library

Library of Congress Cataloging-in-Publication Data
A catalog record for this book is available from the Library of Congress

ISBN-10   0 340 80972 8
ISBN-13   978 0 340 80972 3

1 2 3 4 5 6 7 8 9 10

Commissioning Editor: Georgina Bentliff/Clare Christian
Project Editor: Clare Patterson
Production Controller: Jane Lawrence
Cover Designer: Nichola Smith
Indexer: Laurence Errington

Typeset in 10/12 pts Minion by Charon Tec Ltd, Chennai, India
www.charontec.com
Printed and bound in Italy

What do you think about this book? Or any other Hodder Arnold title?
Please send your comments to www.hoddereducation.com

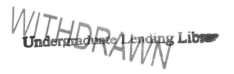

CONTENTS

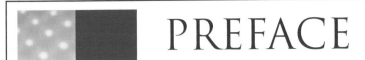

PREFACE

With our advancing understanding of the pathophysiology of diseases, drug therapy is playing an increasingly important role in the treatment and care of patients. The development of new drugs offers the possibility of an effective treatment or cure for patients who, a few years ago, could not be treated, or who were treated only to lessen their symptoms.

The correct use of drugs is a cornerstone in the modern treatment of disease. For medical staff involved in drug treatment, this means an increasing demand for drug knowledge – an understanding of the effects and side effects of drugs, individual responses to drugs, interactions with other drugs, indications for use and contraindications, as well as an understanding of how and why these effects occur. Equipped with the right information, it is possible to judge whether certain changes, expressed through specific symptoms and findings in a patient, are caused by the drug itself or caused by changes in the expression of the disease. Such knowledge is crucial in making treatment decisions, and is one of the main differences between skilled and unskilled medical staff. As a nurse you are close to the patients during your work and are in a unique position to make valuable observations. *Illustrated Pharmacology for Nurses* is a tool to help you combine these observations with your knowledge and skills in order to care for the patient effectively.

Illustrated Pharmacology for Nurses proved a great success when it was first published in 1997 in Norway. In the years that followed the book has been loved by nurse students (and medical students) all over Scandinavia after translation into Danish and Swedish. This edition brings its unique approach to English-speaking students. We hope that you enjoy it.

Good luck in learning and understanding the fascinating subject of pharmacology!

Terje Simonsen
November 2005

ACKNOWLEDGEMENTS

I would like to thank all the staff at Hodder, in particular Clare Patterson, who have made the publication of this book possible. I would also like to thank Jan, Matthew and Amy.

IK

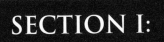

SECTION I: DRUGS AND THEIR USE

1 Drug development

The first drugs were natural products obtained from plants, minerals and animals. Today, most drugs are produced by chemical synthesis or via the use of biotechnology. Nevertheless, natural products are still an important source of some drugs.

AVAILABLE DRUGS

A total of one million drug preparations are available for use worldwide, and some individual national drug registries comprise more than 40 000 preparations. Clearly no single doctor or other health professional can be familiar with all registered drugs. In view of this, the World Health Organization (WHO) has applied both professional and economic criteria to develop a list of essential drugs and vaccines that are considered sufficient to meet most needs in most countries. Familiarity with the WHO list of about 300 drugs enables the professional to have a workable perspective on available drug treatments.

DEVELOPMENT OF NEW DRUGS

New drugs are developed to address medical need, i.e. to treat diseases for which there is no current effective treatment or to improve existing therapy. In addition, most new drugs are produced by commercial pharmaceutical companies. The selection of which candidate drugs to develop will be determined, at least in part, by the projected profit from eventual sales. A high financial return is required to cover the costs of development, manufacture, testing and marketing of the drug, as well as defraying the costs of the majority of new drugs that fail testing.

Many substances that are tested are rejected long before they reach the clinical testing stage, and few out of the many thousands of substances synthesized are put to clinical use. These extensive tests may take up to 12 years and involve costs of around £250–500 million for a new molecular entity to be approved for marketing. The patent on a new molecular entity is of 20 years' duration, and therefore a pharmaceutical company has only eight more years to sell the drug and recoup the expenditure on research and development before competitors can manufacture and sell the same compound.

REQUIREMENTS FOR EVALUATING THE EFFECTS OF DRUGS

Before 1950, few drugs were systematically tested in clinical research trials. In response to the thalidomide disaster of 1963, however, new and stricter requirements were introduced with respect to the testing required before a drug is allowed to be used clinically. A drug must be demonstrated to possess quality (purity of product), safety and efficacy.

The first step of drug development is to identify and synthesize a substance that is expected to have a therapeutic effect. Subsequently these substances undergo laboratory tests to evaluate their physical, chemical and biological properties.

If the results from preliminary tests are promising, the substance (sometimes called the lead compound) enters pre-clinical trials. There are tests to evaluate whether the substance has any toxic effect in the short term (acute toxicity) or longer term (chronic toxicity). In some cases, it is appropriate to estimate the lowest dose that can have a fatal effect. The substance is also tested to see whether it can cause fetal malformations (teratogenic effects) or genetic mutations (mutagenicity). The identification of a potential to cause such serious toxic effects would exclude that lead compound from further development.

Other tests provide data regarding the mode of action of the substance, its effects on various organs, how long the substance remains in the organism, and how it is eliminated from the organism.

Up to this point, tests are conducted in cell cultures or on laboratory animals. One weakness of animal testing is that responses of animals and humans are not directly comparable in all biochemical or physiological systems; there might be drug effects in humans not seen in animals. To improve the likelihood of identifying species-specific effects, it is important to test in both rodents and non-rodents, i.e. obtaining comparable data in two dissimilar animal models.

The collected pre-clinical data are reviewed by a panel of experts in the various disciplines. If they consider that there is sufficient evidence that the lead substance has potential for human benefit at an acceptable risk, then permission is sought to conduct clinical studies.

Box 1.1 The thalidomide disaster

The 'thalidomide disaster' was characterized by a dramatic increase in the incidence of a rare birth defect called phocomelia, a condition involving shortening or complete absence of the limbs. This effect was seen in newborns after the use of thalidomide during the first trimester by pregnant women. Thalidomide was introduced in Europe during 1957 and 1958. Based on animal tests the drug was promoted as a non-toxic hypnotic. The animal model used had different metabolic processes from those in humans. Whilst no apparent toxicity was revealed in animal studies, the drug proved very toxic to the human fetus during early pregnancy. It is estimated that more than 10,000 children were born with severe malformations caused by this drug.

THE FOUR PHASES OF CLINICAL STUDIES

Phases I, II and III are studies carried out before the drug may be marketed for general use. These studies determine whether the drug has sufficient therapeutic effects without significant toxic effects at the doses used. These first three phases are described below but it should be noted that they may overlap. Phase IV studies are post-marketing surveillance studies to monitor the drug once it is in general use.

Phase I: Drug tolerance tests

Phase I is when the drug is tested on human subjects for the first time. Generally, phase I studies involve small numbers (30–80) of healthy young adult volunteers (usually males). The purpose is to ascertain how well the substance is tolerated (i.e. any indication of unwanted side-effects) and to obtain pharmacokinetic data (how the substance is absorbed by, distributed in and eliminated by the subject). Differences in toxic effects between animals and humans are studied. Potential toxic effects are monitored from haematological and biochemical profiles, and by performing liver and renal function tests.

Phase I tests study those effects not revealed by animal research, such as symptoms rather than signs of adverse effects, and guide selection of dosages in further clinical studies. In a minority of cases, phase I tests may be conducted on patients. In the case of particularly toxic drugs, such as anti-cancer agents, it would be inappropriate to give these to healthy subjects, but may be justifiable for patients with a terminal disease for which there is no effective treatment.

Phase II: Therapeutic effect and dose adaptation

Phase II studies are conducted on small groups of patients with the disease under investigation who may benefit from treatment with the new substance. At this stage, the clinical pharmacology of the new substance is investigated in detail. The relationship between dose and therapeutic effect is determined and used to establish the optimal dose regimen – ideally the lowest effective dose which avoids adverse effects.

Phase II studies may be used to build on pre-clinical and phase I data, providing additional information on the mode of action of the test substance and its potential for interaction with other drugs. Additional phase II studies may involve specific groups, such as the elderly, if data indicate that such groups may have a different tolerance or therapeutic response to the test drug compared with the general patient population. If the review of phase II results is favourable, the drug will progress to phase III. A common reason for ceasing development at the end of phase II is lack of expected efficacy.

Phase III: Confirmation of effect on larger groups of patients

Phase III studies are usually conducted on a large number of patients (300–3000) distributed at several regional centres; to ensure sufficient patients, large phase III studies are often conducted at centres in a number of countries. Such a large total of patients is required to give the study sufficient statistical power to detect clinically relevant effects. The testing procedure (the study protocol) is the same at all centres. Selection and allocation of patients to different treatment groups are carried out according to strict scientific criteria in double-blind randomized trials. These trial designs eliminate potential selection bias in conducting the study and ensure that measurement and recording of effects are objective.

The purpose of phase III studies is to confirm the effects discovered in earlier phases, and to find the frequency of adverse drug effects in the target patient population under conditions close to anticipated general use. As phase III studies have larger treated populations and are of longer duration than phase II trials, it is likely that more drug-related adverse reactions will be observed as new events during this phase.

This phase generates the key clinical trial data required for licensing. Studies compare the new substance with placebo, the best available treatment or another leading drug.

At the conclusion of phase III, a report is submitted summarizing results from all the clinical trials. This report is the basis for an application for registration of the substance as a drug. After thorough evaluation of the data by independent experts, the drug may be approved by a regulatory body such as the United Kingdom Committee for the Safety of Medicines (UK CSM), the European Agency for the Evaluation of Medical Products (EMEA) or the US Food and Drug Administration (FDA).

Phase IV: Post-marketing studies

Once approved, the drug may be used to treat patients. However, the effects of a drug continue to be monitored after it has been registered. Clinical trials conducted with registered drugs are termed phase IV studies. Additional trials might be required to enable sales in a particular country, e.g. data comparing efficacy against a comparator drug different from that used in phase III. Any changes in the instructions for use on the registered label must be justified by clinical trial data. These studies would aim to demonstrate that proposed changes do not compromise the efficacy and safety properties of the drug which allowed its original registration. Any claim made about the drug in promotional material must be justified by clinical trial data, and additional clinical trials may be required to support a new claim for the product.

Many phase IV studies are conducted to furnish additional safety data. Severe adverse drug reactions might only occur in a small proportion of the treated population, typically between 1 in 10 000 and 1 in 100 000 patients. As the exposed population in phases I to III would only amount to a total of 10 000 patients, there is a low probability of any of these events occurring prior to registration of the drug. Accordingly, there may be phase IV studies which generate safety data from a large group of patients, e.g. in international multicentre studies set up to ensure sufficient patients to observe rarer events.

Other safety information may be gained by spontaneous reports, such as practitioners using the 'Yellow Cards' supplied at the back of the *British National Formulary* (BNF) to inform of suspected adverse reactions to newly marketed drugs. If new, important information arises about specific patient groups, the range of indication for the drug could be extended. However, such an extension would require submission of a new application to the authorities. Sometimes, permission to sell the drug is withdrawn, or the manufacturers themselves may decide to withdraw the drug from the market if serious adverse drug reactions are discovered. The increase in risk of serious cardiovascular events (coronary heart diseases and strokes) caused by long-term use of COX-2 inhibitors is an example of reporting of unwanted effects obtained in phase IV studies of drugs.

Examples of important treatment regimes established by phase IV studies
- In patients with cardiac failure, it has been shown that the use of angiotensin-converting enzyme (ACE) inhibitors reduces the need for hospital admissions and reduces mortality.
- Use of small doses of aspirin in patients with angina pectoris reduces the risk of myocardial infarction (MI), and that of stroke in at-risk patients.
- Blood pressure-reducing treatment with β-blockers, diuretics, calcium inhibitors and ACE inhibitors reduces the risk of MI and serious cardiovascular episodes in patients with hypertension.
- Insulin treatment in type 1 diabetics reduces the risk of retinopathy and nephropathy.

ETHICS AND DRUG TESTING

USE OF ANIMALS IN MEDICAL RESEARCH

The use of animals in the testing of drugs raises a number of issues. Some people feel that the killing of, or the causing of pain or discomfort to, caged animals to gain drug test information is unwarranted. This could be circumvented by ceasing new drug development or using products that have never been tested in animals. However, people expect improving standards of health care, which require new drugs of greater efficacy, but with no reduction of safety standards. Governments mandate the pharmaceutical industry to develop new drugs and require that tests for efficacy and safety are performed to acceptable procedures. At present, until the development of non-animal systems of sufficient sensitivity and reliability, these legally required data must include animal test data.

In animal testing, however, there are strict legal requirements; the test methods used should cause animals the minimum pain or distress. Even so, some tests will involve some discomfort or distress, in particular when determining toxic doses or in some long-term tests. The onus is on the experimenter to intervene and humanely kill any animal experiencing severe distress. All animals are killed humanely at the end of the experiment and in long-term studies there are pathology examinations in order to determine whether they had developed macroscopic or microscopic organ changes after exposure to the test substance.

There is an emphasis on the 'three Rs' of animal experimentation: refine, reduce and replace, so that new procedures will be developed that will enable testing of drugs that reduces the overall use of animals. One example is the increased use of computer models to simulate reactions between drugs and receptors to enable development decisions.

MEDICAL RESEARCH IN HUMANS

Medical research in humans must be conducted in an ethical manner. It is governed by law and may only proceed after approval from an appropriate independent ethics committee. In a particular area, these are often based in hospitals and, in the UK, are referred to as local research ethics committees (LRECs). Other ethics committees operate nationally. Depending on the scope of the study, it may require both national and local ethics approval for research to proceed. The ethical principles that apply to the use of humans in medical research are stated in the Declaration of Helsinki (from 1952, with subsequent revisions). This states that consideration of the risks and benefits to patients and volunteers overrides scientific considerations; participants in a study should expect at least the possibility of clinical benefit to themselves by consenting to join the trial. It is essential that participation in clinical research is voluntary. The participants must be informed about the nature of the test procedures and the therapeutic and adverse effects of the test drugs. Patients are made aware that they can withdraw from the study at any time, for any reason, without compromising their current or future medical treatment. This information must be provided in oral and written form. If they agree, each participant signs a statement confirming that the trial has been explained, they have understood and are participating voluntarily. This is termed 'giving informed consent'.

Some groups of patients are deemed incapable of providing informed consent: those below the age of adult responsibility or who are incapable of understanding the trial procedures, e.g. due to a mental handicap. In these instances, consent is provided by a parent or other person responsible for that individual. It is a major responsibility of ethics committees to ensure that procedures for obtaining informed consent are appropriate before any clinical trial is permitted to proceed.

Clinical trials are designed to obtain information while minimizing risk to the participants. Particular patient groups may have a greater risk of more severe harm from a drug-related adverse reaction; for example, children and the elderly may be less robust than adults, while exposure of pregnant women introduces an additional risk of harm to the fetus. Consequently, these three groups are routinely excluded from most clinical trials. Women of child-bearing potential are required to use contraception during participation in clinical trials. Any individuals who nonetheless become pregnant during the trial are immediately withdrawn from treatment and there is safety surveillance of the pregnancy to postpartum. Clinical trials are conducted with vulnerable groups when there is a specific need for information to permit use of the drug in those groups. For example, trials may be conducted in children and the elderly but only when the drug already has a strong safety database from adult trials. Clinical trials in pregnant women are only warranted for drugs that are intended to treat complications of pregnancy and where there is strong evidence, e.g. from reproductive studies in animals, that there is a low risk of fetal harm.

NEW MOLECULAR ENTITIES, 'ME TOO' DRUGS AND GENERICS

There is competition between drug companies in developing new drugs and in being able to sell the drug even after the patent protection has elapsed.

NEW MOLECULAR ENTITIES

A new drug (not previously manufactured by others) is called a 'new molecular entity' (NME). NMEs can be protected by patent rules. This means that others cannot manufacture the drug until the patent protection has lapsed. In the UK, patent protection is valid for 20 years from the initial patenting of the original compound. The purpose of patenting a drug is so the developer will have the exclusive right to manufacture it and the opportunity to recover the costs of development and yield a return on investment.

'ME TOO' DRUGS AND GENERICS

'Me too' products refer to the generation of drugs with as few chemical differences from an existing product that can be achieved without infringing patent rights. Here the intention is to capture a portion of an existing market by patients switching to a newer, apparently better product. In fact, the therapeutic benefits of the new drug are likely to be marginal and there is no guarantee that the new product will be cheaper or exhibit the same or lesser side-effects. One of the aims of the UK's National Institute of Clinical Excellence (NICE) committee is to discourage the production of 'me too' drugs by only allowing the use of new drugs in the National Health Service when these show an improvement in efficacy compared with current therapies.

With the lapse of a drug's patent, other companies may then manufacture that drug using the same manufacturing process or another method. These products are referred to as generic drugs and are often sold at considerably lower prices than the NME. Lower prices are possible because the development costs are low and/or the generic manufacturer has an improved synthetic method that reduces production costs. Frequently, once the generic is available, the manufacturer of the NME responds by reducing prices to maintain sales. Generic drugs lead to competition, resulting in lower costs for the individual patient and the authorities alike.

SUMMARY

- The goal of new drug development is to treat diseases for which there is no effective treatment, or to improve existing therapy. Development must also be economically viable, covering costs and yielding a return on investment.
- New drugs undergo thorough tests, particularly with regard to toxicity, safety and quality, before they are permitted in clinical studies.
- Long-term studies on large patient groups may be necessary to discover rare adverse drug reactions and long-term effects.
- The use of animals in drug development is strictly regulated to minimize their suffering.
- The Declaration of Helsinki describes the ethical principles that apply to clinical research in humans. All participants in clinical studies must have given written informed consent before the test procedures begin. Testing of drugs on children, pregnant women, the mentally handicapped and the elderly is rare due to ethical reasons.
- A newly developed drug is referred to as a new molecular entity (NME). 'Me too' is the term for a drug that is manufactured to mimic the properties of an existing product. Once patent protection for a drug has ceased, other companies may manufacture the same product (a generic) which competes for sales with the NME.

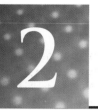

2 Regulation and management of drug therapy and drug errors

Drugs are potent substances that can cause great damage if they are not correctly used and monitored by highly trained personnel. This is the reason why there are laws and regulations closely governing the use of drugs.

REGULATIONS REGARDING THE USE OF DRUGS

In the UK there are several Acts of Parliament that regulate the medical and illicit use of drugs:

- The Medicines Act 1968
- The Misuse of Drugs Act 1971
- NHS Regulations.

The Medicines Act 1968, and subsequent secondary legislation, provides a legal framework for the manufacture, licensing, prescription, dispensing and administration of medicines. In England, the Medicines and Healthcare Products Regulatory Agency (MHRA) is tasked with safeguarding public health and ensuring that appropriate standards are in place to maintain the safety, quality and efficacy of all human medicine. There are similar bodies in Scotland, Northern Ireland and Wales and most other countries.

PROFESSIONAL REGULATIONS REGARDING THE MANAGEMENT OF DRUGS

All health care professionals who are involved in the prescription, dispensing or administration of medication will have explicit standards set out by their professional bodies, e.g. the Nursing and Midwifery Council's (2004) *Guidelines for the Administration of Medicine*. For an in-depth explanation of a health professional's responsibilities in the area of drug administration, these documents should be consulted.

The prescriber's responsibility

Prescription of a drug is, in the majority of cases, a medical responsibility and requires the use of sound clinical and pharmacological knowledge and experience. However, following the Medicinal Products: Prescription by Nurses etc. Act 1992, increasing numbers of nurses are responsible for prescribing from a *Nurse Prescribers' Formulary*. At present, nurse prescribing is found overwhelmingly in the primary care setting, although this will undoubtedly change over time. In 2004, the Nursing and Midwifery Council (NMC) published guiding principles in relation to prescriptions, stating that a prescription should:

- be based wherever possible on informed consent
- be clearly written and indelible
- clearly identify the patient for whom the medication is intended
- clearly state the substance to be administered, together with strength, dosage, timing, frequency of administration, start and finish dates and route of administration
- be signed and dated by the prescriber
- not be a substance to which the patient is known to be allergic.

The nurse's responsibility

The NMC clearly states that registered nurses, midwives or specialist community public health nurses are accountable for their own acts or omissions. They go on to highlight that in administering any medication, or assisting or overseeing any self-administration, nurses must exercise their professional judgment and apply both knowledge and skills to the given situation. The NMC has published key principles in relation to the administration of medication, which suggest that the nurse must:

- know the therapeutic uses of the medicine to be administered, its normal dosage, side-effects, precautions and contraindications
- be certain of the identity of the patient to whom the medicine is to be administered
- check that the prescription, or the label on the medicine dispensed by a pharmacist, is clearly written and unambiguous
- have considered the dosage, method of administration, route and timing of the administration in the context of the condition of the patient and coexisting therapies
- check the expiry date of the medicine to be administered
- check that the patient is not allergic to the medicine before administering it
- contact the prescriber or another authorized prescriber without delay where contraindications to the prescribed medicine are discovered, where the patient develops a reaction to the medicine, or where assessment of the patient indicates that the medicine is no longer suitable
- make a clear, accurate and immediate record of all medicine administered, intentionally withheld or refused by the patient, ensuring that any written entries and the signature are clear and legible.

It is also the nurse's responsibility to ensure that a record is made when delegating the task of administering medicine.

MANAGEMENT OF DRUG THERAPY

A drug is prescribed after careful consideration of its beneficial and harmful effects in relation to the symptoms caused by the disease. To achieve an optimal effect, one must constantly re-evaluate the treatment, and there are both clinical and laboratory tests available to help in this evaluation.

CLINICAL EVALUATION OF EFFECTS AND ADVERSE EFFECTS

The most important element in the evaluation of positive and adverse effects of a drug is a thorough clinical evaluation of the patient. This evaluation requires a good patient history, clinical examination and close observation. Everyone who participates in the treatment is, in his or her own way, responsible for seeing that the best possible results are achieved. Health workers thus have an important task in observing the positive and possible adverse effects of drugs.

In evaluating the benefit of a drug, one must ask whether the drug is necessary and consider the risk of not taking it. The more serious adverse effects that a drug has, the more important it is to come to a rational decision regarding the risk in question.

Observation of the patient

Many patients commence drug therapy during a hospital stay. When evaluating the effects of a particular drug, it is assumed the drug has been taken as prescribed. It is equally important to assess the therapeutic effects of the drug as well as any possible adverse effects; for example:

- Do temperature and C-reactive protein (CRP) fall during treatment of an infectious disease?
- Does urine production increase in a patient who receives diuretics?
- How is the blood pressure altered by antihypertensive medication?
- Do the symptoms improve with treatment for cardiac failure?

Drugs administered by intravenous injection or infusion cause a rapid increase in drug concentration within the blood. With this route of administration, it is particularly important to be aware of any undesired effects immediately after administration. Adverse effects of an allergic nature (anaphylactic shock) can develop quickly. Likewise, there can be disturbances in the heart rhythm with a significant fall in blood pressure, palpitations and loss of consciousness. Some individuals can experience central nervous effects such as dizziness, feelings of being unwell and anxiety, which can be observed by sudden changes in the patient's behaviour.

Within a hospital environment, patients are closely supervised when commencing new drug therapies and all personnel involved in the prescription and administration of drugs should be aware of possible adverse effects. In a primary care setting, patient observation is much reduced, so it is of paramount important that patients and their carers are aware of any possible adverse effects, and of the signs and symptoms of such effects.

Patient history

Some patients are reluctant to disclose information about any unpleasant adverse effects they are experiencing, particularly if no-one asks. In some cases, these adverse effects will result in patients modifying the drug dose or even stopping taking the drug altogether. It is important to obtain a thorough and accurate history from patients with regard to their illness and medication history, as they can often provide valuable information about symptoms such as dizziness, listlessness, dryness of the mouth and constipation when asked. Remember that patients do not always ascribe new problems to their use of drugs.

Clinical examination

The effects of some drugs can be evaluated by clinical examination; some examples of this are as follows:

- The treatment of hypertension is titrated to blood pressure and pulse rate.
- The treatment of cardiac failure is evaluated by the clinical resolution of symptoms such as peripheral oedema and breathlessness (pulmonary oedema).
- The effectiveness of drug treatments for glaucoma can be measured by the determination of intraocular pressure (pressure within the eye).

LABORATORY TESTS

Laboratory tests are an important component in the evaluation of drug therapy. Many drugs have organ-specific effects that cannot be detected by normal observation, patient history or clinical examination. They may, for example, have harmful effects on the bone marrow's production of blood cells, on kidney and liver function, on the central nervous system or on other organs. Laboratory tests can be helpful in discovering such effects before they manifest themselves as clinical symptoms.

X-rays of the lungs before and after drug treatment of pneumonia are very useful in evaluating the effect of antibiotics. Stress electrocardiograms (ECGs) in the treatment of angina pectoris and gastroscopies in the treatment of stomach ulcers can offer similar benefits.

The most frequently used measurements to evaluate benefits and adverse effects, and the improvement or progression of disease are blood tests, as these can demonstrate normal and abnormal values of endogenous substances (clinical chemical analyses). The most commonly used tests measure levels of haemoglobin, leucocytes, platelets, liver enzymes, creatinine, urea and blood sugar. Disturbances in the electrolyte or acid–base balance also provide important information. During treatment with the anticoagulant warfarin, it is useful to measure the clotting tendency of the blood (INR – internationalized ratio) to evaluate its effect and monitor for adverse signs and decide the correct dose.

In a number of chronic diseases and long-term drug therapy, it can often be important to measure drug concentration levels directly to evaluate the need for dose adjustment.

Therapeutic drug monitoring

There are several possible situations where it may be beneficial to directly measure plasma drug concentrations, as follows:

- in conditions where there is a clear correlation between the concentrations of a drug and its effects/adverse effects
- where a concentration range is established for which the majority of users experience the desired outcome without serious adverse effects
- if the drug has serious adverse effects above a certain concentration.

Another possible reason to take measurements is to discover whether a patient is actually taking a prescribed drug (assess compliance).

For these reasons, drug analyses are only performed in a minority of cases. For the majority of drugs prescribed, dosage is modified according to standard dosage regimes and a clinical evaluation of the drug's impact on the development of the disease and any adverse effects.

Drug analyses to monitor drug therapy, or the severity of acute poisoning, are best performed on plasma, as the concentration in blood is the most accurate indicator when evaluating the need to adjust the dose, or whether other measures are required.

Measurement of drug concentration in urine is not suitable, since varying urine volumes will result in a varying concentration of the drug in the urine. In addition, drugs that are metabolized in the liver and which are largely eliminated in the bile through the intestine are not accurately measured in the urine. Blood tests determining plasma drug concentrations are usually taken before the next planned dose (trough levels). This is more thoroughly discussed in Chapter 10.

GROUPS OF DRUGS THAT REQUIRE MONITORING OF CONCENTRATION LEVEL

For drugs with a narrow therapeutic range, i.e. little difference between the concentration that produces the desired effect and that which causes serious adverse effects, drug concentration measurements are important.

Cardiovascular drugs

Digitalis glycosides are a group of drugs that were once the mainstay treatment for heart failure. These drugs have unpleasant and dangerous adverse effects in high concentrations, particularly when plasma potassium levels are low. Several drugs used for treating heart rhythm disturbances can themselves cause life-threatening arrhythmias if they are present in too high a concentration.

Antiepileptics

Antiepileptics have a narrow therapeutic range. They are also the drug group that most affects the elimination of other drugs, by causing enzyme induction or inhibition. Phenytoin demonstrates saturation kinetics when used at high doses, such that a small increase in dosage can result in a considerable rise in plasma concentration. Plasma concentration should be measured following a change in dose or commencement of a drug with the potential for interaction. One such example is the use of antiepileptics with the anticoagulant warfarin. Some antiepileptics can reduce or increase the elimination of warfarin, and lead to either possible haemorrhage or thrombosis.

Antidepressants and psychopharmaceuticals

Standard dosing of tricyclic antidepressants and antipsychotics produces significant individual variations in drug concentration. The differences are associated with the individual's ability to metabolize these drugs. It has been shown that the therapeutic effect diminishes with high concentrations and that the adverse effects increase rapidly. Measurement of drug concentration is therefore important for this drug group. In addition, drug concentration measurements can be used to evaluate compliance to prescription regimes in patients who are known to be non-compliant.

Antibiotics

High concentrations of aminoglycosides damage the kidneys, the auditory nerve and the balance (vestibular) organ over time. It is often important to measure both peak (1 h post-dose) and trough levels (1 h pre-dose), as some antibiotics are dependent on a minimum concentration for effect.

Cytotoxic drugs

Methotrexate is currently the only cytotoxic drug that is measured routinely. However, there is reason to assume that the optimal drug effect on cancer cells is determined by concentrations within certain ranges and at certain stages in the cell cycle. New regimes are likely to be established regarding the dosing of several of the cytotoxics that are currently being used in high concentrations for short periods of time.

DRUG ERRORS

Drug errors can occur at any time from when the drug is prescribed to its administration. At best, mistakes can place patients at risk; at worst, they can be fatal. The cause of drug errors can be attributed to both the health professional and the patient. When using drugs with potent effects, it is even more important to have a raised awareness, in order to avoid potential errors. The same applies when administering drugs to small children, the elderly and unconscious patients.

RESPONSIBILITIES OF HEALTH PROFESSIONALS

Doctors, nurses and other health care professionals can make mistakes in prescribing, preparing and administering drugs. All members of the health care team therefore have a responsibility to reduce the risk of drug errors.

The prescriber

Individuals who prescribe drugs are expected to make a careful assessment of the need for treatment and to be observant when selecting drugs, drug formulations, doses and dosing intervals. The prescriber should also assess whether patients are capable of managing the medication on their own or whether they require help.

Barely legible handwriting and poor user instructions on prescriptions can be sources of error. The name of the drug must be written clearly, using its generic name where possible.

The administrator

Nurses or others who administer drugs to patients are responsible for ensuring that the prescription is followed. Health professionals should be aware of the indications, normal doses and possible adverse effects of any drug they are administering. This will ensure that, if a prescription contains obvious mistakes or indicates unreasonable doses, the error will be highlighted.

Drug calculations

A lack of knowledge about how to calculate drug dosages can result in serious mistakes in the preparation of drugs, particularly intravenous drugs. Therefore, before nurses administer drugs they must be able to perform simple drug calculations, e.g.:

- calculation of the correct dilution required for certain intravenous preparations
- calculation of the volume that must be administered so the patient receives a certain dose of drug per time unit
- calculation of the dose to be administered when it is given in, for example, mg/kg body weight.

Decimal point errors are the most serious mistakes in these calculations and can lead to the patient receiving 10 times too large a dose, or only a tenth of the dose. To minimize the risk of calculation errors, they should always be checked by two people.

Patient observation

The close observation of patients following the administration of medication is an important part of safe drug administration. Poor or a complete lack of observation of a patient for the effects of a drug can mean that dangerous or ineffective treatments are not stopped, and that necessary adjustments are not made. One should observe the patient particularly closely when treating with toxic drugs and when drugs are administered by intravenous injection or infusion.

The reporting of drug errors

It is important that an open culture exists to encourage and support the reporting of drug errors in all areas where drugs are prescribed and administered. It is absolutely crucial that all such errors are reported immediately to protect patient safety.

PATIENT COMPLIANCE

'Compliance' is the extent to which patients follow instructions (the prescribed drug therapy). In relation to drug therapy, the patient is compliant if he or she cooperates fully in taking a prescribed medication following medical recommendations.

Even if a proposed drug treatment is the optimal choice for a disease, it will not be effective if the patient does not cooperate and follow the prescribed instructions for the drug. When dose adjustment or a change of drug is thought necessary, such an evaluation is usually made on the presumption that the patient has taken the drug as prescribed. But if the patient is noncompliant the decision to change treatment will have been made on a false assumption.

Causes of noncompliance

Studies have shown that patients are often noncompliant. There are many possible reasons for noncompliance:

- the patient suffers adverse effects
- the patient does not think the drug is effective
- the patient forgets to take the drug
- the patient believes the disease is cured because the symptoms have abated
- the patient has misunderstood the user instructions
- the patient has run out of the drug
- the patient does not master the administration technique, e.g. inhalation
- the drug formulation is unsuitable
- the drug is unacceptable, e.g. unpleasant taste
- the patient uses many drugs simultaneously (polypharmacy)
- frequent dosages
- the patient has other objections towards the use of a certain drug.

Polypharmacy

The occurrence of disease increases with age. Many elderly patients therefore use several drugs simultaneously (polypharmacy). See Figure 2.1. For some, it can be difficult to remember the different time intervals for taking different drugs. Elderly subjects may sometimes also have difficulty understanding information and following user instructions.

Another group of patients who may be using many drugs simultaneously, and which may lead to noncompliance, are the chronically ill. It is important in this situation to ensure that all drug prescriptions are necessary and to consider stopping a drug where there are no clear indications for its use. This can help to minimize the problems associated with polypharmacy and also to reduce the chances of misuse and adverse effects.

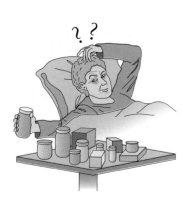

Figure 2.1 Polypharmacy contributes to noncompliance.

If noncompliance is discovered, one must try to ascertain the reason for it, by carefully questioning the patient. If the reason centres on unacceptable adverse effects, other preparations should be considered.

Situations where compliance is important

There are several situations where compliance is of even greater importance than normal:

- when using drugs with a narrow therapeutic range
- when using drugs that may produce serious adverse effects (e.g. cytotoxics, immunosuppressives and anticoagulants)
- with hormone supplementation (e.g. metabolic disease, diabetes, adrenal failure)
- in the treatment of glaucoma and epilepsy
- in the treatment of certain infections, e.g. when treating multidrug-resistant tuberculosis.

Measures to improve compliance

An informed, motivated patient is the best guarantee that a patient will be compliant with the prescribed therapy. It is therefore important to inform patients about why a particular drug has been chosen. This is particularly true if they are likely to experience adverse effects or if they will be expected to take the treatment over a long period of time.

Information

The information about why a particular drug has been chosen should contain the following:

- what drug is to be used
- how the drug is taken
- when the drug is to be administered
- the importance of taking the drug and what happens if it is not taken
- how long the drug is to be used
- what adverse effects can be expected
- the alternatives available.

A patient information leaflet containing all the above points should be included in all drug packaging.

General measures that can improve compliance

- Consider the use of dosette boxes.
- Let relatives, the community nurse or home help dispense the drugs.
- Find a suitable time of the day for administration, e.g. evening doses are not suitable for diuretics.
- Use depot forms to reduce the dosage frequency.
- Use suitable administration aids, e.g. for liquid forms of drugs (measuring cups, graduated syringes).
- Provide patients with written information about the therapy.

SUMMARY

■ Drugs are potent substances that can be harmful if they are not correctly used and monitored by highly trained personnel.

■ There are both legal and professional regulations ensuring the safe use of drugs.

■ Observation, patient history and clinical examination are important in assessing whether a drug has the desired effect.

■ Drug analyses are performed in the following cases:
  – for drugs with a clear correlation between concentration in the blood and effect
  – for drugs with a narrow therapeutic range
  – for drugs with serious adverse effects
  – for assessing whether a patient is taking a prescribed drug (compliance).

■ Drug errors can occur at any time between prescription and administration.

■ Compliance is defined by the patient's ability and will to follow medical advice.

■ Informing the patient about the drug prescribed is one of the most important factors in achieving compliance.

■ Patient compliance decreases with polypharmacy.

3

Classification and nomenclature of drugs

Drugs are classified according to different systems; functional classifications, classifications according to source of origin, chemical classifications and classifications based on generic names. Another classification system is according to prescription, based on the drug's potential for addiction and subsequent abuse.

CLASSIFICATION OF DRUGS ACCORDING TO PRESCRIPTION

In the UK, the regulations controlling the supply of medicines fall into four categories:

- prescription-only medicine controlled drug (POM CD)
- prescription-only medicine (POM)
- pharmacy-only medicine (P)
- general sale list (GSL).

The POM CD category is the most strictly controlled of the four, and the GSL category is the least strictly controlled.

Controlled drugs (POM CD)

These are medicines that have the potential for addiction and subsequent abuse. As stated in the *British National Formulary*: 'The Misuse of Medicines Act (1971) prohibits certain activities in relation to "Controlled Drugs", in particular their manufacture, supply, and possession.' These drugs are graded, fairly broadly, on the basis of their potential to cause harm when they are misused. They are defined in three classes:

- class A drugs, such as cocaine, diamorphine and pethidine, and class B substances prepared for injection
- class B drugs, such as oral amphetamines, barbiturates and pentazocine
- class C drugs, such as androgenic and anabolic steroids, cannabis and benzphetamine.

The Misuse of Drugs Regulations 2001 define the classes of individuals authorized to supply and process controlled drugs. Reference to listing in a current edition of the *British National Formulary* is strongly advised.

Prescription-only medicines (POM)

These are medicines which may only be supplied by a registered pharmacy or dispensing doctor on receipt of a written prescription from a registered medical practitioner. Prescription for these medicines must carry certain information as set out in the *British National Formulary*. POMs tend to be potent agents, where, as in the case of benzodiazepines, there is a risk of addiction or, as in the case of antibiotics, there is a public health issue (i.e. drug resistance). Recent legislation now allows other health care professionals (pharmacists and nurses) who have been trained for the purpose to prescribe POMs under a clear management plan agreed with the doctor. These practitioners are known as supplementary prescribers.

Pharmacy-only medicines (P)

These are medicines that may only be sold from a registered pharmacy under the supervision of a pharmacist. A written prescription from a registered medical practitioner is not necessary, and these medicines are generally supplied by pharmacists in response to patients asking their advice on minor ailments. In recent years, many medicines that had been previously classified as prescription-only have been re-classified as pharmacy-only to allow greater access to medicines where there is a perceived public health benefit (e.g. certain cholesterol-lowering drugs).

General sale list (GSL)

These medicines have the least number of restrictions placed on them and can be sold in most shops or supermarkets without any intervention from a health care professional. These medicines tend to carry a low risk of harm if they are used according to the guidelines that accompany them, e.g. vitamin supplements and mild analgesics. If they are used in larger than recommended doses, they can cause damage. However, for some medicines, such as paracetamol, there is a limit on the number of tablets that may be purchased at any one time.

NOMENCLATURE OF DRUGS

Individual drugs have a generic name. While at one time this may have varied from country to country, the European Directive 92/27/EEC now requires the use of the Recommended International Non-proprietary Name (rINN) for medicines, in order to ensure consistency of recognition. Generally speaking, the British Approved Name (BAN) and the rINN coincided, and where the two differed, the BAN was modified to match the rINN, with the important exceptions of adrenaline and noradrenaline, for which the rINNs are epinephrine and norepinephrine, respectively. Different manufacturers may use different proprietary names, but these will not be used in this text. In Europe the name paracetamol is used while the drug is named acetaminophen in the USA.

SUMMARY

- Medicines are classified according to prescription, as prescription-only medicines controlled drug, prescription-only medicine, pharmacy-only medicine and general sale list.
- Generic drug names should be the same in all countries for consistency of recognition.

SECTION II: FACTORS AFFECTING DRUG ACTION

4 Pharmacodynamics of drugs

Pharmacodynamics is the study of drug effects and how the drugs act to produce these effects.

MECHANISMS OF ACTION OF DRUGS

Drugs are molecules that produce their effects by interacting with target molecules – usually proteins. See Figure 4.1. When a drug binds to a target protein, there is an alteration of (ongoing) physiological processes. The exceptions to this are laxatives

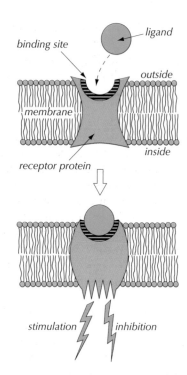

Figure 4.1 Binding between receptor and ligand. When a ligand binds, a receptor–ligand complex is formed, which can trigger or inhibit cellular responses.

which exert their effects via osmotic changes (so-called osmotic laxatives) and antacids which are used in the treatment of dyspepsia.

THE EFFECT OF A DRUG

The effect of a drug can be described at several levels:

- the effect it has on the whole body
- the organ system(s) it targets
- the cell type in the organ system it interacts with
- its molecular target within cells.

For example, suxamethonium chloride is a drug used to achieve muscle relaxation during short surgical interventions and other invasive procedures, e.g. endotracheal intubation. In the context of the above, its effects can be described as follows:

- whole-body effect – paralysis
- organ system targeted – muscular system
- target cell – striated skeletal muscle cells
- molecular target – nicotinic cholinergic receptors.

A single drug may have many effects other than its main therapeutic effect, and in some instances these secondary effects and the responses they produce may not be known in detail.

Ideally, it is desirable that drugs should be as specific as possible. This means that they should produce effects in as few organ systems as possible – other than those in which an effect is required. The treatment can then be controlled to achieve the desired effect.

TARGET PROTEINS AND LIGANDS

In order to understand the actions of a drug, it is necessary to be familiar with the terms 'target protein' and 'ligand'. A target protein is a protein molecule which permits another molecule to bind to it. A ligand is the general term for a substance which binds to a target protein. In its simplest pharmacological context, a target protein would equate to a classic receptor and a ligand to a drug. The drug binding to the receptor results in some alteration of a biological response.

RESPONSES INITIATED BY TARGET PROTEIN–LIGAND INTERACTIONS

The response that is initiated when ligands bind to a target protein can increase, decrease or alter biological processes. The ligand can be a hormone, a neurotransmitter or a drug. In this case, hormones and neurotransmitters would be examples of endogenous ligands (produced in the body), while drugs would be examples of exogenous ligands (not produced in the body). It is generally considered that there are four categories of target proteins, each of which will be described in turn.

Classic receptor. The target protein can be a classic receptor, i.e. a macromolecule (usually a protein) that is an integral part of the cell membrane and to which a drug binds. This ultimately leads to physiological change in the cell. See Figure 4.1. There may be an increase or decrease in an on-going physiological process or a new process may be initiated.

Enzyme. A target protein may also be an enzyme, i.e. a macromolecule whose normal function is to increase the rate at which metabolic reactions proceed in the body. Enzymes are not always bound to cellular membranes. They can be extracellular (plasma and interstitial fluid) or intracellular. When a drug binds to an enzyme, a metabolic reaction can be influenced in that the enzyme activity increases or decreases.

Ion channels. This third group of target proteins may be classified as either ligand-gated or voltage-gated. In the case of ligand-gated ion channels, the target protein forms or is part of an ion channel that spans a membrane. When such a target protein binds a drug, the ion channel can open or close so that the flow of ions across the membrane is altered. In doing so, the potential difference that exists across the cell membrane in which the protein is located may be altered. This in turn may influence a number of physiological processes. In the case of voltage-gated ion channels, the target protein is a macromolecule which forms or is part of an ion channel that once again spans the cell membrane. In this case a drug does not necessarily have to bind to the channel, but interaction with it promotes a physiological response.

Membrane transporters. These target proteins are responsible for transporting molecules across a cell membrane. The molecules transported include a number of endogenous neurotransmitters – this is one way by which neurotransmitters are removed from synapses. These target proteins represent a site of action for a number of important drugs, e.g. selective serotonin reuptake inhibitors (SSRIs).

TARGET PROTEINS AS PART OF A PHYSIOLOGICAL SYSTEM

Although drugs act by binding to target proteins, the effect of the drug is not always obvious. A target protein is a part of a larger, more complicated physiological system that adapts itself to what occurs on a molecular level. Such an adaptation can sometimes occur gradually, so that it takes a long time before the full effect of the drug is achieved. This situation is seen in the treatment of high blood pressure (hypertension).

When treating hypertension, the full effect will not be evident until 2–4 weeks after drug treatment has commenced. This is because it takes time for the blood pressure-regulating mechanisms to adapt to the new lowered pressure. A similar 'delayed' effect is seen in the treatment of depression. Some of the explanation for the delayed effect may be due to the fact that drugs influence the number of target proteins in a particular tissue or organ.

HOW IS THE SPECIFICITY OF DRUG ACTION DETERMINED?

Drug action is specific – ideally, an individual drug will only influence one physiological process. In order to influence such processes, it has already been established that drugs must bind to target proteins. Consider the case of classical receptors. These represent unique proteins – their uniqueness derives from the unique combination of amino acids which form the protein. Within the overall three-dimensional structure of the receptor, there is a specific region to which a drug may bind – the binding site. In order for a drug to bind, its shape must be complementary to the shape of the binding site. Those drugs that have a better fit for the binding site are said, by having a complementary structure to the binding site, to have a high degree of specificity. Thus the specificity of a drug action depends on its affinity to bind to the binding site of its target protein. It is possible to draw an analogy with

Receptor	Receptor subtypes
Cholinergic	Nicotinic and muscarinic
Adrenergic	α (α_1 and α_2) and β (β_1 and β_2)
Dopaminergic	D_1 and D_2
5-Hydroxytryptaminergic	$5\text{-}HT_{1\ (A, B, C, D)}$, $5\text{-}HT_2$, $5\text{-}HT_3$
Histaminergic	H_1, H_2 and H_3

Table 4.1 Examples of classic receptors

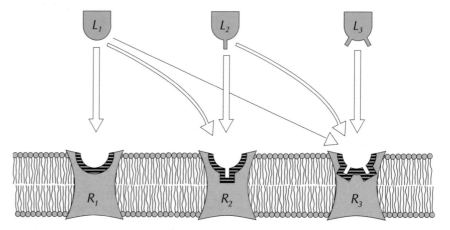

Figure 4.2 **Formation of complexes.** The same ligand can bind to different targets (in this example, classic receptors), but not all the complexes that are formed lead to the same effect. Ligand L_1 fits all receptors, but produces the best response by binding to R_1. L_2 fits R_2 and R_3, but provides the best response in R_2. L_3 only fits R_3.

locks and keys. An individual key (drug) will only open a particular lock (target protein) through the appropriate keyhole (binding site). A key which fails to enter the keyhole will fail to open the lock.

In recent years, it has been possible to distinguish subtypes of a particular receptor. See Table 4.1. By knowing the receptor (or its subtype) it is possible to develop or design drugs that will bind selectively to only one receptor or subtype of receptor.

The receptors (and their subtypes) are distributed differently between different organs. The distribution can also be different within the same organ. For example, the central nervous system has some areas with great densities of receptors that are sensitive to dopamine, while other areas have few such receptors and more receptors that bind other neurotransmitters.

TARGET PROTEINS AND DRUGS

Target proteins are unique, but many have similar properties. By using large doses of a drug that, at normal dosage, acts on a target protein specific for this drug, target proteins with similar properties will also be able to bind the drug. See Figure 4.2. This can therefore result in both desirable and undesirable effects in virtually identical targets since similar (but different) receptors may generate different responses.

The sympathetic division of the autonomic nervous system utilizes the neurotransmitter noradrenaline, which exerts its effects via several different types of adrenergic receptor. The principal adrenergic receptors are termed α- and

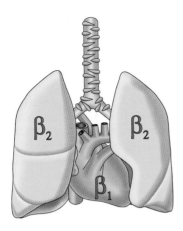

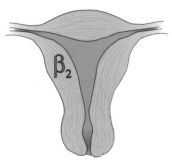

Figure 4.3 Different receptors.
β_1-Receptors in the heart and β_2-receptors in the lungs and uterus have similarities. This means that treatment of disease in, for example, the heart can influence the function in other organs.

β-receptors, each of which has several subtypes. The heart contains β_1-adrenergic receptors. If these are stimulated by released noradrenaline (an endogenous neurotransmitter), the heart rate and blood pressure increase. If they are blocked, then noradrenaline fails to produce an increase in heart rate and blood pressure.

The lungs contain β_2-adrenergic receptors. If these are stimulated, the bronchial muscles will relax and the airways will dilate – hence the use of drugs which activate these receptors in the symptomatic treatment of asthma. Blockage of these receptors therefore may result in bronchial constriction in asthmatic patients. See Figure 4.3.

There are a number of commonly used drugs whose effects are mediated via their interaction with β-receptors. Metoprolol is a drug which specifically blocks β_1-adrenergic receptors – a β-blocker. With normal therapeutic doses, the β_1-receptors in the heart are blocked, but not the lungs' β_2-receptors. With high doses, however, metoprolol will be able to block β_2-receptors in the lungs and thereby compromise ventilation in asthmatic patients.

Terbutaline sulphate acts by stimulating the β_2-receptors in the lungs and airways to produce bronchodilation. Thus this drug is used in the symptomatic treatment of an acute asthma attack. At normal doses, the β_1-receptors in the heart are not influenced to any significant extent. However, with larger doses, the heart's β_1-receptors will be stimulated, resulting in an increased heart rate and palpitations.

The undesirable effects of metoprolol on the lungs, and of terbutaline sulphate on the heart, are examples showing that drugs can both stimulate and block receptors with similar properties.

QUANTIFYING DRUG ACTION: DOSE–RESPONSE CURVES

When a ligand and a target protein bind, a target protein–ligand complex is formed that normally exists for a short time interval (ms). The ligand is then released from the complex and the target protein is ready for a new complex formation. In this way, a target protein will be able to form many complexes in a brief period of time. The more complexes that are created per unit time, the greater the response. The most powerful response is when there are so many ligands present that a new complex can be formed as soon as a target protein is available.

The relationship between concentration of ligand (drug dose) and response is usually plotted as a semilogarithmic graph, which means that only one of the two axes of the graph is in a logarithmic format. It is normal convention to plot the logarithmic values of ligand concentration (drug dose) on the x-axis and the measured response/effect on the y-axis. In most cases, the response produced by a particular ligand concentration is expressed as a percentage of the maximum response achieved with the highest ligand concentration. With this form, the graph is linear between 25 and 75 per cent of the maximum response. The curve will be steepest in the linear area, and here even a small change in the concentration of the ligand will result in a large change in response. See Figure 4.4. This is the customary way to present dose or concentration against response, in part because it is much easier (mathematically) to deal with straight lines as opposed to the curve that would be produced if concentration were simply to be plotted against response.

USEFUL CONCEPTS IN UNDERSTANDING PHARMACODYNAMICS

ADDITIVE AND POTENTIATING EFFECT

By combining two or more drugs, the overall response can be increased. When the overall response is equal to the sum of the responses of the individual drugs, the

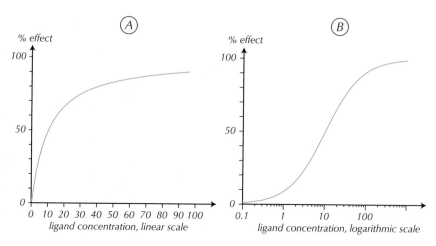

Figure 4.4 **Concentration–response curves.** Response/effect as a function of ligand concentration with a linear scale for the x-axis (diagram A) and with a logarithmic scale for the x-axis (diagram B). By increasing the concentration of the ligand in the region where the semilogarithmic curve is steepest, the greatest increase in response will be obtained. Therefore, the most sensitive dose of a ligand is best visualized on a semilogarithmic plot.

drugs are said to have an additive effect. When it is greater than the sum of the responses of the individual drugs, the drugs are said to have a potentiating effect. See Figure 4.5. Drugs that have inhibitory effects on the central nervous system often have greater effects when they are combined. For example, if a person combines alcohol and opiates, there is a greater inhibitory effect on breathing than when the two substances are taken individually.

REVERSIBLE AND IRREVERSIBLE BINDING

Binding between a target protein and a ligand is usually reversible, i.e. the complex that is formed between the ligand and its target protein dissociates after existing for a short time. If the complex does not dissociate, the binding is irreversible. This means that the target protein is not capable of forming new complexes with other ligands, and that a process is inhibited. See Figure 4.6.

AFFINITY

Different target proteins and ligands can have different affinities for each other. Affinity is a measure of how easily a ligand will bind to a target protein. If two almost identical ligands are present at the same time in the proximity of a target protein, the most complexes will be formed between the target protein and the ligand for which the target protein has the greatest affinity. A simple analogy is that the right hand has greater affinity for gloves that fit the right hand than for gloves that fit the left hand.

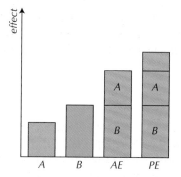

Figure 4.5 **Additive and potentiating effects.** The diagram shows the effects of drugs A and B individually. The total effect can be additive (AE), when it is the sum of A and B, or potentiating (PE), when it is greater than the sum of A and B.

AGONISTS

A ligand that binds to a target protein and evokes a response is called an agonist, and the response produced is termed an agonistic response. Generally, this term applies to drugs which bind to classical receptors.

A number of drugs function as agonists of receptors. For example, morphine is an agonist that acts on opioid receptors. When morphine binds to the opioid receptors on neurons involved in the perception of pain, it results in a potassium

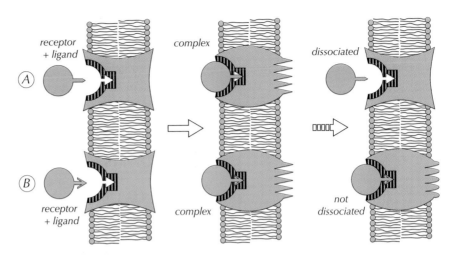

Figure 4.6 **Reversible (A) and irreversible (B) binding.** When the ligand does not dissociate from the target protein (in this case, a classic receptor) after binding, the response mediated by the complex gradually decreases.

channel opening and subsequent efflux of potassium from the neuron. This results in hyperpolarization of the neuron and thus reduced excitability of the cell. The overall effect of this is to abolish, or at least reduce, the number of action potentials reaching the brain and thus produce a reduced perception of pain.

Full agonists and partial agonists

Ligands that can produce a maximum response in a tissue are called full agonists. Those that do not produce a full response, even at very high concentrations, are called partial agonists. In Figure 4.7, A is a full agonist, while B and C are partial agonists. Full and partial agonists may compete for the same receptor in a tissue. By simultaneously administering a full and a partial agonist to a patient, the partial agonist will occupy some of the target proteins otherwise occupied by the full agonist.

Morphine and buprenorphine both bind to opioid receptors and are used as analgesics. Morphine is a full agonist, while buprenorphine is a partial agonist. If morphine is administered first to reduce strong pains, and a short time later buprenorphine is administered to achieve a 'supplementary effect', the buprenorphine will reduce the analgesic effect of morphine by occupying a part of the receptors that the morphine could otherwise have acted upon. If both drugs are administered for pain relief at the same time, then a patient will perceive more pain than if only morphine had been given.

ANTAGONISTS

Some ligands are capable of inhibiting or totally preventing target protein activation by agonists (or partial agonists) by binding to a target protein. These ligands are called antagonists. For example, naloxone is an opiate antagonist that suppresses, and thereby prevents, the action of opiates (e.g. morphine) at opioid receptors. The drug is used to cancel the respiratory depressive effects of opioids following their use in, for example, surgery or after overdoses of heroin. When large doses of opiates have produced unconsciousness and respiratory depression, intravenous administration of naloxone will begin to reverse these effects within 1–3 min. However, the effect of naloxone is short-lived and it is possible that a subsequent relapse into unconsciousness and respiratory depression will occur.

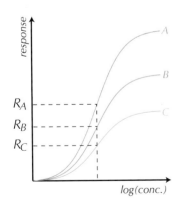

Figure 4.7 **Full and partial agonists.** Drug A is a full agonist, while drugs B and C are partial agonists. For a given drug concentration, the response produced by A (R_A) > R_B > R_C.

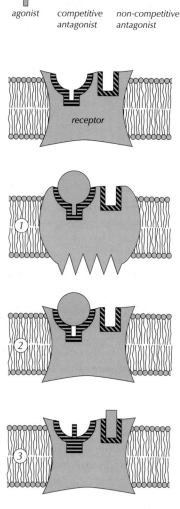

Figure 4.8 **Different ligands.** Ligand A is an agonist that will stimulate the receptor by binding (1). Ligand B is a competitive antagonist that binds to the same binding site as A, but without stimulating it (2). Ligand C binds to another binding site and induces a change in it, such that ligand A or B cannot bind (3). Since ligand C does not compete with A or B, it is a non-competitive antagonist.

Competitive and non-competitive antagonists

If an antagonist competes for the same binding site on a target protein as the agonist, it is termed a competitive antagonist. If the antagonist binds to a region on the target protein other than the binding site, and in doing so causes a change in the target protein such that the agonist cannot bind as effectively as before, the antagonist is termed a non-competitive antagonist. See Figure 4.8. β-Blockers are examples of drugs that act as antagonists.

TARGET PROTEINS AND DRUG ACTION

As indicated earlier, there are a number of target proteins that represent sites for drug action. These are considered below in more detail.

ENZYMES AS TARGET PROTEINS

Some key enzymes also targets for drug action. If the action of these enzymes is inhibited by a drug then there is a change in the resultant biological activity as demonstrated in the following examples. Inhibitors of angiotensin-converting enzymes (ACE inhibitors) are examples of drugs that bind to enzymes. The effects from such drugs are expected in the course of minutes to hours. There are a number of other drugs which exert their effects by binding to and inhibiting the functions of enzymes.

Acetylsalicylic acid (aspirin) has anti-inflammatory, analgesic and antipyretic effects. It acts by inhibiting the enzyme cyclooxygenase, and prevents the formation of prostaglandins and thromboxanes from fatty acids located in cell membranes.

Neostigmine is used in myasthenia gravis to increase the concentration of the neurotransmitter acetylcholine at the motor end-plates. It binds to the enzyme acetylcholinesterase and prevents it from breaking down acetylcholine.

Captopril is a drug that inhibits angiotensin-converting enzymes, and thus conversion of angiotensin-I to angiotensin-II. The latter has a powerful stimulating effect on vascular smooth muscle of arterioles, i.e. it causes the smooth muscle to contract, the consequence of which is an increase in blood pressure. Thus drugs that function as ACE inhibitors are used to lower blood pressure.

Methotrexate inhibits the enzyme dihydrofolate reductase that is necessary to convert folic acid to tetrahydrofolate. Tetrahydrofolate is necessary for DNA synthesis. By inhibiting the conversion of folic acid to tetrahydrofolate, the growth of cancer cells and other cells is inhibited. Of course, it takes time before the effect of methotrexate is observed.

MEMBRANE-BOUND TARGET PROTEINS

Membrane-bound target proteins include classical receptors, ion channels and transport molecules. Membrane-bound receptors have binding sites which project to the extracellular side of the cell and which are linked to an enzyme-active part that projects into the interior of the cell. When a ligand binds to the receptor, changes occur such that the enzymatically active region is activated. See Figure 4.9.

Membrane-bound receptors are also found to be connected to other membrane-bound proteins (G-proteins) that must be activated to initiate cellular responses. Receptors that operate via G-proteins can open ion channels or activate intracellular enzymes. In many cases, the cellular response is amplified by such a reaction. See Figure 4.10.

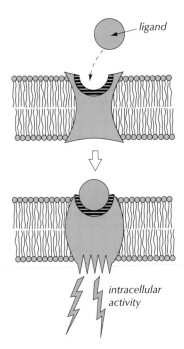

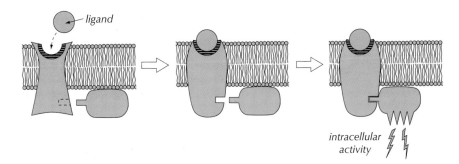

Figure 4.10 **Coupled mechanism.** The reaction between a membrane-bound and an intracellular protein can trigger effects.

Figure 4.9 **Membrane-bound receptor with intracellular enzymatic activity.** When a ligand binds to the outer part of a receptor, the intracellular part is activated.

Receptors that operate via G-proteins produce responses more quickly if the ultimate target of the cellular response is an ion channel as opposed to, say, the activation of an enzyme. This is due to the fact that it takes much longer to initiate changes in metabolism than it does to simply open an ion channel.

Ligand-gated ion channels consist of protein chains that wind their way through the cell membrane, spanning the entire membrane and forming channels or ports that allow ions to pass from one side of the membrane to the other. They are ligand-gated in that a ligand is required to open or close the channel. Examples of such ion channels are those which allow sodium, potassium, calcium and chloride ions to move across the membrane. Receptors for neurotransmitters in synapses are examples of ligand-gated ion channels. In this case, the neuro-transmitter binds to the receptor and, in so doing, opens up ion channels. See Figure 4.11.

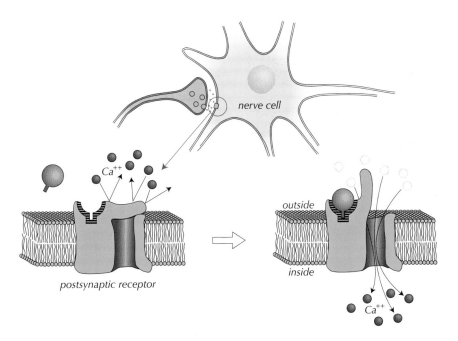

Figure 4.11 **Closed and open ion channel.** When a ligand binds to an ion channel, the channel can be opened so that ions may flow through it. Such a process occurs within milliseconds.

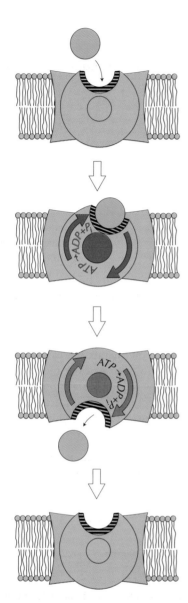

Figure 4.12 **Transport molecule.** The molecule is activated when the ligand binds.

Ion channels are influenced by different ligands. Drugs can block an ion channel or modulate it by increasing or decreasing the permeability for ions. The effect of drugs that open or close an ion channel occurs as soon as the drug is distributed to the tissue where the receptor is found. For example, opioid receptors located in neuronal cell membranes are ligand-gated ion channels. When, for instance, morphine binds to opioid receptors, it opens potassium channels, which allows potassium to leave the neuron. This hyperpolarizes the neuron, effectively switching it off. This effect occurs within minutes of administration.

Transport molecules are found localized to cell membranes. They can transport ions and other molecules into and out of the cell. They can transport molecules against a concentration gradient, or transport those that are slightly lipid-soluble across a membrane. See Figure 4.12. Drugs can act by inhibiting transport molecules.

An example of a commonly used drug which acts by inhibiting a transport molecule is digoxin, which is used to treat heart failure and atrial fibrillation. It inhibits the sodium–potassium-ATPase, a transport molecule, and consequently inhibits the pumping out of sodium from the cardiac muscle cells. This results in an increased intracellular concentration of sodium within the cardiac muscle cells. See Figure 17.26 on p. 252. This in turn activates a sodium–calcium transporter, which results in an increased intracellular concentration of calcium. This causes the cardiac muscle cells to contract more strongly and helps the failing heart.

The effects of drugs that inhibit transport molecules are achieved slower than the effects of drugs that act on ion channels.

INTRACELLULAR TARGET PROTEINS

A ligand can be lipid-soluble and diffuse through the cell membrane where it binds to a target protein – an intracellular protein, e.g. an enzyme (considered earlier in the chapter), or a receptor that regulates gene expression. Drugs that bind to intracellular receptors, e.g. steroids, normally exert an effect by inhibiting the synthesis of other proteins, although they may also promote the synthesis of proteins. This alteration in gene expression requires a considerable amount of time and explains why drugs such as steroids take a considerable time for their effects to be observed.

OTHER MECHANISMS OF ACTION

Some drugs act by altering other properties of membranes. The local anaesthetic lidocaine alters the membrane properties of neurons in such a way that action potentials are inhibited by virtue of the drug physically blocking the sodium channels required for depolarization of the neuron. Acid-neutralizing agents act by increasing pH and thereby reducing the damaging effect of stomach acid on the mucous membrane. Osmotic drugs act by promoting the movement of water.

THE RELATIONSHIP BETWEEN DOSE AND RESPONSE

Even though many people receive the same dose of a drug, not all of them will achieve the same effect. Some may have effect with a low dose, while others require a higher dose. Likewise, some notice adverse effects at lower doses than others.

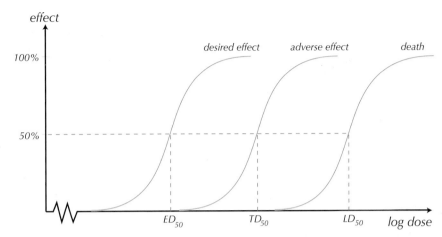

Figure 4.13 **Dose–effect curves.** Curves for effective dose, toxic dose and lethal dose. ED_{50}, TD_{50} and LD_{50} are the effective dose, toxic dose and theoretical lethal dose, respectively, for 50 per cent of users. From the diagram, it can be seen that effect, adverse effect and death will occur at different dosages in different users.

SOME DEFINITIONS

Some terms can help to clarify the understanding of the dose–effect ratio. See Figure 4.13.

Effective dose
The dose that produces the desired effect in 50 per cent of all who use the drug is called the median dose. It is often referred to as the effective dose 50 (ED_{50}).

Toxic dose
The dose that produces a toxic effect in 50 per cent of all who use the drug is called the toxic dose 50 (TD_{50}).

Lethal dose
The dose that results in death in 50 per cent of all who use the drug is called the lethal dose 50 (LD_{50}). This is an experimental term that can only be determined in animal experiments and estimated in humans taking high doses in attempting suicide.

THERAPEUTIC INDEX

If there is a large difference between the dose of a drug that produces the desired effect and the dose that produces a toxic effect, it is said that the drug has a large therapeutic index. This is desirable for all drugs, but in practice, drugs are very different with regard to therapeutic index. See Figure 4.14.

The therapeutic index of a drug may be defined as the ratio between LD_{50} and ED_{50}, i.e. LD_{50}/ED_{50}. Cytotoxic agents, used in cancer chemotherapy, are examples of drugs where there is little difference between the therapeutic and toxic dose. Thus cytotoxic agents are said to have a small therapeutic index.

A high therapeutic index is desirable, and means that a large dose is necessary in order for a person to die from the drug. Penicillin is an example of a drug with a high therapeutic index.

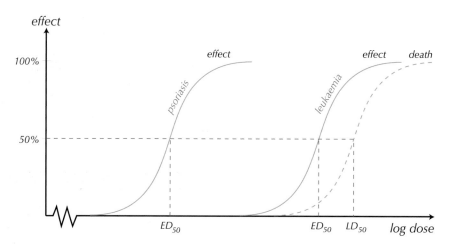

Figure 4.14 **Dose–effect curves for methotrexate.** When using high-dose methotrexate in the treatment of leukaemia in children, large doses are administered to eradicate the cancer cells. With leukaemia, there is little difference between the effective dose and the lethal dose. When using methotrexate to treat psoriasis, small doses are administered. There is a large difference between the effective doses of methotrexate for the treatment of psoriasis and the treatment of leukaemia.

DOSE/CONCENTRATION AND RESPONSE

If two people the same size take the same dose of a drug, they do not always achieve the same concentration of the drug in the blood, since absorption, distribution, metabolism and elimination vary from one person to the next. For most drugs, there is a better relationship between its concentration in the blood and its response than there is between administered dose and response.

RECOMMENDED THERAPEUTIC RANGE FOR A DRUG

Some drugs have a recommended therapeutic range with lower and upper values of the concentration of the drug in blood at which the majority of users can expect a clinical effect with minimal adverse effects. If the concentration falls below the lower limit, the effect diminishes. If it rises above the upper limit, patients may experience adverse effects. This concentration range is called the recommended therapeutic range and is essential information for those who are responsible for controlling the dosage. See Figure 4.15.

As a consequence of individual differences between patients, some will demonstrate an effect at concentrations lower than the recommended therapeutic range, while others will require concentrations above the upper limit. The limits for the recommended therapeutic range require that the patient is receiving monotherapy, i.e. is using only the drug in question. Dose and effect observed are dependent on the condition for which the patient is taking the drug. See Figure 4.14.

For drugs with an obvious relationship between concentration and clinical effect and dose-dependent adverse effects, it can be useful to relate the dosage to the concentration. The concentration of drugs is almost always measured in the blood, even though it is the drug concentration at the site of action that is decisive for the effect. Measurements of drug concentration in blood are used as there is a

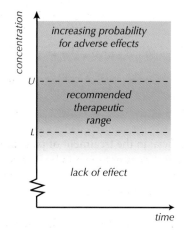

Figure 4.15 **The recommended therapeutic range** for the concentration of a drug indicates the lower (L) and upper (U) limits of concentration at which the majority of users experience effect with a minimum of troublesome or dangerous, dose-dependent adverse effects. Note the use of colours. Below the green range, the effect gradually fades away. In the red range, the possibility of adverse effects increases.

relationship between this and the concentration of the drug at the site of action, and because it is easier to take blood rather than tissue samples for analysis.

For other drugs, the dose is determined according to clinical effects. Some drugs used to treat cardiovascular disease, for example, are administered and titrated against their effects on pulse rate and blood pressure. The anticoagulant warfarin is administered according to its effect on blood coagulation. Drugs with a large therapeutic index can be administered with standard doses without the necessity of taking special measurements.

PLACEBO AND NOCEBO EFFECTS

Drugs are used on the basis of their known pharmacological effects on somatic and psychological conditions. The term 'placebo effect' refers to drugs whose action provides better benefits on the condition being treated than can simply be explained on the basis of the drugs' known pharmacological and therapeutic properties. 'Nocebo effect' is used when the drug produces a worsening effect on the condition being treated, compared with the pharmacological properties indicated.

Every therapeutic intervention instituted implies that someone wants to alter symptoms, complaints or illnesses. It seems, therefore, that patients allow themselves to be influenced by what the prescriber communicates consciously or unconsciously, i.e. a desire for change and improvement. This becomes quite obvious in statements like 'I know this will help' or 'This strong tablet helps against the pain'.

Placebo and nocebo effects are associated with therapeutic measures other than pharmacotherapy. It is known, for example, that specific procedures or experiences that are associated with a treatment can influence the outcome of treatment. A prescriber's behaviour before, during and after a treatment sends important signals to the patient. If a prescriber provides treatment and simultaneously expresses that it is doubtful that it will work, many patients become sceptical and some of the benefits of the treatment are lost. Likewise, a prescriber who exudes confidence in a crisis situation will lessen anxiety more effectively than one who appears uncertain.

It is possible to generalize and state that when positive signals about an effect reinforce the desired effect of a drug, a placebo effect is expressed. However, if signals concerning an effect weaken the desired effect of the drug, a nocebo effect is expressed.

The placebo effect can be particularly beneficial in the treatment of pain, both in surgical and drug treatment. The placebo effect does not seem to be limited to subjective experiences, but also to physiological changes that can be measured objectively. The mechanisms by which a placebo effect may result in physiological changes is unknown.

In all probability, placebo and nocebo effects play a larger role in drug therapy than has previously been acknowledged. The placebo effect was previously regarded as a complicating influence in the development of new therapeutic interventions. Nowadays, when new drugs are tested they are compared against already established drugs and often against placebos (substances with no known pharmacological effects). In this way it is possible to assess whether the pharmacological effect of a new drug is greater than the placebo effect.

There is reason to believe that awareness of placebo and nocebo effects can change the approach to both pharmacological treatment and other therapy regimes. It is possible to imagine that placebo and nocebo effects may be caused by alterations in the release of endogenous ligands like hormones and other biologically active substances that trigger psychological and neurophysiological responses, which act alongside the therapeutic intervention.

With such knowledge, it is possible to imagine that part of the effect some people experience after treatment with homeopathic drugs is the placebo effect. In such an event, this is a favourable utilization of the placebo effect.

SUMMARY

- A drug often produces several effects at the same time. The effect comes from organs that have a sufficiently high concentration of the drug and target proteins, e.g. classical receptors, ion channels and transport molecules, upon which the drug acts. This explains why a drug can produce both desirable and undesirable effects.
- Almost all drugs act by binding to target proteins. The specificity of the target allows only selective drugs to bind to them and exert an effect.
- One drug can reinforce the effect of another by providing an additive or potentiating effect.
- A target protein can have higher affinity for one ligand than for another. This will cause many complexes to be formed per time unit.
- Agonists stimulate a receptor, while antagonists block a receptor.
- Full and partial agonists should not be administered simultaneously to the same patient.
- Competitive antagonists block a receptor by binding to the same receptor as an agonist.
- Non-competitive antagonists block a receptor without binding to the same receptor as an agonist.
- Target proteins can be localized extracellularly, intracellularly, or be bound to membranes in the cell. How rapidly the effects occur depends on how rapidly the drug is distributed to the tissue where the target proteins are found, and how the drug exerts its effects once it has bound.
- The effective dose of a drug is that dose which provides the therapeutic effect. It can vary from person to person. The effective dose also varies according to which effect one wants to achieve.
- The therapeutic index of a drug is a measure of how safe it is with regard to its toxic effects.
- There is a better relationship between concentration of a drug in the blood and response than between the drug's dose and its response.
- The recommended therapeutic range refers to a concentration 'window' for which the majority of the users experience an effect with a minimum of adverse effects.
- Placebo and nocebo effects are mediated by the signals a prescriber expresses in support of a therapeutic measure.

5 Pharmacokinetics of drugs

Pharmacokinetics is the study of the 'movement' or fate of drugs in the body, i.e. what happens to a drug from the time it is administered until it leaves the body. When a drug is prescribed to a patient, the intention is to achieve the therapeutic effect quickly, for an appropriate duration of action and without unpleasant side-effects. It is invaluable to understand how the drug is absorbed into the blood-stream (absorption), how it is distributed about the body (distribution), and how it is eliminated from the body (metabolism and excretion). See Figure 5.1.

IMPORTANT CONCEPTS FOR UNDERSTANDING PHARMACOKINETICS

To understand pharmacokinetics, it can be useful to look at the processes of absorption, distribution and elimination by means of a model in which a fluid

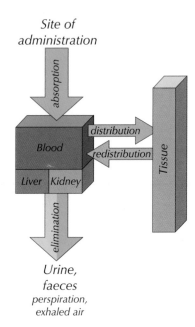

Site of administration

absorption

distribution

Blood

redistribution

Tissue

Liver Kidney

elimination

Urine, faeces

perspiration, exhaled air

Figure 5.1 **Absorption, distribution and elimination.** A drug is absorbed into the bloodstream, distributed to tissue, redistributed to the blood, and then eliminated from it. The liver and kidneys are the two most important organs for elimination.

distributes itself throughout a system of containers (analogous to the distribution of drugs in the different tissues of the body). An important concept is the idea of the 'half-life' of a substance, as this indicates how rapidly a drug is eliminated from the body. The water and lipid (fat) solubility of drugs is important in understanding the drug's movement through different biological membranes, and the drug's distribution in different tissues in the body. Knowledge of the blood supply to the liver and kidneys is vital for understanding how these organs contribute to the elimination of drugs from the body. See Figure 5.1.

DISTRIBUTION OF WATER IN A SYSTEM OF CONTAINERS – A MODEL

In order to clarify the terms absorption, distribution and elimination, one might imagine the body as a system of containers that are connected to each other as shown in Figure 5.2. Container A is the central container to which water is added (analogous to a drug being added to the blood), while B and C represent peripheral containers (analogous to different body tissues such as muscle tissue, fatty tissue and brain tissue). Where B and C are in contact with A, they have an open vertical slit in the wall through which the water can flow. The slit represents the blood's contact with different tissue compartments. The different widths of the slits provide different flow conditions between the containers and are analogous to different blood supplies to different tissues. The central container also has a vertical slit where the water runs out (analogous to the elimination of drugs from the blood).

If water flows into the central container (absorption), it is distributed to B and C at different rates, depending on the width of the slits. Water simultaneously runs out of A (elimination). The water level will rise in the central container as long as water flow exceeds that flowing out and that which is distributed to B and C. When equal amounts of water flow into and out of the central container, the system is said to be in a 'steady state'. When the water level is the same in all containers and no water flows between the central container and the peripheral containers, 'distribution equilibrium' has been achieved.

If the water supply stops, the containers will empty. As the water level sinks in the central container, it will be refilled from the peripheral containers (redistribution). The water level will sink at the lowest rate in the peripheral container with the narrowest slit to A.

A continuous addition of water to the central container is analogous to administering a drug by intravenous infusion at a continuous rate. The different size of the containers is analogous to the body's different tissues having different abilities to bind drugs.

Now imagine that the water flowing into container A contains molecules (drugs) of a substance that can be dissolved in water. Containers B and C are each filled with their own porous material that the water can run through (different body tissues) at different rates with different abilities to bind these molecules. As the water flows through containers B and C, gradually molecules of this substance will be bound in the container having the material with the highest affinity for the molecules. It is possible that the smallest container, C, binds more molecules than B. At distribution equilibrium, however, the water level will be equally high in all the containers. It is the properties of the dissolved molecules and the porous material in the containers that determine how molecules are distributed in the individual containers. This is how it is in the body: different tissues have different abilities to bind different drugs.

The model with the water containers illustrates that absorption, distribution and elimination occur simultaneously. In this process, the concentration of a drug

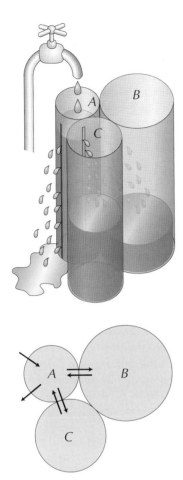

Figure 5.2 **Water container system.** The illustration shows a system of containers where water flows into A at a constant rate (absorption). From the central container, some of the water flows out (elimination), while some is distributed to B and C (distribution). Refer to the text for a more detailed explanation.

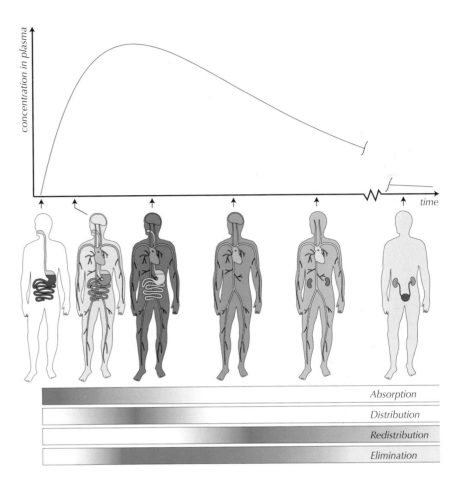

Figure 5.3 **Absorption, distribution and elimination.** These processes occur simultaneously in the organism, but at different rates within a dosage interval. When the concentration is at its peak, the absorption is balanced (to the blood) by distribution and elimination. When all of the drug has been absorbed, absorption stops. When the concentration in the blood is lower than in peripheral tissue, redistribution will be greater than distribution. The illustration depicts the pharmacokinetics of a single dose of drug, eliminated via the kidneys. The intensity of the green colour indicates where in the body most of the drug is located and the rate of the processes within a dosage interval.

is altered over time in the blood and the tissues. Figure 5.3 shows how these processes take place in the human body when a drug dose is administered orally.

Different drugs have different physical properties and will therefore be absorbed, distributed and eliminated at different rates. How long it takes before steady state and distribution equilibrium are established depends on the properties of the different drugs. In this context, a drug's half-life is important.

THE HALF-LIFE OF A SUBSTANCE

The half-life ($t_{1/2}$) of a substance indicates how rapidly it is eliminated from a system, when the elimination rate is proportional to the amount of substance in the system. This may sound difficult, but it is easier to understand in terms of the rate at which water runs out of a container with an open vertical slit in the wall. The half-life for the water in the container is the time it takes to reduce the water's height from one level to half that level. From Figure 5.4 it can be seen that the water level falls rapidly at the beginning, when it is high, but becomes increasingly slower with a decreasing water supply (the curve becomes flatter and flatter). This shows that the rate of elimination is in proportion to the amount of water in the container. Similarly, the rate of drug elimination is proportional to the amount of drug in the system. When the water level is high in the container, a lot of water runs out; when the container is almost empty, the water runs out slowly. For every half-life ($t_{1/2}$), the water level sinks by half the initial value at each half-life. Thus:

- after 0 $t_{1/2}$, 100 per cent remains
- after 1 $t_{1/2}$, 50 per cent remains
- after 2 $t_{1/2}$, 25 per cent remains
- after 3 $t_{1/2}$, 12.5 per cent remains
- after 4 $t_{1/2}$, 6.25 per cent remains
- after 5 $t_{1/2}$, 3.12 per cent remains (96.88 per cent has been eliminated)
- after 6 $t_{1/2}$, 1.56 per cent remains.

If the water is replaced with a viscous fluid (syrup), it will take more time to empty the container if the width of the slit is the same. If the slit is narrowed, it will take more time to empty the container for both water and syrup. It is easy to understand that it is the properties of both the fluid in the container and the container itself that influence how rapidly the container is emptied. The fluid and the container can be compared to a drug that is eliminated from the body. In the same way that different fluids flow out of the container at different rates, different drugs will be eliminated from the body at different rates. This means that every drug has its own half-life, since the half-life is associated with the drug's chemical properties. Some drugs have half-lives of a few minutes, while others may be hours, days or even weeks.

The slit could represent the liver or the kidneys, which are the most important organs for the elimination of drugs. Narrowing of the container's slit can be compared to liver and kidney failure in a patient. It is easy to understand that liver and

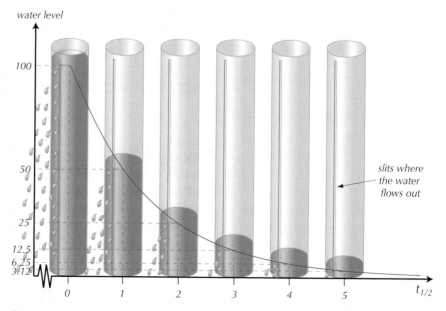

Figure 5.4 **Half–life.** For every half-life, the water level sinks (is eliminated) from one level to half of that level.

kidney failure will lead to an extended half-life of a drug. This must be considered when drugs are to be administered to patients with liver or kidney failure.

In the same way that half-life indicates how rapidly a container empties, the half-life is also important in predicting how rapidly the water level rises when water flows into a container with an open vertical slit in the wall. This is analogous to the way in which drug concentration increases in the body with continuous administration. See Figure 5.11 (p. 47).

WATER AND LIPID SOLUBILITY OF DRUGS

When drugs distribute themselves between different tissues in the body through the processes of absorption, distribution and elimination, they may have to pass through the mucous membrane of the intestine, the walls in small blood vessels and across different cell membranes, i.e. through many different biological barriers. These barriers are lipid bilayers with polar surfaces facing the inside and outside of the cell, and a non-polar middle layer. Within the membranes there are integral proteins with different functions. See Figure 5.5.

The ability of substances to penetrate lipid membranes varies greatly from substance to substance. To understand these processes, it is useful to be familiar with the terms 'water solubility' and 'lipid solubility' (fat-solubility).

Imagine a straight line with, at one end, 100 per cent lipid solubility and 0 per cent water solubility and, at the other end, 0 per cent lipid solubility and 100 per cent water solubility. Different drugs fall somewhere between these extremes, because different drugs have different degrees of water and lipid solubility. The more lipid-soluble a substance is, the more readily it will penetrate a lipid membrane. High lipid solubility is needed by a substance for it to be distributed rapidly from the blood to different tissues, especially across the blood–brain barrier.

Lipid solubility is a function of the size and electrical charge of a drug molecule. Small molecules move more easily across biological membranes than larger molecules. In terms of electrical charge, a molecule could be non-polar (without electrical charge in parts of the molecule or as a whole molecule) or dipolar (one part of the molecule has a negative charge while another part has a positive charge, but the molecule as a whole is neutral – most drugs belong to this group). The drug molecule might be a weak acid or a weak alkali (or base), which dissociates into two ions that have opposite electrical charges. Lipid solubility is greatest for non-polar compounds and least for ionic or polar compounds, with dipolar molecules between these two extremes. See Figure 5.6. Generally speaking, lipid-soluble

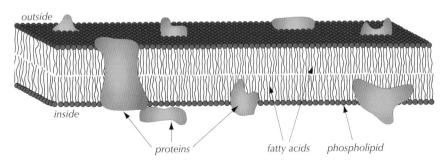

Figure 5.5 **Lipid membrane.** A lipid membrane has two layers, where the fatty acids in the two layers point towards each other and the phospholipid groups lie against the surfaces. All cells have proteins integrated into the membranes.

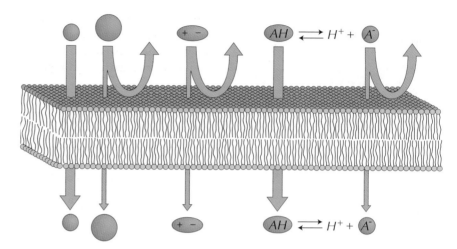

Figure 5.6 **Diffusion through a biological membrane.** Small molecules pass through a membrane more easily than do large molecules. Dipoles pass through more easily than ionized (electrically charged) molecules.

drugs are distributed in fatty tissue, while water-soluble drugs are found in aqueous tissues and interstitial fluids.

Dissociation of weak acids or weak bases depends on the pH (degree of acidity or alkalinity) of the solution. The general rule is that a weak acid is ionized to a greater extent in an alkaline (or basic) solution than in an acidic solution. Conversely, a weak base is ionized to a greater extent in an acidic solution than in an alkaline (or basic) solution. In the ionic form, drugs are more water-soluble and are therefore found in aqueous tissues and interstitial fluids, whilst in their unionized form, drugs are more lipid-soluble, will penetrate membranes more readily and be found in fatty tissues.

An example of a drug with high lipid solubility is diazepam – administered rectally in solution it can be used to stop febrile convulsions in children very quickly. The drug diffuses rapidly through the rectal membrane, is transported via the blood to the central nervous system, where it diffuses across the blood–brain barrier and influences neurons in the central nervous system in such a way that the convulsions stop. The whole process takes only around 1–2 min.

The water and lipid solubility of drugs is crucial in how they are eliminated from the body. The more lipid-soluble a drug is, the more important the liver is in its elimination, while the more water-soluble a drug is, the more important the kidneys are in its elimination. See Figure 5.19. (p. 52).

BLOOD CIRCULATION IN RELATION TO THE LIVER AND THE KIDNEYS

The blood's circulation in relation to the liver and the kidneys is important for understanding what influences the distribution and the elimination of administered drugs.

The liver
Drugs absorbed from the intestine pass to the liver via the hepatic portal vein. From the liver, the blood enters the inferior vena cava. If the liver has a large capacity to metabolize, and thereby eliminate, some of the drug from the blood, a smaller amount

of drug will be passed into the systemic circulation. See Figure 5.7. Drugs that are absorbed from the intestine can be eliminated following this first passage through the liver before they are distributed in the blood to different tissues in the body. This is often referred to as 'first-pass metabolism'.

The kidneys

When blood passes through the blood vessels in the glomerulus, it is filtered by the glomerular membrane of Bowman's capsule of the renal nephron (glomerular filtration), giving rise to the glomerular filtrate. If there is a drug present in the blood, the drug molecules will be filtered in the same way into the tubular system of the nephron. In addition, drugs can be secreted into the tubule of the nephron (tubular secretion), and may or may not be reabsorbed from the tubules of the nephron (tubular reabsorption). If the drug molecules remain in the renal tubules, they will ultimately be excreted in the urine. See Figure 5.8.

ABSORPTION

Absorption of a drug has come to imply absorption into the blood. Absorption largely depends on the form of drug and the site of administration. This is discussed in Chapter 6. Administration of drugs and drug formulations are discussed later in this chapter. Unless the drug has been injected directly into the bloodstream, it will have to pass through membranes before it reaches the bloodstream (see 'Water and lipid solubility of drugs', above). Hence, absorption is also influenced by the different transport mechanisms across the membranes.

SITE OF ADMINISTRATION

The blood supply at the site of administration is important for absorption. It can be compared to a river running through a landscape: the greater the water flow, the faster it will wash away pollution that is deposited in the landscape. When a drug is administered intramuscularly or subcutaneously, it will gradually enter the bloodstream and be moved away fastest from the area with the greatest blood flow.

If there are other substances present at the site of administration, absorption can be affected if these interact with the drug and may lead to either inhibited or increased absorption.

The acid–base status of the tissue at the site of administration is important for whether the drug dissociates or not, and therefore how lipid-soluble it becomes. For example, if there is an infection in the tissue around a tooth, a local acidosis will occur in that tissue. If a dentist administers a local anaesthetic to the nerve of the tooth, the local anaesthetic, which is a weak alkali, will dissociate to a greater degree. As it will have become less lipid-soluble, the local anaesthetic will not diffuse well into the nerve membrane, and consequently there will be less drug available at the site of action and local anaesthesia will not be achieved.

TRANSPORT MECHANISMS ACROSS MEMBRANES

Drugs are transported across membranes by passive diffusion or by different types of active transport. Passive diffusion is largely dependent on the lipid solubility of the drug and its concentration on each side of a lipid membrane. If there is a high concentration on one side and a low concentration on the other, the concentration difference will 'drive' the drug from the side of high concentration towards the side

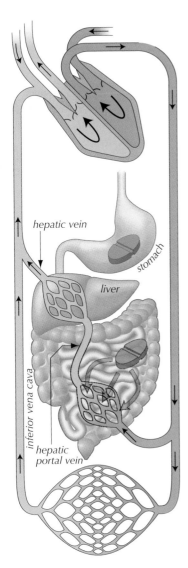

Figure 5.7 The blood's circulation in relation to the abdominal organs. The illustration shows that blood that supplies the intestine passes through the liver before it empties into the inferior vena cava and reaches the systemic circulation. Therefore, drugs that are absorbed from the intestine will exist in high concentration in the blood that reaches the liver via the hepatic portal vein.

hepatic vein

stomach

liver

inferior vena cava

hepatic portal vein

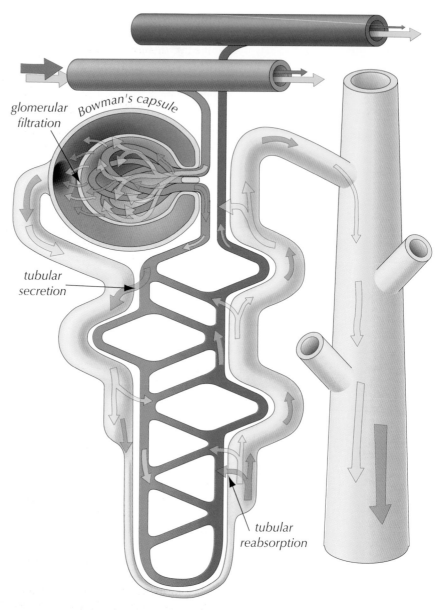

Figure 5.8 **Circulation in relation to a nephron.** In Bowman's capsule, plasma (yellow arrow) is filtered from the arterial blood to the nephron (glomerular filtration). If there are drugs in the blood (green arrow), they will also be filtered across. A drug can also be 'moved' from the blood to the tubular lumen by tubular secretion, and from the tubular lumen back to the blood by tubular reabsorption.

with low concentration. This driving force diminishes as the concentration difference becomes smaller. As the majority of drugs are transported by passive diffusion, the rate of transport is determined by the drug's lipid solubility. See Figure 5.9.

In order to maintain vital functions, the body must sometimes transport molecules against the concentration gradient, i.e. from the side with low concentration towards the side with high concentration. In these cases, transport of the drug molecule is achieved with the help of special transport molecules. See Figure 5.9. This transport is energy-dependent and typically utilizes adenosine

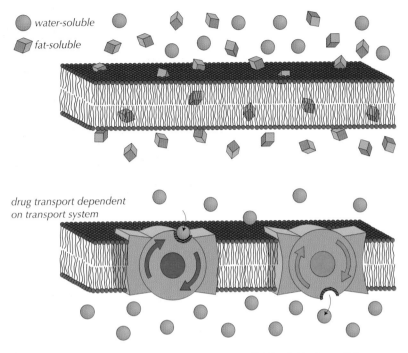

water-soluble

fat-soluble

drug transport dependent on transport system

Figure 5.9 **Transport mechanisms across a membrane.** Lipid-soluble drugs diffuse through the membrane by passive diffusion, while other drugs need the help of specialized transport systems.

triphosphate (ATP) – hence the term 'active transport'. These transport systems can be saturated and reach a maximum in the same way as enzyme-catalysed processes. However, it should be noted that active transport is less relevant for drugs than for nutrients and endogenous substances.

An example of an active transport system is the 'sodium–potassium pump', which pumps sodium out of, and potassium into, cells against their respective concentration gradients.

ABSORPTION AND DRUG CONCENTRATION

As long as the absorption of a drug is greater than its distribution and elimination, the concentration of the drug in the blood will increase. When the distribution and elimination from the blood are greater than the absorption, the concentration of drug in the blood will decrease.

Type of administration
The dosing schedule and the route of administration of a drug are important factors that influence the concentration of a drug in the blood.

Single dose
After an intravenous injection, the drug enters the bloodstream directly and the concentration rises to its peak level almost immediately. Elimination and distribution will start immediately. With intramuscular injection, the drug is absorbed over a longer period, and following oral administration, absorption takes even longer. This results in different absorption curves. See Figure 5.10. The effect of a drug is usually fastest if the route of administration that leads most rapidly to a high concentration in the target organ is used.

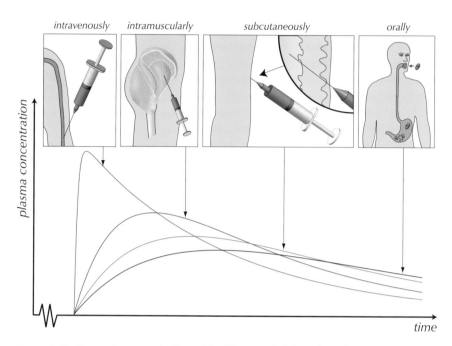

Figure 5.10 **Change in concentration with different administration of a single dose.** The illustration shows how the concentration of a drug changes in the blood according to which route of administration is used when a single dose is administered.

Continuous administration – intravenous infusion

If a drug is administered by a continuous intravenous infusion, the absorption phase will last as long as the infusion continues. When the rate of distribution and elimination equals the infused amount per unit time, steady state is achieved. In the same way that a drug will take five half-lives to be eliminated from the blood, a drug will take five half-lives to achieve steady state following continuous administration. See Figure 5.11.

At the outset, a person has 0 per cent of the drug in the body. For each new half-life ($t_{1/2}$), the increase becomes smaller and smaller, since elimination increases with increasing concentration. Thus:

- after 0 $t_{1/2}$, 0 per cent is accumulated
- after 1 $t_{1/2}$, 50 per cent is accumulated
- after 2 $t_{1/2}$, 75 per cent is accumulated
- after 3 $t_{1/2}$, 87.5 per cent is accumulated
- after 4 $t_{1/2}$, 93.75 per cent is accumulated
- after 5 $t_{1/2}$, 96.88 per cent is accumulated (steady state).

If the infusion rate is increased, it corresponds to a larger amount (dose) of drug per unit of time. Consequently, a new equilibrium is achieved: a doubling of the dose will result in a doubling of the drug concentration in the blood. This is true regardless of the form of administration used (provided that the drug does not saturate the elimination mechanisms or is not eliminated by first-pass metabolism after enteral administration).

Irregular administration – several doses per day

If a drug is administered in 'portions', or by several doses per day, the absorption and subsequent concentration of the drug in the blood will vary between each dose. Initially, the concentration increases for each new dose, if the time interval

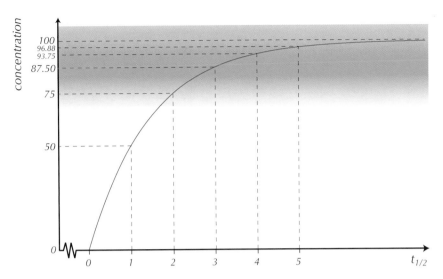

Figure 5.11 **Accumulation of a drug by continuous administration** (intravenous infusion). For each new half-life ($t_{1/2}$), the concentration increases by (100 – the value at the start of each half-life)/2. After $5 \times t_{1/2}$, 96.9 per cent of the anticipated value at steady state is achieved.

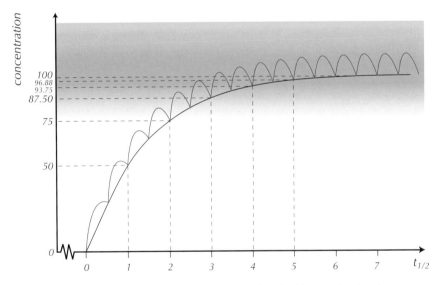

Figure 5.12 **Accumulation of a drug by repeated dosing.** In this case, the drug is administered twice per half-life. Notice that the increase in concentration after each dose is greater in the beginning than at equilibrium. The elimination is less at low than at high concentrations. Therefore, the concentration rises at the beginning and gradually levels off.

between the doses is so short that the drug is not totally eliminated before the next dose is taken. This increase in concentration gradually diminishes, and steady state is eventually achieved, as the rate of elimination of drug increases with increased concentration of the drug.

Once steady state is achieved, the concentration of the drug will only vary between doses. The concentration rises immediately after intake, reaches a peak level, and drops gradually until the next dose is taken. See Figure 5.12.

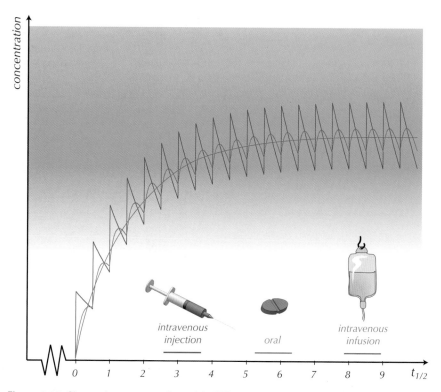

Figure 5.13 **Change in concentration with different forms of administration.** The diagram shows how the concentration of the same drug in the blood changes following three different routes of administration: oral, intravenous injection and intravenous infusion. The same dose is administered per unit of time.

In the case of continuous intravenous infusion, the concentration will remain constant as long as the infusion lasts, once distribution equilibrium has been achieved. With irregular dosing, the changes in concentration in the dosage intervals will be different depending on how the drug has been administered. See Figure 5.13.

Change in the size of a dose

As long as the dose and dosage interval remain constant, the concentration at equilibrium will only vary between each dosage interval. If the doses or the dosage intervals are changed, it will take five times the half-life of the drug before a new steady state is achieved. See Figure 5.14.

DISTRIBUTION

Distribution is taken to mean distribution from the blood to the peripheral tissues. As soon as a drug enters the blood, it will start to be distributed throughout the body. Eventually, distribution equilibrium is achieved in different tissues (as discussed in the example with the water containers, Figure 5.2). At distribution equilibrium, some drug will still be in the blood, while the remainder will be in other tissues. Different drugs will distribute themselves differently between different tissues. How rapidly and the extent to which the drugs are distributed to

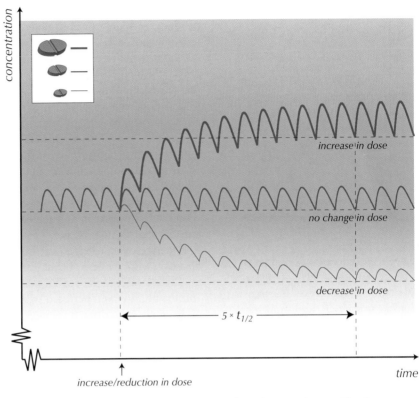

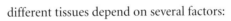

Figure 5.14 **When the dose changes, the value of steady state changes.** The diagram illustrates that from the time a dose change is introduced, it will take five times $t_{1/2}$ before a new steady state is achieved, regardless of whether the dose is increased or decreased.

different tissues depend on several factors:

- the blood circulation and distribution barriers
- the degree of the drug's binding to plasma proteins and tissue protein
- the water and lipid solubility of the drugs (discussed earlier in the chapter).

BLOOD CIRCULATION AND DISTRIBUTION BARRIERS

Different tissues of the body receive different proportions of the cardiac output. The brain, heart, liver, kidneys, lungs and thyroid gland are well perfused tissues. Skin, muscle tissue, fatty tissue and bone tissue are less well perfused with blood. The process of drug distribution depends on the transfer of the drug from the capillary, where, owing to the thinness of the blood vessel wall, there is close contact between blood and tissue.

The capillary wall consists of a single layer of endothelial cells and a basal membrane. In most tissues, there is virtually free passage of substances in the plasma across the capillary wall, with the exception of proteins. See Figure 5.15. In the central nervous system, the endothelial cells have a denser structure than in other tissues. In addition, glial cells cover the vascular wall on the outside, so that the barrier between the blood and the central nervous system (blood–brain barrier) is denser than other blood–tissue barriers. The blood–brain barrier allows only lipid-soluble substances in the blood to diffuse into the cells of the central nervous system. Water-soluble substances have to use special transport systems.

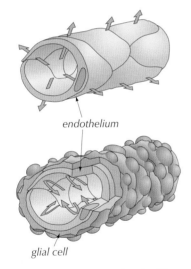

endothelium

glial cell

Figure 5.15 **Blood–tissue barrier.** The barrier between blood and normal tissue, and between blood and the central nervous system. In the central nervous system, the permeability from blood to tissue is less than in other tissues. Glial cells cover the capillaries and form an extra barrier. In addition, the endothelial cells are less permeable for many substances in the central nervous system than in other tissues. This reduces the transport from the blood to the brain, especially of water-soluble drugs.

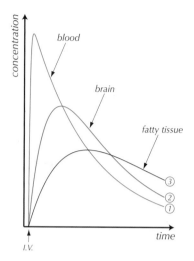

Figure 5.16 Concentration of diazepam in blood, brain tissue and fatty tissue after intravenous injection. Diazepam has high lipid solubility. A large part of the blood is supplied to the central nervous system, which contains a lot of lipid. Thus, the concentration of diazepam in the brain tissue will rise rapidly, while it falls in the blood. Gradually, the diazepam will be redistributed from the central nervous system to other tissue compartments. The diagram is a theoretical representation.

The amount of blood flow to different tissues determines how rapidly the distribution of highly lipid-soluble drugs will occur, while the rate of membrane transport influences how quickly water-soluble drugs are distributed. Imagine that the entire amount of a lipid-soluble drug that is carried in the blood to a tissue crosses the blood–tissue barrier to the tissue. In this case, the better the circulation, the more drug is distributed to the tissue. Conversely, if the blood carries a water-soluble drug to the tissues, the passage of such drugs across the blood–tissue barrier will be less because they are less lipid-soluble. Accordingly, no more of such a drug gets to the tissues regardless of whether the blood flow is great or small, as long as it is the transport across the membrane that limits its distribution.

Drugs that are distributed rapidly to tissues with good circulation can later be redistributed to tissues with poorer circulation. This means that a tissue or organ can have a high concentration shortly after a dose is given, especially after intravenous administration, and thereafter the concentration decreases as the drug is redistributed to other tissues. This is illustrated in Figure 5.16.

A person who receives an intravenous dose of the tranquillizing substance diazepam will fall asleep almost immediately because the concentration of diazepam rapidly increases in the central nervous system (diazepam has high lipid solubility and the brain is well perfused with blood). Gradually, the person awakens as the diazepam is redistributed to other parts of the body, and the concentration in the central nervous system drops.

DRUG BINDING TO PLASMA PROTEINS AND TISSUE PROTEINS

Proteins are found everywhere in the body. There are plasma proteins present in the blood and tissue is composed of protein. Drugs will bind to protein and different proteins will have a different ability (affinity) to bind different drugs (see the example with the water containers, Figure 5.2). Drugs that are bound to particular proteins in certain tissues can achieve high concentration in these tissues simply by virtue of this protein binding.

A drug that is not bound to protein in this way is referred to as 'free drug'. The total amount of a drug in a biological system consists of the sum of free drug and bound drug. How much is free and how much is bound in a tissue vary for different drugs. There will always be a constant ratio between free and bound drugs within the same tissue compartment.

Aminoglycosides are a special group of antibiotics that concentrate in the endolymph in the internal ear (labyrinth) and the organ of equilibrium. It is therefore conceivable that aminoglycosides can damage these organs when they are used in high concentration over a long period.

Suppose there are 1000 drug molecules in the central tissue compartment. Of these, 200 are free molecules, while 800 are bound to plasma proteins. The ratio between free and bound drug is then

$$\frac{200}{800} = 0.25$$

If we then suppose that 600 molecules are distributed from the central tissue compartment to the remaining tissue, we will have a total of 400 molecules remaining in the central tissue compartment. The ratio between free and bound drug will still be 0.25, i.e.:

$$\frac{80}{320} = 0.25$$

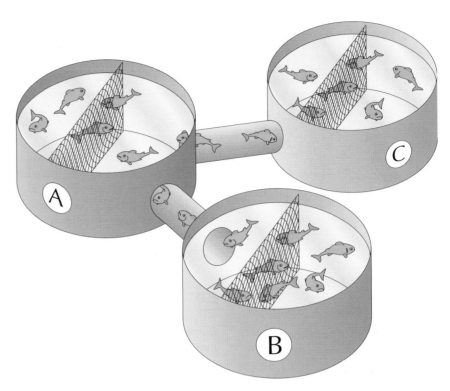

Figure 5.17 **Distribution of fish in fish tanks.** The fish will distribute themselves so that free-swimming fish are equally dense in all the tanks. However, the ratios between free-swimming fish and fish that are trapped in the net are different in the different tanks.

The distribution of the 400 remaining molecules then becomes 80 free and 320 bound. The tissue functions as a depot for drugs that have a high degree of binding to tissue proteins.

When distribution equilibrium is achieved, the concentration of free drug will be the same in all tissue compartments, in the same way as the water level is the same in all containers in our analogous system. See Figure 5.2. The distribution of drugs to different tissue compartments can be compared with the way fish will distribute themselves in large fish tanks if they can swim freely between them. See Figure 5.17. If the fish are put in the central tank, they will rapidly distribute themselves to all the tanks, and most rapidly to that which has the easiest entry. Gradually, the fish distribute themselves in such a way that they are equally dispersed in all the tanks.

However, if there are fish nets in the tanks, some of the fish will get trapped in these. The tank with the net that traps the most fish will, in total, contain the most fish. However, the fish that haven't been caught can swim freely and will distribute themselves equally throughout all the tanks. Thus, there is the same concentration of free-swimming fish in all the tanks, but the ratio between free-swimming fish and trapped fish is different in the different tanks. See Figure 5.17.

In the same way as the tank with the net that catches the most fish will have the highest total concentration of fish, the tissue compartments with the strongest tendency to bind a drug to its proteins will have the highest total concentration of drug.

VOLUME OF DISTRIBUTION

The compartments in which drugs are distributed are called the volume of distribution. The circulating blood volume can be considered as the central compartment,

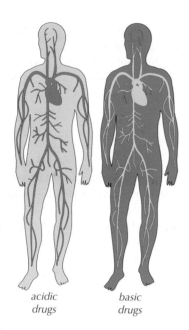

acidic drugs   *basic drugs*

Figure 5.18 Distribution of acidic and basic drugs in tissue. Acidic drugs distribute to proteins in plasma and thereby to the blood. Basic drugs distribute to tissue proteins outside the blood.

and the tissues outside as the peripheral compartment. If all of the drug in the body is in the bloodstream, the volume of distribution is equal to the blood volume (theoretically).

Drugs that are largely confined to the blood system have small volumes of distribution. Acidic drugs have a tendency to bind to albumin, and will therefore mainly be found in the bloodstream. This applies, for example, to phenobarbital (an antiepileptic drug) and the non-steroidal anti-inflammatory drugs (NSAIDs). Basic drugs bind mainly to tissue proteins outside the bloodstream, e.g. tricyclic antidepressants and antipsychotic drugs. See Figure 5.18.

Drugs that are readily distributed from the blood to peripheral tissues tend to have large volumes of distribution, and such drugs can be difficult to remove from the body. During haemodialysis, haemoperfusion or peritoneal dialysis the blood is cleared of drug, but most of it is located outside the bloodstream. There are no effective methods for removing these drugs from the body after a large intake, e.g. after poisoning.

ELIMINATION

Elimination of drugs can occur by metabolism (almost exclusively in the liver) followed by excretion (via urine or bile). The liver and the kidneys are the most important organs for eliminating the majority of drugs. The more water-soluble the drug, the more important the kidneys are in the elimination process. Since many drugs are soluble to a certain extent in both fat and water, they will be partly eliminated via metabolism in the liver and partly via the kidneys. A fraction of some drugs can also be eliminated via perspiration. Anaesthetic gases are eliminated in exhaled air. See Figure 5.19.

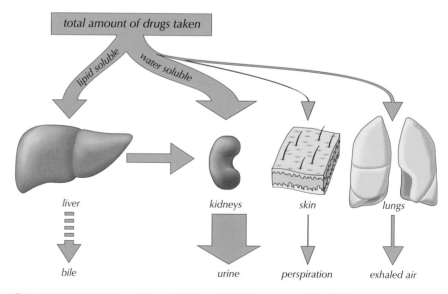

total amount of drugs taken

lipid soluble   *water soluble*

liver   *kidneys*   *skin*   *lungs*

bile   *urine*   *perspiration*   *exhaled air*

Figure 5.19 Elimination of drugs. Water-soluble drugs are mainly eliminated through the kidneys. Lipid-soluble drugs are mainly metabolized, which makes them water-soluble. Thereafter, they are partly eliminated through the bile and partly through the kidneys. For some drugs, elimination via exhaled air will be significant, while elimination via skin perspiration has little effect.

Early in the chapter we explained that the time it takes before a drug is eliminated is determined by the drug's half-life. It is usually estimated to take five times $t_{1/2}$ from stopping the drug administration until the drug is eliminated. As can be seen in Figure 5.20, there will still be a small fraction of drug (3.13 per cent) present after this time.

ELIMINATION BY METABOLISM

Metabolism describes a process whereby the chemical structure (and thereby the properties) of a substance is altered. Drugs that cannot be eliminated unchanged via the kidneys must be metabolized before they can be excreted. Lipid-soluble drugs are eliminated by such a process.

Metabolism of drugs occurs mainly in the liver, but the process can take place in other tissues, including, to a certain extent, by bacteria in the intestinal lumen and in the intestinal membrane. During metabolism, a number of different enzymes, which are located inside the cells, participate in altering the drug molecule. In order to be influenced by the liver's intracellular enzymes, the drugs must enter the liver cells.

First-pass metabolism
Drugs absorbed from the small intestine are transported to the liver by the portal vein. Lipid-soluble drugs, which diffuse easily across lipid membranes, will diffuse

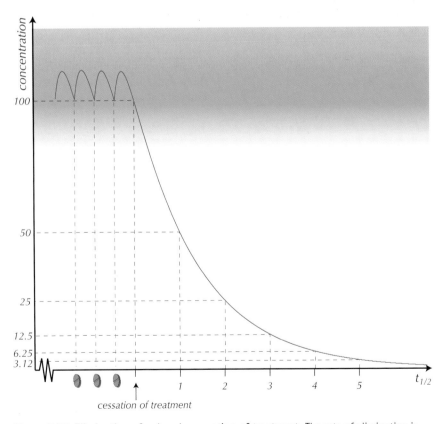

Figure 5.20 Elimination of a drug by cessation of treatment. The rate of elimination is reduced with decreasing concentration. It is estimated that the drug is 'eliminated' from the body after five times $t_{1/2}$, but 3.12 per cent still remains of the concentration present at the end of the last dosage interval.

into the liver cells, where they can be metabolized by various enzymatic processes. This means that drugs that are administered in such a way that they are absorbed from the intestine can be metabolized and thereby eliminated from the blood to a greater or lesser extent on their first passage through the liver, before they pass onwards into the systematic circulation. These types of drugs are said to have been exposed to first-pass metabolism.

Metabolism and biological availability

When a drug is taken orally, some of it can be metabolized by microorganisms in the intestine, and some can be metabolized during transport through the mucosal cells in the intestinal wall. A large portion can be metabolized during first-pass metabolism in the liver. This means that a substance could be absorbed into the blood, but that the drug is eliminated before it reaches the systemic circulation. See Figure 5.21. The same effect can also occur in the lungs before the blood returns to the heart and enters the systemic circulation.

The term bioavailability describes the fraction of an ingested amount of drug reaching the systemic circulation without being metabolized (the fraction that is not eliminated from the pre-systemic circulation), and therefore the fraction of a drug dose the organism can utilize, as follows:

Bioavailability =

$$\frac{\text{(total amount} - \text{amount metabolized before entering systemic circulation)}}{\text{total amount}}$$

Drugs that are exposed to a high degree of metabolism have low bioavailability. For drugs with low bioavailability, the route of administration will be significant. These drugs require higher doses when they are administered via the intestine (enterally) than when they are administered outside the intestine (parenterally).

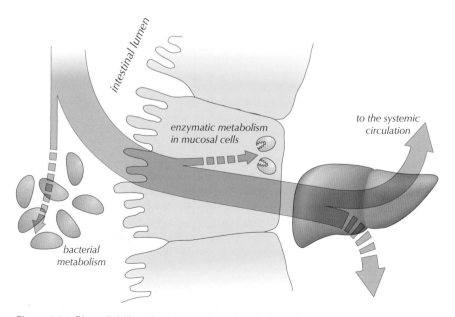

Figure 5.21 **Bioavailability** of a drug can be reduced when microorganisms in the intestine, enzymes in the intestinal mucosal cells or enzymes in the liver metabolize the drugs before they reach the systemic circulation.

Morphine administered as tablets is given in considerably higher doses than when it is administered as an intravenous injection. This is because of the pre-systemic (or first-pass) metabolism of morphine.

Phase I and phase II reactions in the liver

Lipid-soluble substances often pass through two stages, or reaction phases, to become more water-soluble. The first stage is referred to as phase I metabolism where the drug is modified to a reactive metabolite, which in the second stage (phase II) 'fuses together' (conjugates) with another compound to form a water-soluble 'conjugated complex'. See Figure 5.22. The water-soluble conjugated complex can be excreted via the urine or the bile. In some cases, the reactive metabolites may cause harmful effects to the liver cells.

The conjugation process is important both for drugs and for the body's own (endogenous) substances.

Morphine is eliminated after it is conjugated to glucuronic acid. When haemoglobin molecules are broken down, bilirubin is formed which binds to albumin in the blood and cannot be excreted in the urine. In the liver, the bilirubin is conjugated with glucuronic acid. The bilirubin–glucuronic acid complex is excreted with the bile and can thus be eliminated from the circulation.

Paracetamol is metabolized via several steps. One of the metabolites is very toxic to the liver cells, but is conjugated and detoxified by compounds in the liver cells. If a very large dose of paracetamol is taken, the compounds that are used for detoxification are depleted. Thereafter, the toxic metabolites will damage the liver cells. In this way, a large dose of paracetamol may lead to massive damage to the liver cells and death.

Factors affecting the metabolic function of the liver

The metabolic activity of the liver is carried out by enzymatic processes. There is some change with increasing age, but more importantly, if the liver becomes diseased, then its function can be reduced to such an extent that a reduction in the dose of drug becomes necessary. The enzymes can also be affected so that they increase in quantity (enzyme induction) or their activity becomes inhibited (enzyme inhibition). To understand metabolism, it is also important to know that an enzyme's capacity to metabolize drugs can be saturated.

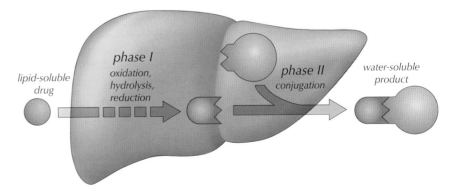

Figure 5.22 Phase I and phase II reactions. Lipid-soluble substances are metabolized in phase I to an intermediate product that is conjugated with another molecule in phase II. The substance thus becomes water-soluble and can be excreted through the kidneys or with the bile. Some substances go directly to phase II, and some become water-soluble after phase I and avoid phase II (not shown in the figure).

Enzyme induction

Enzymes that are active in the metabolism of a drug can be influenced by both drugs and other foreign substances, leading to an increase in the amount of the enzyme. When drug administration leads to increased quantities of an enzyme that participates in the metabolism of drugs, the drug is said to have enzyme-inducing properties, and the phenomenon is called enzyme induction. Enzyme induction leads to increased drug metabolism and thereby reduced drug concentration, and consequently a reduced or absent drug effect. Some drugs can influence enzyme systems to increase the metabolism of the drug itself. Enzyme induction usually occurs over 2–3 weeks, since it takes this length of time to synthesize the enzymes.

Enzyme inhibition

Drugs can also inhibit the enzymes that are responsible for their metabolism, resulting in an increase in drug concentration. When a drug reduces the activity of enzymes that participate in the metabolism of drugs, the drug is said to have enzyme-inhibiting properties, and the phenomenon is called enzyme inhibition. Enzyme inhibition leads to reduced drug metabolism and thereby increased drug concentration, which in turn leads to an increased drug effect (and side-effects). Some drugs can influence enzyme systems to reduce the metabolism of the drug itself.

Drugs with an enzyme-inhibiting effect usually exert their effect soon after intake. The reason for this is that the enzyme activity is inhibited; it is not enzyme synthesis that is reduced. In some cases, however, drugs can inhibit enzyme synthesis. In these cases, it will take time before the inhibiting effect occurs.

Carbamazepine and phenytoin, drugs used in the treatment of epilepsy, are examples of drugs that produce enzyme induction. If someone takes one of these drugs simultaneously with oestrogen-based birth control pills, the metabolism of oestrogen can increase to such an extent that the oestrogen concentration is inadequate to provide a contraceptive effect.

Warfarin is a drug that reduces the blood's ability to coagulate. The enzymes that participate in the metabolism of warfarin are influenced by many different drugs, and their effect on these enzymes can lead to increased concentration of warfarin and fatal bleeding, or alternatively to decreased concentration of warfarin, thus diminishing its effect and allowing blood clots to form.

Another drug, cimetidine, which reduces the production of hydrochloric acid in the gastric mucosa, can inhibit enzymes that participate in the metabolism of many other drugs, and thereby increase the effect of these drugs.

Main groups and subgroups of enzymes

There are many different enzymes that participate in the metabolism of drugs. The enzymes are divided into groups and subgroups. One of the main groups is cytochrome P450, which consists of many virtually identical enzymes (isoenzymes). Isoenzymes of cytochrome P450 are often subject to enzyme induction or inhibition.

Metabolism without saturation of the enzymes – the rule

Drugs are usually administered in doses that, at steady state, do not exceed the liver's ability to metabolize the administered drug at each dosage interval. Thus the concentration is held constant by continuous dosing, and the concentration rises or falls with increased or reduced doses. With doses that do not saturate the enzyme's capacity to metabolize, an increase or reduction in dose will result in an increase or reduction in concentration that is in proportion to the change in dosage. A doubling of the dose results in a doubling of the concentration until a new steady state is established.

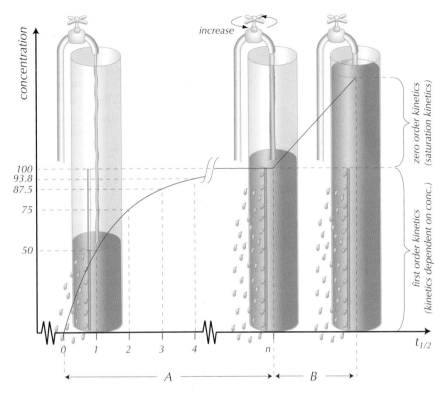

Figure 5.23 The increase in water level in a container during two flow rates. Period A shows an inward flow rate where the level of the water reaches the upper part of the vertical slit in the container when steady state is achieved. Period B shows the situation after a small increase in the flow rate, which leads to overflow of the container; the elimination system has been saturated.

Drugs that do not saturate the enzyme systems when administered in therapeutic doses have non-saturation kinetics, also called first-order kinetics.

Metabolism with saturation of the enzymes – the exception

Some drugs are taken in such large doses that they saturate the enzyme systems that participate in the metabolism. These drugs have saturation kinetics, also called zero-order kinetics. With the use of drugs in such large doses that saturation kinetics occurs, small increases in dosage will cause the drug concentration to increase dramatically, and undesired side-effects can result. This is analogous to the situation where more water flows into a container than can flow out, in which case the water level increases steadily. See Figure 5.23. Phenytoin and acetylsalicylic acid can achieve saturation kinetics when they are regularly administered in high, therapeutic doses.

ELIMINATION BY EXCRETION

The kidneys are the most important organs for elimination by excretion, followed by biliary secretion and excretion via exhaled air.

Elimination via the kidneys

When the blood flows through the arteries in the glomeruli, it is filtered through the glomerular membrane in Bowman's capsule. From filtered blood, approximately

180 L of filtrate is created per day in an adult person. A large part of the filtrate is reabsorbed back into the blood, such that the amount of urine that is finally excreted will be considerably reduced in volume and its composition changed in relation to the initial glomerular filtrate.

Both lipid-soluble and water-soluble drugs are filtered into the renal tubule. In addition, drugs can be eliminated from the blood to the nephron by tubular secretion. Tubular secretion from the blood to the renal tubules occurs primarily by active transport in the proximal tubule. Lipid-soluble drugs are, to a greater or lesser extent, reabsorbed back into the blood by tubular reabsorption. Reabsorption from renal tubule to the blood occurs primarily by passive diffusion in the distal tubule. See Figure 5.8.

Water-soluble drugs will follow the flow of filtrate through the rest of the nephron and be excreted with the urine. Lipid-soluble drugs are subjected to tubular reabsorption to the blood and must circulate through the liver again to be metabolized to water-soluble metabolites before they can be excreted via the kidneys or the bile.

Renal function is impaired with increasing age, with renal disease, and is altered during pregnancy. In serious renal impairment the dose of a drug removed via renal excretion will be considerably reduced.

Tubular reabsorption

Tubular reabsorption is influenced by the pH of the urine. A drug that exists in its ionized form in the glomerular filtrate will have difficulty passing through the wall of the renal tubule. If, on the other hand, it exists in its un-ionized form, it is more lipid-soluble and can pass considerably more easily across the tubule back into the blood.

Weak acids will be ionized at high pH (alkaline urine), and weak bases will be ionized at low pH (acid urine). This can be used to increase the excretion of weak acids and bases when these exist in too high a concentration in the body. The goal is to ionize the drugs, so that they remain in the tubular lumen and are excreted with the urine.

Biliary excretion and enterohepatic circulation

Drugs that have been conjugated in the liver can be excreted in the bile and eliminated from the body via the large intestine. These conjugated drugs can be metabolized further by intestinal bacteria. Since they are generally lipid-soluble, they are reabsorbed from the intestine. After reaching the liver again, the drug will be reconjugated and excreted with the bile once more. In this way, some drugs may 'circulate' in the enterohepatic circulation.

Digoxin is glucuronidated in the liver, and then enters the duodenum via the common bile duct. A little further down the small intestine, the digoxin-glucuronide is hydrolysed and digoxin is reabsorbed to the blood and re-enters the liver – enterohepatic circulation. Morphine, chloramphenicol and stilboestrol also appear in the bile conjugated with glucuronide. These substances are hydrolysed in the intestine, and the active drugs can be reabsorbed into the blood.

CLEARANCE

The 'clearance' of a drug refers to how effectively it is eliminated from the blood. Specifically, it relates to how large a blood volume is cleared of drug per unit time, and it usually has the units litres/hour (L/h) or cm^3/min. As long as elimination mechanisms are not saturated (first-order kinetics), the same blood volume will be cleared per unit time even if the concentration of a substance in the blood varies, i.e. clearance is constant. If the organ that eliminates a substance is affected by disease, clearance will diminish. Clearance is therefore a measure of the organ's ability to eliminate a substance.

SUMMARY

- Pharmacokinetics is the study of the fate of drugs in an organism.
- The site of administration influences the absorption and how rapidly the drug passes into the blood.
- Small and neutral molecules are transported faster across membranes than large molecules or ones that are electrically charged. Most of the absorption occurs in the upper part of the small intestine.
- With continuous dosing, the concentration of a drug in the blood increases at a rate determined by the drug's half-life. With constant dosing, it takes approximately five times the half-life from first taking the drug until steady state is achieved. Likewise, it takes approximately five times the half-life before new steady state is achieved after a change in dosage. It also takes approximately five times the half-life from the time a subject stops taking a drug until it is eliminated from the body.
- Different drugs distribute unevenly in different tissues. Acidic drugs have a tendency to bind to plasma proteins; they are primarily found in the bloodstream and have a small volume of distribution. Basic drugs bind to tissue proteins; they are primarily found outside the blood and have a large volume of distribution.
- At distribution equilibrium, the same concentration of free drug exists in all tissue compartments.
- Lipid-soluble drugs distribute faster and to a greater degree to the central nervous system than water-soluble drugs. Therefore, they cause more frequent central nervous system side-effects than water-soluble drugs.
- Lipid-soluble drugs are metabolized in the liver before they are excreted via the bile or the kidneys. Water-soluble drugs are excreted through the kidneys without undergoing substantial alterations in the liver.
- Drugs that are excreted in the bile may undergo enterohepatic circulation, and be reabsorbed in the blood.
- Drugs that have a large degree of first-pass metabolism (low bioavailability) are administered in different doses by enteral and parenteral administration.
- Some drugs may saturate the elimination mechanisms, thus demonstrating saturation kinetics.
- Some drugs cause enzyme induction; others cause enzyme inhibition.
- The combination of glomerular filtration, tubular secretion and tubular reabsorption determines the rate of drug excretion by the kidneys.
- The renal excretion of weak acids and bases is influenced by the pH of the urine.
- Absorption, distribution, metabolism and elimination occur simultaneously in the organism.

6 Administration of drugs and drug formulations

For a drug to achieve its required effect, a sufficient quantity of drug must be distributed to the site of action and its concentration must be maintained, within certain limits, for the required period of time. Often transport via the bloodstream is required for the drug to reach the site of action, but sometimes it is appropriate to administer the drug locally. Some individuals have difficulty swallowing tablets, some drugs are destroyed by the acidic environment of the stomach, and some drugs might be metabolized by first-pass metabolism, so it can be advantageous to administer the drug in other ways than by mouth.

To meet different needs, drugs can be manufactured in different formulations. The method of administration used is largely determined by the drug formulation chosen.

MAIN ROUTES OF ADMINISTRATION

There are two main routes of drug administration: enteral and parenteral. Administration via an enteral route means that drugs reach the intestine before they are absorbed in the blood. Other means of administration are usually parenteral. See Figure 6.1. The crucial difference between enteral and parenteral administration is that the drug is exposed to varying degrees of first-pass metabolism following enteral administration, because the drug passes to the liver after absorption from the intestine. (For an explanation of first-pass metabolism, see Ch. 5, p. 53.)

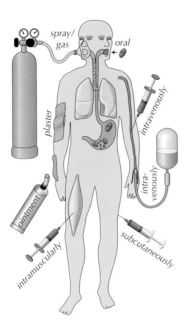

Figure 6.2 **Various routes of administration of drugs.**

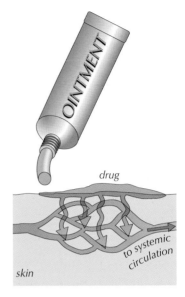

Figure 6.3 **Systemic absorption after local administration.** Drugs that are administered locally can be absorbed in the blood and are distributed to other tissues. With increasing doses that are administered locally, the chances of systemic and adverse effects are increased.

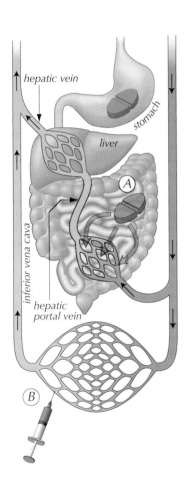

Figure 6.1 **Enteral and parenteral administration.** Following enteral administration, the drug is absorbed and passes through the liver before it enters the systemic circulation. After parenteral administration, the drug avoids first-pass metabolism.

Local administration is used to achieve local effects. It allows the use of lower doses than if the drug were to be administered systemically and so avoids undesired effects in other organ systems. Administration via skin, inhalation, under the eyelid, directly into the joints and vaginally are examples of local administration. Different routes of administration are shown in Figure 6.2.

Local administration is no guarantee that there will not be systemic effects. If the drug is absorbed subsequently into the blood, thereby entering the general circulation, it may produce effects in other organs. See Figure 6.3.

ENTERAL ADMINISTRATION

In enteral administration, the drug enters the body via the mouth (oral administration) or the rectum (rectal administration).

ORAL ADMINISTRATION

Oral administration is the most common form of administration. The drug is swallowed and resides briefly in the stomach before it moves on to the small intestine. For a few drugs, absorption begins in the stomach, but generally most are absorbed in the small intestine. On first passage through the liver, after absorption from the intestine, lipid-soluble drugs will be removed in varying amounts from the blood before reaching the systemic circulation. These drugs are usually given in higher doses when they are administered enterally than when they are administered parenterally.

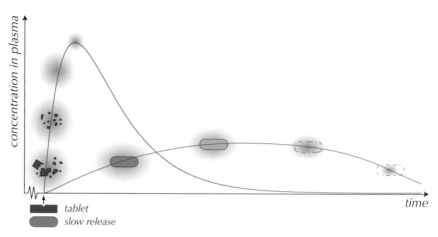

Figure 6.5 Concentration profile of regular tablets and modified-release formulations.
The illustration shows that a regular tablet dissolves quickly and provides quick absorption, while a slow-release form is absorbed over a longer time interval. These forms provide the most uniform change in concentration over time.

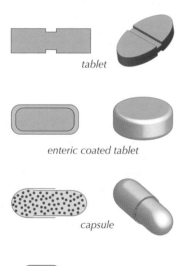

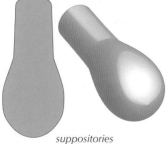

Figure 6.4 Some drug formulations.
Enteric-coated forms have an acid-resistant coating (red) surrounding the active substance and must not be crushed before they are administered.

Any circumstances that reduce intestinal motility will delay the absorption of orally administered drugs. Restriction of parts of the small intestine or diseases of the small intestine may limit the absorption of drugs.

Drug formulations intended for oral administration

Tablets are a compressed mixture of active drugs and additives. They can be loosely or solidly compressed so that they dissolve quickly or slowly after they are swallowed.

Enteric-coated tablets are designed to dissolve after they have passed the stomach and entered the small intestine. Enteric tablets should not be chewed or crushed. This is to avoid destroying an acid-insoluble layer around the outside of the tablet that prevents it from dissolving in the stomach. Enteric forms are principally used for drugs that have a local irritant effect on the mucosa in the stomach, or that are destroyed by the acidic environment there. See Figure 6.4.

Effervescent tablets are tablets designed to dissolve in water.

Capsules consist of drugs in fluid or powder form, enclosed by a gelatine capsule. They can be manufactured to dissolve in the stomach or in the intestine. Some capsules are perforated with a number of small holes to let the contents diffuse slowly and provide delayed absorption. Capsules should be swallowed whole.

Modified-release formulations (e.g. slow release) are drug formulations designed to provide delayed and uniform absorption and avoid frequent dosing. They are used for drugs with short half-lives. See Figure 6.5.

Powders are small-grained forms of the drug.

Granules are preparations consisting of grains 1–2 mm in diameter. They are usually intended to dissolve in water.

Mixtures are drugs in fluid form intended for oral administration.

RECTAL ADMINISTRATION

To achieve this means of administration, the drug is inserted into the rectum. Approximately 50 per cent of the blood from this area bypasses the liver, avoiding first-pass metabolism to some extent. The acidic environment of the stomach and enzymes present in the small intestine are also avoided.

Rectal administration is useful when a drug causes nausea or if the patient is vomiting but may be perceived as an unpleasant experience. In some individuals, the formulation used can cause local irritation in and around the rectum. It is important to place the drug as far into the rectum as possible.

Drug formulations intended for rectal administration

Suppositories are drugs intended for use in the rectum. The drug is mixed with a substance that dissolves at body temperature; on dissolving, the drug is released and is thereafter absorbed across the intestinal mucous membrane.

Enema solutions are liquid preparations intended for use in the rectum. As the drug is presented in solution, absorption can be rapid, which is sometimes useful (e.g. a diazepam enema to treat convulsions in a fitting child).

PARENTERAL ADMINISTRATION

Parenteral administration refers to all routes of drug administration with the exception of oral and rectal administration.

ADMINISTRATION BY INJECTION AND INFUSION

Injection and infusion are used for drugs with poor absorption from the intestine, drugs that are unstable in the gastrointestinal environment, to avoid the first-pass metabolism by the liver, or when a rapid onset of action is required. Patients who cannot receive drugs by oral administration may depend on this form of administration. Injections can be used to achieve local effects, e.g. in joints, and for local anaesthetic effects. Injections tend to be given in a small volume and are delivered in seconds or minutes. Infusions are used when there is a need to use larger volumes over a longer period of time.

Intravenous (i.v.). The drug is injected directly into a vein, which provides immediate and virtually complete entry into the bloodstream. The concentration of drug in the blood will increase quite rapidly following this form of administration, so caution must be exercised as to the rate of administration. It is particularly important to follow instructions with regard to the way in which the drug is to be administered for any drugs that can affect cardiac rhythms or the central nervous system. Also watch for rapidly developing allergic reactions (anaphylactic reactions).

Intra-arterial (i.a.). The drug is injected directly into an artery. It is used for administration of contrast media during special X-ray examinations or to administer a high concentration of cytotoxic drug into a local area/tumour supplied by a specific artery.

Intramuscular (i.m.). The drug is injected directly into a muscle. See Figure 6.6. Muscles have a good blood supply, and the capillary vessels in muscles absorb

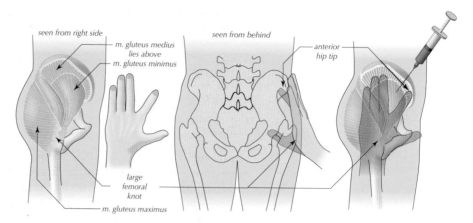

Figure 6.6 **Intramuscular administration.** With this type of administration, the drug is often injected into the large gluteal muscle, a tissue with a good blood supply.

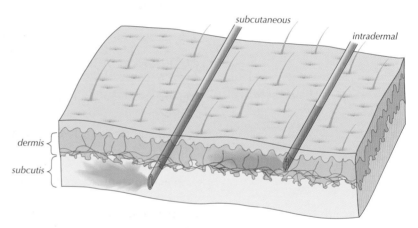

Figure 6.7 **Subcutaneous and intradermal administration.** Following subcutaneous administration, the drug penetrates more deeply than with intradermal administration.

most drugs quickly. Drugs that can irritate the tissue, e.g. diazepam and phenytoin, should not be administered intramuscularly. In pronounced shock, the blood supply to muscles may be so reduced that intramuscular administration does not provide sufficient absorption. In such cases, intravenous administration may be necessary.

Subcutaneous (s.c.). In s.c. administration, the drug is injected under the skin, into the fatty tissue just beneath it. Subcutaneous tissue does not have quite as good a blood supply as muscle, so the concentration of drug in the blood increases more slowly than is seen following i.m. administration. See Figure 6.7.

Intradermal (i.d.) administration means injection directly under the immediate surface of the skin. This form of administration is used in tests of suspected allergens and for BCG vaccination.

Intraspinal. The drug is introduced into the spinal canal/subarachnoid cavity so that it mixes with the spinal fluid and especially influences the nervous system.

This form of administration may be used to achieve an analgesic effect, e.g. before and after surgical intervention (See Figure 25.2, p. 378).

Epidural. The drug is administered into the epidural cavity, i.e. outside the dura, to achieve high concentration around the nerves of the spinal cord. One use of this form of administration is to reduce pain during childbirth. A smaller area is affected by the drug following epidural than is experienced following intraspinal administration.

Intra-articular. The drug is injected into a joint, the purpose being to achieve a high concentration and local effects in structures that are close to joints. As absorption from the synovial fluid occurs slowly, the local concentration can remain high over a long period of time before the drug is absorbed into the bloodstream. Penetration of drugs injected intra-articularly is poor into deeper structures close to the joint.

Intraperitoneal. The drug is injected directly into the abdominal cavity. This form of administration can be used for antibiotics in the treatment of infectious peritonitis and for dialysis fluid in the treatment of peritoneal dialysis.

Intrapleural. The drug is injected directly into the pleural cavity. Certain cytotoxins are injected into the pleural cavity for the treatment of cancers in this part of the body.

Drug formulations intended for injection and infusion

Injection solutions are fluid solutions with a volume of 50 mL or less.

Infusion solutions are fluid solutions with a volume greater than 50 mL. These solutions may have other drugs added to them.

Injection and infusion substances are freeze-dried compounds that have an increased shelf-life as a result. These must be dissolved in sterile solutions.

Infusion concentrates are fluid, concentrated solutions intended to be added to infusion solutions.

Injections and infusions are usually administered intravenously. Infusions can also be administered intraperitoneally (peritoneal dialysis), subcutaneously (insulin) and epidurally (analgesics). It is crucial that perforations of the vessel wall are avoided during intravenous administration, in order to avoid the danger of the injection or infusion leaking out of the bloodstream. This is particularly important when cytotoxic or other potentially toxic drugs are administered. Tissue-irritating substances should be administered into a central vein where the volume of blood gives a greater diluting effect.

Drugs that are given intravenously must be checked rigorously immediately before administration, preferably by two people. The drug must be within the stated 'use by' date, correctly drawn up into the syringe, and the solution should not be discoloured or contaminated in any way. Concentration of drug in the blood increases very rapidly with this form of administration, and serious adverse effects arise if contaminated drugs are used. During an injection, it is important to observe whether the patient's state of consciousness changes, which may occur if there is a disturbance of cardiac rhythm or if an anaphylactic reaction develops.

SUBLINGUAL ADMINISTRATION

Sublingual administration of a drug refers to administration under the tongue. In this case, the drug dissolves quickly and diffuses directly across the mucous membrane lining of the mouth into the capillary network underneath before it moves on to the systemic circulation, without going via the liver, so avoiding first-pass metabolism. Sublingual administration is not regarded as enteral, as absorption does not take place from the intestine, but from the oral cavity.

Drug formulations intended for buccal administration

Lozenges and chewing tablets are tablets that are sucked or chewed to provide a local effect in the mouth (buccal cavity) or in the upper part of the throat (pharynx). This drug formulation is used, for example, to treat fungal infections in the oral cavity. Chewing tablets are also used to neutralize stomach acid.

Buccal tablets are tablets placed under the tongue (sublingually) or chewed to allow the drug to be absorbed through the mucous membrane lining the mouth. This form of administration often results in fast absorption. Buccal tablets are not meant to be swallowed. This form of administration is often used when a rapid effect is needed, e.g. for angina pectoris, or for drugs that are destroyed by stomach acid.

ADMINISTRATION BY INHALATION

Inhalation can take place through the mouth or nose. This form of administration is used to achieve local effects in the lungs or the nasal membrane, or for giving anaesthetic gases. Inhalation is commonly used to administer anti-asthmatic drugs as well as those used for allergies in the respiratory passage.

Drugs for inhalation should be easy to disperse in solution or powder form. Following inhalation through the mouth, the majority of the drug attaches to the mucous membrane in the mouth and throat (buccal and pharyngeal regions), but enough of the drug will reach the lungs to provide sufficient effect, if the correct technique is used. In children under 5 years of age, a 'spacer' into which the drug is sprayed can be used. The child inhales from the spacer and receives the dose in 10–15 inhalations. See Figure 6.8. Before asthmatic patients commence inhalation treatment, they need to be trained in the correct inhalation technique.

Drugs are absorbed well through the nasal membrane into the bloodstream. Examples of administration via this route include oxytocin to increase the milk expulsion reflex in cases of problematic breastfeeding. The migraine drug sumitriptan can be used as a nasal spray since gastric emptying is reduced and tablets provide a delayed effect with migraine attacks. To prevent nightly bed-wetting in older children, an evening dose of desmopressin nasal spray is effective, as the drug has an antidiuretic effect, decreasing the volume of urine produced during the night.

Drug formulations intended for inhalation

Inhalation powders are drugs in finely dispersed powder form administered via an inhaler. The most common means of dispersion is by the use of turbohalers, whereby finely dispersed drug particles move in the air stream generated down into the lungs (See Figure 18.3, p. 270).

Aerosols. In the case of aerosols, the drugs are dissolved in fluid. The fluid is dispersed by gas pressure and is drawn down into the lungs in the air stream.

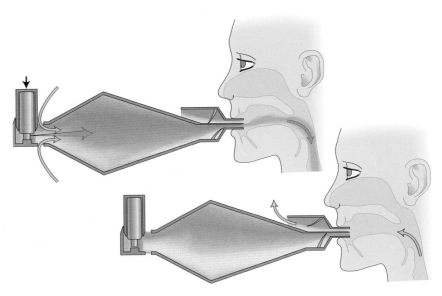

Figure 6.8 **Inhalation using a spacer.** After an aerosol with drugs is sprayed into a spacer, small children can inhale the drug.

Nasal sprays. The finely dispersed particles of fluid are sprayed out of a container and drawn up in the nasal passage. The effects achieved may be local or systemic.

TOPICAL ADMINISTRATION OF DRUGS

Drugs that are administered on to the surface of the skin have a local effect and may be used to treat different types of eczema, psoriasis and skin infections, or they may be used to prevent dehydration of the skin. The drugs are administered in formulations or bases made up of different proportions of oil and water. The greater the proportion of oil, the more effective the preparation is in preventing dehydration. Salve and cream bases are often used to prevent dehydration of the skin in the treatment of different types of eczema. Drugs with anti-inflammatory, moisture-retaining, antiseptic or antibiotic properties can be added to these types of preparation.

Drug formulations intended for topical administration

Ointments are an emulsion of water and oil, where the water is finely dispersed in the oil phase. The active substance can be dispersed in water or oil. Ointments are used on dry parts of the skin. Some individuals feel that ointments have unpleasant cosmetic effects and leave spots on clothing. For this reason, many people choose to use an ointment only at night. See Figure 6.9.

Creams are an emulsion of water and oil where the oil is finely dispersed in the water phase. The active substance can be dispersed in water or oil. Creams are used on moist parts of the skin, e.g. suppurating surfaces, but can also be used on dry parts. Some creams, known as fat creams, have more oil added than usual. Creams are more acceptable cosmetically than ointments and are well suited for daytime use.

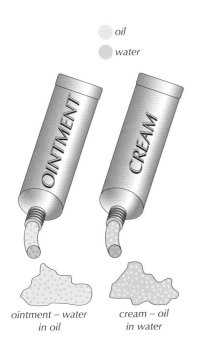

○ oil

○ water

ointment – water in oil

cream – oil in water

Figure 6.9 **Ointment and cream.** In a salve, water is finely dispersed in an oil phase. In a cream, oil is finely dispersed in a water phase.

Liniments are fluid preparations for use on skin and in hair, where the fluid evaporates and allows the drug to remain.

Gels are half-fluid drug formulations comprising substances that evaporate quickly and allow the drug to remain on the skin.

Suspensions are suspensions of solid particles in fluid.

TRANSDERMAL ADMINISTRATION AND DRUG FORMULATIONS

With transdermal administration, the drug is applied to the skin, but the intention is that the drug is absorbed into the bloodstream over a long period. Normally, the skin acts as an effective barrier and not all drugs will be absorbed if they are applied on intact skin. This is why it is important to use additives to ease such transport or to cover the drug and the skin with a watertight plaster. By using the plaster, the skin is softened and the 'barrier' function is reduced.

Drug patches are made in such a way that the drug is absorbed at a constant rate over several hours. The substances in the patch have systemic effects and first-pass metabolism in the liver is avoided. Examples of these patches are nicotine patches and lidocaine patches. The site of application for the patch should be changed each time a fresh patch is applied, to avoid local irritation of the same skin area.

ADMINISTRATION AND DRUG FORMULATIONS OF EYE REMEDIES

Administration of local drugs for the eyes is often in the form of eye drops, but special emulsions and ointments are also used. Drops should be placed in the lower eyelid fold to provide a local effect for infections, analgesic effects, lubricating effects, to dilate or contract the pupils, to improve the drainage of aqueous humour in glaucoma and in the treatment of allergic disorders.

OTHER FORMS OF ADMINISTRATION AND DRUG FORMULATIONS

Vaginal administration of drugs is used to achieve local effects in the vaginal mucous membrane. The indications may be infection with fungi or bacteria. It is possible to treat dry mucous membranes by local administration of hormones using this route. The drugs are administered in the form of pessaries, suppositories or creams that are inserted into the vagina with the help of suitable devices.

SHELF-LIFE OF DRUGS

All drugs must have an expiry date specified on the outside and inside packaging. The expiry date indicates a drug's shelf-life, and specifies the time when the use of a drug should be terminated.

Ampoules and single-dose containers must be discarded after use. All injection preparations that consist of dry substances are to be dissolved immediately before use. Multiple-dose containers should indicate the times for opening. Drugs without preservatives have a shelf-life of 24 h after opening. Preserved drugs have a shelf-life of 4 weeks after opening.

Drugs in solution can become contaminated after opening. In the case of multi-dose ampoules, where drugs are repeatedly drawn through a rubber bung using a needle and syringe, e.g. insulin there is an increased risk of particulate contamination (through the increasing number of perforations of the rubber bung) and microbiological contamination. Some drugs need to be protected against light if they are to be administered by infusion over a long period of time.

MISCIBILITY OF DRUGS IN FLUIDS

As a rule, drugs should not to be added to infusion fluids with buffering properties, such as bicarbonate buffer. Solutions such as sodium chloride and glucose or sterile water are suitable. Check in any instance of uncertainty.

Always note on the label of an infusion container which drugs are added to an infusion fluid, and check the shelf-life on every package of drugs used.

SUMMARY

- There are two different forms of administration: enteral and parenteral. Enteral administration includes oral and rectal administration, while all other forms of administration are considered parenteral.
- The route of administration and the drug formulation determines how quickly a drug enters the bloodstream.
- In the case of intravenous administration, two individuals should check that the correct drug and dose is being administered, that the expiry date has not been exceeded and that the drug is not visibly contaminated.
- Local administration is used to achieve local effects. If a drug is administered locally in large doses, it might be absorbed and produce systemic effects.
- Inhalation is a suitable means of administering drugs used in the treatment of asthma and for allergic disorders in the respiratory passages.
- Local administration on the skin is used for localized skin requirements, especially eczema. Ointment can be used on dry parts of the skin; cream is used on moist parts of the skin, but can also be smeared on dry areas.
- Dry drugs have a longer shelf-life than drugs in solution.
- Fluids with buffer properties should not be used as a solution for dissolving drugs used for injection or infusion.

7 Adverse effects of drugs

An adverse effect is defined as an unwanted and harmful reaction resulting from drugs used therapeutically, prophylactically, diagnostically or to alter physiological functions.

Drugs exert their effects wherever there are substrates or receptors that are influenced by them. This makes it possible for both desired and undesired effects to occur. Ideally, drugs should have a high specificity, that means an effect on the minimum number of different receptors and organs. High specificity allows for a therapeutic effect which largely avoids adverse effects. Effects due to misuse, or which occur as a result of a planned overdose, are not regarded as adverse effects.

It is difficult to assess how frequently adverse effects occur. A common estimate is that approximately 10 per cent of all patients who use prescribed drugs experience adverse effects. For the majority of patients, however, the benefits of therapeutic drug use are greater than the risk of the associated adverse effects.

Adverse effects occur most frequently in the skin, gastrointestinal (GI) tract, cardiovascular system, nervous system, liver and kidneys.

CLASSIFICATION OF ADVERSE EFFECTS

Adverse effects can be classified into dose-related and non-dose-related effects.

DOSE-RELATED ADVERSE EFFECTS

Dose-related adverse effects are associated with the drug's known pharmacological effects and occur when drugs are used in therapeutic doses. In principle, they are predictable. All users will experience these adverse effects if the dose is high enough. Often, an increase in the concentration of the drug due to reduced elimination, or drug interactions which potentiate the effect, can be responsible for such adverse effects.

Desired effect is too strong

Large doses of anticoagulants can cause haemorrhaging. Large doses of insulin can cause hypoglycaemia. Large doses of antihypertensive drugs can cause a pronounced drop in blood pressure, resulting in dizziness, confusion and reduced coronary perfusion, which can trigger angina pectoris or a heart attack. In these cases, the adverse effects can be reduced or abolished by a reduction in dose.

Effects on systems other than the target system

Drugs used to treat asthma that stimulate β_2-adrenoceptors in the bronchi are known to also influence the heart's β_1-adrenoceptors and cause unpleasant palpitations and increase the heart rate. β-Blockers intended to block β_1-adrenoceptors may also block β_2-adrenoceptors in the bronchioles, leading to bronchoconstriction and respiratory problems. (See Figure 4.3, p. 27.) Cytotoxic drugs can cause hair loss and nausea and depress bone marrow function, reducing blood cell production. Renal damage can occur with the use of some antibiotics (aminoglycosides), which act on microorganisms outside the kidneys. To avoid such adverse effects the drug must be discontinued or used in reduced doses.

Effects on hormone synthesis

Drugs that replace hormones secreted by the adrenal cortex will result in downregulation of the body's own hormone production from this organ. If treatment with such a drug is suddenly stopped after long-term use, loss of function can occur because the adrenal cortex has become atrophied and is unable to synthesize sufficient endogenous hormones to maintain normal function.

Adverse effects secondary to the drug's desired effect

Antibiotics that kill or inhibit growth of one microorganism may provide better growth conditions for others. This explains why fungal growth is sometimes observed during treatment with antibiotics. Women are particularly vulnerable to fungal infection in the vagina during antibacterial treatment of urinary tract infections.

NON-DOSE-RELATED ADVERSE EFFECTS

In principle, all effects of drugs depend on the dose that is taken (with a zero dose, there are no effects or adverse effects). When adverse effects are classified as non-dose-related, this means that such effects occur at doses or concentrations that are considerably lower than the standard dose known to produce a therapeutic effect.

Such adverse effects are not predictable, unless a patient has experienced them before. Typically only a few individuals experience non-dose-related adverse effects. Allergic reactions are included in this group.

Allergic reactions

Allergic reactions occur when a patient's immune defence is sensitized by the same or similar compound to which the patient reacts. The reaction can develop during the first exposure to a drug, e.g. following the use of contrast media during radiography, but allergic reactions usually present themselves following the second exposure, once sensitization has occurred. Penicillins, cephalosporins, sulpha drugs and trimethoprim often cause allergic reactions.

'Cross-sensitization' occurs when a person using one drug develops an allergy to another drug. Cross-sensitization between the penicillins and cephalosporins is well known. Cross-sensitization is often associated with similarity in structure between the drugs in question. Some people can experience severe allergic (anaphylactic) reactions to drugs which can become life-threatening. In anaphylactic shock the correct treatment must be administered within minutes if the patient is to survive.

ADVERSE EFFECTS AS A RESULT OF LONG-TERM USE OF DRUGS

Certain types of adverse effects occur gradually and increase with continued use. They are often irreversible (do not disappear when a person stops taking the drug). Long-term use of neuroleptic drugs can cause such adverse effects in the form of involuntary movements (tardive dyskinesia), particularly of mimic muscles.

DELAYED ADVERSE EFFECTS

Delayed adverse effects can occur long after a person has stopped using a drug. For instance, carcinogenic drugs can induce development of malignant disease that does not manifest itself until many years after a person has stopped using the drugs. Immunosuppressive drugs can increase the risk of cancer development having weakened the body's defences against the growth of tumours.

Oestrogens stimulate cell proliferation in the vaginal membrane. There has been much discussion about whether the use of oestrogen leads to an increased risk of vaginal cancer or breast cancer. However, it appears that birth control pills that combine oestrogen and a progesterone can have a protective effect on development of cancer in the vaginal membrane and in the ovaries. The risk of breast cancer is possibly increased in young women who have used the combination pill for many years.

FETAL DAMAGE

Drugs that cause deformities in the fetus as a result of the mother using a drug during pregnancy are said to have a teratogenic effect.

Teratogenic effects are described as being any congenital, anatomical, physiological and psychological defect resulting from the use of drugs. Cytotoxic drugs can damage the fetus as they act on cells during the division phase. Anticoagulants, antiepileptics, aminoglycosides, tetracycline, lithium and anabolic steroids are also suspected of having teratogenic effects. In cases where a pregnant woman needs such drugs, the lowest possible dose to produce the desired effect should be used. Fetal damage and drug use are discussed in more detail in Chapter 26.

DEVELOPMENT OF CANCER

Drugs that are linked to the development of cancer are called carcinogenic. They act by damaging genes. Cancer development can arise in different ways:

■ The alteration from a healthy to a malignant cell is the result of damage to the genetic material, which directly or indirectly leads to mutation or activation of pro-oncogenes (the preliminary stage of cancer genes).

- Special genes that suppress cancer (tumour suppressor genes) can be damaged, allowing cancer to develop.

Cytotoxic and immunosuppressive drugs are gene toxic. Acute myeloid leukaemia and bladder wall cancer are related to the use of cytotoxic drugs. These drugs should be prescribed with care when treating non-malignant disorders. It is believed that immunosuppressive drugs may be indirectly carcinogenic because certain viral infections linked with malignant disease are not suppressed by the immune system.

ADVERSE EFFECTS RELATED TO ORGAN SYSTEMS

Adverse effects most often manifest as changes in organ function. These may be changes in the appearance of the skin, changes in the function of the respiratory, cardiovascular and nervous systems, or changes in bone marrow function and the GI tract. The liver and kidneys are particularly vulnerable, since the concentration of drugs and their metabolites is usually high during drug elimination via these organs.

THE SKIN

Drug-induced adverse effects in the skin often present in the form of rashes and are therefore relatively easy to detect. The rash can vary from small, localized skin changes to severe, life-threatening reactions (Stevens–Johnson syndrome). The most common presentation is itching, erythema and urticaria. Eczema, development of acne, loss of hair and photosensitivity can occur following long-term use of certain drugs.

Skin changes with symmetrical distribution on the right and left sides of the body almost always represent reactions to something a person has eaten or to a parenterally or rectally administered drug. The changes are symmetrical because of the widespread distribution of drug administered systemically.

Itching can be an early sign of adverse effects. If it occurs simultaneously with visible changes in the skin, the chance of it being a drug-induced effect is greater. Erythema is described as red spots on the skin, with or without raised areas, which vary from small to large irregular patches. Erythematous skin changes often present 2–3 days after starting a drug treatment. Urticaria is an allergic reaction that presents as a slight swelling of the skin and mucous membranes, usually with irregular borders. Drug-induced urticaria appears acutely following drug administration. It can be considered an anaphylactic reaction, localized to skin and the mucous membranes. Urticarial symptoms usually disappear quickly after a person stops taking the drug in question. Penicillins, trimethoprim and sulphonamides are the drugs that most frequently cause drug-induced skin rashes.

Photosensitizing refers to an increased sensitivity of the skin to ultraviolet light as the result of an adverse drug effect. Among others, the antibiotic tetracycline, the antipsychotic levomepromazine and the anti-arrhythmic amiodarone can cause this effect. Exposure to sources of ultraviolet light should therefore be avoided by patients using such drugs.

THE RESPIRATORY SYSTEM

Allergic reactions affecting the mucous membranes may well affect the airways within the lungs. There may be marked swelling because of localized oedema, resulting in airway obstruction. Angioedema is swelling of the mucous membrane in the upper airway and mouth, possibly resulting in a life-threatening airway obstruction. Angiotensin-converting enzyme (ACE) inhibitors and some antibiotics are known to cause such anaphylactic reactions.

The use of β-blockers intended to block $β_1$-adrenoceptors may also block $β_2$-adrenoceptors in the bronchioles, leading to bronchoconstriction and respiratory problems.

THE CARDIOVASCULAR SYSTEM

The most common adverse cardiovascular effects are arrhythmias, heart failure and hypotension. These adverse effects can, in turn, lead to a number of secondary effects.

Arrhythmias normally result in a reduced cardiac output, a fall in blood pressure and reduced peripheral circulation. A fall in blood pressure occurs in arrhythmias with a high heart rate, e.g. supraventricular tachycardia, since the ventricles do not have a chance to fill between contractions. Reduced peripheral circulation often manifests itself in the form of cold hands and feet.

Heart failure with a fall in blood pressure can also develop following the use of drugs that reduce the force of contraction of the ventricles (many blood pressure-reducing drugs).

THE GASTROINTESTINAL TRACT

Many drugs can cause adverse effects involving the GI tract. The most common are nausea, vomiting, constipation and diarrhoea. Acid regurgitation, abdominal pains and ulcerations of the mucous membranes also occur relatively frequently. Such unpleasant adverse effects often cause the patient to stop taking the drug.

With nausea, gastric emptying is delayed, resulting in delayed absorption and therefore delayed effects. Vomiting can cause the drug to be removed before it even reaches the small intestine. In these situations, alternative routes of administration such as rectal suppositories may be useful.

Note that drugs should normally be taken between meals to reduce the interaction between drugs and food. Administering drugs together with food, or immediately afterwards however, can reduce some adverse effects. Ulceration of the oesophagus occurs relatively frequently with acetylsalicylic acid, NSAIDs, calcium salts, doxycycline and iron preparations especially when drugs are taken whilst lying down. Drugs should be taken with water while sitting or standing to avoid lodging in the oesophagus and causing local damage.

BONE MARROW

Adverse effects that influence the function of bone marrow are often serious as there can be a reduction in the production of blood cells. The clinical effects are often delayed as these drugs usually affect developing cells and not mature cells. The use of these drugs may cause a great deal of damage before the adverse effects manifest themselves. Close monitoring of haemoglobin, white blood cells and platelets is essential when using drugs known to suppress bone marrow function.

In aplastic anaemia, production of cells in all cell lines is reduced. This is the most serious type of bone marrow depression from drugs, with a high probability of life-threatening complications.

Agranulocytosis is the absence of granulocytes, leading to a situation in which the body's ability to fight infections is considerably reduced. Fever, sore throat and painful aphthous ulcers on the mucous membrane in the mouth are common.

Thrombocytopenia is a disorder characterized by a low platelet count. In cases where there is a serious absence of platelets, a diffuse spreading of small petechial haemorrhages in the skin and bleeding from the nose and gums often result.

Antithyroid drugs such as cabimazole, methimazole and propylthiourcil may suppress the bone marrow. The same is true for the antibiotics chloramphenicol and co-trimazole, and penicillamine used to treat rheumatoid arthritis.

In most cases, stopping the drug in question will result in a gradual return to normal of the haematological profile, but these adverse effects can lead to life-threatening complications.

THE NERVOUS SYSTEM

Adverse effects on the central nervous system normally present in the form of increased tiredness, dizziness, confusion, trembling, headache and convulsions. Mental changes with or without psychoses can also occur. Nausea and vomiting are associated with stimulation of the chemotaxic centre in the brain, effects often demonstrated by opiates and some cytotoxic drugs.

Increased tiredness is seen following the use of almost all drugs that have a suppressive effect on the central nervous system (analgesics, antipsychotics, anti-depressants, hypnotics, sedatives and antiepileptics). Some antihistamines also cause increased tiredness. Drugs that can cause fatigue are always clearly labelled. Alcohol is also known to suppress the function of the central nervous system.

Dizziness often occurs in elderly patients who are treated with antihypertensive drugs or other drugs that cause a reduction in blood pressure. Confusion may result from changes in cerebral perfusion due to low blood pressure. In addition, many drugs that suppress the central nervous system can cause paradoxical reactions in the elderly, in the form of both confusion and increased wakefulness.

Trembling (tremors) is seen with high doses of theophylline and β_2-adrenoceptor agonists used in the treatment of asthma. Headaches are frequently seen with the use of nitrates (nitroglycerine), associated with vasodilatation of cerebral arteries. Convulsions can be a sign of high concentration of several drugs. This is particularly true for tricyclic antidepressants, lidocaine and theophylline.

THE LIVER AND KIDNEYS

The liver and kidneys are particularly vulnerable to drug-induced damage. This is because drugs exist in high concentrations within these organs during elimination.

Drug-induced liver damage manifests itself in different ways, depending on which functions are disturbed. Those that are the result of damage to the liver cells present with elevated levels of intracellular enzymes (transaminases). Those which are the result of damage to the gall function demonstrate elevated alkaline phosphatase. When liver cells are damaged, the ability to conjugate bilirubin (with glu-curonic acid) is reduced. If bile salts are deposited, the bile ducts can become obstructed. Both mechanisms of damage give rise to hyperbilirubinaemia, and have jaundice as a symptom.

Several anaesthetic gases (e.g. chloroform, halothane) are known to cause hepatic necrosis. Antipsychotic drugs such as chlorpromazine are known to damage the liver.

Drugs excreted through the kidneys are usually found in high concentration in the urine and can damage cells in the nephron and the collecting tubule. Drug damage to the kidneys is particularly dangerous in patients who already have reduced renal function. As the elderly often have reduced renal function, dose reduction is often required.

Patients with liver or renal failure should have reduced doses during maintenance treatment with drugs with pronounced hepatic or renal metabolism. Loading doses, however, must be just as high in these patients as in patients without liver and renal failure.

REGISTRATION OF ADVERSE EFFECTS

In the UK, the Committee on Safety of Medicines registers and collates all information regarding adverse events. This makes it possible to highlight adverse effects quickly after a new drug is approved for use. An international collaboration has been initiated for the purpose of registering adverse effects. This collaboration allows adverse effects which seldom occur to be revealed more quickly. Discovering rare adverse effects requires good reporting practices and many people using the drug. There are guidelines for the reporting of adverse effects in the *British National Formulary*.

SUMMARY

- Dose-dependent adverse effects are possible to predict, and will occur in all users with sufficiently high doses. Non-dose-related adverse effects (allergic reactions) are difficult to predict.
- Adverse effects as a consequence of long-term use are often irreversible.
- Delayed adverse effects can appear long after a person has stopped using a drug.
- Drugs that act in the cell's division phase can cause teratogenic effects in the form of structural deformities.
- Drugs can act carcinogenically by activating cancer genes or by damaging genes that suppress cancer.
- Adverse effects on the bone marrow are often serious and can be difficult to discern until long after the damage has been done.
- Adverse effects frequently occur on the skin, in the respiratory and cardiovascular systems and in the GI tract. The liver and kidneys are also vulnerable to adverse effects, as the concentration of drugs and metabolites is often high in these organs.
- Serious adverse effects from new drugs should be reported to the Committee on Safety of Medicines.

8 Drug interactions

Drug interactions occur when the pharmacological profile of one drug is altered by the administration of another drug, resulting in weakened, enhanced or altered effects. This may be due to the fact that some drugs act on the same receptors, modifying each other's effects with no change in drug concentration, a phenomenon known as pharmacodynamic interaction. Drug interactions due to changes in absorption, distribution or elimination, and therefore changes in drug concentration, are called pharmacokinetic interactions. When an unexpected adverse effect occurs in patients using several drugs simultaneously (polypharmacy) such interactions are the likely cause.

Drug interactions manifest themselves to an increasing degree the greater the number of drugs that are being used simultaneously and can be difficult to predict. Patients with reduced renal and hepatic function are particularly at risk, since important physiological elimination processes are frequently influenced by the simultaneous use of several drugs. In the elderly, there are often age-related physiological changes and increased ill health, all of which contribute to increased risk of interactions.

The most clinically important interactions occur with drugs that have a narrow therapeutic range, where the dose must be adjusted precisely in order to avoid serious adverse affects. Such drugs are often metabolized in the liver by enzyme systems. Drugs that influence such enzyme systems usually affect the elimination of other drugs that are metabolized by the same enzymes.

PHARMACODYNAMIC INTERACTIONS

When the effect of a drug is altered by the influence of another drug without the concentration of the drug being altered, a pharmacodynamic interaction exists. The effects of digitalis glycosides, some anticoagulants and centrally acting analgesics, are frequently influenced by pharmacodynamic interactions.

INTERACTIONS DUE TO EFFECTS ON THE SAME RECEPTOR IN THE SAME ORGAN

Agonists and antagonists with affinity for the same receptor compete for binding sites and influence each other's effects. Such interactions can be clinically useful for controlling the effects of certain drugs.

Morphine and other opiates stimulate opioid receptors, resulting in hyperpolarization of nerve cells, blocking impulses thus inhibiting painful stimuli. With the simultaneous use of naloxone, which competes with morphine for opiate receptors, the effect can be cancelled if the concentration of naloxone is sufficient. This is useful in the treatment of opiate overdose. The analgesic effect of morphine is also reduced by the simultaneous use of partial opiate agonists such as buprenorphine. These effects are discussed in more detail in Chapter 4, Pharmacodynamics of drugs.

Another important example is the altered effects of digitalis glycosides with the simultaneous use of potassium-depleting diuretics. The digitalis glycosides digoxin and digitoxin exert their effects by binding to the enzyme Na^+/K^+-ATPase in myocytes. Potassium competes with the digitalis glycosides for the same enzyme to be transported into the heart muscle cells. Diuretics that increase renal excretion of potassium reduce potassium concentration in the blood. When the concentration of potassium is reduced, the digitalis glycosides will be in relative excess and exert a stronger effect because more binding sites become available. Therefore, the same concentration of digitoxin will produce a more potent effect and more adverse effects.

Drugs can also influence the same receptor without any agonist-antagonist effect. In the treatment of type II diabetes, both insulin and glibenclamide are sometimes used simultaneously. Glibenclamide exerts its effect by making insulin receptors more sensitive to the insulin, but does not compete with insulin receptors.

INTERACTIONS DUE TO EFFECTS ON DIFFERENT RECEPTORS IN THE SAME ORGAN

Drugs that exert their effects via receptors in the central nervous system often modify each other's effects. This is true for neuroleptics, antidepressants, narcotic analgesics, tranquillizers/sedatives and muscle relaxants, all of which suppress the central nervous system. These drugs act on different receptors, but enhance each other's effects. Combining these drugs, therefore, can cause confusion, respiratory and cardiovascular depression, lethargy and restlessness. It is important to remember that alcohol enhances the central nervous effect of many drugs because it has a similar (suppressing) effect.

Alcohol can enhance the suppressive effect that opioids have on the respiratory centres within the brain. There are several reports of serious interactions in patients who have consumed alcohol while taking dextropropoxyphene. The latter acts on opiate receptors, while alcohol acts on gamma-aminobutyric acid (GABA) receptors.

INTERACTIONS DUE TO EFFECTS ON DIFFERENT RECEPTORS IN DIFFERENT ORGANS

Simultaneous use of several drugs can influence the effect they have on each other by influencing different physiological mechanisms that contribute to the same final effect.

For example, warfarin reduces the blood's ability to coagulate by inhibiting the synthesis of coagulation factors. Coagulation also depends on the ability of thrombocytes (platelets) to aggregate, which is again influenced by the ability of the thrombocytes to form thromboxanes. Synthesis of thromboxanes is inhibited by acetylsalicylic acid (ASA) and by the non-steroidal anti-inflammatory group of drugs (NSAIDs). The resultant effect of combining warfarin with ASA or a NSAID-type drug is an increased risk of bleeding from mucous membranes and internal organs. While the drugs are often used individually, it is important to take great care when combinations of these types of drugs are used.

PHARMACOKINETIC INTERACTIONS

When the concentration of a drug is altered as a result of the use of another drug, a pharmacokinetic interaction exists. The causes can be altered absorption, distribution or elimination.

Drugs that often exhibit pharmacokinetic interaction are those with a central nervous site of action, anticoagulants, oral hypoglycaemics, antiepileptics, oral contraceptives, antiarrhythmics, digitalis glycosides, antihypertensives, theophylline and lithium.

INTERACTION BY ABSORPTION

Most drugs are absorbed after they leave the stomach and arrive at the small intestine. Drugs that delay gastric emptying will therefore influence absorption. With delayed absorption, the plasma concentration of a drug that is taken intermittently will be lower.

Atropine and tricyclic antidepressants have anticholinergic effects and are known to reduce intestinal motility. Therefore drugs taken simultaneously remain in the stomach longer. This effect is useful in tricyclic antidepressant overdoses where gastric lavage many hours after the overdose has been taken will often still yield significant amounts of the ingested drug.

Nausea and vomiting, leading to delayed gastric emptying, often is part of a migraine attack. Delayed gastric emptying leads to delayed duodenal absorption of drugs and thereby to a delay in the therapeutic effects of drugs taken to reduce the migraine attack. Metoclopramide reduces nausea and thereby maintains gastric emptying, allowing analgesics to be taken simultaneously and rapidly absorbed.

Drugs can also influence each other's absorption due to the formation of complexes. If insoluble complexes are formed, these can pass through the small intestine without being absorbed. For example, antacids that are used to relieve dyspepsia (indigestion) contain ionized aluminium, calcium and magnesium. These ions form complexes with tetracyclines and iron and can lead to reduced absorption of tetracyclines and iron if the drugs are taken simultaneously with antacids. Calcium in milk can also reduce the absorption of iron and tetracyclines. The absorption of kinolones (urinary tract antibiotics), osteoporosis drugs and thyroid hormone can also be influenced in the same way.

The formation of complexes can, however, be clinically useful. Activated charcoal will form complexes with many drugs, rendering them insoluble. Activated charcoal is therefore a useful treatment for oral overdoses of many drugs.

The simultaneous intake of food and drugs can influence absorption. It is therefore a general rule that drugs should be taken at fixed times between meals.

This can prevent fluctuations in absorption and in the concentration of the drug in the blood.

However, it is important to note that some drugs need to be taken together with food. Among other reasons, this is to reduce adverse affects such as nausea and irritation of the mucous membrane in the stomach. This is particularly true for acidic drugs. For example, NSAIDs should be taken with food to prevent damage to the mucous membrane in the oesophagus and stomach.

INTERACTION BY DISTRIBUTION

When drugs are absorbed into the blood, elimination and distribution to other tissues begins. After the distribution equilibrium is reached, the ratio between the quantity of drug that is inside and outside the bloodstream will be constant. Factors that influence the degree of binding to plasma or tissue proteins can influence this relationship.

Acetylsalicylic acid displaces methotrexate from plasma albumin and also reduces renal elimination. A combination of these drugs gives rise to an increased concentration and effect of methotrexate.

Altered binding to plasma proteins

Almost all drugs bind to plasma proteins. The degree of binding varies from a few per cent to almost 100 per cent. Drugs that have high degree of binding to plasma proteins are mainly found in the bloodstream and have a small volume of distribution, e.g. warfarin.

If a person uses two drugs with a high degree of binding to the same plasma proteins, each will influence the other's binding. Since it is the free drug that is effective, an alteration in the concentration of free drugs can lead to an altered effect. However, it is important to remember that it is the concentration of free drug in the target organ that determines the degree of effect. In practice, such a displacement mechanism rarely causes problems. This is because metabolism and elimination increase when the concentration of free drug increases. This quickly reduces the concentration of free drug in the blood, and the concentration of free drug in the target organ is only slightly influenced. If such displacement occurs simultaneously with inhibition of elimination, the effect will be noticeable (poisoning). See Figure 8.1.

Bilirubin is a decomposition product from red blood cells. Bilirubin and sulphonamides (urinary tract antibiotics) or acetylsalicylic acid can displace each

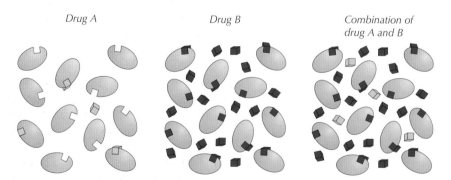

Drug A *Drug B* *Combination of drug A and B*

Figure 8.1 **Drug displacement.** Drug A is bound to plasma proteins. Following administration of drug B some of drug A may be displaced from binding sites resulting in an increase in the free drug concentration of drug A.

other from plasma proteins. This mechanism is of particular importance in new-borns who have a high concentration of bilirubin due to decomposition of fetal haemoglobin. With the use of sulphonamides or acetylsalicylic acid in newborns with hyperbilirubin (neonatal jaundice), the value of free bilirubin can be so high that the bilirubin crosses the blood–brain barrier, causing irreversible damage to the central nervous system.

INTERACTION BY ELIMINATION

Drugs often influence enzymatic processes in the liver. By so doing, a drug can influence the metabolism of another drug that is used simultaneously. Drugs can also influence transport across the tubule cells in the kidneys.

Interaction by metabolism

Lipid-soluble drugs are metabolized before they can be secreted out across the kidneys or with the bile. This mainly occurs by enzymatic processes in the liver. Many drugs are metabolized by the same enzymes, and two or more drugs can influence each other's metabolism if they compete for the same enzymes.

Some drugs increase the amount of enzyme. With such enzyme induction, the metabolism of drugs by the induced enzyme system may be greatly increased, possibly reducing its therapeutic effect.

The anti-tuberculosis drug rifampicin is a strong enzyme inducer that influences the metabolism of many other drugs. The effect of induction normally reaches its peak 1–3 weeks after a person starts to take the drug. Phenobarbital, phenytoin and carbamazepine are other drugs known to cause enzyme induction.

Other drugs inhibit the effect of certain enzymes systems. Enzyme inhibition can lead to reduced metabolism of many drugs, often resulting in a prolonged effect. Enzyme inhibition can result within hours of taking a known enzyme-inhibiting drug.

Dextropropoxyphene has a strong inhibiting effect on the metabolism of carbamazepine. A patient with epilepsy whose condition is controlled with carbamazepine can demonstrate a considerable increase in the plasma concentration of carbamazepine if the analgesic dextropropoxyphene is used simultaneously. Other drugs with enzyme-inhibiting effect include antidepressants, neuroleptics, cimetidine, erythromycin, verampamil, sodium valproate and disulfiram.

Chronic alcohol abuse leads to the induction of several enzymes. As long as a person has alcohol in the body, however, the metabolism of alcohol will tax a substantial part of the enzyme activity. The metabolism of some drugs is inhibited in this way. If a chronic alcoholic abstains after a period of drinking, he or she will have increased metabolism of drugs that are metabolized by the induced enzymes, until the inducing effect of alcohol has subsided.

Interactions can also manifest themselves when people stop treatment with a drug that has inducing or inhibiting effects on other drugs they continue to use. For example, if a patient is taking the anticoagulant warfarin and simultaneously uses rifampicin, enzyme induction takes place and the metabolism of warfarin increases. If the patient stops taking rifampicin and continues the warfarin, the metabolism of the latter will be reduced. The concentration of warfarin thus increases, resulting in possible bleeding as an adverse effect.

Tobacco can also cause enzyme induction. If a chronic smoker who uses theophylline stops smoking, the enzyme-inducing effect of tobacco stops. The metabolism of theophylline is thus reduced and its concentration increases greatly. A reduction in dose becomes necessary to avoid adverse affects.

Interaction by excretion

The most important organs for excretion are the kidneys. Drugs are eliminated via the kidneys by glomerular filtration and tubular secretion.

Probenecid inhibits the tubular secretion of penicillin and cephalosporins. Simultaneous treatment with probenecid is used in some cases to prolong the effect of penicillins. NSAIDs inhibit the tubular secretion of lithium and thereby increase lithium concentration.

Tubular reabsorption is the movement of a substance from the tubular lumen back into the blood. By varying the pH of urine, it is possible to influence the degree of dissociation of certain drugs that are acids or bases. Increased dissociation (ionization) contributes to increased elimination because the drugs do not travel across the tubular wall and back into the blood, but remain in the tubular lumen and are eliminated with the urine.

Alkalinization of the urine results in the dissociation of acids and increased secretion of acidic drugs. This causes the drug plasma concentration to fall more quickly. In cases with poisoning by acetylsalicylic acid and phenobarbital, it is beneficial to alkalinize the urine to increase the secretion of these drugs. Acidification of the urine is less important than alkalinization. It can, however, increase the secretion of amphetamine, which is a weak base.

SUMMARY

- The most important cause of pharmacodynamic interactions is polypharmacy.
- Pharmacodynamic interactions occur when one drug influences the effects of another without altering the concentration of that drug.
- Pharmacokinetic interactions result when the concentration of a drug is altered as a consequence of the use of another drug.
- Enzyme induction and enzyme inhibition are the most important causes of clinically important pharmacokinetic interactions.
- Displacement from plasma proteins and simultaneous reduced elimination can lead to toxic concentrations.
- Alkalinization or acidification of the urine influences the renal elimination of acids and bases.

9 Individual variations in drug responses

If the same dose of a drug is administered to different people, there can be variations in the response produced. This difference in response between people is known as interindividual variation. A change in response in the same patient is called intraindividual variation. It is important to be aware of and consider the factors that contribute to variation in interindividual and intraindividual responses to drugs.

FACTORS DETERMINING INTERINDIVIDUAL RESPONSES

The most important causes of individual variations in drug responses are genetic differences, presence of diseases, drug interactions, age, and body weight.

GENETIC DIFFERENCES

Just as genetic differences between individuals are the causes of many external differences, so they are also the causes of many internal differences. Among these is the ability to metabolize drugs. Since genetic traits are inherited, these differences may exist between different ethnic groups, but also among individuals within a particular ethnic group.

Genetic differences are primarily associated with differences in enzyme activity and therefore differences in the ability to metabolize drugs. As it is mainly lipid-soluble drugs that are metabolized, the greatest differences are found among such drugs.

Tricyclic antidepressants are an example of a drug group where there can be large individual differences in the ability to eliminate the drug. In a study of one of these drugs, it was discovered that in one subject the lowest concentration measured

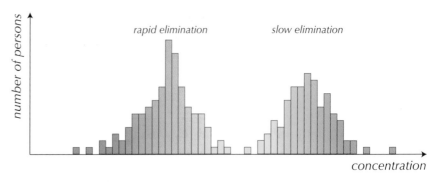

Figure 9.1 Genetic-associated differences in metabolism. If many people take the same dose of tricyclic antidepressants per kg body weight, the drug concentration in the blood of the participants may distribute into two groups: people with a fast metabolism have the lowest concentration, while people with a slow metabolism have a higher concentration. Different people who take the same drug need different doses to achieve the same drug concentration.

in blood was 40 nmol/L, while in another the highest concentration was 1400 nmol/L, despite using the same dosage per kilo body weight in all subjects. See Figure 9.1. This is true for many other drugs.

People with fast elimination of a particular drug will need larger doses than those who have a slower elimination rate. People who have a slower elimination of a drug will need smaller doses than those who have a faster elimination.

A minority of individuals have a genetically low concentration of the enzyme pseudocholinesterase in the blood. Pseudocholinesterase breaks down suxamethonium, a peripherally acting muscle relaxant which is used for brief surgical interventions. People with such deficiency will have delayed breakdown of suxamethonium and longer paralysing effect on the muscles (ventilation) than is expected after a standard dose. After administration of this drug, these people must have their ventilation supported for a longer period of time than those people with normal levels of the enzyme.

Genetic differences can contribute to variations in receptor density in organs and also to differences in the configuration or shape of receptors, both of which may cause different individual responses to a drug.

The condition familial hypercholesterolaemia, for example, is found in both heterozygous and homozygous forms. In the heterozygous form, the liver cells have a reduced number of low-density lipoprotein (LDL) receptors, while in the homozygous form, the liver cells completely lack these receptors. LDL receptors bind and remove LDL cholesterol from the circulation, thereby reducing the concentration of cholesterol in the blood. Drugs that increase the number of LDL receptors on the liver cells (statins) have a reduced effect in heterozygous familial hypercholesterolaemia and no effect in people with homozygote familial hypercholesterolaemia, since they do not possess the genes that code for these receptors.

Genetic variations in drug metabolism are being discovered for more drugs. Using modern techniques, it is possible to evaluate an individual's capacity for specific drug metabolism (genotyping) or their efficiency in metabolizing different drugs (phenotyping). This provides an opportunity to match the dose of a drug to an individual, which may be of value when using drugs with a narrow therapeutic index, using drugs in high doses (e.g. cytotoxics in cancer chemotherapy) and for drugs that inhibit the immune defence in individual patients.

PRESENCE OF DISEASE

Renal failure will cause reduced elimination of water-soluble drugs, while liver failure causes reduced elimination of lipid-soluble drugs. Heart failure can lead to reduced blood circulation to the kidneys and liver, and to reduced elimination of both types of drug. Failure in the organ that eliminates a drug results in an increased half-life for the drug, and an increased concentration if the doses are not reduced.

Disease may also modify the response produced by a particular concentration of drug. For example, a given dose of insulin may result in a smaller reduction of plasma glucose when given to a diabetic with a high plasma glucose concentration than when given to one with a moderately elevated plasma glucose concentration. The sensitivity for the blood pressure-reducing effect of angiotensin-converting enzyme (ACE) inhibitors is greater in hypertensive patients with heart failure than in those with hypertension without heart failure.

DRUG INTERACTIONS

The most important drug interactions are associated with enzyme induction and enzyme inhibition. The former leads to increased drug metabolism and consequently a reduction in effect. When the effect of a particular drug deteriorates 1–3 weeks after initial administration, or after administration of a second drug, it is necessary to consider enzyme induction as a possible explanation. If this is the case, then, to maintain the desired effect, the dose must be increased.

An example of enzyme induction involves the administration of carbamazepine (a drug used to treat epilepsy) to a patient who is receiving warfarin (an anticoagulant). The carbamazepine may increase the synthesis of those enzymes that metabolize warfarin, and thereby result in a reduction in its anticoagulant effect.

In the case of enzyme inhibition, the activity of the enzymes that metabolize a particular drug is inhibited. This inhibition may be caused by the drug itself or by taking a second drug. Enzyme inhibition leads to an increased drug concentration and may result in an increase in both desirable and undesirable effects. For example, the administration of cimetidine (a drug used to inhibit gastric acid secretion in the treatment of peptic and duodenal ulcers) reduces the metabolic elimination of theophylline (used in the treatment of asthma) with the risk of a considerable increase in the concentration of theophylline, and thereby an increased risk for adverse effects.

Drug interactions are discussed in more detail in Chapter 8.

AGE

The age of a patient can have an effect on that individual's response to drugs. For example, in neonates, especially premature babies, the functions of the liver and the kidney are poorly developed. During the first month there is a gradual 'maturation' of the liver function. It takes 6 months after birth before the kidneys' tubular functions reach full capacity in relation to body weight. Metabolism and elimination of drugs will not be as effective during this period. See Figure 9.2.

Neonates have a less efficient skin barrier compared with older children, resulting in an increased absorption of drugs via this route. They also have a more permeable blood–brain barrier, which increases the distribution of some drugs from the blood across to the central nervous system.

Elderly subjects may have a reduced renal function and disease-associated failure in other organs. See Figure 9.2. The elderly can have a greater reaction than

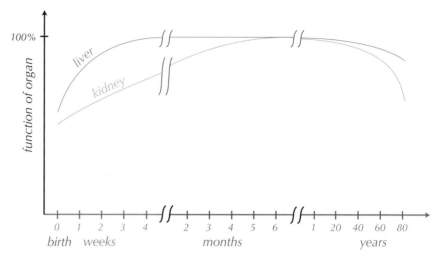

Figure 9.2 **Organ function – elimination.** Liver function is not fully developed until approximately a month after birth, whilst it takes 6 months before renal function is fully developed. In old age, there is a physiological decline in renal function, while liver function stays relatively stable.

younger individuals to many drugs that affect physiological processes modulated by the central nervous system. This is probably because of their reduced ability to compensate for alterations in physiological processes caused by drugs and is particularly evident in the effects induced by sedatives and analgesics. The elderly are often more susceptible to adverse effects than younger people.

As the liver and the kidneys are the most important organs in respect of the elimination of lipid-soluble and water-soluble drugs, respectively, it is necessary to consider the dosages of a drug when it is to be given at these two extremes of age. Administration of drugs should start with low doses, which should be gradually increased until the desired effect is achieved. Drugs for children and the elderly are discussed in Chapters 27 and 28.

BODY WEIGHT

With different body sizes, a drug has different distribution volumes in which to be distributed. A small body needs a smaller dose than a larger body to achieve the same drug concentration. Children will receive lower doses than adults. For some drugs, particularly cytotoxic agents, the dose is adjusted according to the estimated body surface area.

FACTORS DETERMINING INTRAINDIVIDUAL RESPONSES

The response to fixed doses of a drug can change with time in the same patient, and may be either reduced or increased. This change in response may be due to altered elimination of drugs or altered physiological adaptation.

ALTERED ELIMINATION OF DRUGS

The elimination of a drug may be altered by the influence of other drugs, as described above and in Chapter 8. A change in response may also be associated with disease progression or regression and with changes in the drug-eliminating organs, as discussed above.

ALTERED PHYSIOLOGICAL ADAPTATION

Desensitization is the loss of effect of a drug that is continuously administered to a patient. When desensitization develops over days to weeks, it is known as the development of tolerance. When it develops during minutes or hours, it is called tachyphylaxis.

The mechanisms that lie behind desensitization can be partly explained by the regulation of receptors. With downregulation, the number of receptors in a tissue is reduced, and the effect of the same concentration of drug in the tissue is also reduced. To maintain the same effect, the concentration of the drug must be increased.

Tolerance to drugs is particularly pronounced for psychological effects, and less so for physiological effects. In the case of substances that suppress the central nervous system (e.g. alcohol and opioids), tolerance to their intoxicating effects develops quickly, but this is not the case for all their physiological effects. This is particularly true for heroin: the use of increasing doses to maintain the intoxicating effect leads to an increasing depressive effect on the ventilatory centre in the brain stem and can cause death from respiratory failure. In the case of substances that stimulate the central nervous system (e.g. amphetamine and cocaine), tolerance to the intoxicating effects also develops, but the user does not become tolerant to the stimulating effects on the heart, which, with increasing doses, can lead to acute heart failure and sudden death.

An example of physiological tolerance involves the use of β-blockers. An increase in the numbers of β-receptors is well known with β-blockers, which are used to treat hypertension. The drugs act by blocking the effect of noradrenaline on β_1-receptors in the heart. The reduced effect of noradrenaline leads to an increase in the number of receptors (upregulation) upon which the noradrenaline acts. If a patient suddenly stops treatment with β-blockers, the noradrenaline will have more receptors available upon which it can act, resulting in a rebound hypertension, i.e. a rise in blood pressure that exceeds the values before treatment with β-blockers started.

Tachyphylaxis, the rapid development of desensitization to a drug, is found particularly with the use of positive inotropic drugs, i.e. drugs that increase the heart's force of contraction, such as dopamine. Dopamine is used for acute heart failure, but normally only for a few days, as its stimulatory effect rapidly diminishes.

SUMMARY

■ Differences in response can occur as interindividual responses and intraindividual responses.

■ The most important causes of differences in response to standard doses are as follows:
- *Genetic differences.* These differences are important for drugs that are modified or metabolized in the liver. Differing ability for the biotransformation of drugs is the most important component, but genetic-associated differences in receptors are also important.
- *Disease.* With organ failure, the elimination of some drugs will be reduced. This results in an extended half-life for a drug. The concentration of the drug will be increased if the doses are not reduced.
- *Drug interactions.* With drug interactions, the most important causes of changes in drug response are associated with enzyme induction and enzyme inhibition. The possibility of drug interactions increases with the increasing number of drugs that are used simultaneously.
- *Age.* Metabolism and elimination are reduced early in life. Organ failure, resulting in reduced elimination, increases with increasing age.
- *Weight.* A standard dose to a large body results in reduced concentration in the target organ compared with a small body.

■ Tolerance is the term used to describe the phenomenon of reduced effect of a drug that develops in days to weeks.

■ Tachyphylaxis is the term used to describe the phenomenon of reduced effect of a drug that develops in minutes or hours.

10 Dosing of drugs

Drugs exert their effects by binding to target proteins at the site of action (in the target organ). Generally, an increased concentration of the drug provides an increased effect. There is generally a good correlation between the concentration of a drug in the target organ and the effect, as there is between the concentration of a drug in the blood and the concentration of that drug in the target organ when distribution equilibrium is achieved. Consequently, there is usually a correlation between the concentration of drugs in the blood and effects. This is the rationale for monitoring the concentration of drug in the blood in order to decide if the dose is to be changed. The value is usually expressed as the plasma concentration of the drug, as once the blood sample has been collected, it is the amount in the plasma that is measured.

Even if there is a correlation between the concentration of a drug in the plasma and the effect, some individuals require a high concentration in the plasma (and at the site of action) in order to obtain a satisfactory effect, while others may obtain the same effect at considerably lower concentration. At high concentrations, the risk of adverse effects increases. At low concentrations, this effect may diminish or disappear.

When determining doses and dosage intervals of a drug for a patient, it is important to consider how high a concentration of drug is needed and how much this can fluctuate between the peak concentration and the trough concentration (just before the next administration of the drug). As a general rule, most drugs should be administered in doses and at dosage intervals that are appropriate for the individual user.

USE OF STANDARD DOSES OR INDIVIDUALLY ADAPTED DOSES

Drugs that are tolerated at high concentrations before adverse effects occur can be administered in standard doses to adults. This means that everyone receives the same dose whether they are female or male, young or old, have high or low body weight, or have much or little body fat. By using standard doses, the concentration of drug in the blood can vary from patient to patient. When using drugs with a narrow therapeutic range (i.e. a small margin between doses that produce effects and those that produce adverse effects), it is important to use individually adapted dosages. See Figure 4.15 (p. 34). In children and the elderly, it is particularly important to evaluate doses and dosage intervals carefully. Newborns have incomplete function with regard to drug elimination. The elderly can have physiological organ failure or diseases resulting in failing organ function and, thereby, in impaired pharmacokinetic conditions. Such conditions may make individual dosing necessary.

VARIATION IN DRUG CONCENTRATION BETWEEN DOSES

The plasma concentration of a drug varies between each dose. The variation is greatest for drugs with short half-lives, but plasma concentration also depends on the route of administration and the drug formulation. Following oral administration, the plasma concentration of the drug is likely to be at its highest 1–3 h after ingestion, depending on how rapidly absorption occurs. After intravenous injection, the concentration in the blood will be at its highest immediately after the injection is completed. The concentration of a drug is at its lowest immediately before the next dose is administered. With continuous intravenous infusion, the concentration of the drug in the blood will be constant when a steady state is achieved.

With frequent and small doses, the concentration will vary less than with large doses and long dosage intervals. However, it is troublesome to take a drug several times a day. To avoid frequent administration of drugs with short half-lives, manufacturers produce slow-release forms. In this way, the active drug is gradually released into the blood, and the concentration varies less than if someone were to take the same dose of a drug formulation that gives rapid absorption. See Figure 10.1.

Drugs that produce dose-dependent adverse effects are often better tolerated if the individual starts with small doses, gradually increasing them until a full dose is achieved. This is particularly pronounced for drugs that produce anticholinergic adverse effects (e.g. dryness in the mouth) and for those that lower blood pressure.

MAINTENANCE DOSES

During the long-term use of some drugs, it is customary to prescribe fixed doses with virtually identical long intervals between doses. Doses are taken to maintain the plasma concentration and are called maintenance doses. With a dosage of 1×1, there will be 24 h between each dose. With a dosage of 1×3, there will be 8 h between each dose. With dosages that are more frequent than twice a day, the dosage intervals will, in practice, often vary during the course of the day. The night intervals are often longer than the day intervals, giving rise to skewed concentration during the day and night. See Figure 10.2.

If one or more doses are forgotten during maintenance treatment, it will result in variation in the plasma concentration of the drug, which could result in periods of time during which there is no therapeutic effect. See Figure 10.3.

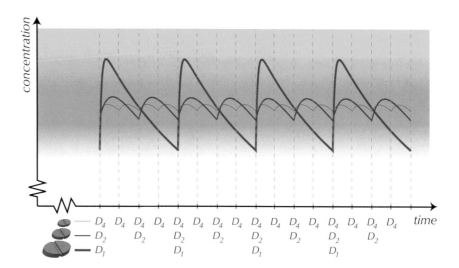

Figure 10.1 **The concentration of a drug varies between each dose.** D_1, D_2 and D_4 designate the points in time for drugs that are administered once, twice and four times daily, respectively. If a drug is administered in small doses with short intervals, the variation in concentration will be less than with large doses and long intervals. In the three cases, the same quantity of drug is administered per day. Notice that the average concentration is the same for the three routes of administration.

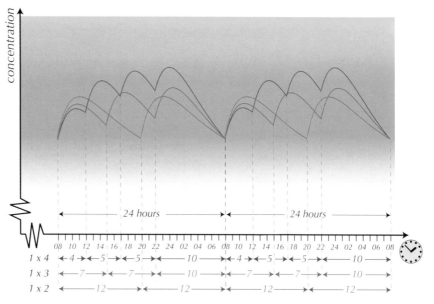

Figure 10.2 **Different dosage regimes.** With dosage regimes where patients take a drug more than twice a day, the last dose will seldom be taken after 10 pm. The morning dose is seldom taken before 8 am. The nightly dosage interval is therefore long compared with the intervals during the day. This results in variation in plasma concentration, with the highest value usually experienced late in the evening and the lowest usually experienced before the morning dose is taken.

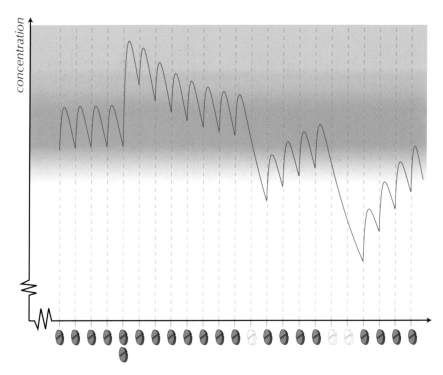

Figure 10.3 **Variation in concentration.** The concentration will vary if a person takes an extra or a double dose or forgets several doses.

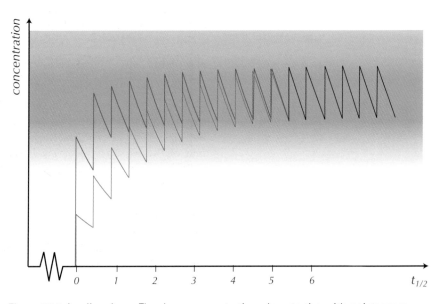

Figure 10.4 **Loading doses.** The plasma concentration when starting with maintenance doses (red curve), and when starting with loading doses (green curve). By administering larger doses at the beginning, one can rapidly achieve the desired concentration.

LOADING DOSES

To achieve high plasma concentrations rapidly, a drug can be administered in large doses when commencing treatment (loading doses), and maintained thereafter using smaller maintenance doses. This is important when trying to achieve a rapid effect for drugs with long half-lives. See Figure 10.4.

When treating an individual with the analgesic drug methadone (which has a half-life of between 24 and 48 h), steady state is achieved after 5–10 days using maintenance doses. If the dose is doubled for the first two days, a steady state is achieved more rapidly. Loading doses are also used with doxycyclin (double the first dose) and with other drugs that have long half lives, in emergency treatment when a rapid effect is needed.

CORRECT TIME FOR DRAWING BLOOD SAMPLES TO DETERMINE PLASMA CONCENTRATION OF DRUGS

To determine the concentration of a drug in blood, the sampling time is important. At the sampling time the concentration of the drug should have reached steady state (after about five half-lives). The blood sample should be drawn as close to the trough value as possible, i.e. immediately before the next planned dose. In some cases, it is appropriate to draw blood samples before steady state is achieved, in order to have an early idea of the concentration at steady state.

In other cases, it may be necessary to measure both the lowest and highest concentrations within a dosage interval. This applies, for example, when using aminoglycoside antibiotics, which have a toxic effect at high concentrations. Here, the peak plasma concentration (about 1 h after ingestion) and the trough plasma concentration are determined. The dose should be sufficiently low as to avoid a toxic effect, but high enough to achieve the required therapeutic effect.

It is particularly important to take samples at the correct time for drugs that vary considerably during the dosage interval and for those with a narrow recommended therapeutic range. Drugs with a short half-life (e.g. theophylline) vary more than drugs with a long half-life (e.g. phenytoin). Large doses and long intervals result in greater variation than small doses and short intervals. This is clearly shown in Figure 10.1. If the dosage intervals within each day are uneven, or if someone takes an additional dose or forgets some doses by mistake, the concentration may well vary in an adverse way. This is shown in Figures 10.2 and 10.3.

If there is a change in dose, it will take approximately five half-lives for that drug before a new steady state is established, in which case it would be sensible to wait to take new samples after changing a dose until at least three half-lives have elapsed (at which point 87.5 per cent of the change has taken place) (see 'Half-life of a substance', Ch. 5, p. 39).

Samples for drug analysis without information about the time of the last dose or sampling time are unsuitable for evaluating any need for a change in dose.

DRUG DOSE IN ORGAN FAILURE

When organ failure is present, especially renal or liver failure, the dose must be adapted to ensure the patient receives the lowest possible effective dose with minimal adverse effects. Similarly, if the patient suffers from any disease of the gastrointestinal tract or heart failure, drug doses may need to be changed from standard to individual dosing. These organs play an important role in pharmacokinetics, and hence the fate of the drugs in an individual. Also, disease in some other organs may make the patient more sensitive to the drug. Depending on which organ system is affected, it can have a considerable impact on the dose of drug used.

RENAL FAILURE

Renal function diminishes with increasing age. With reduced renal function, there is often a reduction in glomerular filtration and tubular secretion. The elimination rate for drugs and metabolites that are excreted through the kidneys will be reduced, increasing the risk of overdose and adverse effects. At the same time, the risk of drug damage to the kidneys increases, which could further exacerbate renal failure.

It is especially important to be careful with dosing of aminoglycosides. Quantitative measurements may be valuable in deciding the right doses. In diabetics with reduced renal function, oral hypoglycaemic drugs should be replaced with insulin. Drugs excreted by renal elimination or with active metabolites that are eliminated renally should be replaced, e.g. ranitidine, metoclopramide, digoxin, atenolol, trimethoprim, non-steroidal anti-inflammatory drugs (NSAIDs), citalopram and lithium.

LIVER FAILURE

The liver has significant reserve capacity with regard to the metabolism of drugs. However, any disease that damages the liver cells (hepatocytes) can cause drugs to be metabolized less effectively than would usually be the case. In these cases, drugs would have an increased bioavailability because their first-pass metabolism is reduced.

This results in slower metabolism, of both the original parent drug and its metabolites, and the drug's half-life will be extended. For this reason, it may be necessary to administer drugs in reduced doses when liver disease is present.

Morphine has pronounced metabolism in the liver and a bioavailability of approximately 20–30 per cent in patients with healthy livers. This means that following an oral dose of 50 mg, 10–15 mg morphine will reach the systemic circuit. In patients with pronounced cirrhosis of the liver, the liver's metabolic capacity will be considerably reduced. Thus, the morphine may pass virtually unaffected into the systemic circulation in these patients.

DISEASE IN THE GASTROINTESTINAL TRACT

In the oesophagus, narrowing of the lumen or the presence of dry mucous membranes or oesophageal diverticulitis may result in tablets and capsules getting stuck and causing sores. The osteoporosis drug alendronic acid, doxycyclin, NSAIDs and 5-aminosalicylic acid (ASA) can all cause irritation and sores in the oesophagus. In these conditions, it is important that the drugs be taken with water or given in liquid form. Because of their reduced swallowing function, it is also important to give drinks to patients who take their drugs while lying down.

Drugs that are taken orally are mainly absorbed in the small intestine. Conditions such as pyloric stenosis will delay the movement of a drug from the stomach into the small intestine. In consequence, any delay in reaching the main site of absorption will delay the absorption of the drug. Similarly, if an individual suffers from nausea and vomiting, the drug will be lost from the body, leaving very little available for absorption. Conversely, slower transport through the small intestine can result in increased absorption. This applies to drugs that are not completely absorbed under normal conditions, such as digoxin.

Diarrhoea and different types of malabsorption can cause the absorption of drugs to be less effective, especially for drugs with limited absorption (e.g. lithium). The same is true if there has been surgical removal of parts of the small intestine.

Drugs with anticholinergic effects (e.g. narcotic analgesics, antidepressants) will delay gastric emptying and decrease intestinal motility, and may cause greatly delayed absorption.

Patients who have taken an overdose of drugs with anticholinergic effects (e.g. antidepressants or antipsychotics) have considerably delayed absorption. The drugs can remain in the stomach for a long time without reaching the small intestine, where absorption occurs. Even if these patients present for treatment hours after ingestion, it is important to remove any remaining drugs from the stomach.

HEART FAILURE

In right ventricular failure, the 'pumping' function of the right ventricle fails. The blood is congested in the systemic circulation, with the development of oedema and reduced peripheral circulation. This will result in reduced circulation in the liver and kidneys, and eventually in reduced elimination of drugs.

In left ventricular failure, the blood is congested in the pulmonary circulation. In addition, hypotension and reduced systemic circulation can occur, with poor blood perfusion of the liver and kidneys.

Each condition, in its own way, will influence the choice and dosage of drugs. With advanced right-sided heart failure, substantial congestion and development of oedema in the liver and intestine can occur. This can reduce the absorption of drugs from the intestine, including those that are necessary to treat the failure. The temporary use of injections may be necessary for a short period, until the usual function of the intestine has been restored and the drugs can again be taken orally.

DOSING IN CASES OF ORGAN FAILURE

In order to achieve an effect, a certain drug concentration is needed in the target organ. This is also true for individuals with failure in the organ that eliminates the drug. Therefore, the starting dose or loading dose should not be reduced in cases of organ failure. The maintenance dosage, however, should be adapted to the functional reduction of the eliminating organ. Without a reduction in dose, the drug concentration will rise until a new steady state is achieved, or as long as the organ failure increases. See Figure 10.5.

To reduce the daily dose for individuals with reduced liver or renal function, the individual doses should be reduced while maintaining the dose intervals. Drugs with a narrow therapeutic range should have their individual doses reduced and their concentration in serum determined, if possible, while simultaneously monitoring the therapeutic effect.

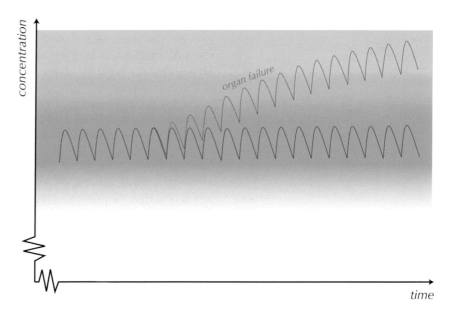

Figure 10.5 **Organ failure.** Failure in the organ that eliminates a drug leads to reduced elimination and a rise in its concentration. The dose must be adapted to the failure. As the failure worsens, the concentration of the drug rises if the dose is held constant. This is analogous with the slit in container A in Figure 5.2 (p. 39) becoming narrower. Thus, the water level rises and a new equilibrium is established.

SUMMARY

- The concentration of a drug varies between each dose, depending on the length of the dosage intervals, the route of administration and the drug's half-life.
- Maintenance doses are used to maintain the effect.
- Loading doses are used to achieve a rapid effect.
- Blood samples for monitoring the concentration of drug in the blood should normally be drawn at trough value (immediately before the next planned dose) and at steady state in order to evaluate the need for a change in dose.
- Absorption is delayed with delayed gastric emptying. With rapid intestinal passage, the absorption of digoxin may be insufficient, but most drugs are completely absorbed, even with rapid intestinal passage.
- Heart failure can lead to reduced circulation in the liver and kidneys and cause organ failure, which leads to reduced elimination.
- Renal failure occurs more often than liver failure. Drugs with pronounced degrees of first pass metabolism should be administered in reduced doses with liver failure.
- Many elderly individuals may have renal failure.
- The half-life of a drug increases when there is failure in the organ that eliminates the drug.
- When organ failure is present, it may be necessary to adapt the dose to the degree of the organ failure. The loading dose or starting dose should not be reduced when organ failure is present. It is the maintenance dose that should be reduced.

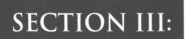

SECTION III: PHARMACOLOGY OF ORGAN SYSTEMS

Structure and function of the nervous system

The nervous system consists of specialized cells with an ability to generate and conduct electrical impulses along a nerve cell and to transmit the impulse to other nerve cells, or to sense organs and effect organs. Together with the endocrine system, the nervous system controls the body's functions, by the release of chemical signal substances called transmitter substances or transmitters. Drugs, some food substances, natural stimulants and intoxicating substances can alter the nerve cells' ability to generate, conduct and transmit signals. The ways in which drugs can modify the actions of the peripheral nervous system are relatively well understood but there is still a great deal to be learnt about drug action in the central nervous system.

ANATOMY AND PHYSIOLOGY OF THE NERVOUS SYSTEM

The nervous system functions as a unit, but is usually divided into the central nervous system and the peripheral nervous system. The central nervous system consists of the brain and the spinal cord. The peripheral nervous system forms a communication link between the central nervous system and all the sense and effector organs. It consists of a motor (efferent) division, which carries information away from the central nervous system to effector cells, and a sensory (afferent) division, which returns information to the central nervous system. Figure 11.1 shows the relationship between the central nervous system and the peripheral nervous system. It is useful to look at the components of the nervous system before detailing their functions.

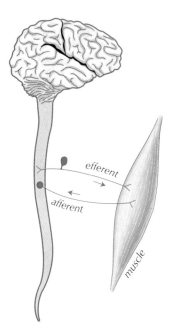

Figure 11.1 Relationship between the central nervous system and the peripheral nervous system.

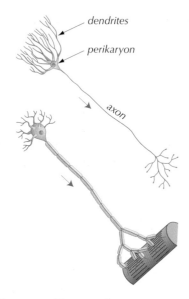

Figure 11.2 **Diagram of a neuron.**

COMPONENTS OF THE NERVOUS SYSTEM

The nervous system consists of neurons (nerve cells) and neuroglial cells (often just called glial cells). The neurons are able to generate nerve impulses and are characterized by their ability to conduct impulses quickly across long distances. See Figure 11.2. The glial cells serve a variety of functions, including protection and maintenance of nerve cells, and control of the neuronal environment. The region around the nucleus is called the cell body or soma (body). The cell body has two types of process leading off from it: dendrites and axons. The dendrites are heavily branched and primarily receive signals and transmit them to the cell body. Axons are long processes that primarily transmit signals away from the cell body. Each cell has only one axon, but this can branch out with connections to several thousand other cells. Because the dendrites and axons are branched, one cell can receive and send signals from and to many other nerve cells. This structure provides the nervous system with the ability to establish neuronal networks and achieve very complicated control functions.

Some axons have a fatty (myelin) sheath around them. This myelin sheath is formed by specialized glial cells (Schwann cells), and its presence greatly speeds up the transmission of impulses along the axon. In addition to increasing the speed of the impulse conduction, these Schwann cells help to maintain the neurons and control the composition of surrounding tissue fluid.

SYNAPSES AND TRANSMISSION OF INFORMATION

An axon ends in many small swollen nerve ends (boutons) that are very close to other neurons, or effector cells, nearly touching but not quite. This is called a synapse and the small gap between them is termed the synaptic cleft. The part of the neuron before the synaptic cleft is described as the presynaptic part and the part of the neuron or effector cell after the synaptic cleft is termed the postsynaptic part of the synapse. See Figures 11.3 and 11.4. In the synapse, information is transferred across the synaptic cleft by chemical signalling substances, called neurotransmitters. Neurotransmitters are stored in presynaptic vesicles and are released into the synaptic cleft when the presynaptic axon is depolarized. The neurotransmitter diffuses across the synaptic cleft and binds to receptors on the

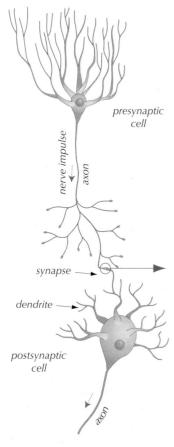

Figure 11.3 **Relationship between a presynaptic cell and a postsynaptic cell.**

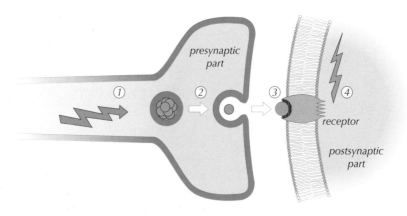

Figure 11.4 **Synapse.** An action potential (1) stimulates the release of neurotransmitters from the presynaptic cell (2). The neurotransmitters diffuse across the synaptic cleft and bind to specific receptors on the postsynaptic cell (3). The binding to the receptor triggers a response (4).

postsynaptic membrane. Binding between the neurotransmitter and receptor is very brief and transmits stimulatory or inhibitory signals further along the neural network. The sum of all the signals a cell receives will determine whether the cell transmits the impulse further or not.

Neurotransmitters

The biochemistry of a synapse determines the way in which neurotransmitters are synthesized, released, how they bind to receptors and how they are removed from the synaptic cleft. Not all of these steps occur in all synapses. In discussing different nerve pathways, the most important points will be given for each type of synapse.

Drugs can influence all of these processes, with the exception of the physical movement (diffusion) of neurotransmitters across the synaptic cleft. Agents that affect the nervous system often exert their effect by influencing the amount of neurotransmitter in the synaptic cleft or the synapse's ability to transmit impulses further. See Figure 11.5.

Membrane potential, excitability and impulse conduction of a nerve cell

There are different concentrations of different ions inside and outside a cell. Close to the inner side of the cell membrane, there is a surplus of negative ions in relation to the outside. This arrangement means that there is a potential difference of approximately 60 millivolts (mV) between the inside and outside of a cell. This potential difference is referred to as the cell's membrane potential. The membrane potential in the cell's resting phase is called the resting potential.

The membrane potential can be changed from its resting potential when released neurotransmitters bind to postsynaptic receptors, which causes a change in ion flow across the membrane, and hence changes the charge on the inside and

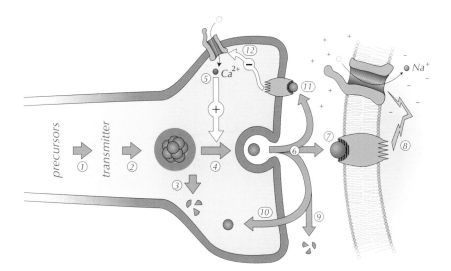

Figure 11.5 Schematic diagram of the biochemistry of a synapse. Synthesis of neurotransmitters (1) and storage in presynaptic vesicles (2). (3) Enzymatic breakdown of surplus neurotransmitters. (4) Release of neurotransmitters into the synaptic cleft. An influx of calcium (5) increases the release of neurotransmitters from presynaptic vesicles. Diffusion of neurotransmitters across the synaptic cleft (6) and binding to a postsynaptic receptor (7), which triggers a response (8). Inactivation of neurotransmitters can occur by enzymatic breakdown (9), or uptake into the presynaptic neuron (10). Binding to a presynaptic receptor (11) results in inhibition of the Ca^{2+} influx (12).

outside of the cell. See Figure 11.5. When the membrane potential, or the voltage, is changed in the positive direction, it can result in a brief opening of voltage-controlled ion channels, so that ions flow across the cell membrane from areas of high concentration to those of low concentration. If Na^+ channels open, permitting the entry of Na^+ ions, a positive charge flows into the cell and the voltage changes further in the direction towards and above zero. The cell changes from a polarized to a depolarized state, a process known as depolarization. Immediately after a depolarization, K^+ flows quickly out of the cell, leading to repolarization. A depolarization and subsequent repolarization is referred to as an action potential. After the repolarization, the potential difference between the inside and outside of the cell is then restored to the resting level. See Figure 11.6.

If the binding of neurotransmitter results in the voltage across the membrane becoming more negative, it will stabilize the cell and reduce the possibility of triggering an action potential.

The lower the resting potential, the more powerful the stimulus that is required to trigger an action potential and propagate an impulse along the nerve axon. Cells with a high resting potential need only a small stimulus to trigger a depolarization. Such cells are described as excitable. Use of drugs that influence the resting potential is an important mechanism for regulating impulse propagation in the central nervous system.

Impulse propagation along an axon occurs when the electrical membrane potential is continuously altered along the membrane, so that new action potentials are continuously created in the direction of the nerve impulse. Voltage-gated Na^+ channels are found all along the membrane of the axon. As long as these channels are stimulated to

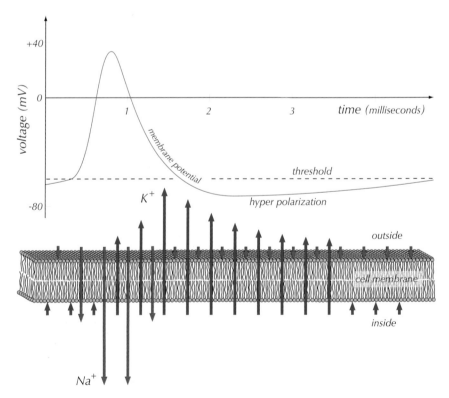

Figure 11.6 Voltage change across the cell membrane during an action potential. The illustration shows how the cell's membrane potential is altered when an action potential is triggered, and the accompanying ion flow across the membrane.

open by a sufficient voltage, impulse propagation continues. When the impulse reaches a presynaptic nerve end, neurotransmitters will be released into the synaptic cleft to carry the impulse across to the next neuron or effector cell. Drugs that inhibit voltage-gated Na^+ channels reduce the possibility of propagating an action potential further and may be used as local anaesthetics or in the treatment of epilepsy.

For the cell to be able to accomplish depolarization and repolarization continuously, the ionic balance is maintained by energy-dependent ion pumps. During the resting phase, Na^+ is pumped out of the cell and K^+ is pumped in, by a sodium–potassium pump (Na^+/K^+-ATPase), which requires ATP as an energy source. Digitalis, which is used in cardiac failure, acts by inhibiting Na^+/K^+-ATPase in heart cells.

Many drugs and intoxicating substances that suppress activity in the nervous system act by reducing the resting potential of the cell. This can occur by influencing gamma-aminobutyric acid (GABA)-controlled Cl^- channels, or by direct inhibition of voltage-gated Na^+ channels (see Ch. 12). By inhibiting Ca^{2+} channels, the release of neurotransmitters into the synapse is reduced and the possibility of triggering further action potentials is reduced. See Figure 11.5.

THE PERIPHERAL NERVOUS SYSTEM

The motor division of the peripheral nervous system is usually divided into the somatic nervous system (voluntary) and the autonomic nervous system (involuntary). In both these systems, neurons conduct impulses from the central nervous system to an effector organ (efferent pathways). In the central nervous system, there are input (afferent) and output (efferent) pathways that communicate with the peripheral nervous system. These make it possible to influence the activity of effector organs, and ensure that they are adapting to the body's changing needs.

SOMATIC NERVOUS SYSTEM

In the somatic nervous system, impulses from the central nervous system are conducted directly to skeletal muscles via one motor neuron. Each muscle cell receives signals from one nerve cell, but each nerve cell forms many synapses. At each synapse there are a large number of receptors that can bind neurotransmitters. If enough neurotransmitters are bound to the receptors, the muscle cell responds with a contraction. Figure 11.7 illustrates the principles of the somatic nervous system.

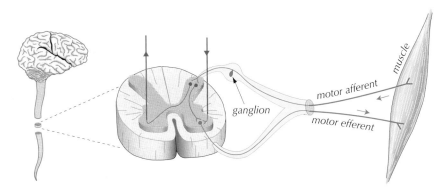

Figure 11.7 **Schematic diagram of the somatic nervous system.** There is one continuous fibre in the efferent nerves of the somatic nervous system. The nucleus of the afferent branch lies in ganglia.

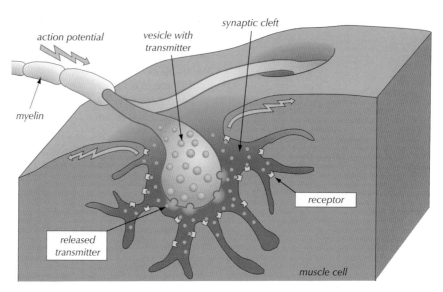

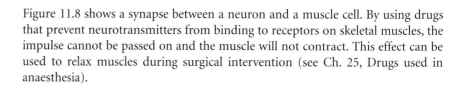

Figure 11.8 **Synapse between a neuron and a muscle cell.** An axon forms many synapses with a muscle cell. At each synapse there are a large number of receptors that can bind the neurotransmitter substance.

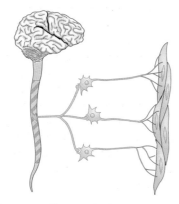

Figure 11.9 **Neurons in the sympathetic nervous system** originate in the thoracic and lumbar regions of the spinal cord.

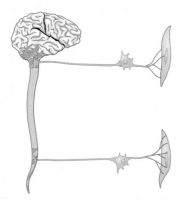

Figure 11.10 **Neurons in the parasympathetic nervous system** originate in the cranial and sacral regions of the spinal cord.

Figure 11.8 shows a synapse between a neuron and a muscle cell. By using drugs that prevent neurotransmitters from binding to receptors on skeletal muscles, the impulse cannot be passed on and the muscle will not contract. This effect can be used to relax muscles during surgical intervention (see Ch. 25, Drugs used in anaesthesia).

AUTONOMIC NERVOUS SYSTEM

The autonomic nervous system carries impulses from the central nervous system to effector cells, which can be glands, the heart, smooth muscle in arteries, intestinal organs and a number of other structures. Unlike the somatic neuron, the autonomic neuron is made up of two neurons. These form synapses in autonomic ganglia. The preganglionic fibre has the cell body in the central nervous system. The postganglionic fibre has its cell body in the autonomic ganglia, and the postganglionic nerve cell sends its axon to the effector cell.

The autonomic nervous system is itself divided into two parts: the sympathetic and parasympathetic systems. During stress, the impulse traffic increases in the sympathetic division. At rest, the impulse traffic increases in the parasympathetic system. The activities of these two systems often have opposite effects on effector organs. Together, they contribute to a balance in the activity of the effector organs, instantly adapting to the needs of the body. In this way, homeostasis is maintained. See Figures 11.9 and 11.10. Neurotransmission across autonomic ganglia is affected by drugs only to a small extent.

Sympathetic nervous system

Efferent preganglionic neurons in the sympathetic nervous system end in ganglia on each side of the spinal cord, and in sympathetic ganglia in the abdominal cavity. They have their origin from the central nervous system in the thoracic and lumbar segments of the spinal cord. Postganglionic neurons run from the sympathetic ganglia to their target organs. See Figures 11.9 and 11.11.

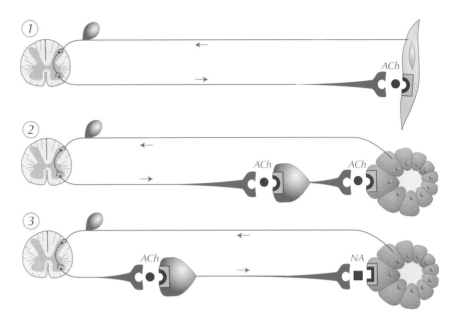

Figure 11.11 Somatic nerves (1) are one continuous neuron from the central nervous system (CNS) to the target tissue that they innervate. In contrast, autonomic nerves are in two sections. There is a neuron from the CNS to the first 'break'. This is known as the **preganglionic neuron**. There is then a second neuron from the 'break' to the target tissue, known as a **postganglionic neuron**. As a rule, in parasympathetic nerves (2), the preganglionic neuron is long and the postganglionic is short. The opposite is the case for the sympathetic nerve (3) where the preganglionic neuron is short and the postganglionic is long. Because of the break (**synaptic cleft**) between the two neurons and between the neuron and the target tissue, there has to be a way of transmitting the information. This is achieved by a chemical that diffuses across the cleft, termed a **neurotransmitter**. There are many chemicals that fulfil this function in the body. In the peripheral nervous system, the focus is on two neurotransmitters: **acetylcholine (ACh)** and **noradrenaline (NA)**.

Preganglionic neurons form synapses with many postganglionic sympathetic neurons, innervating large numbers of organs and tissues. Because of this anatomical construction, the activity of the sympathetic system will be widely spread, which is important when the sympathetic nervous system is activated in a crisis ('fight or flight' situation). This response is enhanced by the release of adrenaline from the adrenal medulla. The sympathetic nervous system is particularly important for controlling blood circulation by regulating cardiac function and smooth muscle tone in arterioles. Different drugs may modulate the activity in the sympathetic nervous system.

Parasympathetic nervous system

Parasympathetic efferent nerve neurons emerge from the cranial and sacral regions of the spinal cord. Preganglionic neurons end in parasympathetic ganglia, located close to the target organ. Figure 11.10 shows neurons in the parasympathetic nervous system. This system is particularly important for the control of smooth muscles in the digestive tract. The activity of the parasympathetic system is greatest in resting situations. Different drugs may modulate the activity in the parasympathetic nervous system.

NEUROTRANSMISSION IN THE PERIPHERAL NERVOUS SYSTEM

Neurotransmission is the chemical means by which the nerve impulse is carried across the synaptic cleft. The peripheral nervous system has two main neurotransmitters: acetylcholine and noradrenaline. Neurotransmitter release from the presynaptic neuron is triggered by the nerve impulse. The neurotransmitter then diffuses across the synaptic cleft and binds to specific receptors on the postsynaptic membrane. Neurotransmitters that are released into the synaptic cleft will be metabolized by enzymes in the synaptic cleft or taken back up into the presynaptic neuron (re-uptake). Drugs may act by inhibiting these enzymes and uptake mechanisms by blocking or stimulating the postsynaptic receptors.

Acetylcholine

Acetylcholine is the transmitter in all ganglionic synapses in the autonomic nervous system, and at effector cells in the parasympathetic and somatic nervous systems. See Figure 11.11. Acetylcholine is metabolized by the enzyme acetylcholinesterase, which is located in the postsynaptic membrane close to the receptors.

Cholinergic receptors

Receptors that are stimulated by acetylcholine are called cholinergic receptors. These are divided into muscarinic and nicotinic receptors. Acetylcholine released from the nerve terminals of postganglionic parasympathetic neurons binds to muscarinic receptors and can be selectively blocked by atropine. There are several subgroups of muscarinic receptors.

Nicotinic receptors are located in autonomic ganglia, in the adrenal medulla and postsynaptic motor end-plates of skeletal muscle. Nicotinic receptors in ganglia and motor end-plates have different sensitivities for blocking drugs. This explains the selective effect of muscle relaxants on motor functions rather than autonomic functions. Figure 11.12 illustrates the biochemical processes in a cholinergic synapse.

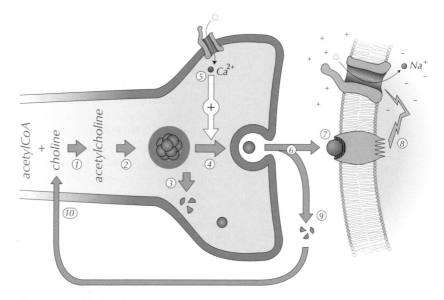

Figure 11.12 Biochemistry in a cholinergic synapse. Acetylcholine is synthesized from choline and acetyl-CoA (1) and is stored in presynaptic vesicles (2). The different processes are explained in Figure 11.5 (p. 101).

Drugs that increase the activity at cholinergic synapses are called *cholinomimetics*, while those that block cholinergic receptors are called *anticholinergics*.

Cholinomimetics

Cholinomimetic drugs can be categorized into two subgroups:

- drugs that stimulate the receptors, i.e. either nicotinic or muscarinic agonists
- drugs that inhibit the enzyme acetylcholinesterase, preventing it from breaking down acetylcholine – known as anticholinesterases.

This latter group has an indirect effect in that the consequence of their use is accumulation of acetylcholine in the synapse.

Generally speaking, muscarinic agonists have little use in clinical medicine. One exception to this is pilocarpine, a muscarinic agonist used in the treatment of glaucoma. It stimulates muscarinic receptors, causing the muscles of the pupil of the eye to contract, improving the outflow and absorption of the aqueous humour.

Anticholinesterases, such as neostigmine, are mainly used for their nicotinic effect on the motor end-plates of skeletal muscle in the treatment of myasthenia gravis, a neurological disease (see Ch. 12, Drugs used in neurological disorders). They are also used after surgical procedures to counteract the effect of muscle paralysis, when drugs have been administered to block impulse transmission from somatic nerve neurons to skeletal muscles to cause relaxation (see Ch. 25, Drugs used in anaesthesia).

Anticholinergics

Anticholinergic drugs are muscarinic antagonists. Atropine and scopolamine are the most commonly used. The purpose of these drugs is to counteract effects that are the result of parasympathetic stimulation, especially mucus secretion in the airways. Different tissues have different sensitivities to muscarinic antagonists. In low doses, they decrease the activity of salivary glands, mucus-producing glands in the airways and sweat glands. At higher doses, the pupils are dilated, the ability of the lens of the eye to accommodate is reduced, and tachycardia can occur as a result of blocking parasympathetic input to the heart. Still higher doses will inhibit parasympathetic control of smooth muscle in the gastrointestinal tract and bladder. The secretion of stomach acid is most resistant to anticholinergics.

Atropine is used during anaesthesia to reduce vagal tone, thus preventing bradycardia and increased bronchial secretion of mucus. Anticholinergics are also used to treat motion sickness.

Noradrenaline/adrenaline

Noradrenaline is the main neurotransmitter of effector organs in the sympathetic nervous system (however, some postganglionic sympathetic nerves, e.g. to sweat glands, are cholinergic). The adrenal medulla can be regarded as a postganglionic, sympathetic neuron without projections. During stress, adrenaline is released from the adrenal medulla and is distributed by the blood. Adrenaline acts on the same receptors as noradrenaline. Noradrenaline and adrenaline are both metabolized by the enzymes monoaminoxidase (MAO) and catechol-O-methyltransferase (COMT). MAO is found in the presynaptic nerve terminal, the synaptic cleft and the postsynaptic membrane, while COMT is found in the synaptic cleft and the postsynaptic membrane. By using drugs that inhibit MAO or COMT, the breakdown of adrenaline and noradrenaline is reduced, which causes increased adrenergic effects. Noradrenaline's action is modulated by reuptake of the neurotransmitter into the presynaptic neuron. Blocking the re-uptake by use of drugs

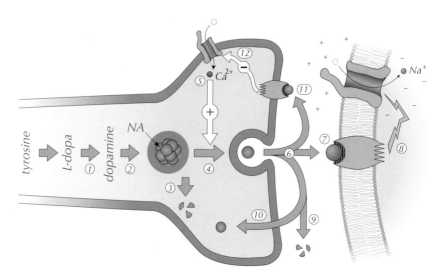

Figure 11.13 Biochemistry of an adrenergic synapse. Noradrenaline (NA) is synthesized from tyrosine via L-dopa and dopamine (1) and is stored in presynaptic vesicles (2). The different processes are explained in Figure 11.5 (p. 101).

leads to accumulation of noradrenaline in the synapse, causing increased sympathetic effects.

Adrenergic receptors
Noradrenaline, which is released at the synapse, and adrenaline, which is distributed by the blood, act on two main types of receptors: the α- and β-adrenoceptors. Both receptors serve glands, smooth muscle and cardiac muscle. α_1-receptors are localized postsynaptically and stimulation leads to increased activity in the effector cells. β_1-adrenoceptors are mainly found in the heart and β_2-adrenoceptors are mainly found in bronchial smooth muscle and uterine smooth muscle. Drugs that act by blocking β_1-receptors cause a slower heart rate, less powerful contraction of the heart and dilation of small arteries. Drugs that act by stimulation of β_2-receptors cause relaxation of smooth muscle in bronchi and the uterus. Figure 11.13 illustrates the biochemical processes in an adrenergic synapse.

Drugs that partially or totally imitate the effects of noradrenaline and adrenaline are called *sympathomimetics*. Drugs that block adrenoceptors are called *sympatholytics*.

Sympathomimetics
Adrenaline and noradrenaline are the most important sympathomimetics. They are endogenous, but can also be used as drugs. Metaraminol stimulates α- and β_1-adrenoceptors and leads to an increased force of contraction in the heart and constricts the small arterioles that regulate the blood pressure. Such drugs are used for serious hypotension and cardiac failure. Salbutamol and terbutaline are selective β_2-agonists used in asthma and chronic bronchitis to achieve bronchodilation.

Cocaine and amphetamines are also sympathomimetics. Cocaine inhibits the uptake of noradrenaline, whilst amphetamines increase the release of noradrenaline into the synaptic cleft. Both increase the amount of noradrenaline within the synaptic cleft and thus have an indirect sympathomimetic effect.

Sympatholytics

Drugs that block α- and β-receptors are called adrenoceptor antagonists. They reduce muscle tone in arterioles and thus reduce peripheral resistance and therefore blood pressure. β-blockers are divided into selective β_1-blockers, which are cardioselective, and non-selective β-blockers, which block both β_1- and β_2-receptors. The cardioselective β_1-blockers cause less vasoconstriction than the non-cardioselective ones. They are preferred for treatment of hypertension in diabetics, as they do not suppress the hypoglycaemic response, and in asthmatics, because they do not block β_2-receptors in the lungs, and therefore does not lead to bronchial constriction.

THE CENTRAL NERVOUS SYSTEM

The central nervous system regulates and integrates all mental, physical and autonomic activities. Between its different parts, there are abundant neuronal networks that provide a good opportunity for coordination of higher functions. If the communication between any of the different networks is broken, some functions will suffer, as occurs for example in Parkinson's disease. Even though there has been considerable progress in understanding neurobiology in recent years, we still know little about how emotional and intellectual functions occur in the central nervous system.

The cerebral cortex

The size, thickness and degree of folding of the cerebral cortex are among the most characteristic anatomical features in humans when compared with other animals. It is also the structure that forms the foundation for behavioural and other functional differences. Also found in the cerebral cortex are areas associated with perception of touch, pain and temperature difference, in addition to sight, hearing and smell, and areas that provide us with a foundation for rational treatment of all the impulses we receive. The cerebral cortex has numerous connections with other parts of the central nervous system. These connections are necessary for the integration of sensory and motor information.

Drugs can modulate the activity in the cerebral cortex by influencing the impulses in these connections.

Deeper areas in the brain

The deep brain nuclei are collections of neuronal nuclei that send out axons to different parts of the central nervous system and form pathways or neuronal networks where different functions are controlled. These networks have good communications with the cerebral cortex. The nuclei are developmentally older than the cerebral cortex and are involved in mediating more primitive and basal functions for survival. Areas are found here that regulate heart activity, respiration, basic emotion and instinctive behaviour and movements.

Many drugs act by inhibiting or stimulating the activity in the brain's deep nuclei. For example, drugs used to treat Parkinson's disease, depression, nausea and hypertension, as well as intoxicating substances and centrally acting analgesics modulate the activity in these areas.

Spinal cord

Descending pathways from the brain end at neurons in the spinal cord, and ascending neurons end in the brain. Afferent and efferent neurons between the spinal cord

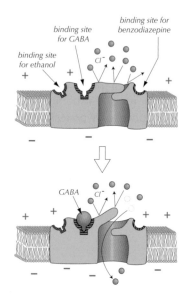

Figure 11.14 Model for activity at the gamma-aminobutyric acid (GABA) receptor complex.

and effector organs connect with each other via interneurons and, in this way, form spinal loops. Some of the control functions in relation to the effector organs occur at the spinal level, i.e. in the loop between the effector organ and spinal cord. Other functions are controlled via the ascending and descending pathways.

NEUROTRANSMISSION IN THE CENTRAL NERVOUS SYSTEM

Many different neurotransmitters and receptors are used to coordinate the functions of the central nervous system. A characteristic feature of neural transmission involves networks of inhibitory neurons that can modulate total activity. Release of neurotransmitters from these neurons leads to hyperpolarization and thereby stabilization of the neurons with which they form synapses. The neurotransmitters in these neurons are called inhibitory neurotransmitters. There are also excitatory neurotransmitters. The most important groups of neurotransmitters in the central nervous system are amino acids, monoamines and peptides.

Amino acids

Amino acids are neurotransmitters in pathways where there is very rapid neurotransmission. The nerve cells in these rapid pathways have few branches connecting to a small number of other nerve cells. GABA is one of the key inhibitory neurotransmitters in the brain. GABA hyperpolarizes neurons by increasing the Cl^- flow into cells. Alcohol, benzodiazepines and barbiturates enhance the effect of GABA. These are more thoroughly discussed in Chapter 13, Drugs with central and peripheral analgesic effect. Figure 11.14 shows a model for activity at the GABA receptor complex.

Another amino acid, glycine, is also an inhibitory neurotransmitter in the spinal cord. Glutamate is the most important excitatory transmitter, and depolarizes neurons by increasing the Na^+ entry into cells.

Monoamines

Monoamines are neurotransmitters involved in slower regulatory nerve pathways. The neurons in these pathways synapse with many different areas of the brain, thus influencing a large number of neurons in many parts of the central nervous system. They have considerable impact on the level of consciousness, sleep phases, attention, mood and motivation. Parkinson's disease, depression, migraines and schizophrenia are central nervous system disorders where disturbances in monoamine transmission are suspected to play a considerable role. The biochemical disturbances found in these diseases show the importance of control via monoamine pathways. Dopamine, noradrenaline and 5-hydroxytryptamine (5-HT or serotonin) are important monoamines in the central nervous system.

Noradrenaline

Noradrenaline is found in the central nervous system as well as in the peripheral nervous system. The biochemical processes occurring at the synapses are very similar in both the central and peripheral nervous systems. Noradrenergic pathways have their cell bodies in the pons and the medulla oblongata. The neurons project to the cortex, hippocampus and hypothalamus. The effects are mostly inhibitory and mediated via β-receptors. Amongst other effects, these pathways control mood (depression), reward, sleep arousal and blood pressure regulation. Some antidepressants act by inhibiting the uptake of neurotransmitters into the presynaptic neuron or by inhibiting the enzymes COMT or MAO, thereby reducing the metabolism of noradrenaline. Both effects result in more noradrenaline in the synaptic cleft and increased noradrenergic effects.

Dopamine

Dopamine is both a neurotransmitter and a precursor of noradrenaline and adrenaline. There are three important pathways in the central nervous system where dopamine is the most important neurotransmitter (dopaminergic pathways):

- the *nigrostriatal* pathway, concerned with motor control
- the *mesolimbic* pathway, concerned with behaviour and feelings
- the *infundibular* pathway, concerned with endocrine control.

Dopamine also stimulates the chemoreceptor trigger zone in the medulla oblongata, and is therefore associated with nausea and vomiting.

The influence of dopaminergic transmission is central in the drug treatment of Parkinsonism and psychoses. Antidopaminergic drugs that inhibit the chemoreceptor trigger zone are effective against some types of nausea, e.g. that caused by cytotoxic drugs. Several different dopamine receptors have been characterized.

5-Hydroxytryptamine

5-Hydroxytryptamine (5-HT), also referred to as serotonin, is formed from the amino acid tryptophan. In the central nervous system, the transmitter is important for control of the sleep–wake cycle, appetite, body temperature, pain perception, nausea and vomiting, and aggressive behaviour.

As with noradrenaline, 5-hydroxytryptamine is also important in depression. Depression can be alleviated by increasing the levels of serotonin in certain areas of the central nervous system. This occurs by inhibiting the reuptake of 5-HT in the synaptic cleft. The biochemistry of 5-HT in the neuron is illustrated in Figure 11.15.

5-Hydroxytryptamine stimulates 5-HT receptors, of which there are several different subtypes. 5-Hydroxytryptamine antagonists are used in the treatment of migraines and nausea induced by cytotoxic drugs.

Acetylcholine

Acetylcholine operates as a neurotransmitter in the central nervous system in the same way it does in the peripheral nervous system. The substance is found in many

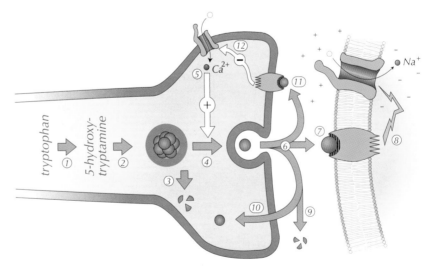

Figure 11.15 **Biochemistry in a 5-hydroxytryptamine synapse.** Synthesis, storage, release and reuptake of 5-hydroxytryptamine resembles corresponding mechanisms for noradrenaline. 5-hydroxytryptamine is often stored together with peptide hormones. The different processes are explained in Figure 11.5 (p. 101).

pathways, including the basal ganglia, which are important for control of skeletal muscles. The effects are mediated via nicotinic and muscarinic receptors. Acetylcholine is also probably important for learning, short-term memory and attention.

Drugs that inhibit the breakdown of acetylcholine in the central nervous system are used in the treatment of Alzheimer's disease.

Peptides

Peptides are short chains of amino acids. They are found as neurotransmitters in central neurons and nerve endings and probably play a role similar to that of monoamines, by influencing other nerve pathways. Many different peptides also exist as neuromodulators, i.e. they are released in parallel with neurotransmitters, and in this way can modify the effect triggered by a neurotransmitter.

Nitric oxide

Although nitric oxide (NO) does not satisfy the usual criteria for a transmitter substance, it is released as a response to increases in intracellular calcium. NO is produced in a matter of seconds. It is a gas at body temperature and influences neuronal activity, increasing GMP activity that leads to both inhibitory and excitatory effects.

THE NERVOUS SYSTEM AND DRUGS

Drugs can modulate many physiological processes controlled by the nervous system. This is the case with epilepsy, Parkinson's disease, psychiatric disorders, Alzheimer's disease, pain, regulation of blood pressure, nausea and vomiting, dizziness, when a neuromuscular blockade is required, and other conditions. Treatment of these conditions is discussed in Chapter 12, Drugs used in neurological disorders and Chapter 13, Drugs used in psychiatric disorders. It is likely that drugs with more specific effects against localized processes in the central nervous system will be developed in the future.

SUMMARY

- The nervous system functions as a unit, but is usually divided into the central nervous system and the peripheral nervous system. The central nervous system consists of the brain and the spinal cord. The peripheral nervous system forms the communication link between the central nervous system and sensory and effector organs.
- The nervous system has neurons and glial cells. Neurons have a cell body, dendrites, which carry information to the cell body, and an axon, which carries information away from the cell body. Contact between two neurons occurs at a synapse.
- An action potential stimulates release of neurotransmitters from the presynaptic terminal. The transmitter diffuses into the synaptic cleft and binds to receptors. Receptor binding triggers a response, e.g. depolarization of a postsynaptic nerve cell, or hyperpolarization of a cell so that impulses are not transmitted further.
- The nerve cells have a potential difference of approximately $-60\,mV$ between the inside and the outside. Opening of voltage-controlled Na^+ channels causes depolarization and propagation of the action potential.
- Drugs can influence neurotransmitter function at the synapse, and thereafter the conduction of impulses in nerve cells.

- The peripheral nervous system has a voluntary somatic element and an involuntary autonomic element. The autonomic nervous system innervates glands, heart and smooth muscles. It is divided into the sympathetic and parasympathetic nervous systems. The sympathetic nervous system originates in the spinal cord between level T_1 and L_2 and causes a widespread 'fight or flight' reaction. The parasympathetic nervous system originates from the cranial and sacral parts of the spinal cord. The activity controls the 'at rest' functions.

- Acetylcholine is the neurotransmitter in somatic motor neurons, in autonomic ganglia and in effector organs of the parasympathetic nervous system. Acetylcholine binds to cholinergic receptors. The main types are muscarinic and nicotinic receptors.

- Noradrenaline is a neurotransmitter acting on effector organs in the sympathetic nervous system. Noradrenaline binds to α- and β-adrenoceptors.

- In addition to noradrenaline and acetylcholine, the central nervous system also contains the neurotransmitters dopamine and 5-hydroxytryptamine. These bind to specific receptors. Dopamine controls coordination of musculoskeletal movements, mood, behaviour and endocrine control. 5-Hydroxytryptamine controls the sleep–wake cycle, appetite, temperature, pain perception, nausea and vomiting.

- The central nervous system also contains amino acids such as glutamate and gamma-aminobutyric acid (GABA). Glutamate is an excitatory neurotransmitter, while GABA is an inhibitory neurotransmitter.

- Peptides are also neurotransmitters in the central nervous system, as is nitric oxide (NO), a gas.

- Drugs can alter function in the nervous system by influencing biochemical processes in the synapses or by influencing the ability of the axon to conduct nerve impulses.

12 Drugs used in neurological disorders

The majority of neurological disorders cause disturbances in impulse traffic within the nervous system or between the nervous system and effector organs. Some disorders are degenerative, i.e. the tissue is destroyed, while others are functional, i.e. the function is disturbed without visibly altering or damaging anatomical structures. As a rule, damaged or degenerated neural tissue cannot be repaired. In the peripheral nervous system, however, a damaged axon can regenerate, but if cell bodies are destroyed, the neuron will die and no new neurons can completely replace the function. The central nervous system, on the other hand, has a certain amount of plasticity, where an adjoining healthy area can partially undertake the functions of a damaged area.

The complex construction and important functions of the nervous system explain why damage to it, or disease therein, results in significant loss of function. It is difficult to find drugs with a sufficiently specific effect such that this can be achieved on selected processes without considerable simultaneous undesirable effects.

EPILEPSY: A DISEASE WITH RECURRING SEIZURES

Epilepsy is characterized by recurring seizures of episodic high-frequency discharges of action potentials from groups of neurons in the brain. The diagnosis requires that seizures be caused by central nervous system dysfunction.

Symptomatic epileptic seizures are considerably more common than the disease itself, and can be provoked by fever in small children (febrile convulsions), concussion, meningitis, encephalitis and poisoning, and during abstinence periods in abusers of alcohol and other intoxicating substances. Low blood sugar and disturbances in electrolyte balance are other causes of epileptic seizures. People who have these types of provoked seizures are not considered to have epilepsy.

PATHOPHYSIOLOGY OF EPILEPSY

Epileptic discharges are triggered by an imbalance between excitatory and inhibitory impulses. The impulses spread from a local starting point to other parts of the brain. The seizures can be caused by both extracranial and intracranial conditions. Extracranial causes can be long-term sleep deprivation, ingestion of drugs or intoxicating substances, or physical or psychological stress. It is also known that high-frequency flashes of light can trigger seizures, so-called photosensitive epilepsy. Intracranial conditions may be injury after trauma, infection or tumour. In many patients, however, no special anatomical or functional causes for the epilepsy have been identified.

The starting focus and the degree of spreading determine the symptoms, which can vary from a minor attention disturbance to a fully developed seizure with generalized convulsions that last for several minutes. If the motor cortex is involved, the person experiences convulsions, and if the hypothalamus or somatosensory cortex is involved, the person may experience peripheral autonomic effects. If the reticular formation in the brain stem is affected, then the level of consciousness is affected. Abnormal electrical activity during a seizure can be recorded using an electroencephalogram (EEG). Characteristic clinical symptoms and EEG traces make it possible to diagnose and classify epilepsy.

CLASSIFICATION OF SEIZURES

Clinically, there is a distinction between generalized seizures, partial seizures and status epilepticus. See Figure 12.1.

Generalized seizures
In generalized seizures the impulses spread in both hemispheres simultaneously. They can be brief without convulsions (petit mal) or last for several minutes with tonic-clonic convulsions (grand mal). Partial seizures start in confined regions of the brain and may be triggered by muscle cramps or sensory experiences such as smells, sounds, tastes or lights.

Partial seizures
These are divided into simple (consciousness remains unaffected) and complex (loss of consciousness) seizures.

Status epilepticus
This refers to prolonged epileptic seizures or recurring seizures where the patient does not recover in between. Status epilepticus of generalized tonic-clonic seizures is a serious condition that requires immediate treatment and hospital admission.

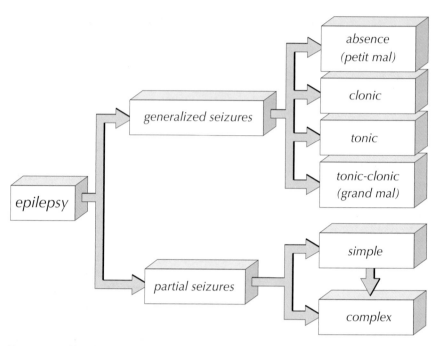

Figure 12.1 **Classification of epileptic seizures.**

Frequent triggering of neuronal activity results in brain oedema and cell death. Status epilepticus lasting more than 60 min is life-threatening.

DRUGS USED TO TREAT EPILEPSY

Drug treatment of epilepsy aims to make the patient seizure-free, or to reduce the strength and frequency of the seizures. This can be done by reducing the excitability of the parts of the central nervous system that trigger seizures. This can be achieved by influencing gamma-aminobutyric acid (GABA) transmission, inhibiting the opening of voltage-controlled Na^+ channels, or by inhibiting the opening of Ca^{2+} channels.

Increase of GABA transmission

Gamma-aminobutyric acid is an inhibitory transmitter that binds to GABA receptors and leads to opening of Cl^- channels and an increased influx of Cl^- ions in the neuron. This results in a more negative membrane potential (i.e. stablization of the membrane). GABA transmission can increase in three ways:

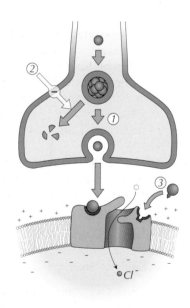

Figure 12.2 **Increase of gamma-aminobutyric acid (GABA) transmission.** (1) Increased release of transmitter substance. (2) Reduced presynaptic breakdown of transmitter substance. (3) Use of drugs that stimulate the GABA-receptor complex.

- increased release of GABA from presynaptic neurons (process 1)
- increased postsynaptic effects of GABA by inhibition of GABA transpeptidase, the presynaptic enzyme that breaks down GABA (process 2)
- through the use of drugs with GABA agonist properties (process 3). See Figure 12.2.

Benzodiazepines and vigabatrin both enhance the effects of GABA transmission.

Inhibition of Na^+ channels

Drugs can reduce the electrical excitability in neurons by preventing Na^+ ions from leaking across the membrane into the nerve cell. Thus, the neuron is not depolarized, remains electrically stable, and action potentials are not generated.

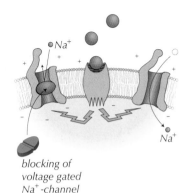

*blocking of
voltage gated
Na⁺-channel*

Figure 12.3 Blocking of Na⁺ channels.
By blocking Na⁺ channels, Na⁺ ions are
inhibited from leaking across the membrane
into the inner part of a nerve cell.

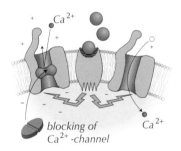

*blocking of
Ca²⁺-channel*

Figure 12.4 Inhibition of Ca²⁺ channels.
By blocking of Ca²⁺ channels, Ca²⁺ ions are
inhibited from leaking across the membrane
into the inner part of a nerve cell.

See Figure 12.3. Some drugs specifically block Na^+ channels in neurons that generate action potentials repeatedly, i.e. the higher the frequency, the more effective the block. In this way, a selective inhibition is achieved of the epileptic focus. This is the most likely mechanism of action for phenytoin, carbamazepine, valproate and lamotrigine.

Inhibition of Ca²⁺ Channels
A third mechanism for reducing excitability is to reduce Ca^{2+} ion flow across membranes in thalamic neurons. A reduced Ca^{2+} content in the neuron will reduce the release of neurotransmitters, hence reducing the possibility of triggering action potentials. Ethosuximide and valproate achieve their response by influencing the operation of Ca^{2+} channels. Figure 12.4 shows this mechanism.

CHOICE OF ANTIEPILEPTIC DRUGS

Different drugs are used to treat different types of seizure. In clinical practice, monotherapy, i.e. using one drug, is the first choice, and this empirically renders seizure-free 70–80 per cent of patients with a relevant type of seizure. Treatment commences with a low dose, which is gradually increased. If the disease is not maintained by monotherapy, combination therapy with two or more antiepileptic drugs may be necessary. Antiepileptic drugs are also called antiepileptics.

GENERAL PROPERTIES OF ANTIEPILEPTIC DRUGS

For antiepileptics to act, they must pass through the blood–brain barrier and be distributed to the central nervous system. Antiepileptics are designed to be as lipid-soluble as possible. The high lipid solubility also means that elimination occurs primarily in the liver. For this reason, antiepileptics can affect or be affected by enzyme induction and inhibition. Several antiepileptics have their own enzyme-inducing or inhibiting effect. This means that they influence the hepatic metabolism of other drugs that are metabolized by the same enzymes. Antiepileptics have a high level of binding to plasma proteins, which means that the plasma concentration of these drugs will be affected by anything that alters the concentration of plasma proteins. It is advisable to monitor drug concentration in plasma when a patient is receiving combination therapy.

Antiepileptics have a depressant effect on the central nervous system and can cause sedation. These drugs are potentially dangerous if the person taking them operates a motor vehicle or heavy machinery. With successful long-term treatment, the majority of patients may still be able to drive a car provided they have been seizure-free for 2 years.

ANTIEPILEPTIC DRUGS AND PREGNANCY/BREASTFEEDING

Many antiepileptics drugs are teratogenic. However, a pregnant woman who is having recurring generalized convulsive seizures can also have a negative effect on the fetus she is carrying. As a rule, epileptics who wish to become pregnant should continue to use antiepileptics, but monotherapy is recommended together with the lowest possible doses that provide protection against convulsions. Using valproate in the first trimester in doses that result in high plasma concentrations increases the risk of neural tube defects in the child. Use of supplements of folic acid reduces this risk. To counteract the risk of neural tube defects adequate folate supplements are advised before and during pregnancy. Patients should therefore be advised about supplements of folate before planning conception. Some recommend giving all women of fertile age with epilepsy daily supplements of multivitamins containing folate. This is particularly important when using valproate and carbamazepine.

Women who use antiepileptics can usually breastfeed their child, but if it appears that the child is being sedated, the drug dose should be reduced or breastfeeding should be discontinued.

OLDER ANTIEPILEPTIC DRUGS

Treatment of epilepsy has long been based on certain key drugs, including phenytoin, carbamazepine, valproate, ethosuximide and phenobarbital.

Phenytoin

Phenytoin has a strong anticonvulsive effect and is used for many forms of epilepsy. It is also used for heart arrhythmias caused by digitalis poisoning and as a prophylactic against seizures during neurosurgical interventions. Because of its complicated pharmacokinetics (saturation kinetics and pronounced ability for interactions), the drug is used less in prophylactic treatment.

Mechanism of action and effects. The effect is attributed to blockade of voltage-controlled Na^+ channels. The cell requires a stronger stimulus to trigger a depolarization and spread the nerve impulses. This reduces the tendency for seizures caused by spontaneous depolarization of excitable cells.

Pharmacokinetics. Phenytoin is metabolized in the liver. The drug is an enzyme inducer and will also increase the quantity of enzymes metabolizing the drug itself, leading to a lower concentration of phenytoin during the first weeks. At high therapeutic concentrations, the drug-metabolizing enzymes are saturated, such that the elimination does not keep pace with the intake. Under these conditions, even a small increase in dosage will result in a considerable increase in the plasma concentration of phenytoin. Phenytoin demonstrates a high degree of protein binding to albumin. With any reduction in the albumin concentration, a larger percentage of the total concentration of phenytoin exists as a free/active drug than with normal albumin. This should be taken into consideration when adjusting doses on the basis of phenytoin in plasma.

Phenytoin is affected by many other drugs. Cimetidine, for example, will inhibit phenytoin metabolism. Phenytoin, by acting as an enzyme inducer, increases the metabolism of carbamazepine, warfarin and theophylline.

Adverse effects. Many of the adverse effects exhibited by phenytoin, e.g. sleepiness, nystagmus, ataxia, confusion and diplopia (double vision), are dose-dependent. Hyperplasia of gums, hirsutism, skin eruptions/rashes and megaloblastic anaemia also occur.

Carbamazepine

Carbamazepine is used for generalized seizures of tonic-clonic type and for partial seizures. Carbamazepine also has an analgesic effect in the treatment of trigeminal neuralgia (acute deep-seated pain in the facial area that is innervated by the trigeminal nerve).

Mechanism of action and effects. Mechanism of action is by blockade of voltage-controlled Na^+ channels. The analgesic effect in trigeminal neuralgia most likely occurs because the impulses in afferent fibres are inhibited. See Figure 12.5.

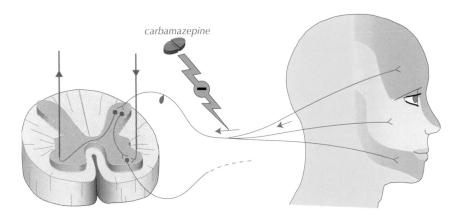

carbamazepine

Figure 12.5 **Carbamazepine's effect in the treatment of trigeminal neuralgia.** It is assumed that carbamazepine acts by blocking Na$^+$ channels in the afferent neuron, inhibiting most of the impulses before they reach the cerebral cortex.

Pharmacokinetics. Carbamazepine is metabolized in the liver and is a strong inducer of drug-metabolizing enzymes. When the drug metabolism increases, the elimination rate will increase. A consequence of this is that the half-life of the first single dose is approximately 30 h, while subsequent doses are reduced to about 15 h. With simultaneous use of carbamazepine, the concentrations of phenytoin and warfarin are reduced in serum. Alcohol also inhibits the metabolism of carbamazepine. Dosing is determined on the basis of determination of plasma concentration.

Adverse effects. Adverse effects are concentration-dependent and resemble those found with phenytoin. Diplopia, nystagmus, fatigue, ataxia, dizziness and headache are the most common. Bone marrow depression has been reported in some subjects, and liver toxicity in others.

Other older drugs

Valproate
Valproate is used for different types of epilepsy. The mechanism of action is blockage of voltage-controlled Na$^+$ channels and Ca^{2+} channels. In addition, the inhibitory effect of GABA on Cl$^-$ channels increases. Valproate is well absorbed and metabolized in the liver. The adverse effects are sleepiness and hair loss. Liver damage occurs most frequently in combination with other antiepileptics. Transient thrombocytopenia occurs in some subjects. Valproate is an enzyme inhibitor and interacts with many other drugs. Valproate metabolism can be induced by other antiepileptics.

Ethosuximide
Ethosuximide is a primary drug for treatment of absence seizures (classic petit mal), but does not protect against motor seizures. The mechanism of action is by inhibition of Ca^{2+} channels. It is well absorbed, metabolized in the liver and has a very long half-life (approximately 50 h). The adverse effects are nausea and anorexia, and sometimes sleepiness.

Phenobarbital
Phenobarbital is an old antiepileptic that has been prescribed much less frequently in recent years. The primary indication is generalized tonic-clonic seizures, myoclonias and partial seizures. The mechanism of action is enhancement of the effect of GABA on Cl$^-$ channels. It is readily absorbed and metabolized in the liver. The

adverse effects are concentration-dependent drowsiness, concentration difficulties and hyperactivity. Phenobarbital has a considerable potential for interaction with other drugs by inducing drug-metabolizing enzymes. Because it has a tendency to sedate, it should be used with caution in children.

Primidone

Primidone is metabolized to phenobarbital and has a similar mode of action.

Benzodiazepines

Benzodiazepines especially diazepam, are used to treat both epileptic seizures and febrile convulsions. The mechanism of action is enhancement of the effect of GABA on the Cl^- channels. Benzodiazepines have potential for misuse. Drug interactions are less significant with this group.

Clonazepam

Clonazepam is a benzodiazepine derivative that is used in the treatment of generalized and partial seizures in children and adults. Clonazepam is well absorbed and is metabolized in the liver. Sedation is the most important adverse effect. Other benzodiazepines are mainly used to treat anxiety and insomnia.

NEWER ANTIEPILEPTIC DRUGS

Whilst there has been little development of new antiepileptics for a few decades, the following drugs have been developed more recently:

Lamotrigine

Lamotrigine is effective for both generalized and partial seizures. The mechanism of action is blocking of voltage-controlled Na^+ channels. The adverse effects are concentration-dependent. The most common are double vision, dizziness, drowsiness, headache, nausea and irritability. In rare cases, there may be serious adverse effects to the skin. Interactions are less important with this group, but valproate inhibits the metabolism of lamotrigine.

Vigabatrin

Vigabatrin is used in treating partial epilepsy that is resistant to treatment. The mechanism of action is inhibition of GABA metabolism. The adverse effects are dizziness, sleep problems, concentration difficulties and visual disturbances.

Gabapentin

Gabapentin increases the synthesis of GABA, but the mechanism is unknown. It is used as a supplementary medicine when other antiepileptics lack effect.

Felbamate

Felbamate is used in treating partial seizures that are resistant to treatment. The mechanism of action is probably through an increase of GABA effects. The preparation has rare, but serious, adverse effects such as blood dyscrasias and liver toxicity.

Topiramate

Topiramate acts both by inhibiting Na^+ channels and by increasing the GABA transmission. It is used as a supplement when other antiepileptics are ineffective.

Levetiracetam

Levetiracetam has an unknown mechanism of action, but probably increases the GABAergic effect and Ca^{2+} channel effects. It is effective for partial-onset seizures.

Increase of GABA transmission
Phenobarbital, Diazepam, Gabapentin, Clonazepam, Vigabatrin
Inhibition of Na$^+$ channels
Phenytoin, Carbamazepine, Lamotrigine, Oxcarbazepine, Topiramate, Valproate
Inhibition of Ca^{2+} channels
Ethosuximide, Valproate
Other
Levitiracetam

Table 12.1 Drugs used to treat epilepsy

Levetiracetam lacks any of the typical serious side effects of the older antiepileptics involving the liver or bone marrow. It does not have any known interaction with the other antiepileptics or other drugs.

TREATMENT STRATEGY WITH EPILEPSY

There is a difference between prophylactic treatment and treatment of acute seizures.

Prophylactic
Treatment should not be started after the first seizure unless epileptic activity can be established by EEG measurements. Treatment starts with small doses that are gradually increased, in order to reduce the risk of adverse effects. Monotherapy is advised, as the risk of adverse effects and interactions increases with the simultaneous use of several drugs. Attempts to discontinue antiepileptic drugs should be by a gradual reduction in dose in order to reduce the risk of triggering seizures. Pregnancy in patients with epilepsy requires referral to a specialist.

Acute tonic–clonic seizures and status epilepticus
For acute seizures, intravenous or rectal administration of a benzodiazepine or intravenous administration of phenytoin is recommended. Large doses of benzodiazepine can cause respiratory depression, a particular problem in tonic-clonic seizures where ventilation is already poor. Large doses of phenytoin can cause a fall in blood pressure and disturbance of cardiac rhythms. Status epilepticus requires specialist treatment and can require general anaesthesia to stop the seizures.

Drugs used in the treatment of epilepsy are listed in Table 12.1.

PARKINSON'S DISEASE: FAILURE IN DOPAMINERGIC TRANSMISSION

Parkinson's disease is a progressive neurological disorder characterized by diminished control over voluntary muscles. The aetiology is unknown, but there may be a link with viral infections. The disease often manifests itself between the ages of 50 and 60 years.

The three main symptoms are:

- tremors – involuntary, rapid, repetitive movements, usually of the 'pill-rolling' type, most intense at rest
- rigidity – stiffness in the muscles, with passive resistance against movement

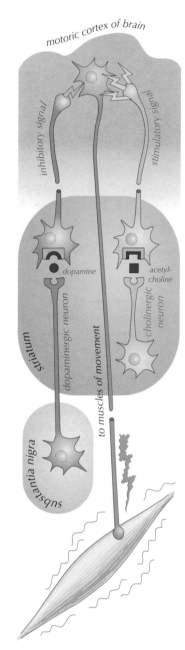

Figure 12.6 **Parkinson's disease.** In Parkinson's disease, dopaminergic neurons degenerate, leading to reduced release of dopamine and deteriorating motor function.

■ hypokinesia ('little movement') – this manifests itself in problems in both starting and stopping movements coupled with movements that are executed very slowly.

Patients with Parkinson's have little facial expression (a mask-like facial expression) and have a characteristic forward-stooping gait with small steps. They may eventually show signs of dementia.

By 'Parkinsonism', we mean Parkinson-like symptoms, secondary to other disorders or as adverse effects from the use of drugs, particularly antipsychotics.

PATHOPHYSIOLOGY OF PARKINSON'S DISEASE

Voluntary movements are controlled by the sum of efferent impulses from the motor cortex to the muscles. However, the activity in the efferent impulses is modulated by impulses from other neuronal networks. These modulating networks are found in the basal ganglia. The basal ganglia are a functional collection of subcortical nuclei which also communicate with the motor cortex. The substantia nigra and striatum are examples of structures which comprise the basal ganglia.

Dopamine and acetylcholine are two of the transmitters in the basal ganglia. Dopaminergic neurons run from the substantia nigra to the striatum. Cholinergic pathways are used by interneurons in the striatum. Parkinson's disease is a degenerative disorder in the basal ganglia, characterized by loss of dopaminergic neurons in the substantia nigra, a region in the basal ganglia. Symptoms first appear when 80–90 per cent of the neurons are destroyed. There is a gradual surplus of activity in cholinergic neurons. This lack of inhibitory input to the striatum gives rise to a reduced inhibitory output from the basal ganglia. The result is a gradually deteriorating effect on motor functions. See Figure 12.6.

As the number of dopaminergic neurons degenerate in the substantia nigra, the number of dopaminergic receptors in striatum seems to increase, a purely compensatory mechanism. The impulse traffic seems to be dependent on the presence of a number of dopaminergic neurons that release dopamine. With increasing loss of dopaminergic neurons, there is a progression of symptoms.

DRUGS USED TO TREAT PARKINSON'S DISEASE

The principle of treatment is to restore the balance between dopaminergic and cholinergic activity. This can be accomplished by increasing dopaminergic activity or reducing cholinergic activity. Drug therapy, however, cannot prevent the development of the disease, but improves the quality of life for most patients.

Drugs that increase dopaminergic activity

One treatment goal is to increase the dopamine content in the synapses of the nigrostriatal pathways. This can be done by adding dopamine, by using dopamine agonists, or by inhibiting the metabolism of dopamine.

Levodopa

Dopamine cannot be used in its pure form, since it barely crosses the blood–brain barrier. Levodopa is a precursor of dopamine that crosses the blood–brain barrier and is subsequently metabolized to dopamine by the enzyme dopa decarboxylase in dopaminergic neurons.

Mechanism of action and effects. In the central nervous system, administered levodopa that is metabolized to dopamine in the dopaminergic neurons will have

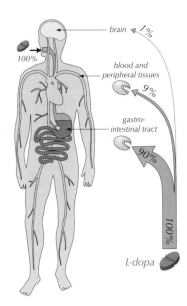

Figure 12.7 **Levodopa.** When using levodopa, only 1 per cent of an oral dose reaches the central nervous system.

the same effect as endogenous dopamine. This can restore the balance between activity in dopaminergic and cholinergic pathways, and improves not only the hypokinesia, but also the tremors and rigidity. The difficulty is to find the dosage and dosage frequency that produce an appropriate physiological concentration of dopamine in the basal ganglia. Levodopa is effective in the early stages in the majority of Parkinson's patients. However, the effect is a short-term one and diminishes after 3–5 years. The explanation may be that, after a while, there are probably only a few remaining working dopaminergic neurons available to metabolize levodopa to dopamine.

Pharmacokinetics. Levodopa is absorbed by dopaminergic neurons and metabolized there to dopamine. The metabolism of levodopa to dopamine also occurs in peripheral tissue. If dopamine is administered in the doses needed to influence the dopamine level in the substantia nigra, it causes a number of unwanted peripheral effects on other dopaminergic receptors, as approximately 1 per cent of an oral dose of levodopa reaches the central nervous system. See Figure 12.7.

By combining levodopa with decarboxylase inhibitors such as carbidopa and benserazide, the peripheral metabolism of levodopa is considerably reduced and smaller doses of levodopa can be used. The decarboxylase inhibitors do not cross the blood–brain barrier. By administering a combination of levodopa and dopa decarboxylase inhibitors, fewer peripheral effects of dopamine are observed and there is an increased concentration of dopamine in the substantia nigra. See Figure 12.8.

Levodopa has a short half-life, which partly explains the fluctuations in effect. Some amino acids in food compete with levodopa for absorption in the intestine, and transport of amino acids across the blood–brain barrier influences the distribution to the central nervous system. For this reason, the drug should be taken between meals. By using controlled-release formulations, fluctuations in levels of levodopa are reduced in both plasma and brain tissue.

Adverse effects. Treatment with levodopa involves several dose-dependent adverse effects as a consequence of the high concentrations of dopamine in the central nervous system. The most important are involuntary movements, followed by postural hypotension, psychological symptoms such as confusion, mania, agitation, hallucinations and paranoid thoughts. Dopamine stimulates dopamine receptors in the chemoreceptor trigger zone and can cause nausea and vomiting. An unpleasant adverse effect is the on–off phenomenon, when the symptoms of the disease suddenly set in and then disappear. This phenomenon is most apparent when treatment with levodopa becomes less effective, usually after several years. There is good control of movement in the so-called 'on phase', but it is important to note that the majority of patients are more troubled by the hypokinesia than by the involuntary movements. In the 'off phase', the Parkinson-like symptoms return. The phenomenon is probably connected with the dose-dependent diurnal variation in dopamine levels. The most important peripheral adverse effects are rhythm disturbances with tachycardia and ventricular extrasystoles. Metabolic products of dopamine cause brown-coloured saliva and urine.

Amantidine

Amantidine (originally an antiviral drug) also acts by increasing the release of dopamine from the nerve endings and by preventing reuptake from the synaptic cleft. The drug is less potent than levodopa, briefer and without any effect on tremors. Amantidine is more effective than anticholinergic drugs in treating rigidity and hypokinesia. The adverse effects resemble those seen with levodopa. In addition,

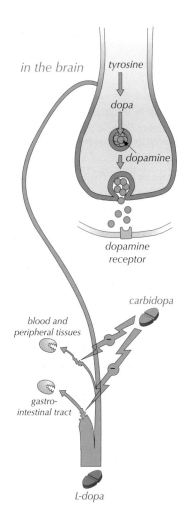

Figure 12.8 Combination of decarboxylase inhibitors and levodopa. By combining carbidopa with levodopa, a smaller dose of levodopa is needed to achieve the desired effect.

there is marbling on the thighs and ankle oedema. Amantidine can be used in combination with levodopa.

Bromocriptine, cabergoline, lisuride, pergolide, pramipexole and ropinirole

These drugs are dopamine agonists that bind to dopamine receptors in the central nervous system. The effect is similar to that of dopamine, but the clinical effect is weaker than that of levodopa. They can be combined with levodopa in more advanced disease and help to reduce the on–off symptoms. The most common adverse effects are nausea, vomiting, dizziness and fatigue. Mental disturbances seem to be exacerbated with use of bromocriptine. All but lisuride have been associated with retroperitoneal and pericardial fibrotic reactions. Patients should be monitored for dyspnoea, persistent cough, chest pain and cardiac failure. Lung function tests should be considered.

Selegiline

Selegiline inhibits monoamine oxidase B (MAO-B). (See Figure 12.9.) The drug thereby reduces the metabolism of dopamine, while the metabolism of 5-hydroxytryptamine (5-HT) and noradrenaline are only slightly influenced (as they are metabolized by MAO-A) (see Ch. 13). The drug can be combined with levodopa, enhancing its effect. By combining selective MAO-B-inhibitors early in the course of the illness with levodopa, it seems that the Parkinson-like symptoms progress more slowly than without it. In addition, the same effects can be achieved with lower doses of levodopa.

The adverse effects are similar to those seen with the use of levodopa. It is important to be aware of potential interactions, especially with antidepressants, which are metabolized by MAO-A and COMT. With large doses of selegiline, the selective effect on MAO-B is lost, and hypertensive crises can occur because MAO-A and COMT are inhibited and noradrenaline and 5-HT are not metabolized.

Entacapone

Entacapone prevents the breakdown of peripheral levodopa by inhibiting the enzyme catecol-*O*-methyltranspherase (COMT), allowing more levodopa to reach the brain. By using the drug as an adjunct to levodopa with decarboxylase inhibitor, the concentration of levodopa will be more stable and the dose may be reduced. The drug is used when the patient is experiencing 'end-of-dose' motor fluctuations, which means that control of voluntary muscles is lost at the end of a dose interval. Side-effects are caused by too strong dopamine effects (involuntary movements, psychotic signs, nausea and vomiting).

Drugs that reduce the cholinergic effect

Anticholinergics reduce the cholinergic effect by blocking cholinergic receptors in the central nervous system. In principle, different anticholinergics have the same effect.

Biperiden, orphenadrine and benzatropine

Anticholinergic drugs block cholinergic receptors in the striatum and alter (restore) the balance between dopaminergic and cholinergic pathways that coordinate movements. These drugs are most effective in treating tremors, and are less effective in treating hypokinesia. Anticholinergics are the only treatment alternatives for antipsychotic drug-induced parkinsonism. There may be adverse effects on the central nervous system, such as confusion and hallucinations. Peripheral adverse effects are urine retention, dryness of the mouth and constipation. All adverse effects are predictable consequences of anticholinergic treatment and reflect inhibition of

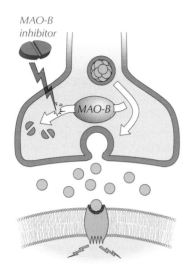

Figure 12.9 **MAO-B-inhibitor.** By inhibiting the enzyme MAO-B that metabolizes presynaptic dopamine, the amount of dopamine in the synapse will increase.

activity in the parasympathetic nervous system. The drugs must be administered with caution to the elderly because of increased occurrence of glaucoma, prostate hypertrophy and cardiac arrhythmias in this age group. See Figure 12.10.

TREATMENT STRATEGY IN PARKINSON'S DISEASE

As neuronal degeneration continues, the treatment is somewhat different in the early and late phases. In the early phase, in the youngest patients, the lowest effective dose of levodopa is used together with a supplement of selegiline or bromocriptine. In elderly patients, monotherapy is used, with the lowest effective dose of levodopa.

In the late phase, the therapy is levodopa, using controlled-release formulations, highly soluble tablets and individually adapted dosage intervals. The purpose is to avoid large fluctuations in levels of dopamine. Bromocriptine or other dopamine agonists can be combined with levodopa.

The most important adverse effects are hallucinations, paranoid thoughts, nightmare-like dreams and disrupted sleep. Such adverse effects are probably connected with increased dopamine effects in other parts of the central nervous system. Reduction in the evening dose can help with nocturnal problems.

All patients should be offered physiotherapy, which should improve mobility and prevent restriction of the degree of movement in the joints. Rhythmic gymnastics to music have a preventive effect on rigidity and hypokinesia and promote social well-being.

Drugs used in the treatment of Parkinson's disease are listed in Table 12.2.

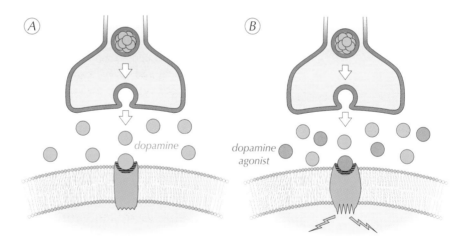

Figure 12.10 **Dopamine agonist.** By taking a dopamine agonist, it is possible to compensate for 'missing' dopamine.

Dopaminergic drugs
Levodopa with dopa-decarboxylase inhibitors, Amantidine, Bromocriptine, Entacapone, Cabergoline, Lisuride, Pramipexole, Ropinirole, Selegeline
Anticholinergic drugs
Benzatropine, Biperiden, Procyclidine, Orphenadrine, Trihexyphenidyl

Table 12.2 Drugs used to treat Parkinson's disease and parkinsonism

MIGRAINES: EPISODIC, STRONG HEADACHES

A migraine is defined as an episodic, strong headache that lasts from 4 to 72 h. The headache can be throbbing and unilateral, often accompanied by nausea and vomiting. Many patients suffer discomfort from light or sound (photo/phonophobia). Aura symptoms may be present before the seizure, e.g. flicker, scotomata and aphasia. Between 5 and 10 per cent of the population suffer from migraine, with twice as many female sufferers as males. The most common age of onset is around 40 years, but the disease can also be found in childhood.

PATHOPHYSIOLOGY OF MIGRAINES

There is great uncertainty surrounding the mechanisms that lie behind migraines, especially the pain-triggering mechanisms. The classical pathophysiological theories claim that the cause of the pain is a reduction in the blood supply to the brain preceding a migraine attack, with subsequent dilatation of the arteries in the meninges. Reduced cerebral circulation has been demonstrated at the start of a seizure, but after approximately 1 h, the cerebral blood flow is normal during the pain period. Nor are the headaches assumed to originate from stimulation of sensory nerve terminals in the meninges or in the large cerebral arteries. There is little evidence to support the hypothesis that vasoconstriction followed by vasodilatation is the source of pain. Other theories suggest changes in the cortex, where a neuronal inhibition slowly spreads with electrolyte changes that initiate reduced cerebral blood flow. Yet others claim that disturbances in peptide transport in meningeal blood vessels are the cause.

Recent theories relate to changes in 5-HT metabolism. The concentration of 5-HT in blood falls during a migraine episode and levels of the 5-HT metabolite, 5-hydroxyindole acetic acid (5-HIAA), in urine increase. It is claimed that release of 5-HT causes constriction of cerebral vessels and is the cause of aura symptoms such as visual and speech disturbances. The direct cause of the pain associated with a migraine attack is unclear.

DRUGS USED TO TREAT MIGRAINES

Drug treatment of migraines involves the use of many different classes of drugs either to alleviate attacks or to prevent their occurrence. The most effective drugs are 5-HT receptor agonists and antagonists. It may seem paradoxical that both agonists and antagonists are effective for the same condition, but until the disease and the drugs' mechanisms of action are better understood, clinicians and scientists have to accept these apparent contradictions.

Alleviating seizures
Alleviating seizures with medication should start as soon as the symptoms appear. The purpose is to reduce the phase which, by unknown mechanisms, contributes to the pain. During a migraine attack, many people experience nausea. In this case, gastric emptying is reduced such that orally administered drugs have delayed absorption and thereby delayed effect. To counteract the gastric retention, it is sometimes beneficial to take a dose of metoclopramide at the start of the migraine attack.

Triptans
Triptans are agonists on 5-HT$_1$ receptors found in the smooth muscle of cranial arteries. They act by constricting blood vessels and are currently considered the

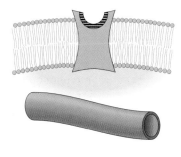

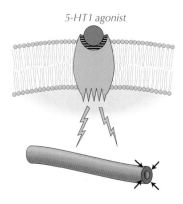

5-HT1 agonist

Figure 12.11 **5-HT₁-agonists.** By stimulating these receptors cerebral arteries constrict.

most effective agents for alleviating seizures. Effects occur approximately 20 min after injection, and about 1–2 h after oral administration. Sumatriptan and zolmitriptan are examples of drugs in this group. See Figure 12.11.

The most common adverse effects are pain at the injection site, a tingling sensation and a warm and heavy pressure in the chest and neck region. Some patients have increased blood pressure, probably as a result of increased peripheral resistance. Caution should be exercised in patients with angina pectoris as triptans can cause vasoconstriction in coronary arteries. Because of this risk, triptans should not be taken until at least 1 day after taking ergotamines. Correspondingly, ergotamines should not be taken until at least 6 h after taking triptans. To avoid an overly potent effect, the drugs should not be combined with MAO inhibitors, selective serotonin reuptake inhibitors (SSRIs) or lithium.

NSAIDs and paracetamol

Many migraine attacks can be treated using 'over the counter' drugs such as NSAIDs and paracetamol. It is important that a sufficient dose is taken as early as possible during the development of the attack.

Ergotamine

Ergotamine produces peripheral vasoconstriction by stimulation of α_1-adrenoceptors in blood vessels. The drug is also a partial agonist. If used, ergotamine should be administered as soon as possible after an attack starts. Adverse effects are nausea and vomiting, and long-term, heavy use of ergotamine preparations can lead to rebound headaches and peripheral vasoconstriction. The drugs should not be administered to pregnant women because of their ability to initiate uterine contractions.

Prophylactic treatment

Prophylactic treatment is indicated if an individual suffers two or more migraine attacks per month. The goal is to reduce both the frequency and intensity of the attack. Patients should keep a migraine journal, and the effect of drug intervention should be evaluated after 2–3 months' use. After 6–12 months, it may be worth stopping treatment. Many patients can manage for a long period of time without prophylactic treatment.

β-blockers

Propanolol, metoprolol, nadolol and timolol may be used. The mechanism for the prophylactic effect of β-blockers on migraines is unknown, but many individuals experience both reduced frequency and reduced intensity of attacks. β-blockers are discussed in Chapter 17, Drugs used to treat diseases in the cardiovascular system, p. 223.

Pizotifen

Pizotifen is a 5-HT₂ receptor antagonist. It can cause fatigue and sleepiness and it is therefore common to start with a small dose. Some patients experience weight gain owing to an increased appetite. Because some antimuscarinic effects, urinary retention and constipation may occur.

TREATMENT STRATEGY WITH MIGRAINES

The frequency and intensity of migraine attacks vary considerably. Some patients benefit from rest and sleep in a dark and quiet room.

Drugs alleviating seizures
Triptanes
Almotriptan, Eletriptan, Frovatriptan, Naratriptan, Rizatriptan, Sumatriptan, Zolmitriptan

Ergotamine
Ergotamine

Prophylactic drugs
Betablockers
Propanolol, Metoprolol, Nadolol, Timolol

Others
Pizotifen, Amytryptyline, Sodium Valproate

Table 12.3 Drugs used to treat migraines

Treatment of attacks should first be attempted with paracetamol or aspirin (see Ch. 14, Drugs with central and peripheral analgesic effects, p. 161). If these do not have sufficient effect, naproxen or diclofenac may be tried. Short term use of NSAIDs have relatively limited adverse effects and can be effective for many patients if they are taken early in the course of treatment. Metoclopramide can be used together with both paracetamol and NSAIDs. If NSAIDs do not produce a sufficient effect, it may be appropriate to try triptans.

With particularly troublesome pain, patients sometimes find that the drugs themselves can cause headaches (drug-induced headaches). When this occurs, a 'detoxification period' may become necessary where all medication is stopped and the migraine treatment is reinstated at a later stage.

Prophylactic treatment
Patients should be offered prophylactic treatment in cases where there are two or more attacks per month. Initially, β-blockers are used, but patients should try stopping these after approximately 6 months, when they may find that the reduced attack frequency continues to last. If the attacks return, treatment is resumed. If there is poor response to β-blockers, pizotifen may be used. Other alternatives are to initiate trials with antidepressants or the antiepileptic drug valproate.

Drugs used in the treatment of migraine are listed in Table 12.3.

ALZHEIMER'S DISEASE

Alzheimer's disease is usually manifested in individuals after the age of 60. The disease is characterized by a gradual and irreversible cognitive decline, which occurs as a consequence of atrophy of the cerebral cortex. The symptoms are insidious in their onset, progressing from apathy, diminished problem-solving skills and loss of short-term memory to agitation and aimless activity and ultimately apraxia and global loss of cognitive ability. Symptoms of depression occur in 50 per cent of patients. Patients suffering from Alzheimer's disease have changes in central neurotransmitter function, particularly dysfunction of the cholinergic system. There is also evidence of increased levels of the neurotransmitter glutamate, which contributes to neuronal injury.

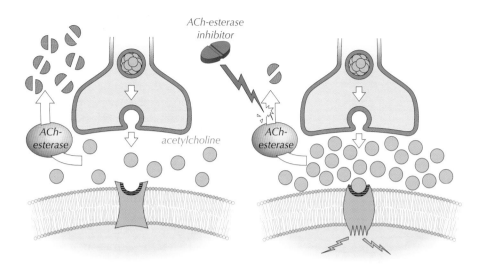

Figure 12.12 **Inhibition of acetylcholinesterase.** By inhibiting acetylcholinasterase, the enzyme that breaks down acetylcholine, the amount of acetylcholine present in the synaptic cleft will increase.

DRUGS USED TO TREAT ALZHEIMER'S DISEASE

There has been considerable debate as to the benefit of drug treatment of Alzheimer's disease.

Centrally acting inhibitors of acetylcholinesterase are used to prevent the breakdown of acetylcholine thereby increasing the concentration of acetylcholine in the brain. The inhibitory neurotransmitter glutamate is an agonist at N-methyl-D-aspartate (NMDA) receptors. Blockade of the NMDA receptor reduces glutamate neurotransmission. Treatment is palliative as no therapy is currently available to cure the disease.

Centrally acting inhibitors of acetylcholinesterase

Donepezil, galantamine and rivastigmine are reversible inhibitors of acetylcholinesterase, which leads to increased levels of acetylcholine in the synaptic cleft of central nervous system neurons. See Figure 12.12. The drugs are used in the earlier, more moderate stages of the disease. Side effects are related to the increased levels of acetylcholine and include dizziness, tiredness, fatigue, nausea, vomiting, anorexia, diarrhoea and urinary incontinence. Less frequently, patients may suffer from duodenal and gastric ulcers, and convulsions.

NMDA receptor antagonist

Memantine acts by blocking the NMDA receptor and so reduces glutamate neurotransmission thereby slowing neuronal degeneration. The drug is used to treat the latter, moderate to severe stages of the disease. Side effects include confusion, headache, hallucinations, tiredness and dizziness.

Centrally acting inhibitors of acetylcholinesterase
Donepezil, Galantamine, Rivastigmine

NMDA-receptor antagonist
Memantin

Table 12.4 Drugs used to treat Alzheimer's disease

MYASTHENIA GRAVIS

Myasthenia gravis is a rare autoimmune disease with antibodies directed against acetylcholine receptors in the motor end-plates of skeletal muscles. By destroying these receptors, the response from muscles will diminish when the neurotransmitter is released into the synaptic cleft.

The key symptom is increased fatigue in the muscles. The onset of the disease is often revealed by fatigue of the extraocular muscles. After a while, there is weakness in the facial muscles, and difficulty with chewing and swallowing. Eventually the muscles of respiration are affected and the condition becomes life-threatening if it remains untreated.

The aim of treatment is to increase the acetylcholine concentration in the synaptic cleft at the motor end-plates by using drugs that inhibit the breakdown of acetylcholine, e.g. acetylcholinesterase inhibitors such as pyridostigmine. The adverse effect of these drugs is an excessive cholinergic effect in the parasympathetic system. Treatment can also be with gulcocorticoids and immunosuppressive drugs, e.g. azathioprine, ciclosporin and corticosteroids, in order to suppress the autoimmune response that is destroying the acetylcholine receptors. Immunosuppressive drugs are described in Chapter 22, Drugs used in allergy, for immune suppression and in cancer treatment, p. 333.

Drugs used in the treatment of myasthenia gravis are listed in Table 12.5.

Acetylcholinesterase inhibitor drugs
Edrophonium, Neostigmine

Immunosuppressant drugs
Azathioprine, Ciclosporin, Corticosteroids

Table 12.5 Drugs used to treat myastenia gravis

SUMMARY

- Epilepsy is characterized by recurring seizures of episodic high-frequency discharges caused by permanent intracranial disease or injury. The seizures can be generalized or partial. Antiepileptics act by influencing GABA transmission, by inhibiting the opening of voltage-controlled Na^+ channels or by inhibiting the opening of Ca^{2+} channels. Monotherapy is preferable when treating epilepsy.
- Antiepileptics are lipid-soluble and can cross the blood–brain barrier. They are eliminated by liver metabolism and can be affected by enzyme induction and inhibition. The majority demonstrate a high level of binding to plasma proteins.
- Antiepileptics are potentially teratogenic drugs. Epileptics who are pregnant should use antiepileptics, but in low doses.
- Phenytoin blocks voltage-gated Na^+ channels; it displays saturation kinetics and causes enzyme induction.
- Carbamazepine blocks voltage-controlled Na^+ channels; it increases its own metabolism in the liver by enzyme induction.
- Valproate inhibits voltage-gated Na^+ channels and Ca^{2+} channels. Liver damage can develop.
- Ethosuximide inhibits Ca^{2+} channels.
- Phenobarbital enhances GABA effects on Cl^- channels and is a powerful inducer of drug metabolism.

- Benzodiazepines such as diazepam enhance GABA effects on the Cl^- channel.
- Newer drugs, e.g. lamotrigine and vigabatrin, have been developed to enhance the effects of GABA and, to some extent, Na^+ channel inhibition. They are good supplementary medicines to antiepileptics.
- The use of folic acid before and during pregnancy reduces the risk of neural tube defects in the fetus.
- Parkinson's disease is caused by failure in dopaminergic transmission in nigrostriatal pathways. The main symptoms are tremors, rigidity and hypokinesia. Pathophysiologically, the balance between dopaminergic and cholinergic pathways is disturbed. The treatment is either administration of dopamine or anticholinergic treatment.
- Dopamine is administered as the precursor levodopa plus a DOPA decarboxylase inhibitor. Levodopa treatment has serious adverse effects, and the therapeutic effect of its use diminishes over time.
- Amantidine increases the release of dopamine.
- The effect of bromocriptine is similar to that of dopamine.
- Selegiline inhibits monoamine oxidase B and reduces the metabolic breakdown of dopamine.
- Biperiden, orphenadrine and benzatropine are anticholinergics. These are the only treatment alternatives for parkinsonism that has been induced by antipsychotic drugs.
- Migraines are episodic strong headaches; research links such attacks to changes in the 5-HT metabolism. The mechanisms that trigger the pain are unknown.
- Ergotamine and dihydroergotamine cause vasoconstriction via α_1-adrenoceptors.
- Sumatriptan is a selective 5-HT agonist on 5-HT_1 receptors; its effect is vasoconstriction and effective pain relief.
- Prophylactic migraine treatment is indicated in patients suffering two or more migraine attacks per month. β-Blockers and the 5-HT receptor antagonist pizotifen may be used.
- Alzheimer's disease is characterized by degenerative changes in the brain. The clinical presentation is associated with deficiency in acetylcholine levels and an increased level of glutamate. Treatment is by drugs that increase the amount of acetylcholine in brain synapses and by drugs inhibiting the NMDA receptor to reduce the effect of glutamate.
- Myasthenia gravis is a autoimmune disease with antibodies directed against acetylcholine receptors in the motor end-plates of skeletal muscles. Treatment is by drugs that inhibit the breakdown of acetylcholine, e.g. acetylcholinesterase inhibitors such as pyridostigmine.

13 Drugs used in psychiatric disorders

It is difficult to differentiate between 'normal' and 'abnormal' behaviour. It also is difficult to provide a good pathophysiological description of psychiatric illnesses. For this reason it is difficult to make a correct psychiatric diagnosis. Without the correct diagnosis, it is not possible to establish the appropriate treatment. To overcome the diagnostic problem, different criteria have been used to diagnose mental illness and disorders. The diagnostic system used by most experts today is the DSM-IV (*Diagnostic and Statistical Manual of Psychiatric Disorders*, 4th revised edition). In this system, the diagnoses are criterion-based, i.e. a certain number of symptoms and conditions must be fulfilled before a diagnosis can be made. DSM-IV does not attempt to explain the causes of a condition. The system has proved to be useful regardless of whether one is seeking psychological, biological or social explanations for the illness.

Despite the difficulty of describing the pathophysiological processes in psychiatric illnesses, it has been helpful to focus on 'disturbances' in biochemical processes of the central nervous system, related to three main diagnoses:

- **anxiety and sleep disturbances**, where drug treatment aims to enhance the inhibitory effect of the neurotransmitter gamma-aminobutyric acid (GABA) – benzodiazepines are an example of drugs used for this purpose
- **psychosis**, where drug treatment is directed at overactive dopamine pathways in parts of the central nervous system – drugs with anti-dopaminergic activity are used here
- **depression**, where drug treatment is directed towards a reduced concentration of noradrenaline or 5-hydroxytryptamine (5-HT, the same as serotonin) in parts of the central nervous system. Drugs that inhibit the reuptake of these neurotransmitters, or that inhibit the enzymatic breakdown of these transmitters in the synaptic cleft, are used.

Using this approach rational drug treatment regimes have been established, but not without adverse effects.

ANXIETY AND SLEEP DISTURBANCES

Anxiety and sleep disturbances are amongst the most frequently occurring psychiatric conditions. Anxiety is an unpleasant experience or fear of something unknown, and is often a sub-symptom of a number of different psychiatric conditions such as depression and psychosis. Anxiety can also be associated with pain, breathing difficulties or discomfort. There are a number of well-defined anxiety syndromes where specific pharmacotherapeutic treatment is established. OCD (obsessive compulsive disorder) or compulsive syndrome is one of them. Another common anxiety illness is panic anxiety with recurring anxiety attacks. Situation-conditional anxiety, such as social phobia, and various specific phobias such as post-traumatic stress syndrome and maladaptive stress reaction also manifest themselves with anxiety as one of the main symptoms. Possible underlying physical or psychiatric illness should be precluded before pure symptomatic anxiety treatment is commenced.

Sleep disturbances are generally divided into difficulties in falling asleep, poor quality of sleep or premature awakenings. For difficulties in falling asleep, it is best to avoid stimulant drinks (e.g. coffee and tea) and large meals before bedtime. Anxiety and other psychiatric disorders frequently contribute to sleep disorders.

PATHOPHYSIOLOGY OF ANXIETY AND SLEEP DISTURBANCES

Anxiety and sleep disorders are different clinical syndromes, but tend to be discussed together because the drugs used to treat the disorders are often the same.

In severe anxiety, there is increased activity in the sympathetic nervous system, resulting in an increase in heart rate, blood pressure, sweating and tremors. Many patients experience dryness of the mouth, as parasympathetic activity is suppressed. It is important to explain to patients that these symptoms naturally accompany anxiety.

The role of GABA is important in understanding the mode of action of anti-anxiety (anxiolytic) drugs and sedatives. GABA binds to $GABA_A$ receptors. These are Cl^- channels and increase the Cl^- flow into the cell, thereby hyperpolarizing the postsynaptic membrane. This causes inhibition of impulse traffic and reduced anxiety and wakefulness. See Figure 13.1.

Areas of the central nervous system believed to be related to anxiety have an abundant supply of GABAergic neurons and $GABA_A$ receptors, as well as neurons that release other transmitters. Electrical stimulation of such an area (i.e. the amygdala) causes release of GABA, inhibition of impulse transfer to other parts of the brain and reduction of anxiety. Benzodiazepine receptors are distributed in the central nervous system in a similar way to $GABA_A$ receptors, and are found in high density in the amygdala, especially in the parts that distribute anxiety-conditioned fear reaction in experimental animals.

Considerable research has been conducted to find an endogenous ligand for the benzodiazepine receptor on the GABA receptor complex, the body's own 'benzodiazepine'. Neurosteroids can bind to the $GABA_A$ receptor at a different site and act as endogenous anxiolytics.

The neurophysiological basis for sleep is complicated, and many parts of the brain participate in sleep control. Stimulation of areas in the brain stem (especially the central pons and parts of the reticular formation) can induce sleep. Injuries in the same

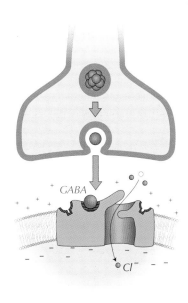

Figure 13.1 **The gamma-aminobutyric acid (GABA) receptor complex.** Cl^- ions flow into the cell, the resting potential becomes more negative and the cell is hyperpolarized. GABA therefore has a suppressive effect.

areas prevent sleep. Acetylcholine, noradrenaline and 5-HT are also assumed to play a role in inducing sleep, but GABA, dopamine and a number of neuropeptides influence the sleep-inducing activity in the cholinergic neurons in the pons.

DRUGS USED TO TREAT ANXIETY AND SLEEP DISTURBANCES

Drugs that are used to suppress anxiety are called anxiolytics. Drugs that are used to induce sleep are called hypnotics. All anxiolytics generally have a suppressive effect on the central nervous system, which is undesirable when solely treating anxiety, but very useful for sleep disturbances.

The development of benzodiazepines has provided drugs with specific effects on anxiety and sleep. At one time, barbiturates and similar agents with characteristics similar to those of general anaesthetics were used. However, these drugs have many adverse effects, including impaired coordination of motor function, strong sedative effects and the danger of dependence. For several anxiety syndromes, drugs in the SSRI group have been used with good results. See further information in the section on depression (p. 139).

Anxiolytics and hypnotics

Benzodiazepines are probably the most regularly used drugs against anxiety and sleep disturbance. However, because of their great potential for abuse, their use has become more limited and new agents with other effects have been developed. For certain conditions, antihistamines are used for sleep disturbances, especially for patients with drug abuse problems.

Benzodiazepines

Benzodiazepines have similar mechanisms of action to anxiolytics and hypnotics. Grouping them into anxiolytics and hypnotics is based around pharmacodynamic and pharmacokinetic differences, but the division is not always clear-cut. Benzodiazepines with a slow onset of effect and a long half-life are best suited to be anxiolytics. Diazepam and oxazepam belong to the anxiolytics group. Drugs that are quickly absorbed and quickly distributed to the central nervous system have a rapid effect and are probably best for sleep problems. See Figure 13.2. This latter group have the greatest potential for abuse. Nitrazepam, flunitrazepam and midazolam belong to the hypnotics group. Lorazepam is used both as an anxiolytic and a hypnotic drug.

Mechanism of action and effects. Benzodiazepines bind to the GABA receptor complex in the central nervous system and act by enhancing the binding of GABA. Figure 13.3 shows that the GABA receptor has several binding sites. One is the binding site for GABA, another for benzodiazepines. Benzodiazepines do not

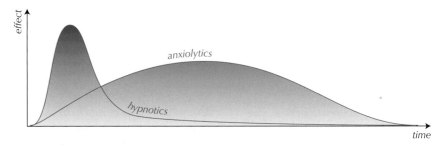

Figure 13.2 **Anxiolytics and hypnotics.** Anxiolytics are slower acting than hypnotics and last longer. The differences are not as clear-cut as the illustration suggests.

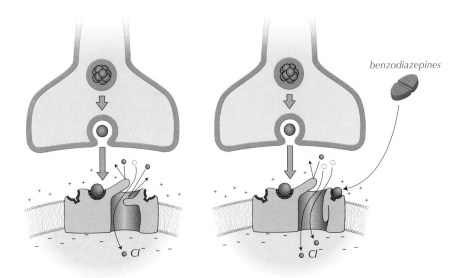

benzodiazepines

Figure 13.3 **The mechanism of action of benzodiazepines** is to bind to the gamma-aminobutyric acid (GABA) receptor complex and enhance the effect of GABA.

themselves open the Cl⁻ channel, but when they are bound, the effect of GABA increases on the channel. It has been shown that benzodiazepines increase the number of channels that open at a given concentration of GABA. In this way, the influx of Cl⁻ ions into the cells increases, consequently the neuronal membrane becomes hyperpolarized. The hyperpolarization causes the neurons to require a stronger stimulus to depolarize. This leads to inhibition of activity in areas of the central nervous system associated with anxiety and wakefulness.

This action is useful for treatment of muscle cramps, and these drugs can be used to treat both febrile convulsions and epileptic seizures. The relaxing effect on spastic muscles is probably exerted by presynaptic inhibition of neurons that run from the spinal cord to skeletal muscles.

Pharmacokinetics. All benzodiazepine preparations are absorbed almost entirely from the intestines. They are relatively rapidly distributed to the central nervous system and eliminated from the central nervous system into the blood after a short time. The rate of elimination is important for waking in that the drug concentration in the brain falls below the limit for sleep effects after a single dose.

Benzodiazepines are eliminated by metabolism in the liver. Many of the metabolites are pharmacologically active. The half-life of the parent agent and metabolites is long, e.g. 20–100 h for diazepam and 36–200 h for some of its metabolites. With once a day dosing, the majority of benzodiazepines will accumulate. Consequently, as with sedatives, these are best suited to short-term use.

Adverse effects. Drowsiness (hangover), disorientation, impaired memory and impaired learning function frequently occur with large doses. Perception and ability to coordinate are also impaired, such that ability to drive safely may be diminished.

Very large doses of benzodiazepines are needed to commit suicide, but in combination with other agents that suppress the central nervous system, e.g. alcohol, antipsychotics, opioids or antidepressants, benzodiazepines can cause respiratory failure and circulatory collapse, as their inhibitory effects are greatly enhanced.

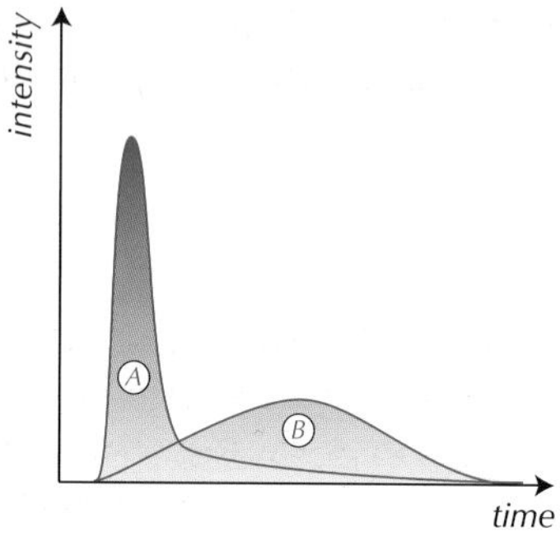

Figure 13.4 **Abstinence.** Agents with a short half-life cause the most intense abstinence-related problems while the abstinence-related problems last longer for drugs with a longer half-life. A has a shorter half-life than B.

Anxiolytics
Alprazolam, Buspirone, Diazepam, Oxazepam
Hypnotics
Flunitrazepam, Midazolam, Nitrazepam, Zolpidem, Zopiclone

Table 13.1 Drugs used to treat anxiety and sleep disorders

Flumazenil can be used as an antidote for benzodiazepine poisoning. Acute overdose of benzodiazepines is described in Chapter 30, Poisoning.

Tolerance and dependence. Tolerance to benzodiazepines develops gradually during treatment of sleep problems, while treatment for anxiety does not appear to require an increase in dose to maintain a therapeutic effect. However, both psychological and physical dependence can occur after 2–4 weeks at therapeutic dose levels. When treatment is stopped after continuous use, abstinence symptoms in the form of anxiety, restlessness, sleep problems and irritability may be experienced and can be serious in some cases. Withdrawal of treatment after long-term use of high doses should be gradual. The abstinence symptoms are more marked following withdrawal of drugs with a short half-life, but last longer for drugs with a long half-life. See Figure 13.4.

Other anxiolytics and hypnotics

Zolpidem and zopiclone
Zolpidem and zopiclone differ chemically from benzodiazepines, but appear to bind to the GABA receptor complex and enhance the effect of GABA. The effect resembles that of benzodiazepines with regard to impact on anxiety, sleep problems and drug dependence. Zolpidem appears to lack muscle-relaxant and anticonvulsive effects. Interactions with agents that suppress the central nervous system (e.g. alcohol) are the same as for benzodiazepines. The half-life is approximately 4 h, which indicates that these drugs are probably well suited for use in sleep disorders.

Buspirone
Buspirone is a partial agonist at 5-HT$_1$ receptors and increases the content of 5-HT in 5-HT neurons; however, the effects are not apparent until after a couple weeks' use and a maximum effect gradually appears during the course of approximately 4 weeks. Because of this slow onset, buspirone has little sedative effect and is not well suited for use in sleep problems, but is effective for anxiety, usually associated with depression. There does not appear to be a high risk of dependence. The effects are not enhanced by other central nervous system drugs or alcohol, but simultaneous use of other drugs that also increase the content of 5-HT in the synaptic cleft may cause adverse effects, including increased blood pressure.

Drugs used in the treatment of sleep and anxiety are listed in Table 13.1.

PSYCHOSES

Psychoses are serious psychiatric disorders described as distorted perceptions of reality. They manifest themselves in the form of hallucinations, delusions, thought disturbances, restlessness and aggression.

Psychoses are divided into several subgroups, depending on their cause and how they present clinically. Drugs that reduce the problems associated with psychoses are called antipsychotics. The drugs that are in current use do not have a curative effect, but increase the possibility that the patients can function within society in more acceptable ways.

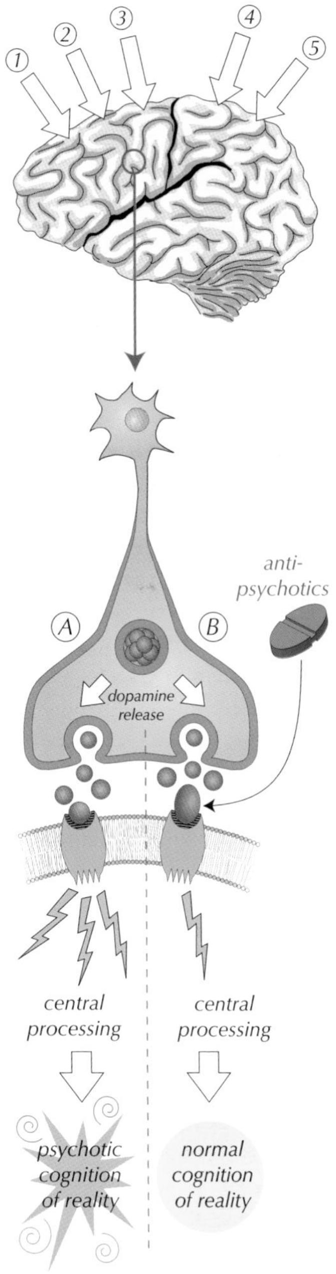

PATHOPHYSIOLOGY OF PSYCHOSES

Organically based psychoses are secondary to other illnesses or injuries. They can be caused by organic brain disease, infections, circulatory disorders or intoxication with drugs, alcohol or other narcotic agents. With these psychoses, the underlying disease needs to be treated. Functional psychoses include schizophrenia, manic-depressive disorder, special paranoid psychoses and reactive psychoses. Research in animal models have shown that psychological effects may have caused changes in neurotransmitter receptors that may be correlated to altered behaviour. This lends support to theories that emotional disturbances are partly associated with environmental influences.

The causes of psychoses are not completely known. However, research suggests that patients with schizophrenia have disturbances in dopaminergic function in areas of the brain associated with complex mental and emotional functions. Numerous observations regarding dopamine's role in these areas have given rise to the dopamine hypothesis for psychoses, and in particular for schizophrenia. The theory is based on overactivity in dopaminergic pathways. Five main types of dopamine receptor (D_1–D_5) have been established in the central nervous system. These are divided into two subgroups. D_1-type comprises D_1 and D_5, and D_2-type comprises D_2, D_3 and D_4. The theory of overactivity of dopamine arises from observation of the effects of antidopaminergic drugs on psychotic conditions, particularly drugs that block D_2 receptors and achieve an antipsychotic effect. This antipsychotic effect can be reversed by drugs that increase the dopamine concentration, such as levodopa or amphetamines.

Figure 13.5 illustrates a simple way of explaining that while what triggers a psychotic reaction can have many causes, the condition manifested will be the result of some disturbance in dopamine metabolism.

DRUGS USED TO TREAT PSYCHOSES

The clinical symptoms of psychoses are often divided into positive and negative symptoms. Positive symptoms include hallucinations and delusions; negative symptoms are social withdrawal and emotional apathy. Antipsychotics tend to be more effective in treatment of the positive rather than the negative symptoms.

Antipsychotics
Antipsychotics are divided into two main groups, classical and atypical. The newer atypical antipsychotics have a different profile of adverse effects compared with the classical drugs. Antipsychotics are also classified as high-dose preparations, transitional preparations and low-dose preparations, based on the dose that must be administered to achieve a therapeutic effect. The drugs in the three groups are broadly similar with regard to antipsychotic effects, but have different profiles with regard to their specific inhibitory effect, sedative effect and extrapyramidal adverse effects.

Mechanism of action and effects. All antipsychotics that are used today have the ability to block D_2 receptors. See Figure 13.6. There is often a good correlation between receptor binding and the ability to alleviate psychotic symptoms.

Figure 13.5 **Psychotic perception of reality.** Different central nervous system influences can result in increased dopamine release. (1) Brain disease; (2) infection; (3) circulatory disturbances; (4) intoxication; (5) mental influence. Antipsychotics inhibit dopamine-associated stimulation.

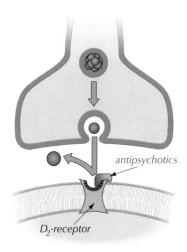

Figure 13.6 Antipsychotics block D$_2$ receptors.

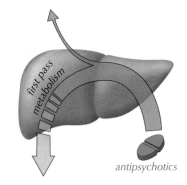

Figure 13.7 Antipsychotics have a considerable degree of first–pass metabolism.

The most distinctive clinical effect of antipsychotic drugs is the alleviation of hallucinations, delusions and thought disturbances. In addition, there is a non-specific sedative effect and a specific depressive effect. The non-specific sedative effect causes a general tiredness, which often diminishes over time. The specific depressive effect inhibits agitation, hyperactivity and aggression without necessarily causing drowsiness. Chronic schizophrenics who lack initiative and apathy can experience some reversal of these symptoms. With agitation and psychotic depression, there is an antidepressant effect.

Pharmacokinetics. There is variable absorption of different antipsychotics, and several are exposed to a considerable degree of first-pass metabolism. See Figure 13.7. All are quickly distributed to the central nervous system as well as to other parts of the organism. They are lipid-soluble and have a large volume of distribution.

Adverse effects. Antipsychotics act by inhibiting dopamine receptors that have widespread distribution in the central nervous system. Consequently, there are a number of dose-dependent central nervous system adverse effects that have been reported. However, only in large doses do these drugs become dangerous.

Many users demonstrate adverse extrapyramidal effects and tardive dyskinesia, as a result of disturbances in nerve pathways from the brain stem to the spinal cord and on to skeletal muscle. These symptoms manifest themselves in poor coordination of both fine and gross motor movements and in uncontrolled movements, particularly of facial muscles. It can take several months before extrapyramidal adverse effects develop, and they may be exacerbated over the years with chronic use of antipsychotics. Tardive dyskinesia is often irreversible, especially in the elderly. Akathisia is a condition where the symptoms consist of tension, panic, irritability and impatience, allied to movements like shuffling of the feet while sitting and pacing about while standing. Many patients have problems continuing with antipsychotics when they experience these types of symptoms. β-Blockers such as propranolol can improve these symptoms.

Antipsychotics cause frequent Parkinson-like problems by exerting an inhibitive effect on dopamine receptors in the same areas as those associated with Parkinson's disease. Atypical antipsychotics such as clozapine and risperidone are least likely to demonstrate these Parkinson-like adverse effects. Generally, however, these adverse effects can respond well to anticholinergic drugs. Blocking D$_2$ receptors in the vomiting centre results in a considerable antiemetic effect. Dopamine inhibits the secretion of prolactin via stimulation of D$_2$ receptors. By blocking the receptors with antipsychotics, the concentration of prolactin in serum increases. This leads to enlargement of mammary glands and sometimes milk production, in both men and women.

Almost all antipsychotics suppress activity in the parasympathetic nervous system by blocking muscarinic receptors, leading to dryness of the mouth, constipation and urinary retention. Some blocking of α$_1$-adrenoceptors in arterioles causes dilatation of peripheral blood vessels and a tendency for hypotension to occur. All of the drugs can cause neutropenia. Agranulocytosis is most common after treatment with clozapine. It is important to monitor the haematological profile, preferably weekly, during commencement of therapy and monthly after the first 4 months.

An even closer haematological follow up is needed for the treatment with clozapine.

Most antipsychotics rarely cause 'Neuroleptic malignant syndrome', which may be fatal if not treated promptly. See Box 13.1.

Acute overdose with antipsychotics is described in Chapter 30, Poisoning, p. 440.

Box 13.1 Neuroleptic malignant syndrome

Neuroleptic malignant syndrome is a potentially fatal syndrome associated primarily with use of neuroleptic agents which are in turn associated with dopaminergic receptor blockade and sympathetic dysregulation. Clinical features include diffuse muscle rigidity, tremor, high fever, diaphoresis, labile blood pressure, cognitive dysfunction and autonomic disturbances. Serum creatinine phosphokinases (CPK) level is often increased.

Treatment strategy. The choice of drug is determined as much on the basis of potential adverse effects as on the therapeutic value. The duration of the treatment varies with diagnosis and severity of the condition. Patients with predominantly negative symptoms should initially try low doses, the treatment lasting at least 2 years.

Depot preparations are useful for patients who are not capable of cooperating or who forget to take their medicine. In addition, it is an alternative for patients who do not receive a sufficiently high concentration after oral administration.

Determination of plasma concentrations of antipsychotics can provide useful information, especially where there is a lack of effect with standard doses or in patients with reduced liver function, e.g. elderly patients, pregnant and breastfeeding women, and children. Often, medicines are not taken as prescribed, or there may be unexpected adverse effects in relation to the dose. Antipsychotics may interact with other drugs that affect the central nervous system. Elderly patients with psychotic reactions often respond well to antipsychotics. However, patients with dementia, confusion or behaviour problems have less clearly documented responses.

Drugs used in the treatment of psychoses are listed in Table 13.2.

Low-dose antipsychotics
Flufenazin, Flupentixol, Haloperidol, Olanzapine, Pimozid, Risperidone

Transitional-dose antipsychotics
Pericyazine, Zuclopenthixol

High-dose antipsychotics
Klorpromazin, Chlorpromazine, Clozapine, Levomepromazine, Quetiapine, Tioridazin

Table 13.2 Drugs used to treat psychoses

DEPRESSION

After anxiety and sleep problems, depression is one the most frequently occurring psychiatric disorders. There has been an increase during the last 10 years, especially of mild and medium to serious depression. The age of onset appears to have dropped and is now below 18 years of age in the majority of patients with bipolar disease. Depression is often a lifelong disease with recurrent episodes, sometimes leading to suicide.

Depression is characterized by a general feeling of misery, pessimism and apathy. Many patients suffer from low self-esteem, feelings of guilt and feelings of inadequacy. The patients have reduced decision-making ability due to loss of motivation. Mental activity is sluggish and often the patients will engage in little physical activity. Many experience sleep disturbance and reduced appetite. In some individuals, their symptoms alternate between those of depression and mania, termed bipolar disease. Mania is the diametrical opposite of depression. See Figure 13.8. The patients are in excessively high spirits, enthusiastic, filled with self-confidence and are very

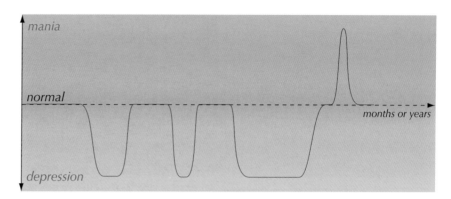

Figure 13.8 **Depression and mania.** With bipolar disease, the mood swings from depressive to manic.

active physically. They are often impatient and irritable. Bipolar disease occurs more frequently in young patients, and the clinical picture is compounded with symptoms such as anxiety and agitation.

The most frequently used drugs are agents that increase the content of noradrenaline and 5-HT in synapses in parts of the central nervous system.

PATHOPHYSIOLOGY OF DEPRESSION

Modern theories of causal relations for depression attempt to explain the disorder as incidents that lead to neurobiological changes. The monoamine theory maintains that depression stems from a defective monoaminergic transmission in the central nervous system, with regard to too little noradrenaline and 5-HT in some central nervous synapses. The theory is based on the observation that antidepressants such as tricyclic antidepressants (TCAs) and monoamine oxidase (MAO) inhibitors increase monoaminergic transmission. Correspondingly, it was observed that patients who received reserpine became depressed. Reserpine acts by depleting the stores of monoaminergic transmitters.

It has been maintained that the drug effect on the mood is largely an effect on 5-HT neurotransmission, while psychomotor stimulation is associated with an increase in noradrenaline neurotransmission.

There are a number of flaws in the monoamine theory. Some drugs that increase the concentration of monoamines do not have an antidepressant effect. Conversely, other antidepressants have an effect without influencing monoaminergic transmission. Neither can the monoamine theory explain the slow onset of the therapeutic response.

DRUGS USED TO TREAT DEPRESSION

Most antidepressants in clinical use directly or indirectly increase the concentration of noradrenaline or 5-HT in the synaptic cleft. They exert their effect by preventing reuptake in the presynaptic neuron, or by reducing enzymatic breakdown in the synaptic cleft. Based on these modes of action, the main antidepressant drugs are TCAs, which block the reuptake of both noradrenaline and 5-HT; selective serotonin reuptake inhibitors (SSRIs), which selectively block the reuptake of serotonin, i.e. 5-HT; MAO inhibitors, which inhibit the enzyme that breaks down noradrenaline and 5-HT; and atypical antidepressants with other mechanisms of action.

Acute overdose with antidepressants is described in Chapter 30, Poisoning, p. 440.

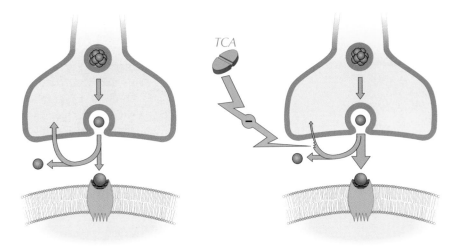

Figure 13.9 **Mechanism of action for tricyclic antidepressants.** The drugs inhibit the reuptake of both nonadrenaline and 5-HT. The synaptic degradation of nonadrenaline and 5-HT is not affected. See also Figure 11.15 on p. 111.

Tricyclic antidepressants

Tricyclic antidepressants, such as imipramine or amitriptyline, derive their name from three aromatic rings in the molecule. This drug group has been the basis of drug treatment of depression, but their usage has been reduced following the introduction of SSRIs.

Mechanism of action and effects. Tricyclic antidepressants inhibit the reuptake of both noradrenaline and 5-HT in nerve terminals. See Figure 13.9. This results in an increase of the neurotransmitter in the synaptic cleft. There is relatively little difference among the classical tricyclic antidepressants in their ability to inhibit the reuptake.

Most tricyclic antidepressants also inhibit one or more types of neurotransmitter receptors. These include muscarinic receptors, histamine receptors and α-adrenergic receptors. This influence provides an explanation of some of the antidepressant effect, as well as adverse effects such as the anticholinergic effect. One theory for the antidepressant effect states that the number of monoamine receptors, α_2- and β-adrenoreceptors is downregulated after chronic antidepressant treatment.

A positive clinical response is seen in 60–70 per cent of patients with depression who receive TCA treatment. Tolerance is developed to a small extent. Patients may benefit from treatment over a long period of time.

Pharmacokinetics. Therapeutic doses of TCAs are absorbed quickly and completely in the small intestine. 25–75 per cent is metabolized in the liver following first-pass metabolism, so bioavailability is low. TCAs are completely metabolized, some to active metabolites.

In some populations, individuals may lack a subgroup of enzymes (CYP2D6) that metabolize TCAs. Such patients become extremely sensitive to standard doses because they receive a high concentration of the drugs in serum (see Figure 9.1 on p. 84).

There is an established correlation between plasma concentration and therapeutic effect of nortriptyline and several other TCAs. With a considerably elevated plasma concentration, however, the effect diminishes. See Figure 13.10. Because of individual differences in metabolism, determination of plasma concentration is useful in the management of treatment and control of toxicity.

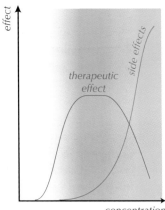

Figure 13.10 **Therapeutic window.** In concentrations above a certain value, the effect diminishes while the adverse effects quickly increase.

Adverse effects. Many patients experience anticholinergic effects such as dry mouth, blurred vision, constipation, urinary retention and postural hypotension. All of these effects are associated with antagonism of muscarinic receptors in the parasympathetic nervous system.

Antidepressants have a narrow therapeutic index. Overdose with suicidal intent can occur in depressed patients, especially when psychomotor inhibition is reduced during the initial phase of antidepressive treatment. Intoxication with TCAs is potentially life-threatening, with symptoms of respiratory depression, ventricular rhythm disturbances and coma. Large doses cause considerable anticholinergic effects, with delayed gastric emptying as one of the consequences. Tablet remnants can remain in the stomach for some time and so absorption is delayed. Hence, in overdose, it can still be useful to perform gastric lavage, even hours after ingestion.

Interactions. Two important mechanisms increase the effects and adverse effects of TCAs. Drugs that act by inhibiting the removal of the neurotransmitter from the synapses, by selectively inhibiting the reuptake of 5-HT or inhibitors of the enzyme MAO can dramatically increase the concentration of the neurotransmitter in the synapse. See Figure 13.11. They can produce a syndrome consisting of confusion, agitation, cramps, hyperreflexia, increased sweating, tremor, diarrhoea and fever. TCAs must not be combined with MAO inhibitors.

Dosing. Initially, the patient must be carefully dosed, increasing the dose in small increments after 3–4 days and reaching the maximum dose after approximately 2–3 weeks. The doses used by elderly patients must be lower than those used by younger patients.

Selective serotonin reuptake inhibitors (SSRI) and selective noradrenaline reuptake inhibitors (SNRI)

These drugs are of more recent origin than the TCAs, but are used by many patients with a number of depressive disorders. They have a somewhat different spectrum of adverse effects than TCAs and a lower acute toxicity.

Mechanism of action and effects. The monoamine reuptake inhibitors inhibit selectively the reuptake of 5-HT or noradrenaline into presynaptic nerve ends. See Figure 13.11. The clinical effect is almost the same as for TCAs with a slow onset of effects. The sedative effect is less than for TCAs. The drugs have also proved to be effective in treating panic disorders and bulimia.

Pharmacokinetics. The monoamine reuptake inhibitors are slowly metabolized in the liver, and some into active metabolites. Elimination is slow, and it takes time before the therapeutic concentration is established. Because of the long half-life, it takes time for the steady state/therapeutic concentration to be reached.

Adverse effects. The adverse effects of SSRIs and SNRIs are more readily tolerated than those of TCAs, primarily because they do not have anticholinergic or cardiovascular adverse effects. They are well suited to elderly patients. These drugs do not cause weight gain, and the acute toxicity is low. Conversely, SSRIs often cause nausea, anorexia and insomnia, and aggression and violence have been observed. Reduced libido occurs in both sexes, and men experience ejaculation disturbances. These adverse effects are often stated as the main reason when patients decide to stop treatment.

In the period after treatment has ceased, many patients experience problems such as dizziness, headache, irritability, coordination disturbances and nausea. These abstinence-like symptoms can be reduced by gradual withdrawal of the drug.

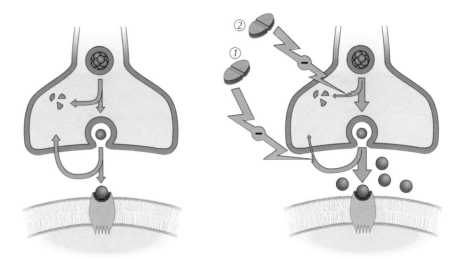

Figure 13.11 **Interactions.** Combinations of drugs that inhibit the reuptake of 5-hydroxytryptamine (1) and the presynaptic breakdown via monoamine oxidase (MAO) (2) can lead to a dramatic increase of 5-HT in the synapses and produce effects related to excess 5-HT.

Because of an increase in aggression, violence and suicides by teenagers treated with monoamine reuptake inhibitors, great care is advised before prescribing these drugs to young people.

Interactions. Selective serotonin reuptake inhibitors inhibit the metabolism of a number of drugs such as TCAs, antipsychotics, propranolol, warfarin, cimetidine, phenytoin and theophylline. To avoid effects due to excessive levels of 5-HT, they must not be combined with MAO inhibitors. See the section on TCAs (p. 141).

> **Box 13.2 The serotonin syndrome**
>
> The serotonin syndrome is an adverse drug interaction characterized by altered mental state, autonomic dysfunction, and neuromuscular abnormalities. It is most frequently caused when combining serotonin reuptake inhibitors and monoamine oxidase inhibitors (MAOs), but may also be the result of combining TCAs and MAOs, leading to excess serotonin availability in the CNS.

Monoamine oxidase inhibitors
There are two forms of the MAO enzyme (MAO-A and MAO-B). These are influenced to various degrees by enzyme inhibitors.

Moclobemide
Moclobemide is a reversible and specific MAO-A inhibitor that increases 5-HT, nonadrenaline and dopamine in the synaptic cleft by a reduction of presynaptic breakdown of these transmitters. By inhibiting MAO the amount of neurotransmitter in the synaptic cleft is increased. MAO-A inhibitors have a good antidepressant effect. There are generally few adverse effects. However, older MAO inhibitors, such as tranylcypromine, inhibit tyramine breakdown in the liver leading to higher levels of tyramine, which is an indirectly acting sympathomimetic. The consequence is the potential for a severe hypertensive crisis and patients

should strictly avoid foods with high tyramine content such as mature or ripe cheeses, concentrated yeast extract products, game and broad beans. MAO inhibitor drugs should not be combined with SSRIs because of the risk of serotonin syndrome.

Atypical antidepressants

Mianserin and mirtazapine-blocking of α_2 receptors
Mianserin probably increases the release of noradrenaline by blocking presynaptic α_2-receptors. Blockade of α_2-receptors results in increased influx of Ca^{2+} in presynaptic neurons and increased release of transmitters from presynaptic vesicles into the synapse. For an explanation see Figure 17.14 on p. 235.

Clinically, mianserin has an antihistamine effect with good sedation and a good anxiolytic effect. Because of these properties, the drug is well suited for depressed patients with anxiety, restlessness and sleep problems. Because of the small anticholinergic effect, the drug is also suited for use in elderly patients. Mianserin has a lower toxicity than tricyclic antidepressants.

Lithium
Lithium (Li^+) is a monovalent cation like Na^+ and K^+. However, it is not pumped out of the cells as quickly as sodium and thus has a tendency to accumulate intracellularly. Lithium influences the metabolism of noradrenaline and 5-HT and reduces the release of monoamines after depolarization. Biochemically, lithium inhibits hormone-induced synthesis of cyclic AMP, but it is uncertain how the therapeutic effect occurs.

Patients with manic-depressive disorders particularly benefit from prophylactic treatment with lithium.

Lithium is absorbed quickly and is eliminated through the kidneys with a half-life of 1–2 weeks. There is a very narrow therapeutic index for lithium. Kidney disease or sodium deficiency reduces the elimination rate and increases the toxicity. Diuretics have a similar effect when they are combined with lithium. Because of lithium's potential toxic effect, the patients should have their lithium plasma concentration monitored very closely. Patients with reduced kidney function are particularly susceptible to overdose. Adverse effects are nausea, vomiting, diarrhoea, listlessness and tremors. Lithium passes into the breast milk and breastfeeding is not advised. The acute toxicity of lithium is described in Chapter 30, Poisoning.

Drugs used in the treatment of depression are listed in Table 13.3.

Tricyclic antidepressants
Amitriptyline, Doxepin, Cloimipramine, Nortriptyline, Trimipramine

Selective serotonin reuptake inhibitors
Citalopram, Fluoxetine, Fluvoxamine, Paroxetine, Sertraline

Selective noradrenaline reuptake inhibitors
Reboxetine, Venlafaxine

Selective inhibitors of monoamine oxidase A
Moclobemide

α_2-receptor antagonists
Mianserin, Mirtazapine

Lithium
Lithium

Table 13.3 Drugs used to treat depression

ATTENTION DEFICIT HYPERACTIVITY DISORDER (ADHD)

Attention deficit hyperactivity disorder (ADHD) is a behaviour disorder of children and adolescents, which may affect up to 3% of the population. Sufferers exhibit inattentiveness, motor unrest, learning disorders, hyperactivity and occasionally incontinence. Some ADHD sufferers can become subject to drug abuse. Whilst reports vary, males are four times more likely to display ADHD behaviours than females. The cause is uncertain, though evidence suggests that in ADHD there is weak inhibitory control of the limbic system as a consequence of fronto-limbic dysfunction, possibly through a disorder of the right frontal cortex. A 70 per cent increase in dopamine re-uptake transporter has been reported in the same area of the brain. The dopamine D_4 receptor is also thought to be associated with ADHD.

DRUGS USED TO TREAT ADHD

Psychostimulant drugs, such as dexamphetamine and methylphenidate and the sympathomimetic atomoxetine are, rather surprisingly, effective. They do not cause a worsening of symptoms but, paradoxically, improve self-control, time spent on tasks and general attentiveness. Better adjustment to school and home life has also been demonstrated. These drugs are often used as part of a comprehensive treatment programme for children and adolescents when remedial measures alone are insufficient. Psychostimulant drugs are effective in 70 per cent of cases. Serotonin and SSRI drugs appear to be ineffective in the treatment of ADHD.

Mechanism of action and effects. The mechanism of action of these drugs is not entirely clear. They act on noradrenergic and dopaminergic systems by inhibiting the re-uptake of noradrenaline and dopamine. Increase in the levels of both these neurotransmitters in the prefrontal cortex increases, in turn, its inhibitory effect on the limbic system. As plasma level must be maintained, slow release preparations are used to prolong the time of drug release, thereby prolonging duration of action of the drug. Some evidence indicates that nicotinic cholinergic receptors are ineffective in ADHD. The use of nicotine, delivered via transdermal patches has been shown to improve symptoms of the disorder.

Side effects and contraindications
The side effects of the psychostimulant drugs are related to the enhanced effects of noradrenaline and dopamine and include insomnia, restlessness, irritability and excitability, nervousness, night terrors, euphoria, tremor, dizziness, headache, dependence and tolerance and sometimes psychosis. Their use is contraindicated in hypertension and caution is advised regarding their use in epileptic subjects.

Psychostimulant drugs
Atomoxetine, Dexamphetamine, Methylphenidate

Table 13.4 Drugs used to treat ADHD

SUMMARY

- Anxiety and sleep disturbances are effectively treated with benzodiazepines, which enhance the effect of GABA. For sleep problems, drugs with a short duration of action are used. In anxiety, drugs with a longer duration of action are used. Benzodiazepines have potential for abuse.

- Psychoses are characterized by distorted perceptions of reality. Antipsychotics act by inhibiting the effect of dopamine on dopamine receptors. The therapeutic effect is virtually the same for the different drugs. The drugs have different degrees of non-specific sedative effect and a specific inhibitory effect on agitation, hyperactivity and aggression. Adverse effects are tardive dyskinesias, ataxia and Parkinson-like effects, and possibly hypotension as well.

- Depression is characterized by a general feeling of misery, apathy and pessimism. Many patients have low self-esteem and great feelings of guilt. The monoamine theory maintains that the disorder is caused by too little noradrenaline and 5-HT in some synapses in the central nervous system.

- Antidepressants primarily act by inhibiting the reuptake of both noradrenaline and 5-hydroxytryptamine (TCAs), or only of 5-HT (SSRIs). Moclobemide inhibits the breakdown of noradrenaline and 5-HT by inhibiting the enzyme monoamine oxidase.

- TCAs have anticholinergic adverse effects and cause delayed gastric emptying when taken in large doses. There is high acute toxicity with overdose.

- SSRIs have less acute adverse effects than TCAs. TCAs and SSRIs must not be combined with MAO inhibitors because of the risk of the development of effects due to 'serotonin syndrome'.

- Psychostimulant drugs, such as dextroamphetamine and methylphenidate, are used to treat ADHD.

Drugs with central and peripheral analgesic effect

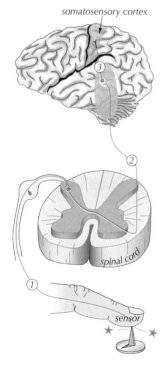

Figure 14.1 The afferent pathway to the somatosensory cortex. (1) Primary neuron; (2) secondary neuron; (3) tertiary neuron.

Stimuli that give rise to different sensory modalities such as touch, pressure, pain and temperature are carried to the somatosensory cortex in afferent pathways consisting of three neurons. The primary afferent neuron carries an action potential from a sensory receptor to the dorsal horn of the spinal cord or the medulla oblongata. The secondary neuron carries the action potential further from the dorsal horn to the thalamus. The tertiary or third-order neuron carries the action potential from the thalamus to the somatosensory cortex. See Figure 14.1.

PAIN

Pain is a subjective, unpleasant sensory and emotional experience that occurs in association with tissue damage or the threat of tissue damage, or which is described as though it is caused by tissue damage. Experiencing and interpreting pain largely depends on previous experiences and a person's physical condition at the time the pain is experienced. Altered states of mind, e.g. anxiety and depression, also influence the perception of pain. In this way, our experiences and physical condition contribute towards modulation of the pain experience.

ANATOMY, PHYSIOLOGY AND PATHOPHYSIOLOGY OF PAIN

Different sensory modalities are carried in different types of afferent neurons to the dorsal horn of the spinal cord. Pressure and touch are carried in thick (Aα and

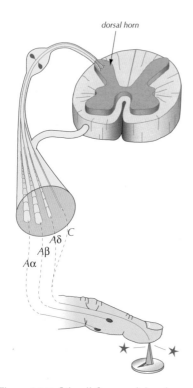

Figure 14.2 **Stimuli from peripheral nerve ends.** The sensations of touch and pressure are carried in thick myelinated fibres (Aα and Aβ) and medium-thick fibres (Aγ – not shown in the figure), while stimuli from nociceptors are carried in thin myelinated (Aδ) and thin unmyelinated fibres (C), to the dorsal horn of the spinal cord.

Aβ fibres) and medium-thick myelinated nerves (Aγ fibres). Pain is carried in thin myelinated (Aδ fibres) and thin unmyelinated nerves (C fibres). See Figure 14.2. The receptor endings of pain-conducting neurons are called nociceptors (pain sensors). Nociceptors are dendritic endings of sensory neurons that are activated by stimuli that have caused, or have the potential to cause, tissue damage if the stimulus persists.

NOCICEPTORS

Nociceptors are activated by the release of chemicals from cells which have ruptured as a consequence of tissue damage. Such chemicals include protons, 5-HT or serotonin from platelets, histamine from mast cells and a whole variety of other substances which are known to activate, or in some cases sensitize, nociceptors to other substances. Other nociceptors will respond to mechanical or thermal stimuli. Those nociceptors that respond to mechanical and thermal stimuli tend to have an increased threshold for activation.

Nociceptive endings are found in the skin, muscles, viscera and other structures. They transmit action potentials to the dorsal horn of the spinal cord. There, the action potential is passed to a second-order neuron, which crosses over to the opposite side of the spinal cord before travelling up to the thalamus. In the thalamus, the action potential is transmitted to a third-order neuron which terminates in the somatosensory cortex. It is the somatosensory cortex that perceives the localization and intensity of the pain. The different qualities of pain, e.g. piercing, cutting, prickling, aching, etc., are called the modalities of pain. Nociceptive afferent pathways also have projections to other higher centres, such as the hypothalamus, amygdala and the reticular formation, all of which are important centres for processing somatosensory information and for the association of this information with previous pleasant or unpleasant experiences that are related to pain. See Figure 14.3. The perception of pain can also be initiated by other neural mechanisms when there is damage to the nervous system and in disease states such as anxiety and depression.

NON-DRUG MODULATION OF PAIN

The perception of pain may be influenced by both descending neural activity and neural activity in other non-nociceptive neurons. Within the central nervous system there are neurons that utilize neurotransmitters such as the encephalins and endorphins. These substances act as endogenous analgesics. These neurotransmitters have the ability to hyperpolarize neurons, which means that, when these neurons are activated, there is a reduced perception of pain. A model has been formulated to explain how nociceptive information may be modulated within the central nervous system – the so-called gate control theory.

The gate control theory

The gate control theory postulates that in the spinal cord there are neural mechanisms which are able to open and close 'gates' for afferent stimuli arising from nociceptors. By opening a gate, the afferent impulses will be transmitted to the secondary neuron. Alternatively, when a gate is closed, nociceptive information will not be transmitted to the secondary neuron, and not reach the somatosensory cortex. The gate control theory proposes that the activity of interneurons in the spinal cord influences the opening and closing of such 'gates'. The depolarization of these interneurons results in the release of endorphins and hyperpolarization

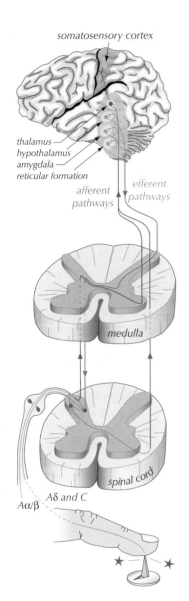

somatosensory cortex

thalamus
hypothalamus
amygdala
reticular formation

afferent
pathways

efferent
pathways

medulla

spinal cord

Aδ and C

Aα/β

Figure 14.3 **Afferent and efferent neural activity associated with pain.** The figure illustrates how pain impulses are carried from nociceptors in peripheral tissue to the central nervous system. Refer to the text for a more detailed explanation.

of the presynaptic primary afferent neuron in the dorsal horn, which corresponds to closure of the gate. Pain impulses that are carried in Aδ or C fibres stimulate the second-order neuron at the same time as the interneuron is inhibited. See Figure 14.4.

The neural activity in the interneurons can also be increased by stimulation of afferent fibres that transmit the sensations of pressure and touch from the same region from which the nociceptive signal has arisen. This explains why mechanical stimulation of a corresponding tissue area to the pain provides pain relief. For example, women in childbirth experience reduced labour pains when the skin over the lumbar region is massaged. It is possible to explain the pain relief provided by transcutaneous electrical nerve stimulation (TENS) using this model.

Influence of previous experience of pain on current pain

The gate control theory helps to explain how previous pain experiences may influence the experience of pain. Efferent pathways from higher centres in the brain have fibres that synapse in the dorsal horn of the spinal cord. This descending efferent neural pathway releases neurotransmitters that may stimulate the interneuron, which then release endorphins and hyperpolarize the presynaptic primary neuron. By hyperpolarizing the presynaptic primary neuron the transmission of the afferent signals to the secondary neuron will be inhibited and fewer nociceptive signals will reach the thalamus. Such a process reduces the perception of pain because fewer afferent nociceptive stimuli reach the somatosensory cortex.

The opposite situation may also occur. The recognition of a set of circumstances that gave rise to strong, uncontrollable pain may result in inhibition of the interneuron. In doing so, it will result in an increased number of nociceptive signals reaching the somatosensory cortex and increased perception of pain. See Figure 14.4.

LOCALIZATION OF PAIN

Different tissue areas have different densities of nociceptors. Areas with many nociceptors will transmit the most precise information of the origin of the pain. Sharp, stabbing and cutting pains are usually easier to localize than pains of aching, throbbing and rupturing character. Inflammation in an area gives rise to diffuse pain that is difficult to localize precisely.

The skin is the organ containing most nociceptors per unit area. Therefore, pain from the skin can be described precisely with regard to both localization and modality. This is particularly true for pain in the face and hands. Acute joint pains can normally be precisely described, while chronic joint pains and pain from muscles and bones are experienced diffusely.

Pain from internal organs is most often experienced diffusely and is less easy to localize. With pain from internal structures, there is also usually simultaneous pain perception from certain skin areas – although there is no tissue damage to the skin. For example, cardiac pain coincides with a perception of pain in the neck, jaws and radiating outwards in the left arm. Pain from the bile duct system can be experienced in the skin over the right shoulder. Pain that is experienced from somewhere other than the organ from which it originates is known as 'referred pain'.

Referred pain

Referred pain can be described by two possible mechanisms. Firstly, a single nociceptive afferent neuron may terminate in both the skin and internal organs. Nociceptive stimuli from the organ will thus be experienced as pain from the corresponding surface tissue. Alternatively, different afferent pain fibres from an organ and other

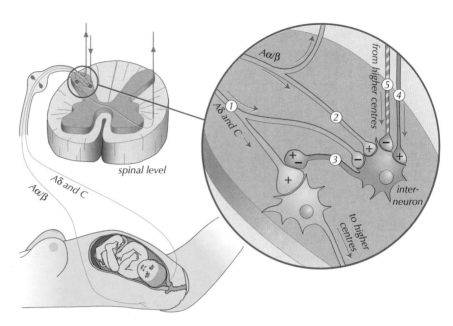

Figure 14.4 **The gate control theory.** Afferent stimuli from nociceptors are carried in primary afferent neurons (1) to second-order neurons in the dorsal horn, which transmit the impulse to higher centres. An inhibitory impulse is simultaneously sent to the interneuron. Signals from touch and pressure receptors in corresponding areas to the pain are carried in thick myelinated Aα and Aβ fibres, which stimulate interneurons (2). Stimulation of the interneuron leads to depolarization and release of endorphins that hyperpolarize the primary neuron in the dorsal horn and inhibit transmission of the signal (3). In this way, the impulse traffic to higher centres is reduced. Modulation from higher centres (experience) can probably stimulate and inhibit interneurons, and in this way modulate the experience of pain (4 and 5).

surface tissue structures may terminate on a common second-order neuron in the dorsal horn of the spinal cord, which in turn transmits nociceptive information to higher regions of the CNS. This phenomenon is called 'somatovisceral convergence', and explains why a person can experience pain in a surface structure when it actually arises from an internal organ. See Figure 14.5.

ACUTE PAIN AND CHRONIC PAIN

The body's interpretation of and reaction to pain are largely determined by whether the pain is acute or chronic. Acute pain is perceived as a danger signal that something is wrong. Such pain is accompanied by anxiety and autonomic reactions such as tachycardia, an increase in blood pressure and dilated pupils. In principle, it results in avoidance reactions and measures that preserve health by removal from the danger.

Chronic pain is not perceived as an acute danger signal. Because of constant and persistent pain, the body does not respond with measures to evade the situation. This type of pain may cause depression rather than anxiety, and generally results in inactivity and isolation. There are normally few or no visible reactions from the autonomic nervous system. Chronic pain can diminish the health of the individual.

If impulses from nociceptors continuously stimulate neurons in the dorsal horn over a long period of time (persistent pain), neurons may be damaged and

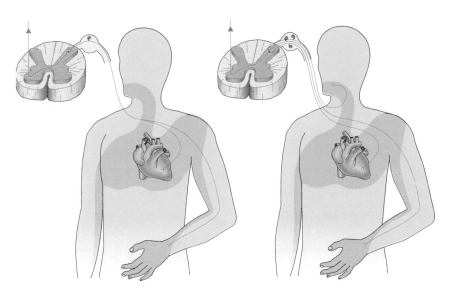

Figure 14.5 **Referred pain.** The illustration shows two possible models for the phenomenon of 'referred pain'. Refer to text for a detailed explanation.

neuronal function may be altered. It is assumed that this type of damage explains why long-lasting pain can persist even after the initial pain stimulus has ceased. Such an observation indicates that the pain should be treated early, so that no permanent neuronal damage in the dorsal horn is established, which could result in the maintenance of pain.

Analgesic treatment should be based on whether the pain is acute or chronic and on the patient's prognosis. With acute, severe pain, it is possible to use pain-relieving drugs (analgesics) in the short term, which, if used for longer periods, may cause dependency. With chronic pain, such drugs must be used more selectively. Problems of dependency become less important in the treatment of terminally ill patients. Under all circumstances, it is necessary to provide pain relief with both a combination of drugs and non-drug therapies. Adequate pain treatment requires knowledge of the cause of the pain.

Nociceptive pain

Pain that is attributable to potential or real tissue damage is associated with direct stimulation of nociceptors. Nociceptive stimuli that are carried in the Aδ fibres are experienced as sharp, stinging or prickling, short-lasting pain – so-called epicritical pain. Nociceptive stimuli that are carried in the C fibres are experienced as deep, aching and often throbbing pain – so-called protopathic pain. Nociceptive pain can be treated with peripherally or centrally acting analgesics.

Neurogenic pain (neuropathic pain)

Neurogenic pain is attributable to damage in the central or peripheral nervous system. A common form of neurogenic pain is that experienced in association with herpes zoster (shingles), also called post-herpetic pain. Another common form of neurogenic pain is the kind that appears in association with sensory neuropathies, e.g. as a result of diabetes. A further example is seen after strokes that affect the thalamus, where considerable neurogenic pain may develop.

Pain can also be induced by trauma or surgery which can cause the formation of neuromas ('nodes'), where a nerve is damaged. In such cases, the pain is perceived as originating in structures which the damaged nerve originally innervated. Phantom pains and trigeminal neuralgia are further examples of neuropathic pain. TENS can reduce neurogenic pain where there is still some functional nerve activity.

Neurogenic pain is difficult to treat with drugs, but can be reduced with the use of local anaesthetics (post-herpetic pain), tricyclic antidepressants (pain after strokes, post-herpetic pain) and antiepileptics (trigeminal neuralgia).

Psychogenic versus organic pain

Psychogenic pain is described as pain that arises or exists because of mental disorders in the absence of any known physical damage. The diagnosis requires the absence of an organic basis for the pain. Purely psychogenic pains are very rare, and include unexplainable pain in association with psychotic disorders.

Pain of unknown origin

Pain of unknown origin, or idiopathic pain, includes several different pain conditions, e.g. fibromyalgia (muscle pain of unidentifiable origin). It has been suggested that, in such cases, there is a defect in the central pain-modulating systems.

SITES OF ACTION FOR THE MODULATION OF NOCICEPTIVE STIMULI

- Reduced sensitivity of nociceptors (peripherally acting analgesics)
- Blockage of nociceptive afferent impulses in sensory nerves (local anaesthetics)
- Modulation of synapses processing nociceptive information (centrally acting analgesics)
- Inhibition of the perception of nociceptive information in the somatosensory cortex (general anaesthetics)
- Therapeutic (and non-therapeutic) measures to modify accompanying disorders such as anxiety and depression.

The most important mechanism for modulation of pain is the use of drugs that reduce pain, i.e. analgesics. Analgesia means 'absence of pain'. It is common to divide analgesics into those that act centrally and those that act peripherally. Such a division is based on the mechanism and site of action for the drugs.

CENTRALLY ACTING ANALGESICS

Drugs that reduce the pain experience by binding to receptors in the central nervous system are regarded as centrally acting analgesics. They have an effect on all forms of nociceptive pain, but are less effective with pain of neurogenic and psychogenic origin. Antidepressants and anxiolytics can enhance the analgesic effect of centrally acting analgesics.

Opioids

All substances that have morphine-like effects by acting on opioid receptors and that can be reversed with naloxone (an opioid antidote) are regarded as opioid compounds. The term opiates refers to substances with molecular similarity to morphine and is thus more limited than the term opioids. The opioids inhibit neural activity at the level of the spinal cord, and probably in the thalamus, by hyperpolarizing neurons involved in the processing of nociceptive information. See Figure 14.6.

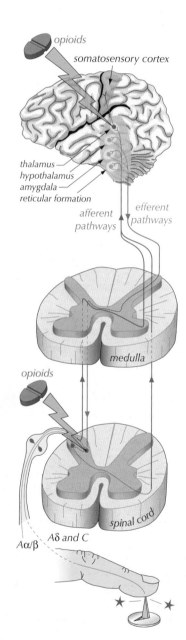

Figure 14.6 Centrally acting analgesics. Opioid analgesics inhibit neural activity to the somatosensory cortex by hyperpolarization of neurons that convey nociceptive information at the spinal level and in the thalamus.

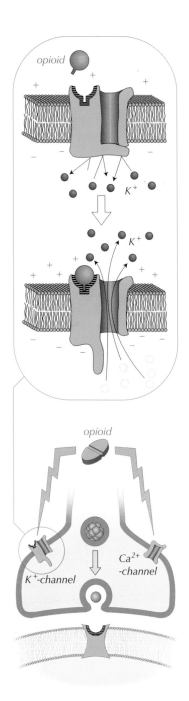

Figure 14.7 Mechanism of action of opioids. Opioid analgesics hyperpolarize neurons by increasing the efflux of positive potassium ions from the cell. Additionally, the influx of calcium is inhibited, which leads to a reduced release of neurotransmitter and therefore a reduction in nociceptive neural information (not shown in the figure).

Mechanism of action and effects. Opioid analgesics mediate their analgesic effects via opioid receptors in the central nervous system. When opioids bind to their opioid receptors, the efflux of potassium ions increases. This makes the cell more negative on the inside, i.e. the cell becomes hyperpolarized. See Figure 14.7. Simultaneously, the influx of calcium in the neuron is reduced. A hyperpolarized nerve cell requires a stronger stimulus to trigger depolarization. This means that the release of transmitter substances between neurons involved in the transmission of nociceptive information is also reduced. This results in fewer pain stimuli reaching the somatosensory cortex where the pain is experienced, i.e. 'less' pain is felt.

Endogenous substances such as endorphins bind to opioid receptors and exert morphine-like effects. These substances appear to be released in increased quantities when a person who is exposed to pain has some control of the situation which is resulting in production of pain. For example, the release of endorphins is probably increased during potentially painful endurance events such as running a marathon race. If a person is exposed to a painful situation over which they have no control, the release of endorphins seems to decrease and the pain is experienced more strongly. These mechanisms are probably connected to efferent pathways from higher centres for consciousness and experience. Different receptors have been shown to be responsible for different opioid effects. See Box 14.1.

The central and peripheral effects of opioid administration are shown in Box 14.2.

Different opioid analgesics have different effects on different receptors. Tolerance and dependency develop quickly, especially with intravenous and intramuscular use. The use of centrally acting analgesics in the absence of pain (i.e. opioid abuse)

Box 14.1 Opioid receptors and effects of their stimulation

- μ/δ receptor – analgesia, euphoria (pleasant, intoxicating-like effect), respiratory depression, sedation, dependence and myosis
- κ receptor – analgesia at the spinal level
- σ receptor – dysphoria (unpleasant, intoxicating-like effect) and hallucinations

---

Box 14.2 Central and peripheral opioid effects

Central nervous effects
- Analgesia – of all types of pains
- Euphoria – lessens anxiety and fear and gives a feeling of well-being
- Sedation – reduced level of wakefulness
- Respiratory depression – reduced sensitivity for CO_2 in the respiratory centre
- Cough suppression – reduced activity in the cough reflex centre
- Nausea – stimulation (reduced inhibition) of the nausea centre
- Pupil constriction (myosis) – parasympathetic stimulation
- Reduced urine production – stimulation of antidiuretic hormone (ADH) secretion

Peripheral effects
- Constipation – reduces gastrointestinal motility
- Hypotension – dilation of peripheral vessels
- Itching – release of histamine

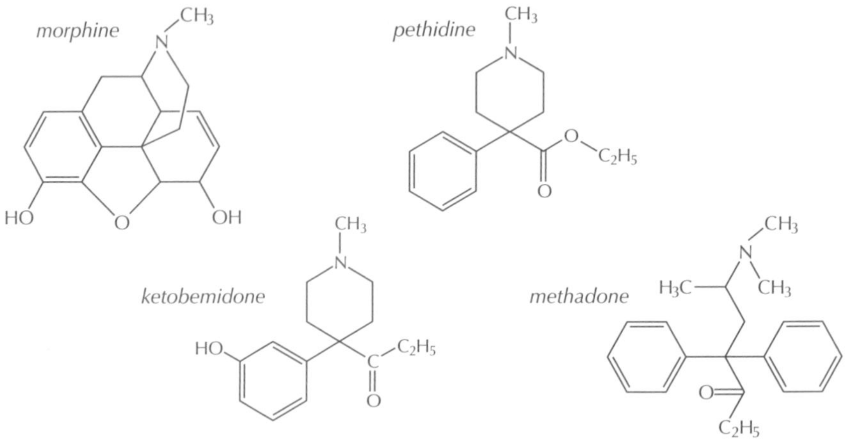

Figure 14.8 Molecular structures of some strong opioid analgesics. Morphine, pethidine, ketobemidone and methadone.

increases the danger of dependence compared with their use in the treatment of strong pain.

Strong opioid analgesics

Morphine

Morphine is the prototype opioid analgesic and should be the first drug of choice when a powerful analgesic is required. Morphine is used for acute pain associated with heart attacks, surgical intervention and the chronic pain experienced by patients with terminal illness. Morphine has the ability to contract some smooth muscles and is therefore not the first choice drug for the relief of pain associated with gallstones and kidney stones. A typical dose (5–10 mg i.v.) provides pain relief for 3–5 h. Depot preparations result in a relatively steady state plasma concentration and produce a longer-lasting analgesic effect. Figure 14.8 demonstrates the molecular structure of some strong opoid analgesics.

Pethidine

Pethidine has similar indications for use as morphine, but has less spasmogenic smooth muscle activity. It is therefore better suited than morphine to pain relief associated with gallstones or renal calculi, where there is a need to dilate a muscular hollow tube where stones have lodged. Pethidine has a shorter duration of action than morphine and is sometimes used in the treatment of labour pain. Because of its shorter duration of action, there will be less neonatal respiratory depression.

Methadone

Methadone has a similar effect to morphine. With repeated doses, the half-life will increase, resulting in a relatively steady state plasma concentration, which provides a long-lasting analgesic effect. It is used for severe pain in patients with a poor prognosis. Methadone is also used, to a certain extent, as a substitute for heroin in the rehabilitation of heroin addicts. The use of methadone in association with intoxicating substances is discussed in more detail in Chapter 29, Drugs of abuse.

Medium–strong opioid analgesics

Buprenorphine and pentazocine

Buprenorphine and pentazocine are partial agonists and antagonists. This means that they have an analgesic (i.e. opioid agonistic) effect when they are administered alone

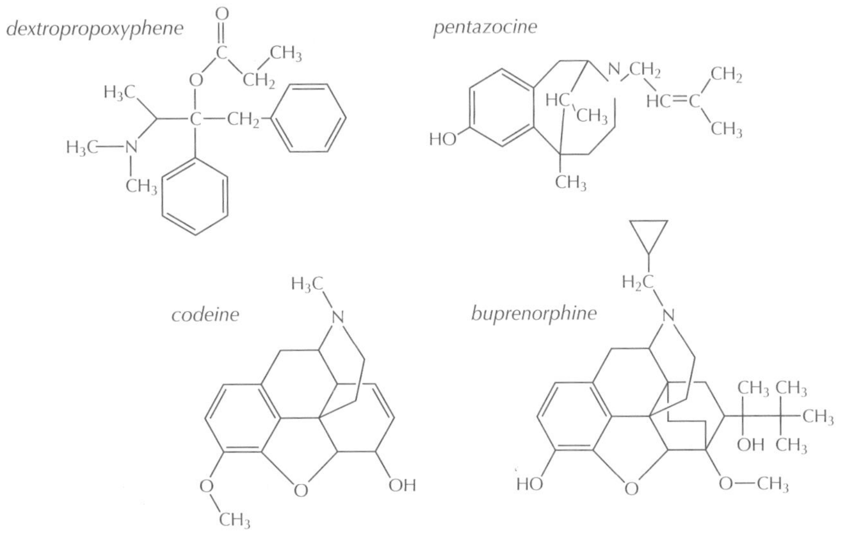

Figure 14.9 Molecular structures of some medium–strong opioid analgesics. Buprenorphine, pentazocine, codeine and dextropropoxyphene.

and an antagonistic effect when administered together with a pure agonist like morphine. In this way they can reduce the effect of other opioid analgesics when they are administered in conjunction with these, i.e. they have an antagonist effect and prevent the other opioid from exerting its full effect. It is advisable therefore not to administer a pure opioid agonist in conjunction with an opioid partial agonist/antagonist. Figure 14.9 demonstrates the molecular structure of medium-strong opoid analgesics.

Codeine

Codeine is often used in combination with paracetamol or acetylsalicylic acid (aspirin). It has both an analgesic and a cough-suppressing effect. Approximately 10 per cent of the codeine is metabolized into morphine in the body.

Dextropropoxyphene

Dextropropoxyphene resembles codeine. The duration of action of an individual dose increases if several doses of the drug are given successively when compared with the duration of effect of a single dose. With long-term use, a metabolite accumulates that has a toxic effect on the liver.

Tramadol

Tramadol is an opioid that causes a small reduction in the neuronal reuptake of serotonin and noradrenaline. It has the same analgesic qualities of codeine but has a slower effect. It also has less of a constipating effect than other opioids. Figure 14.9 demonstrates the molecular structure of some medium-strong opoid analgesics.

Adverse effects of opioids. Nausea, drowsiness and constipation often occur with the use of opioids. In large doses, respiratory depression is seen. Drowsiness and respiratory depression are intensified by other substances that suppress the central nervous system. For this reason, the combination of opioids with alcohol, tranquillizers or sedatives can have life-threatening effects.

Elimination. Methadone and codeine are different from other opioids in terms of their bioavailability. They have a bioavailability of 70–80 per cent, while the remaining opioid analgesics have a low bioavailability, of around 30–35 per cent,

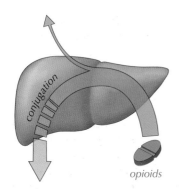

Figure 14.10 **Opioids are conjugated in the liver.** The majority have pronounced first-pass metabolism, and therefore low bioavailability.

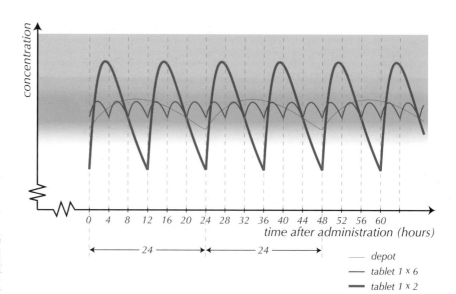

Figure 14.11 **Plasma concentration levels with different dosage regimes.** When using tablets, the dosage must be more frequent (4–6 times daily) or larger doses must be administered with the possibility of adverse effects and reduced effect at the lowest plasma concentrations of each dosage interval. Depot forms with oral administration of opioids provide the possibility for dosing once or twice a day and more stable plasma concentration during the dosage interval.

due to pre-systemic metabolism in the liver. See Figure 14.10. Morphine-like drugs are conjugated in the liver with glucuronic acid and are excreted into the intestine in bile. Conjugated opioids can be metabolized by bacteria so that the morphine released can be reabsorbed back into the plasma. Conjugated compounds are eliminated in the urine.

Pregnancy and breastfeeding. Considerable caution should be taken when using opioids during pregnancy, especially during the final stage, due to the possibility of the fetus developing a dependence for opioids. Neonates have an immature liver, and thus reduced ability to conjugate morphine-like drugs, so there is an effective increase in the half-life of the drug. For this reason, the effect of these drugs will last longer in neonates than in others. Thus when analgesia is required during childbirth, pethidine, which has a short half-life, is the drug of choice.

Dosing of opioids. Opioids have low bioavailability when administered orally. Therefore, patients with chronic pain require frequent and large doses to maintain the analgesic effect. Large, single doses increase the possibility of adverse effects, particularly immediately after the drug has been given, when the plasma concentration reaches its peak. Depot preparations result in a more stable plasma concentration and give a longer duration of analgesia. See Figure 14.11. Methadone has a

Strong opioid analgesics
Methadone, Morphine, Oxycodone, Pethidine
Medium–strong opioid analgesics
Codeine, Dihydrocodeine, Tramadol
Partial agonists
Buprenorphine, Pentazocine

Table 14.1 Centrally acting analgesics

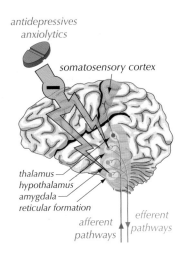

antidepressives
anxiolytics

somatosensory cortex

thalamus
hypothalamus
amygdala
reticular formation

afferent pathways

efferent pathways

Figure 14.12 Antidepressants reduce the experience of pain. The figure shows possible sites of action of antidepressants and anxiolytics in reducing the pain experience. By inhibiting the impulse traffic in the efferent neurons that inhibit the interneurons, the release of endorphins is increased. This results in inhibition of nociceptive impulses. See also Figure 14.4 (p. 150).

high bioavailability and a long half-life, and is used in terminally ill patients with chronic pain. The elderly are particularly susceptible to opoid side-effects and should receive lower doses.

ANTIDEPRESSANTS AND ANXIOLYTICS FOR PAIN

When used in conjunction with antidepressants or anxiolytics, the effect of analgesics is increased. The gate control theory explains this phenomenon, in that these drugs decrease the activity in efferent neurons from higher centres in the central nervous system that have an inhibiting effect on the interneurons of the dorsal horn of the spinal cord. Thus, the release of endorphins and other neurotransmitters is increased. This effect is shown in Figures 14.4 and 14.12.

Tricyclic antidepressants have a place in the treatment of psychogenic pain. They are also used in the treatment of pain after strokes and post-herpetic pain. Generally, the doses required are less than those required to treat depression. Antidepressants and anxiolytics are discussed in more detail in Chapter 13, Drugs used in psychiatric disorders.

PERIPHERALLY ACTING ANALGESICS

Inflammation leads to sensitization of nociceptors. Analgesics that inhibit nociceptive stimuli before they reach the central nervous system are regarded as peripherally acting analgesics. The use of peripherally acting analgesics is therefore related to inflammation. The purpose of peripherally acting analgesics is to reduce the synthesis of substances that are created by inflammation and which result in sensitization of the nociceptors. The enzyme cyclooxygenase has a central role in this sensitization process. Peripherally acting analgesics display differing degrees of analgesic activity together with antipyretic and anti-inflammatory effects. See Figure 14.13.

Peripherally acting analgesics are used in the treatment of musculoskeletal pain, headache, pain associated with menstruation and pain associated with mild trauma. Their antipyretic (temperature-reducing) effects are used in the treatment of febrile conditions with temperatures above 39.5°C. Their anti-inflammatory effects are used for the treatment of acute inflammation and for the treatment of rheumatic conditions.

NON-STEROIDAL ANTI-INFLAMMATORY DRUGS

Non-steroidal anti-inflammatory drugs (NSAIDs) are those that inhibit the activity of the enzyme cyclooxygenase and include, amongst others, acetylsalicylic acid (aspirin), ibuprofen, indometacin and piroxicam. Two cyclooxygenase enzymes (COX-1 and COX-2) have been identified. COX-1 is found in small quantities in almost all tissues and is necessary for a number of physiological functions, such as the regulation of platelet aggregation and a protective effect on the mucous membrane of the stomach. COX-2 is generated acutely in inflamed tissue. However, it also has an additional role in the maintenance of the renal circulation.

Mechanism of action and effects. Tissue trauma that leads to inflammation results in the release of arachidonic acid from membrane phospholipids. Arachidonic acid is an unsaturated, long-chain fatty acid that is found in all cell membranes of the body. Cyclooxygenase converts arachidonic acid to prostaglandins and thromboxanes,

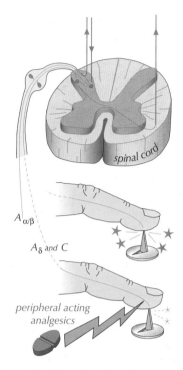

Figure 14.13 Peripherally acting analgesics inhibit the synthesis of nociceptor-sensitizing substances in inflamed tissue – in doing so they reduce activation of nociceptors and generation of nociceptive impulses. See also Figure 14.4 (p. 150).

which, among other things, sensitize nociceptors. The effects of NSAIDs are mediated via inhibition of cyclooxygenase. See Figure 14.14. The inhibition of cyclooxygenase occurs in one of two ways:

- irreversible inactivation of the enzyme (e.g. acetylsalicylic acid)
- fast, reversible, competitive inhibition (e.g. ibuprofen and piroxicam).

Analgesic effect. A number of prostaglandins sensitize not only peripheral nociceptors but also nociceptors in the central nervous system, thus enhancing even weak pain stimuli. This explains why an inflamed area has a lowered pain threshold to pressure and touch. NSAIDs reduce pain from inflamed tissues by inhibiting the synthesis of prostaglandins, but they have a poor analgesic effect with other types of pain.

Antipyretic effect. The normal body temperature is regulated via a 'thermostat' located in the thermoregulatory centre of the hypothalamus. When infections take hold, toxins from microorganisms stimulate the formation of prostaglandins, which can influence the 'thermostat' so that the body temperature is 'set' higher. Because NSAIDs inhibit the creation of these prostaglandins, the disruption of the thermostat will be reduced and body temperature will return to its normal value.

Anti-inflammatory effect. With inflammation, cyclooxygenase metabolizes arachidonic acid to form prostaglandins and thromboxanes. The enzyme lipoxygenase metabolizes arachidonic acid to form leukotrienes.

Prostaglandins contribute to an acute inflammatory response by producing a vasodilation, increased blood vessel permeability and a reduction in the aggregation of platelets. Thromboxanes have almost the opposite effect.

Leukotrienes produce chemotactic factors which result in the migration of neutrophils, granulocytes, monocytes, macrophages and mast cells.

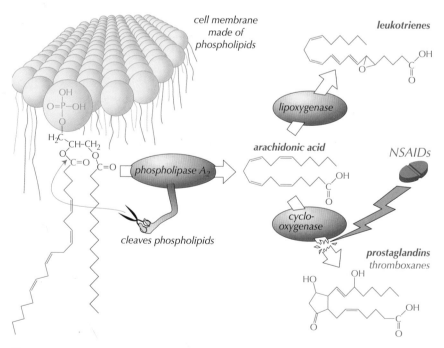

Figure 14.14 Non-steroidal anti-inflammatory drugs (NSAIDs) inhibit the enzyme **cyclooxygenase,** thereby reducing the synthesis of prostaglandins and thromboxanes.

NSAIDs inhibit cyclooxygenase, but not lipoxygenase. By inhibiting the synthesis of prostaglandins, vasodilation is inhibited. As a consequence, the acute inflammatory response becomes limited.

Antiplatelet effect. Thromboxanes promote platelet aggregation and adhesion. Most NSAIDs inhibit the formation of thromboxanes, resulting in an increased bleeding time. Therefore, these drugs should not be used in conjunction with other drugs that interfere with the haemostatic response, e.g. anticoagulants and fibrinolytics.

Effect on the mucous membrane of the intestines. Prostaglandins inhibit the synthesis of hydrochloric acid in the parietal cells of the stomach mucosa. By inhibiting the synthesis of prostaglandins with NSAIDs, acid secretion increases, thus increasing the risk of acid-related inflammation of the stomach and duodenal mucosa. See Figure 19.4 on p. 282.

Effect on renal blood flow. Prostaglandins contribute to the maintenance of blood flow in the kidneys, producing a vasodilatory response, especially with a simultaneously high level of noradrenaline and angiotensin-II. Chronic use of NSAIDs inhibits the synthesis of prostaglandins and can therefore cause renal damage because renal blood flow is reduced. Renal damage by NSAIDs is most likely with users who, for various reasons, have reduced renal blood flow. In patients with latent cardiac failure, treatment with NSAIDs can reduce renal function further and give rise to fully developed cardiac failure. This happens because the secretion of renin increases and contributes to an increased production of angiotensin-II, which further causes increased sodium retention, thereby increasing the circulating fluid volume. See Figure 17.19 on p. 241.

Pharmacokinetic aspects

Non-steroidal anti-inflammatories display a high degree of binding to plasma proteins, such that only a small proportion of a given dose is free to exert a pharmacological effect. By increasing the dosage, the binding sites on the plasma proteins become saturated, therefore effectively increasing the concentration of free drug more than anticipated and thus possibly causing unwanted adverse effects.

NSAIDs are eliminated mostly as inactive metabolites after metabolism in the liver. Acetylsalicylic acid displays saturation kinetics. Therefore, even a moderate increase in dosage can have a toxic effect if the dose is so high that elimination is saturated.

Specific COX-2 NSAIDs

Specific COX-2 NSAIDs selectively inhibit the COX-2 enzyme. The benefit of these drugs was thought to be a reduction in some of the adverse effects experienced with nonspecific NSAIDs, like gastric inflammation with ulceration and bleeding and inhibition of blood platelet aggregation. Specific COX-2 NSAIDs have proved to be as effective as nonspecific NSAIDs in the treatment of musculoskeletal inflammatory

---

Non-specific COX inhibitors
Aceclofenac, Acetylsalicylic acid (Aspirin), Dexketoprofen, Diclofenac, Diflunisal, Fenbufen, Fenoprofen, Flurbiprofen, Ibuprofen, Indometacin, Ketoprofen, Ketorolac, Meloxicam, Nabumetone, Naproxen, Piroxicam, Sulindac, Tenoxicam
Specific COX-2 inhibitors
Etoricoxib

Table 14.2 Peripherally acting analgesics

problems, with a reduction in gastric adverse effects. However it is suspected that the use of specific COX-2 NSAIDs increases the risk of thromboembolic diseases (myocardial infarction and stroke) and serious skin reactions (toxic epidermal necrolycis and Stevens-Jonsons syndrome), which has resulted in withdrawal of some of the drugs in this group and warnings about usage. Use of specific COX-2 NSAIDs by people with an increased risk of thromboembolic diseases should be avoided.

There seems to be a dose-dependent increase in risk of these serious adverse effects, which has led to recommendations that the lowest effective dose is used for as short a time as possible, when needed. The drugs should not be used for the treatment of pain shortly after coronary bypass surgery. The thromboembolic adverse effect is a 'class-effect', which means it is associated with all NSAIDs.

Indications for use of NSAIDs. Non-steroidal anti-inflammatories are used for the relief of mild-to-moderate pain associated with acute inflammation. In the case of severe pain, the need for opioids can be reduced with the simultaneous use of NSAIDs.

The effective treatment of pain associated with chronic inflammatory connective tissue diseases often requires higher doses than does treatment of pain associated with acute inflammation. In chronic inflammatory connective tissue diseases, NSAIDs can promote joint functionality and contribute to the toleration of other treatment methods. Acute attacks of gout, dysmenorrhoea and acute migraines can also be treated with NSAIDs. When used for the treatment of migraines, the best responses are seen if NSAIDs are given at the onset of an attack.

NSAIDs are generally the first line of treatment of pain associated with kidney stones and gallstones. NSAIDs are also now part of several postoperative pain regimes. Pain due to skeletal metastases of cancer responds well to NSAIDs.

Paracetamol is recommended when there is a need to reduce elevated temperatures.

Adverse effects. The most common adverse effects are dyspeptic abdominal pains with haemorrhaging from the gastrointestinal mucosa, nausea and vomiting. The adverse effects can be somewhat reduced by using enteric-coated forms of NSAIDs. In these forms, the tablet is coated with a gelatine capsule that dissolves after it has passed into the intestines, where it has a less damaging effect on the mucosa. The drugs should be used with caution by patients with ulcers, haemophiliacs and patients using other drugs that increase the danger of haemorrhaging. Patients over 65 years are a clear risk group for adverse gastrointestinal effects.

Allergic skin reactions are the most frequent adverse effects after adverse gastrointestinal effects. Renal damage can occur with long-term use due to the loss of the vasodilating effect of prostaglandins.

In susceptible allergic subjects, parenteral use of NSAIDs can occasionally trigger severe asthma attacks. In rare cases, bone marrow depression and damage to liver cells are also seen. See Figure 14.15. See also the specific adverse effects mentioned with specific COX-2 NSAIDs.

Pregnancy and breastfeeding. The use of NSAIDs reduces the possibility of pregnancy occurring because implantation of a fertilized egg in the endometrium is dependent on a critical prostaglandin level in the woman. These drugs should be used with great caution during the last stage of pregnancy due to the danger of haemorrhaging in the fetus and mother during the birth process.

Prostaglandins are necessary to maintain the patency of the ductus arteriosus in the developing fetus. This is a shunt which provides a direct link between the pulmonary artery and the aorta in the fetus. The use of NSAIDs in the latter stages

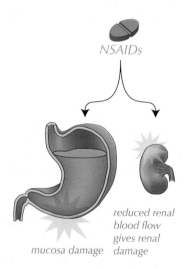

NSAIDs

mucosa damage

reduced renal blood flow gives renal damage

Figure 14.15 **Adverse effects of non-steroidal anti-inflammatory drugs (NSAIDs).**

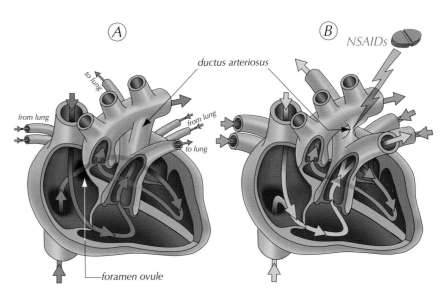

Figure 14.16 **Fetal and adult circulation.** In fetal life, the blood flows through the ductus arteriosus to avoid blood flow through the pulmonary vessels (A). The use of non-steroidal anti-inflammatory drugs (NSAIDs) at the end of pregnancy can cause the ductus arteriosus to close before the birth (B), and thus lead to the development of acute pulmonary hypertension in the developing fetus.

of pregnancy can cause the ductus arteriosus to close before the birth, because the synthesis of prostaglandins is inhibited. This will prevent the blood that is pumped from the right ventricle from being delivered into the aorta (via the ductus arteriosus). Instead, it will be delivered into the pulmonary circulation of the fetus. However, the pulmonary circulation is incapable of receiving this quantity of blood, since the lungs and vessels in the pulmonary circulation are 'compressed' in fetal life. See Figure 14.16.

During the latter stages of pregnancy prostaglandins contribute to the maturation and softening of the cervix which aids labour and delivery. The use of NSAIDs inhibits the formation of prostaglandins and therefore may have a harmful effect when used during the the latter stages of pregnancy.

OTHER PERIPHERALLY ACTING ANALGESICS

Paracetamol
Paracetamol (acetaminophen) is another example of a peripherally acting analgesic. Since paracetamol has little anti-inflammatory effect, it is common to exclude this drug as a NSAID, although some work has shown it to possess anti-inflammatory properties. It is the drug of choice in the treatment of mild-to-moderate pain in children aged under 16 who should not be prescribed aspirin.

Properties. Paracetamol has both antipyretic and analgesic effects, but has poor efficacy in pain due to inflammatory processes. Therefore, paracetamol is not considered to be a NSAID. The mechanism of action of paracetamol is unclear.

Adverse effects/caution. There are few adverse effects associated with a normal dosage. However, in the case of overdose and with intoxication, paracetamol can cause serious liver damage. Poisoning with paracetamol is discussed in Chapter 30, Poisoning.

Elimination. Paracetamol is metabolized in the liver with a half-life of 2–3 h. Large doses (>10 g in adults) may cause acute liver damage which may be life-threatening.

Pregnancy and breastfeeding. If analgesics are needed during pregnancy, paracetamol is recommended as the first choice.

SUMMARY

- Pain (nociception) is a subjective experience that is associated with actual or potential tissue damage. Pain impulses are conducted in afferent neurons to the somatosensory cortex, where the conscious experience takes place. Acute pain and chronic pain result in different responses in the people who experience the pain. The gate control theory explains modulation of the pain experience.
- Opioid analgesics bind to receptors in the central nervous system and inhibit the release of transmitter substances. Partial opioid agonists should not be given simultaneously with pure agonists. Opioid analgesics can cause serious respiratory depression and dependence. Sedation, nausea and constipation are common adverse effects. Opioid analgesics do not relieve elevated temperatures or have any effect on inflammation.
- NSAIDs act by inhibiting the synthesis of prostaglandins and thromboxanes that are formed from arachidonic acid. Different NSAIDs have different degrees of analgesic, antipyretic and anti-inflammatory effect. The most common adverse effects are dyspeptic pains, nausea and vomiting. Nonspecific NSAIDs inhibit the aggregation of the platelets and increase the tendency towards haemorrhage. NSAIDs do not cause dependence or abstinence when treatment ceases.
- The use of specific COX-2 inhibitors increases the risk of thromboembolic disease when used in high doses over long periods of time.
- Paracetamol lacks an anti-inflammatory effect. The drug is recommended as an analgesic for mild-to-moderate pain, and as needed to reduce elevated temperatures. Acetylsalicylic acid and paracetamol cause life-threatening poisoning in large doses.

15 Drugs used in inflammatory and autoimmune joint diseases

Rheumatic joint diseases and gout are characterized by chronic inflammation primarily in the joints but also in other structures. Phagocytic cells are recruited to the inflamed area and contribute to tissue damage by the release of toxic mediators.

Rheumatoid arthritis, juvenile rheumatoid arthritis and Bechterew's disease (ankylosing spondylitis) are autoimmune diseases, each with a varying degree of inflammation and structural changes in cartilaginous surfaces and the synovial membranes.

RHEUMATIC JOINT DISEASES

PATHOPHYSIOLOGY OF RHEUMATIC JOINT DISEASES

All joints with a certain amount of movement have cartilaginous surfaces that slide against each other and which are enclosed by a joint capsule that is partially lined by a synovial membrane. Rheumatic joint disorders are characterized by inflammation and proliferation of the cells of the synovial membrane and damage to other structures near the joints as the disease progresses. Affected areas have increased activity of phagocytic cells which cause tissue damage by the release of lysosomal enzymes and toxic oxygen metabolites. The result is destruction of cartilage and bone together with inflammation and hypertrophy of the synovial membrane. See Figure 15.1.

Non-drug treatments are important for this patient group, as drugs form only part of the total treatment programme.

Rheumatoid arthritis

Rheumatoid arthritis is a chronic, inflammatory, autoimmune disease with a multifactorial aetiology. The disease process takes place in the synovial membrane, cartilage, ligaments, tendons and bone tissue of the joints. As the disease progresses and structural damage increases, there is pain, misalignment and decreased function of the joint.

The characteristic symptom is persistent, symmetrical joint inflammation (arthritis) of more than 6 weeks' duration. There is an elevation of the plasma concentration of C-reactive protein (CRP) and other acute-phase proteins. These are

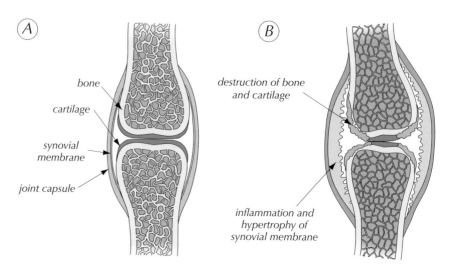

Figure 15.1 **Healthy and inflamed joints.** (A) shows a joint with normal joint structures; (B) shows typical changes with cell proliferation of the synovial membrane and destruction of cartilage.

proteins released in response to inflammation, and their levels correlate well with the severity of the disease. Within the patient group there are large individual differences in how quickly the disease progresses.

Juvenile rheumatoid arthritis
Juvenile rheumatoid arthritis presents before 16 years of age. It is a heterogeneous disease group with several subtypes and a variety of different symptoms and findings. Growth disturbances are often associated with juvenile rheumatoid arthritis.

Bechterew's disease (ankylosing spondylitis)
In Bechterew's disease, the iliosacral and vertebral joints become ossified. The ligamentum flava (a ligament that connects adjacent vertebrae and which runs ventrally across the spinal column) becomes ossified and shrinks, so that the spinal column curves forward and restricts rotational movement of the vertebral joints. Treatment aims to reduce pain and counteract the stiffness and misalignment of the vertebral column.

DRUGS USED TO TREAT RHEUMATIC JOINT DISEASES

When considering the use of drugs in the treatment of different rheumatic disorders, it is important to ensure that the diseases are chronic and of an inflammatory and autoimmune nature. Drugs with anti-inflammatory actions will tend to relieve pain and increase joint functionality. Drugs that inhibit the activity of phagocytic cells and cells that release toxic mediators (DMARDs – disease-modifying antirheumatic drugs) can slow or temporarily inhibit development of the disease.

Drug treatment therefore aims to:

■ relieve pain and symptoms and increase joint functionality
■ limit or stop inflammation and prevent structural destruction of the tissue.

Drugs that relieve pain and symptoms
Non-steroidal anti-inflammatory drugs (NSAIDs) have both anti-inflammatory and analgesic effects. Glucocorticoids have anti-inflammatory and immunomodulatory

effects. These effects occur after short-term use. Paracetamol can provide adequate analgesia when the disease is in remission.

NSAIDs

Non-steroidal anti-inflammatory drugs are used for their anti-inflammatory properties. They inhibit cyclooxygenase, an enzyme which metabolizes arachidonic acid to prostaglandins and thromboxanes. Inflammatory symptoms are reduced; there is moderate pain relief and increased joint functionality. Patients taking these drugs are able to tolerate training and physical mobilization better than without them. NSAIDs do not modulate the disease process, do not prevent tissue destruction and do not bring about remission. Figure 14.14 (p. 158) shows how NSAIDs prevent synthesis of prostaglandins and thromboxanes. NSAIDs are more thoroughly discussed in Chapter 14, Drugs with central and peripheral analgesic effect. See Table 14.2 (p. 159) for an overview of NSAIDs.

Glucocorticoids (steroids)

Many patients with rheumatic disease experience dramatic improvement of symptoms after using glucocorticoids (e.g. methylprednisolone, cortisone and betamethasone). These drugs do not inhibit progression of the disease in the long term since the condition worsens when treatment is stopped. Because of the many, and sometimes serious, adverse effects, glucocorticoids are used only in serious cases of rheumatic disease, and often in combination with other drugs.

Mechanism of action and effects. The glucocorticoids bind to specific receptor proteins in the cell's cytoplasm. The receptor–steroid complex migrates into the cell's nucleus and binds to specific regions of DNA, resulting in a change in gene activity. The products of gene activity then have a variety of cellular effects.

Glucocorticoids are anti-inflammatory in that some of the products of gene expression inhibit the modification of the gene transcription and thereby alters the synthesis of regulatory proteins affecting cellular functions. In this way the enzyme phospholipase A_2, which is responsible for the release of arachidonic acid from membrane phospholipids, is inhibited. Thus, production of prostaglandins, thromboxanes and leukotrienes is inhibited, and the influx of phagocytic cells to the inflamed area is reduced. This helps considerably to reduce the inflammatory response in autoimmune diseases such as rheumatoid arthritis. See Figure 15.2.

Adverse effects. The glucocorticoids also have a number of other actions, some of which are adverse effects. These are dose-dependent and are related to biochemical and physiological effects. See Box 15.1.

Glucocorticoids used in the treatment of rheumatic diseases are listed in Table 15.1.

Drugs that can limit the progress of disease (disease-modifying antirheumatic drugs or DMARDs)

Some antirheumatic drugs can delay or arrest the progress of disease for long periods, but none of them contributes to total healing of the damaged structures. These drugs do not act by inhibiting cyclooxygenase and do not have an analgesic or direct anti-inflammatory effect. Their effect appears weeks to months after use. The drugs are used with particularly aggressive forms of disease and when further disease progression is anticipated. Some patients experience such serious adverse effects to these drugs that they have to cease the treatment.

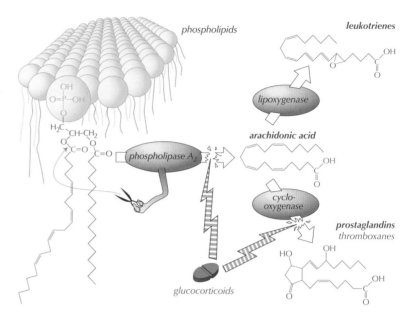

Figure 15.2 **Glucocorticoids have an anti–inflammatory effect.** Glucocorticoids lead to an increase in the synthesis of lipocortin, a protein that inhibits phospholipase A_2 (broken green arrow). Thus, less arachidonic acid is released from the cell membrane's phospholipids. In this way, the production of prostaglandins, thromboxanes and leukotrienes is inhibited. In addition, glucocorticoids inhibit the synthesis of cyclooxygenase-2, which is involved in inflammatory responses. See also Figure 21.10 on p. 321.

Box 15.1 Adverse effects of glucocorticoids (steroids)

- Changes in body shape – effect of changed fat distribution
- Atrophy of skin and connective tissue – catabolic effect on connective tissue
- Osteoporosis – catabolic effect on bone tissue and reduced production of collagenous connective tissue
- Myopathy – catabolic effect on muscle proteins
- Growth inhibition in children – the epiphyseal discs are closed before full linear growth is attained
- Reduced glucose tolerance – high blood sugar provides only a weak stimulus to insulin secretion
- Gastrointestinal haemorrhage – increased secretion of hydrochloric acid by stimulation of parietal cells in the mucosa of the stomach
- Increased risk of infection – inhibition of the immune system
- Pituitary gland/adrenal failure – inhibition of adrenocorticotrophic hormone secretion from the pituitary gland, such that stimuli to the adrenal cortex are reduced

---

NSAIDs
See Table 14.2 (p. 159)

Glucocorticoids
Cortisone, Hydrocortisone, Methylprednisolone, Prednisolone, Triamcinolone

Table 15.1 Drugs that relive pain and symptoms in inflammatory and autoimmune joint diseases

Chloroquine and hydroxychloroquine

Chloroquine and hydroxychloroquine are generally the primary choice of drugs in the treatment of malaria. In rheumatic disorders they are used for modifying the disease progression in moderate forms of disease.

Mechanism of action and effects. The mechanism(s) of action of these drugs in the treatment of joint disorders is not fully established. However, they produce effects which contribute to the suppression of the inflammatory response, including:

■ inhibition of the migration of leucocytes and proliferation of lymphocytes to and in the inflamed area
■ reduction in the release of lysosomal enzymes and formation of toxic oxygen metabolites in phagocytic cells
■ an inhibitory effect on phospholipase A_2, which results in a reduction in the formation of arachidonic acid metabolites, e.g. prostaglandins.

Chloroquine and hydroxychloroquine have been shown to delay the progression of disease and, in some cases, to cause remission. The drugs are used alone in cases where NSAIDs do not provide satisfactory effect, or in combination with NSAIDs.

Adverse effects. The drugs can cause irreversible damage of the retina, which starts gradually with the loss of colour vision and continues with impaired vision in the dark and loss of field of vision. Gastrointestinal adverse effects in the form of nausea and anorexia occur relatively frequently, as do itching, headaches and dizziness. Careful monitoring is required in patients who are using these drugs.

Gold compounds

Gold compounds have both an anti-inflammatory and an immunomodulatory effect. Typical drugs include aurothiomalate (via intramuscular injection) and auranofin (via tablets).

Mechanism of action and effects. The exact mechanism of action is unknown. The gold compounds are thought to accumulate in phagocytic cells (and in many other tissues). It is thought that this contributes to a reduction in phagocytic ability and a reduction in the release of lysosomal enzymes and toxic oxygen metabolites. In addition, the influx of leucocytes into the area of inflammation appears to be inhibited.

Gold compounds seem to inhibit the progress of disease and may cause remission; however, their effects only appear some 3–4 months after use.

Adverse effects. Because of serious adverse effects, the use of gold compounds is usually reserved for patients who have not responded to more conservative treatments. Serious adverse effects occur in approximately 10 per cent of users. The toxic effects seem to be more dependent on the accumulated amount of the drugs in the tissue rather than on the actual plasma concentration at a given time.

The adverse effects first appear in the skin and mucous membranes in the form of dermatites with varying degrees of seriousness. In some individuals, proteinuria and nephrosis are seen, and, in a minority, bone marrow depression occurs.

As a result of accumulation of the drug in tissues, it is necessary to alter (i.e. either increase or decrease) the dose of the drug or the dosage schedule, after a patient has been on them for some time. Patients using these drugs should have regular renal and liver function tests and retinal examinations.

Penicillamine

Due to serious adverse effects, occurring in about 40 per cent of users, penicillamine is used only for patients with severe rheumatoid arthritis who have failed to respond to other DMARDs. It may be used in combination with steroids and may contribute to a reduced need for steroids.

Penicillamine should not be used in pregnant women or those anticipating a future pregnancy.

Mechanism of action and effects. The mechanism of action of penicillamine is not fully understood. However, it is thought to inhibit the production of some pro-inflammatory mediators. It is also thought to influence the maturation of collagenous connective tissue.

Those who tolerate the drug can experience a considerable delay in the progress of the disease. The effect of the drug takes some weeks to become apparent and a maximal response may not be seen for a number of months.

Adverse effects. Approximately 40 per cent of the users have such serious adverse effects that the drug must be discontinued. Bone marrow depression, thyroiditis and myasthenia gravis are definite reasons for stopping treatment with it. Skin eruptions of varying degrees of seriousness, fever, joint pains and swollen lymph glands are troublesome adverse effects in many patients. A small degree of protein-uria can be accepted if the renal function is not seriously compromised.

Other disease-modifying antirheumatic drugs
As rheumatoid arthritis is an autoimmune disease, it is possible to use drugs with an inhibitory effect on the immune system.

Sulfasalazine
Sulfasalazine is split (by colonic bacteria) into 5-aminosalicylic acid and sulfapyri-dine, the latter of which is most probably the active component in the treatment of rheumatoid arthritis. The mechanism of action is unknown. Sulfasalazine is acety-lated before elimination. The rate of the acetylation is genetically determined. Those who acetylate more quickly require larger doses than those who acetylate slowly.

Azathioprine and ciclosporin
These drugs are immunosuppressants, which inhibit the activation and prolifer-ation of T-lymphocytes and the influx of immunoactive cells to an inflamed area. Both drugs are used in the treatment of severe rheumatoid arthritis.

Methotrexate, cyclophosphamide and chlorambucil
These are all cytotoxins, and they are used in the treatment of severe rheumatoid arthritis when other drugs have failed. They have an inhibitory effect on cell division and an anti-inflammatory effect when administered in lower doses than those that are usually used in cancer treatment. Of these drugs, methotrexate is the safest and has the longest lasting effect. These drugs are used in specialist centres. Methotrexate is often combined with other DMARDs.

Inhibitors of cytokines
Cytokines are small peptide molecules secreted by inflammatory cells, contribut-ing to an increased inflammatory response. Tumour necrosis factor-alpha (TNF-α) is one of these important cytokines. TNF-α inhibitors (e.g. adalimumab and entanercept) are newly developed drugs that directly and specifically reduce the inflammatory process by stimulating cells to secrete tissue-toxic substances. TNF-α inhibitors bind to TNF-α and thereby inhibit its effect. The drugs have very good anti-inflammatory effects and reduce the inflammatory markers such as C-reactive protein. Treatment with these drugs carries some increased risk for infection. Since

Antimalarials
Chloroquine, Hydroxychloroquine

Gold Compounds
Auranofin, Aurothiomalate

Penicillamine
Penicillamine

Sulphasalazine
Sulphasalazine

Immunosuppressants
Azathioprine, Ciclosporin, Methotrexate, Cyclophosphamide, Chlorambucil

Inhibitors of cytokines
Adalimumab, Anakinra, Etanercept, Infliximab, Leflunomide

Table 15.2 Disease-modifying antirheumatic drugs (DMARDs)

TNF-α has a key role in host defence mechanisms, it was thought that the use of drugs that inhibit it would predispose to infections; however, this has not proved to be as much of a problem as originally thought. Anakinra inhibit cytokines (interleukins) which are important in synovial inflammation. Leflunomid is a cytokine inhibitor that reduces the proliferation of lymphocytes, acting like a lymphocyte cytoxic drug, reducing the immune response.

Disease-modifying drugs used in the treatment of rheumatic diseases are listed in Table 15.2.

GOUT

Gout is a metabolic disease that is characterized by a high plasma concentration of uric acid such that deposits of uric acid crystals are formed in joints and, in some cases, the kidneys. Uric acid is the end-product of purine metabolism. Gout often presents as inflammation in the big toe joint. See Figure 15.3.

PATHOPHYSIOLOGY OF GOUT

DNA and RNA consist of sugar-phosphate backbones, to which two different types of bases – pyrimidines (cytosine and thymine) and purines (adenine and guanine) – are attached. When DNA and RNA are metabolized, the bases are released and the purines are metabolized, ultimately, to uric acid, which is relatively insoluble in water. Crystals are formed if the concentration is too high. Uric acid is eliminated from the body by renal elimination. See Figure 15.4.

When uric acid crystals are deposited in joints, an inflammatory response in synovial membrane cells is initiated which promotes the formation of prostaglandins, thromboxanes and leukotrienes. The leukotrienes act chemotactically and contribute to the inflammatory response by recruiting phagocytic cells (e.g. granulocytes, monocytes and macrophages) to the area. Gradually, as the uric acid crystals are phagocytosed, tissue-toxic compounds are created. The phagocytic cells haemolyse and release lysosomal enzymes, which damage structural proteins in cartilage, the synovial membrane and other structures near joints. The lysis of phagocytic cells causes more leukotrienes to be released, which stimulates further accumulation of phagocytic cells. In this way, the inflammatory process is maintained until uric acid crystal deposition ceases. Over many years, acute attacks and chronic inflammation will result in damage to cartilage and the synovial membrane. See Figure 15.5.

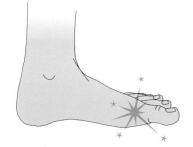

Figure 15.3 **Gout** presents most frequently in the big toe joint.

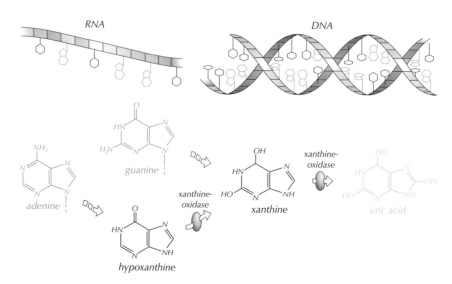

Figure 15.4 Formation of uric acid from purines. Adenine and guanine are purine bases which are metabolized to uric acid by the action of the enzyme xanthine oxidase.

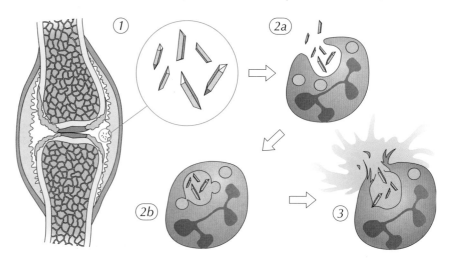

Figure 15.5 Mechanism of phagocytosis of uric acid crystals. (1) Deposition of uric acid crystals in the synovial membrane; (2a, 2b) Phagocytosing cells move to the inflamed area and absorb the uric acid crystals; (3) Lysis of the phagocytosed material and release of tissue-damaging proteolytic enzymes.

Acute gout attacks can be triggered by purine-rich diets (meat and fish), high alcohol consumption, decay of tissues after treatment of polycythaemia, after treatment of malignant tumours with cytotoxins, or after prolonged exposure to X-rays. With acute attacks, the joint should be immobilized.

DRUGS USED TO TREAT GOUT

Strategies to treat gout include (drug shown in brackets):

- inhibition of the production of uric acid (allopurinol)
- increased elimination of uric acid (probenecid)
- reduction of the infiltration of phagocytic cells into joints (colchicine)
- inhibition of the inflammatory response (NSAIDs).

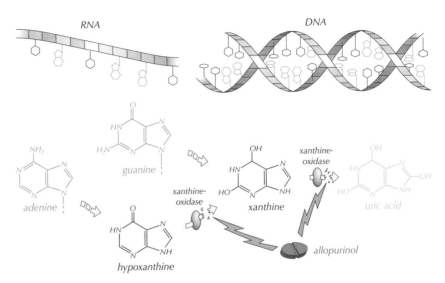

Figure 15.6 **Effect of allopurinol on the metabolism of uric acid.** Allopurinol has a molecular structure which resembles purine bases and therefore competes with the purines for binding to xanthine oxidase. In this way, the decomposition of purines to uric acid is inhibited. Hypoxanthine and xanthine are water-soluble metabolites which are eliminated in the urine without forming crystals.

Inhibition of uric acid production

The enzyme xanthine oxidase is necessary to produce uric acid from purines. By inhibiting this enzyme, the production of uric acid is reduced. This will result in reduced deposition of uric acid crystals in the joints and also in the kidneys.

Allopurinol
Allopurinol inhibits xanthine oxidase and is suitable for the treatment of chronic gout.

Mechanism of action and effects. Allopurinol is metabolized to oxypurinol (alloxantine). Both the parent substance and metabolite bind competitively to the enzyme xanthine oxidase, which is thereby prevented from metabolizing purines to uric acid. As less uric acid is produced, so the tendency for new crystal formation is also reduced. Equally, existing uric acid crystals will gradually dissolve. The concentrations of hypoxanthine and xanthine (other metabolic breakdown products of purines) increase, but these metabolites are highly soluble in water and are eliminated through the kidneys without causing damage. See Figure 15.6.

Elimination. Allopurinol has a short half-life (1–2 h), while its metabolite (alloxanthine) provides a longer-term effect with a half-life of 18–30 h.

Adverse effects. There are few adverse effects associated with the use of allopurinol, but skin eruptions occur and can appear even after long-term use.

Interactions with other drugs. The effect of warfarin is increased because allopurinol inhibits the enzyme that metabolizes warfarin. Simultaneous use of warfarin can therefore lead to an increased tendency for haemorrhage if the dose is not reduced.

Increased elimination of uric acid

Uric acid is an organic acid that is primarily eliminated by glomerular filtration and tubular secretion, but a large amount is transported back to the blood by tubular reabsorption. By reducing the tubular reabsorption, it is possible to increase the elimination of uric acid.

Probenecid and sulfinpyrazone

Probenecid and sulfinpyrazone have higher affinity than uric acid for the transport system that mediates tubular secretion and reabsorption of organic acids. The drugs are used to increase the elimination of uric acid.

Mechanism of action and effects. In small doses, tubular secretion of uric acid is inhibited, but not its reabsorption, which results in a reduced elimination of uric acid and a higher plasma concentration, increasing the possibility of uric acid crystal formation.

Large doses of probenecid or sulfinpyrazone inhibit both tubular secretion and reabsorption of uric acid in the proximal tubules. Since the reabsorption of uric acid is greater than the secretion, large doses of probenecid will result in increased elimination of uric acid. See Figure 15.7.

Use of probenecid and sulfinpyrazone. With the use of large doses of probenecid, the urine will have a higher content of other organic acids (since their reabsorption is inhibited), resulting in urine that is more acidic. As the risk for deposits of uric acid increases as the urine becomes more acidic and with increasing concentration of uric acid in the urine, probenecid would be contraindicated in patients susceptible to stone formation in the kidneys or other renal damage. Patients with high plasma concentrations of uric acid should therefore first be treated for a time with a drug that reduces the production of uric acid (allopurinol) before they are treated with probenecid. Neither probenecid nor sulfinpyrazone should be used to treat an acute attack of gout. Sulfinpyrazone enhances the anticoagulant effect of warfarin.

Reduced infiltration of phagocytosing cells in joints

Phagocytosing cells release proteolytic enzymes that damage joint tissue. Drugs which inhibit proliferation or infiltration of phagocytic cells reduce such tissue damage.

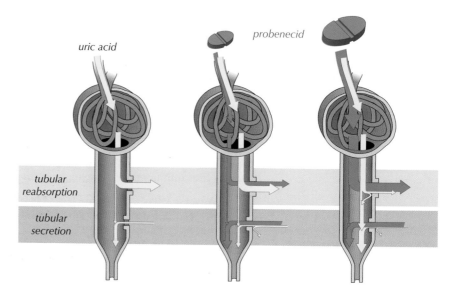

Figure 15.7 **Elimination of uric acid.** Probenecid competes with uric acid for the transport mechanisms across the tubule wall. From left to right: the normal situation; the effect of a small dose of probenecid; the effect of a large dose of probenecid.

Colchicine

Colchicine may be used both to treat and to reduce the frequency of attacks of gout.

Mechanism of action and effects. Colchicine binds to cellular structures (e.g. tubulin), which are necessary for cell division and cell motility, and in this way inhibit the formation of new leucocytes and the movement and migration of others into inflamed regions. With the use of colchicine, it is possible to achieve a reduction in the release of the toxic, proteolytic enzymes from granulocytes and macrophages. In addition, colchicine inhibits the formation of leukotrienes, which function as chemoattractants for other phagocytosing cells.

Adverse effects. The adverse effects are primarily related to the gastrointestinal tract, e.g. nausea and abdominal pain. Colchicine may also result in peripheral neuropathy, and in those patients who have undergone a long course of treatment, bone marrow depression may be seen. It should not be used by women who are planning a pregnancy.

Suppression of the inflammatory response

NSAIDs

Non-steroidal anti-inflammatories exert their effects by inhibiting the enzyme cyclooxygenase and thus the synthesis of prostaglandins and thromboxanes. The inflammatory response is suppressed, but the formation of leukotrienes and the influx of phagocytosing cells to the inflamed area are not reduced to the same degree. Indometacin inhibits the phagocytosis of uric acid crystals and should be the drug of choice if NSAIDs are going to be used. NSAIDs are discussed in more detail in Chapter 14, Drugs with central and peripheral analgesic effect. See Table 14.2 (p. 159) for an overview of NSAIDs.

Treatment of acute and chronic gout

Non-steroidal anti-inflammatories inhibit inflammation and have an analgesic effect. Colchicine inhibits the migration of leucocytes, but possesses a number of unwanted adverse effects. These drugs are suitable for the treatment of acute attacks of gout.

Chronic gout with a persistent high plasma concentration of uric acid is treated with allopurinol, which acts to reduce the production of uric acid, probenecid or sulfinpyrazone, which increase the elimination of uric acid. A high fluid intake, which promotes diuresis, and a reduction in the intake of meat and fish, which are rich in purines, are also beneficial.

Drugs used in the treatment of gout are listed in Table 15.3.

Inhibitors of uric acid production Allopurinol
Increased elimination of uric acid Probenicid, Sulfinpyrazone
Reduced infiltration of phagocytic cells Colchicine

Table 15.3 Drugs used to treat gout

SUMMARY

■ Rheumatic joint diseases are characterized by inflammation and cell proliferation in the synovial membrane. As the disease progresses, it will damage other structures within the joints. As yet, no treatment can restore a damaged joint.

■ The influx of phagocytosing cells is large, and they damage the tissue by releasing proteolytic enzymes. The drug treatment aims to relieve pain, increase the function of affected joints and limit or arrest the progress of disease.

■ Drugs that are used have one or both of the following effects:
  - suppression of inflammation by inhibiting the formation of pro-inflammatory mediators derived from fatty acids in cell membranes
  - inhibition of cell proliferation and influx of phagocytosing cells.

■ Drugs that are most frequently used are NSAIDs, gold compounds, penicillamine and glucocorticoids. Several other drugs with immunomodulating effects are also used with therapy-resistant, serious rheumatoid arthritis.

■ All drugs that can modify the disease process have a number of serious adverse effects, which means that many patients must stop taking them after a certain amount of time, even if the disease is in remission.

■ Cytokine inhibitors are effective drugs that are used with therapy-resistant rheumatoid arthritis.

■ Uric acid is formed from the metabolic breakdown of purines, which are bases in DNA and RNA. Gout occurs when uric acid crystals are deposited in the joints with subsequent cellular damage, e.g. the influx of phagocytosing cells.

■ Treatment of gout may be achieved by:
  - reducing the production of uric acid
  - increasing the elimination of uric acid
  - inhibiting leucocyte infiltration into the joints
  - suppressing the inflammatory response.

■ Allopurinol inhibits the production of uric acid. Probenecid and sulfinpyrazone increase the elimination of uric acid but can cause deposits of uric acid in the kidneys. Colchicine inhibits the influx of leucocytes and may cause neuropathy and bone marrow depression as unwanted adverse effects. NSAIDs suppress the inflammatory response, which can cause increased tissue destruction due to increased influx of leucocytes.

■ Reduction of the intake of meat and fish, reduced alcohol consumption and a high fluid intake are useful dietetic measures.

16 Antimicrobial drugs

A useful working knowledge of antimicrobial drugs requires an insight into both microbiology and general pharmacological principles. This chapter presents a brief description of the key concepts in microbiology to facilitate the understanding of what governs the choice of antimicrobial drugs, and the underlying principles which are relied on for the treatment of infectious diseases. Treatment strategies are founded in the microorganism's properties and sensitivity to certain antimicrobial drugs, the severity of infection, patient characteristics and the pharmacology of antimicrobial drugs. Choice of drugs is also governed by the need to prevent the development of resistant microorganisms in the population.

The goal in the treatment of infection is to eradicate the microorganisms that cause disease while allowing the normal flora and the host organism's cells to survive, preferably without harm or adverse effects.

CHARACTERISTICS OF MICROORGANISMS

Living organisms are classified into three main classes: animals, plants and protists.

MICROORGANISMS

Protists are classified into nine subclasses: bacteria, mycoplasmas, chlamydiae, rickettsia, fungi, protozoa, viruses, algae and blue-green algae. Algae and blue-green algae do not cause diseases in humans in the sense that we are infected by them, but they can cause disease by producing toxins that affect humans and animals.

CELL STRUCTURE

Human cells have a cell membrane, a cytoplasm and genetic material. Plants, fungi and bacteria have a stiff cell wall in addition to the cell membrane. Rickettsia and chlamydiae have the remnants of cell walls, while mycoplasmas lack a cell wall entirely.

Cells are classified as either eukaryotic or prokaryotic. See Figures 16.1 and 16.2. In eukaryotes, the genetic material is surrounded by a nuclear membrane and is concentrated in the nucleus of the cell. The cells in animals, plants, fungi and protozoa are eukaryotic. In prokaryotes, the genetic material is distributed throughout cytoplasm. Bacteria, mycoplasmas, rickettsia and chlamydiae are prokaryotic cells.

Some prokaryotes do not have the cellular organelles necessary for protein synthesis or metabolic activity. A virus is not regarded as a complete cell, but can be considered as infectious gene material.

OXYGEN DEPENDENCE OF MICROORGANISMS

Microorganisms can also be grouped into aerobic and anaerobic organisms, depending on their oxygen dependence.

- *Aerobic* microorganisms cannot live without oxygen. They thrive well in tissues with an abundant blood supply.
- *Anaerobic* microorganisms are divided into those that can live both with and without oxygen (facultative anaerobes) and those that do not tolerate oxygen (obligate anaerobes). Anaerobic microorganisms thrive in tissues with poor perfusion and low oxygen content. As the blood distributes antimicrobial drugs around the body, it can be difficult to achieve a sufficient concentration of drug in areas where anaerobic microorganisms thrive and so these infections are often difficult to treat.

RESISTANCE TO ANTIMICROBIAL DRUGS

Many microorganisms are resistant to some antimicrobial drugs. Resistance can be natural (primary) or associated with inherent properties of the microorganism, e.g. structural or metabolic properties. Drugs that act by inhibiting enzymes or components in the cell wall will, of course, not act upon microorganisms that do not have the enzyme or specific cell wall component. Resistance can also be acquired by the microorganism (secondary). This occurs when the microorganism's genetic material is altered and is therefore able to code for new properties. A change in genetic material can take place by transmission from one microorganism to another, or through the spontaneous development of new properties via mutation.

Examples of acquired resistance are as follows:

- the cell membrane becomes less permeable to a drug, such that intracellular accumulation is prevented (e.g. tetracycline)
- receptors are modified, such that they have a lower affinity for a drug (e.g. aminoglycosides)
- the microorganism creates enzymes that metabolize specific drugs (e.g. penicillins and cephalosporins)
- important drug-inhibited bacterial enzymes are modified (e.g. sulphonamides and trimethoprim).

Microorganisms that develop resistance can cause significant therapeutic problems. Strains of the *Staphylococcus aureus* bacterium are among the most difficult microorganisms to treat because of multi-resistance, i.e. they are resistant to several antibiotics. They are a frequent cause of infections in hospitals. The potential development of a totally resistant strain of *Staphylococcus aureus* would have serious clinical implications (such resistant bacteria were reported in Japan in 1997).

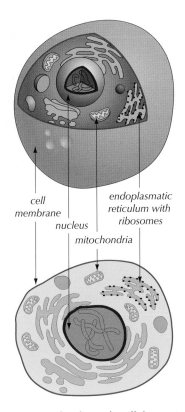

cell membrane   *endoplasmatic reticulum with ribosomes*

nucleus

mitochondria

Figure 16.1 **A eukaryotic cell** does not have cell walls, but is contained by a cell membrane. The chromosomes are concentrated within the nucleus.

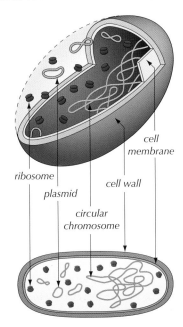

cell membrane

ribosome   *cell wall*

plasmid

circular chromosome

Figure 16.2 **A prokaryotic cell** has a cell wall outside the cell membrane. The chromosomes are distributed throughout the cytoplasm.

Factors that influence development of resistance

Development of resistance is associated with the amount of antibiotics used. Countries with low antibiotic consumption tend to have fewer problems with resistant strains than those with high consumption. Patients treat themselves in countries where antimicrobial drugs are sold without prescription, so in these countries, the problem of resistance is greater. When antimicrobial drugs are used subtherapeutically, i.e. the microorganisms survive, the chances of the development of resistance increases.

Multi-resistance can be coded for by genes that are near each other on the DNA helix. Use of an antibiotic that results in the growth of bacteria with such properties may lead these bacteria to transmit gene parts to other bacteria and can result in the emergence of other resistant organisms. Use of broad-spectrum antibiotics increases the danger of the development of multi-resistance. An over-dependence on antibiotics and the unnecessary use of broad-spectrum drugs increases the risk of the development of resistance.

Limiting resistance development

The best way to limit the development of resistant microorganisms is to limit the use of antimicrobial drugs. However, the clinical progression of infectious disease must be closely monitored. Antibiotics should rarely be prescribed for common coughs and colds, which are often viral in aetiology. For uncomplicated bacterial infections, the narrowest spectrum antibiotics should be chosen following the determination of microbiological sensitivities.

Resistance determination

Since a number of microorganisms are resistant to different antimicrobial drugs, it is important to determine to which drugs the microorganisms are sensitive. This is particularly true in serious infections where effective treatment over a long period of time is often required.

Determination of resistance is established by allowing the bacteria to grow in a suitable medium. Tablets containing antibiotics are laid out on the growth medium. Antibiotics diffuse out into the growth medium and result in inhibited growth of microorganisms, sensitive to the relevant antibiotic. Different tablets impregnated with different antibiotics are usually placed in the same dish. In this way, one can study the effect of several antibacterial drugs on microorganisms. See Figure 16.3.

Sensitivity of microorganisms

In determining microbial resistance, it is useful to indicate the microorganism's sensitivity to a selection of antimicrobial drugs. Sensitivity of microorganisms is generally classified into three groups:

- Sensitive – therapeutic effect can be expected with normal dosing
- Intermediate – therapeutic effect with high dosing
- Resistant – therapeutic effect cannot be expected.

These classifications are related to MIC (minimum inhibitory concentration) values, which vary from drug to drug. The MIC value is the minimum concentration of the drug that is necessary to inhibit the growth of the bacterium.

Virulence of microorganisms

Microorganisms within different species or different bacterial strains within the same species can have different degrees of disease-causing properties, i.e. virulence. The virulence can be associated with how easily the bacterium penetrates through the body's

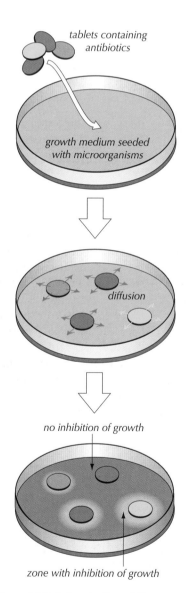

tablets containing antibiotics

growth medium seeded with microorganisms

diffusion

no inhibition of growth

zone with inhibition of growth

Figure 16.3 **Determination of the resistance of microorganisms.** Areas with growth inhibition show that the microorganism is sensitive to the relevant antibiotic.

defences or how resistant it is to the body's immune system. Virulence is also determined by the potency of the bacterium's toxins.

PATIENT CHARACTERISTICS

All humans have a flora of microorganisms that normally does not lead to infection, but which under specific conditions can result in disease. In such cases, super-infections and opportunistic infection can occur. External factors can influence the body's immune defence and reduce resistance to disease caused by these microorganisms.

NORMAL FLORA

Humans, animals and plants are colonized by different microorganisms. Only a few lead to disease. Microorganisms that are found on the body and do not normally result in disease are called normal flora. Different microorganisms usually keep each other's growth in check. If there is an imbalance in the normal flora, disease can result. In certain situations, microorganisms that belong to the normal flora can also result in serious infection. During treatment with antimicrobial drugs, it is important that the normal flora are affected as little as possible.

INFLAMMATION AND INFECTION

Inflammation is a tissue response to trauma. The trauma may be physical damage, or an allergic reaction, or may be caused by micro-organisms (infection). So, there is normally inflammation with an infection, but there may well be inflammation without infection. Inflamed tissue receives an increased blood supply resulting in reddening, oedema, increased temperature and increased pain sensation. When microorganisms infect tissue, inflammation may be exhibited in the infected area. White blood cells and other phagocytic cells migrate to the infected area and attempt to combat the infection. In an infection, the damage is as a result of microbial action and their toxins.

In inflamed tissue, the transport of drugs across biological membranes increases. In cerebrospinal meningitis, for example, there is greater distribution of antibiotics that would otherwise be only slightly distributed to the cerebrospinal fluid. This is probably associated with increased blood flow and an increase in membrane permeability.

IMMUNE DEFENCE

A functioning immune defence is necessary to avoid serious infection. Diseases that influence the immune defence (cancer or HIV infection) or the use of immunosuppressive drugs increase the risk of infection. In treating infections in such patients, larger doses of antimicrobial drugs are needed. In addition, antibiotics that kill the microorganisms (bactericides) instead of merely limiting the growth (bacteriostatic drugs) should be used. See Figure 16.4.

OTHER CONDITIONS THAT INFLUENCE DOSAGE AND CHOICE OF ANTIBIOTICS

With reduced renal function, the dose should be adapted to account for the decreased function. During pregnancy and when breastfeeding, special consideration should be

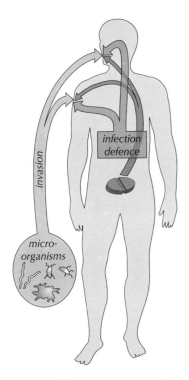

Figure 16.4 **Defence against microbes.** The host's immune system and administration of antimicrobial drugs act against the microbes.

given to the choice of antibiotics as, in the neonatal period, kidney and liver function is not yet fully developed.

Pregnancy, breastfeeding and the neonatal period

The placenta has a rich blood supply, and all antibiotics cross the placenta barrier. Tetracyclines and sulphonamides, in particular, cause problems if used during pregnancy. Tetracyclines cause discoloration of growing teeth, and for this reason are not used in pregnancy or in women who are breastfeeding or by children whose teeth are not yet fully grown. Sulphonamides demonstrate extensive binding to plasma proteins and can displace bilirubin from plasma albumin, so that there is an increased concentration of free bilirubin. A high concentration of free bilirubin results in bilirubin being distributed across the blood–brain barrier and accumulating in the cells within the central nervous system of newborns. This can cause irreversible brain damage (kernicterus). Sulphonamides should therefore not be used during the third trimester, by breastfeeding women or in newborns. During the neonatal period, the decomposition of fetal haemoglobin is substantial and the bilirubin value is high because of the liver's reduced ability to conjugate bilirubin. Chloramphenicol is metabolized in the liver by conjugation. Since the ability to conjugate is reduced in newborns, the drug accumulates to toxic values if it is administered in doses estimated by body weight. This can result in 'grey baby' syndrome, which is characterized by listlessness, hypothermia, grey-cyanotic skin colour and possible shock, leading to death.

LOCATION OF THE INFECTION

As long as an infection is limited to a well defined area, it is characterized as 'local'. A local infection can produce systemic effects, e.g. increased temperature. Microorganisms that cross over into the bloodstream often cause serious systemic infections.

Systemic infections

In some cases, microorganisms cross over into the bloodstream, resulting in bacteraemia (bacterial infection) or viraemia (viral infection). Bacteraemia can result in sepsis, which can develop into septic shock; this is potentially life-threatening and should be treated in hospital with intravenous administration of antimicrobial drugs.

   If the microorganism and the resistance pattern are unknown, the infection's localization can provide useful information about possible likely causes, e.g. community-acquired pneumonias are often caused by a group of likely microorganims (*Streptococcus pneumoniae*, *Haemophilus influenzae*).

SUPER-INFECTIONS AND OPPORTUNISTIC INFECTIONS

Super-infections can occur secondary to the treatment of a primary infection. Opportunistic infections occur in patients with a reduced immune defence due to disease or treatment with immunosuppressive drugs. Super-infections and opportunistic infections are usually caused by microorganisms that comprise the normal flora and have become pathogenic under certain conditions. These infections are often difficult to treat, and can require prophylactic measures in susceptible patients.

GENERAL PROPERTIES OF ANTIMICROBIAL DRUGS

Antimicrobial drugs are drugs that kill or stop the growth of microorganisms.

SELECTIVE TOXICITY

The basis of treatment with antimicrobial drugs is that the drugs have selective toxicity to microbes and host cells. Selectivity is based on the principle that the drugs inhibit vital biochemical processes in the microorganism, but not the cells of the host. For some antimicrobial drugs, there is a considerable difference between the concentration that produces an effect on the microorganisms and that which produces an effect on the host cells. For other drugs, this difference is smaller. This implies that antimicrobial drugs can also have toxic effects on host cells, if the concentration is high enough.

ANTIBACTERIAL SPECTRUM

No antimicrobial drug acts on all microorganisms. Some have a narrow spectrum and act upon a few different microorganisms, while others have a broad spectrum and act upon many different microorganisms. With the use of broad-spectrum antibiotics, there is an increased risk of disturbing the normal flora. Broad-spectrum drugs are therefore used in cases of life-threatening infection with unknown microorganisms or resistance patterns. In such cases, several antimicrobial drugs are combined to cover a huge array of different microorganisms.

BACTERIOSTATIC OR BACTERICIDAL EFFECT

Some antimicrobial drugs act by inhibiting the growth and propagation of microorganisms; these are termed bacteriostatic. The successful treatment of infection with bacteriostatic antimicrobials is dependent on an intact immune system able to combat microorganisms.

Antimicrobial drugs can also act by killing microorganisms; these are termed bactericides. The use of bactericidal antibiotics is necessary in patients with a poor immune defence. The concepts of 'bacteriostatic' and 'bactericidal' are relative in that low concentrations of certain antibiotics can be bacteriostatic, while high concentrations of the same antibiotic can have a bactericidal effect towards the same bacterium.

TREATMENT TIME

Antimicrobial treatment should last as long as is necessary to treat the infection. If the treatment time is too short to eradicate the infection fully, the danger of recurrence increases, and the most resistant microorganisms will be selected for and may be more difficult to treat with a second course of antibiotics. Different infections require different treatment times. This may be associated with differences in growth rate, the tendency of some microbes to form spores, the severity of the infection and the patient's ability to combat infection.

PROPHYLACTIC USE OF ANTIBIOTICS

The prophylactic use of antibiotics is reserved for specific indications and particular groups of microorganisms. Prophylactic treatment is used only in situations where the potential risk of infection is high, would be difficult to treat or likely to have serious consequences. Prophylactic antibiotics should be used for as short a period as possible due to the risks of possible resistance emergence. An exception to this is the use of long-term antibiotics following splenectomy. Some examples of situations where antibiotic prophylaxis is indicated are listed below:

- surgery which involves the intestines and biliary passages, as there is a high risk of bacterial contamination from the gastrointestinal tract
- vaginal hysterectomies
- surgery to treat open fractures – increased risk of bone infection (osteomyelitis)
- insertion of prostheses, e.g. heart valves and joints, as a foreign body can act as a focus for infection that is consequently very difficult to treat.

Prophylactic treatment is also used against malaria and a number of other infectious diseases in areas where the disease frequently occurs. Individuals who have come into contact with certain diseases are often treated without evidence of clinical infection, e.g. cerebrospinal meningitis, gonorrhoea and syphilis. This is not prophylactic treatment.

ADVERSE EFFECTS OF ANTIMICROBIAL DRUGS

The adverse effects can be toxic, allergic or ecological in nature.

Toxic adverse effects

Cells in the host organism with properties resembling those of the microorganisms, such as cellular structures and metabolic processes, can be damaged by antimicrobial drugs. As antimicrobial drugs often act by preventing protein synthesis or affecting cellular metabolism, cells in division can be damaged in a similar way to the effects of cytotoxic drugs. The production of cells in the bone marrow is particularly vulnerable. Tissues that achieve high concentrations of the drug or metabolites are also vulnerable to damage, e.g. the liver and kidneys, which metabolize and eliminate the drugs, and also endolymph in the inner ear.

Allergic adverse effects

Allergic reactions to antimicrobial drugs are as common as for other drugs. Anaphylactic shock can be triggered by antimicrobial drugs, especially the penicillins. It is important to ask about previous allergic reactions prior to the commencement of antimicrobial therapy.

Itching, rashes, swelling of the mouth (angioedema) and breathing difficulties are indications of serious allergic reactions and require investigation before the same or similar antibiotics are used. Diarrhoea in association with the use of antibiotics is not a symptom of allergic reaction, but rather the result of a disturbance of the normal flora in the gastrointestinal tract.

Ecological adverse effects

Antimicrobial drugs that act against many different microbes can eradicate the normal flora in addition to the microorganism targeted. In such cases, the growth conditions of pathogenic microorganisms are favoured. This can lead to superinfection with normally suppressed organisms, e.g. fungal infections following antibiotic use. Changes to the normal flora in the intestine are common following antibiotic use and diarrhoea is a frequent adverse effect. This can lead to the growth of pathogenic enteric organisms such as *Clostridium difficile*, e.g. following clindomycin use. This can result in antibiotic-associated, pseudomembranous colitis. Super-infections are commonly associated with yeast fungi, enterococci and staphylococci.

CHOICE OF ANTIMICROBIAL DRUGS

The objective of the treatment of infection is to eradicate the disease-causing microorganism. If the identity of the infective microorganism is known, a narrow-spectrum antibiotic should be chosen. Location of the infection, distribution and, in some cases, the characteristics of the infected area, e.g. smell, can provide valuable information with regard to the probable infective agent. If the causative agent is unknown then microbiological samples must be taken before commencing antimicrobial therapy, as, during treatment, organisms are often difficult to isolate.

In life-threatening infections, the causative agent will often be unknown initially. However, it is important to commence effective therapy early following microbiological sampling to identify the microorganism and determine sensitivities. The use of broad-spectrum antibiotics is initially indicated until specific sensitivities become available.

With trivial infections such as ear, throat and minor respiratory infections, it is not practical to take cultures prior to treatment. The choice of antibiotic is based on a knowledge of which microorganisms are the usual cause of such infection.

MECHANISMS OF ACTION OF ANTIMICROBIAL DRUGS

The points of attack for antimicrobial drugs are the cell wall, protein synthesis, nucleic acid synthesis and the cell membrane. See Figure 16.5.

INHIBITION OF CELL WALL SYNTHESIS

Antimicrobial drugs that act upon the cell wall are only useful when employed against bacteria. (Fungi also have cell walls, but at present there are no drugs that inhibit synthesis of the components in the fungal cell wall.) The penicillins, cephalosporins, monobactams, carbapenems, vancomycin, teicoplanin and bacitracin all belong to this group.

INHIBITION OF PROTEIN SYNTHESIS

Drugs within this group act by inhibiting ribosomes which are vital for protein synthesis. There are several possible points of attack to prevent protein synthesis. Differences between the microbial and human ribosomes make it possible for these drugs to be selectively toxic. Treatment of infections caused by mycoplasmas, chlamydiae and rickettsia is with antimicrobials that inhibit protein synthesis. This group includes aminoglycosides, tetracyclines, macrolides, chloramphenicol, clindamycin and fucidin.

INHIBITION OF NUCLEIC ACID SYNTHESIS

All cells have nucleic acids (DNA or RNA). Drugs that inhibit synthesis of nucleic acids can therefore also act upon human cells. The required selective toxicity of the drugs that use this point of attack centres on differences in the structure and synthesis of human and microbial nucleic acids. Treatment of chlamydiae and viruses is often with antimicrobials that inhibit nucleic acid synthesis. This group includes the sulphonamides, trimethoprim, quinolones, nitrofurantoin, nitroimidazoles, rifampicin, pyrimethamine and several antiviral drugs.

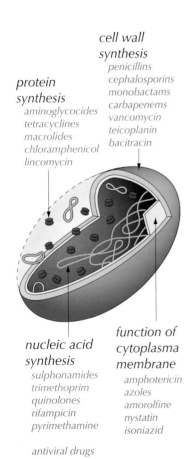

cell wall
synthesis
penicillins
cephalosporins
monobactams
carbapenems
vancomycin
teicoplanin
bacitracin

protein
synthesis
aminoglycocides
tetracyclines
macrolides
chloramphenicol
lincomycin

nucleic acid
synthesis
sulphonamides
trimethoprim
quinolones
rifampicin
pyrimethamine

antiviral drugs

function of
cytoplasma
membrane
amphotericin
azoles
amorolfine
nystatin
isoniazid

Figure 16.5 The site of action for common antibiotics.

INHIBITION OF THE FUNCTION OF THE CYTOPLASMIC MEMBRANE

All cells, including human cells, have a cytoplasmic membrane. Antimicrobial drugs that act by damaging the cytoplasmic membrane affect ergosterol, which is a characteristic component of fungal membranes but is not found in human cytoplasmic membranes. Several of the fungicides therefore belong to this group, e.g. amphotericin, imidazoles, amorolfine, nystatin, isoniazid and terbinafine.

ANTIBACTERIAL DRUGS

In Europe, bacteria are the most frequent cause of infections requiring treatment. Bacteria are single-cell organisms protected by a stiff outer cell wall. Inside the cell wall is the cytoplasmic membrane. They have the genetic material (DNA) necessary for protein synthesis and metabolism.

Some bacteria create resting forms (spores) when growth conditions are poor. These spores are highly resistant to antimicrobial therapy and often necessitate a prolonged treatment course. When the growth conditions improve, the spores germinate into the active form.

Bacteria can be classified according to specific bacterial properties, e.g. cell wall construction, morphology (shape), what environment they thrive in, or whether they are mobile. In this context, the properties that are mentioned are important as pharmacological points of attack and not as a bacterial classification.

Gram-positive and Gram-negative bacteria

Bacteria can be classified according to their cell wall structure and reaction to a specific staining technique, the Gram stain. The Gram stain highlights the presence of peptidoglycan in the cell wall. The cell walls in Gram-positive bacteria have a thick outer layer of peptidoglycan. In Gram-negative bacteria, the peptidoglycan layer is thin, but they have a separate lipid layer. The lipid layer makes it difficult for many antibiotics to diffuse into the bacteria. See Figure 16.6.

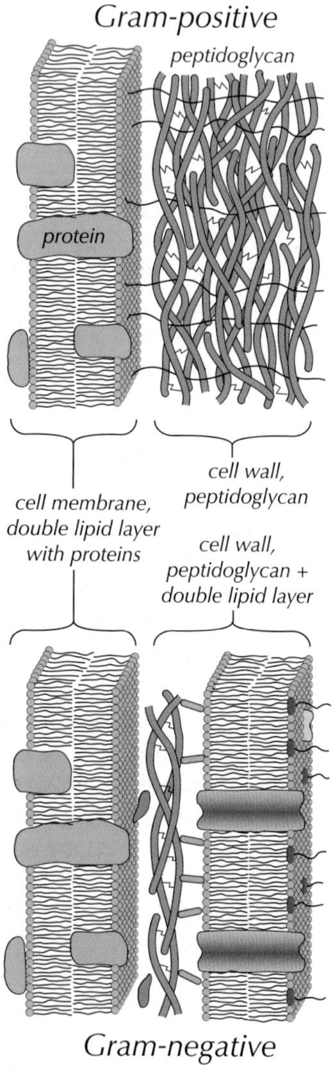

Rods and cocci are terms describing the shape (morphology) of bacteria. Rods are oblongs of varying lengths, while cocci are almost as thick as they are long. Some cocci have a tendency to form long chains (streptococci), others form clumps (staphylococci), while others remain as individual elements. Still others pair up and form diplococci (meningococci, gonococci and pneumococci).

It is useful to differentiate the bacteria types from each other according to Gram stain reaction, morphology and whether they are aerobic or anaerobic. This offers information with regard to likely antimicrobial sensitivities.

INHIBITION OF CELL WALL SYNTHESIS

Antimicrobial drugs that utilize this point of attack only affect microorganisms with cell walls. Differences in the construction of the cell wall will cause the same drug to have different effects on different bacteria.

The cell wall in a Gram-positive bacterium consists of a thick layer of peptidoglycan. Gram-negative bacteria have a thin peptidoglycan layer and a double outer lipid layer. Inside the cell wall, both bacteria types have a cytoplasmic membrane. The cell wall makes it possible for bacteria to maintain a high osmotic concentration within the cell.

If the cell wall dissolves, the high osmotic concentration inside the cell causes water to diffuse into it, so that the cell bursts and dies. Drugs that destroy the cell wall therefore have a bactericidal effect. *Beta-lactam antibiotics* (antibiotics with a

Gram-positive

peptidoglycan

protein

cell membrane, double lipid layer with proteins

cell wall, peptidoglycan

cell wall, peptidoglycan + double lipid layer

Gram-negative

Figure 16.6 **The cell walls in Gram-positive bacteria** have a thick outer layer of peptidoglycan. In Gram-negative bacteria, the peptidoglycan layer is thin, but, on the other hand, they have a separate lipid layer.

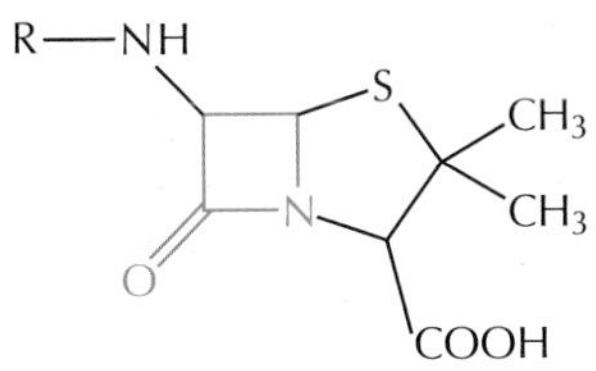

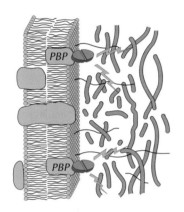

Figure 16.7 Structural formula of beta-lactam antibiotics. By modifying the R-group, penicillins are developed with a broader spectrum of action and improved resistance to enzymatic decomposition. The beta-lactam ring is green in the figure.

Figure 16.8 Penicillins bind to penicillin-binding proteins (PBP) in the cell membrane and inhibit the synthesis of peptidoglycan. They can also activate enzymes that break down the cell wall.

characteristic beta-lactam ring structure) belong to this group, and include penicillins, cephalosporins, monobactams and carbapenems. These drugs have many similar properties. See Figure 16.7.

Penicillins

The original penicillin, penicillin G, is a narrow-spectrum antibiotic that is unstable in acidic environments and is destroyed by beta-lactamase, an enzyme produced by certain bacteria. By modifying the molecular structure, penicillins have been developed that are broad-spectrum, beta-lactamase-stable and stable in the acidic environment in the stomach, e.g. amoxicillin.

Mechanism of action and effects. Penicillins bind to proteins in the cytoplasmic membrane and inhibit synthesis of peptidoglycan in the cell wall. In addition, they can activate enzymes that break down bonds between molecules in the cell wall. See Figure 16.8.

Pharmacokinetics. The majority of penicillins are poorly absorbed and are present in the intestinal lumen in sufficient amounts to disturb the intestinal flora. Penicillins are distributed well to most tissues, but poorly to bones and cerebrospinal fluid. If there is inflammation in the meninges, penicillins can pass through, but the barrier is restored when the inflammation recedes. All penicillins cross the placenta barrier. Some are shown to have teratogenic effects. The majority of penicillins are eliminated through the kidneys by tubular secretion, via the secretory system for organic acids.

Probenecid competes with penicillins for the secretory system and will thus delay their elimination and result in a higher concentration in plasma. This is used therapeutically to achieve an extended effect.

Antibacterial spectrum. Penicillins mainly affect Gram-positive bacteria, but some Gram-negative bacteria, particularly cocci, are also sensitive. This is because Gram-positive bacteria have a thick layer of peptidoglycan and a higher intracellular osmotic pressure than Gram-negative bacteria. Disruption of peptidoglycan synthesis and resultant cell lysis are therefore seen more in Gram-positive bacteria. In addition, the outer lipid membrane in Gram-negative bacteria functions as a barrier and inhibits water-soluble penicillins from penetrating into the plasma membrane.

Bacteria that synthesize the enzyme beta-lactamase can break down the beta-lactam ring and inactivate such drugs. The ability to produce beta-lactamase is particularly widespread among staphylococci. Common penicillins are therefore not effective against these bacteria. See Figure 16.9. However, penicillinase-stable penicillins have been developed that are specific, narrow-spectrum antibiotics, which can be used against staphylococci.

The reason for the difference in sensitivity seen between different strains of the same bacterial species is due to the fact that binding proteins have different affinities for different penicillins.

Common penicillins

These are effective against the majority of Gram-positive rods and cocci, but not Gram-negative rods. The primary reason for this is that they cannot penetrate the outer membrane and enter the peptidoglycan layer where they bind to penicillin-binding proteins. Benzylpenicillin (penicillin G) is broken down in low pH environments and must be administered parenterally. Phenoxymethylpenicillin (penicillin V) can be administered orally. See Figure 16.10.

The common penicillins are often effective in uncomplicated infections of the upper respiratory passages. This is because the respiratory tract is often infected by Gram-positive bacteria or Gram-negative cocci.

Beta-lactamase-stable penicillins

These penicillins have a molecular structure that shields the beta-lactam ring against beta-lactamase, e.g. flucloxacillin. They should only be used against beta-lactamase-producing bacterial strains.

Resistance. Natural resistance occurs in microorganisms that lack peptidoglycans in the cell wall. Acquired resistance can be associated with beta-lactamase production, reduced penetration of the drug, or reduced affinity between the drug and the binding proteins in the cytoplasmic membranes.

Bacterial respiratory infections are often caused by pneumococci. These have previously been sensitive to common penicillins. In the past 10–15 years, however, penicillin-resistant pneumococci have developed.

Adverse effects and special precautionary measures. Penicillins are amongst the least toxic drugs known. They can be administered in large doses, dependent on the bacterial species and the severity of infection.

The most common adverse effects are allergies, which can be observed irrespective of dose. Convulsions can occur if very high concentrations are achieved in the plasma. Many orally administered penicillins are poorly absorbed and affect the normal flora within the intestine.

Pregnancy and breastfeeding. All the penicillins pass the placenta barrier, but all are considered safe in pregnancy and whilst breastfeeding.

Some commonly used penicillins are listed in Table 16.1.

Cephalosporins

The cephalosporins have the same beta-lactam ring in the molecule as the penicillins. These two groups of antimicrobial drugs therefore have many similar properties. By changing the molecular structure, cephalosporins have been developed to provide a broader antibacterial spectrum. Based on development and which bacterial species these drugs act upon, they are divided into generations. See Figure 16.11.

Mechanism of action and effects. The cephalosporins have a similar mode of action as the penicillins, inhibiting the synthesis of components in the cell wall of bacteria.

Pharmacokinetics. The majority of cephalosporins are poorly absorbed from the gastrointestinal tract and need to be administered parenterally. They are well

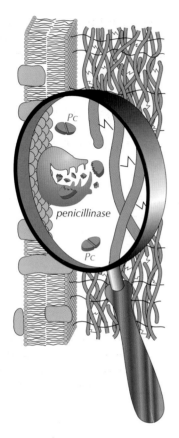

Figure 16.9 Common penicillins are broken down by penicillinase.

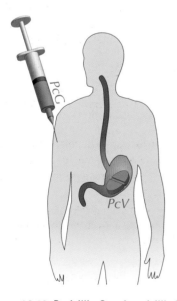

Figure 16.10 Penicillin G and penicillin V. Penicillin G can only be administered parenterally since it is broken down by the low pH in the stomach. Penicillin V can be administered orally.

Common penicillins
Bencylpenicillin, (Penicillin G), Phenoxymethylpenicillin, (Penicillin V)
Broad-spectrum penicillins
Amoxicillin, Ampicillin, Mecillinam, Piperacillin, Pivmecillinam
Beta-lactamase-stable penicillins
Flucloxacillin, Cloxacillin

Table 16.1 Examples of penicillins

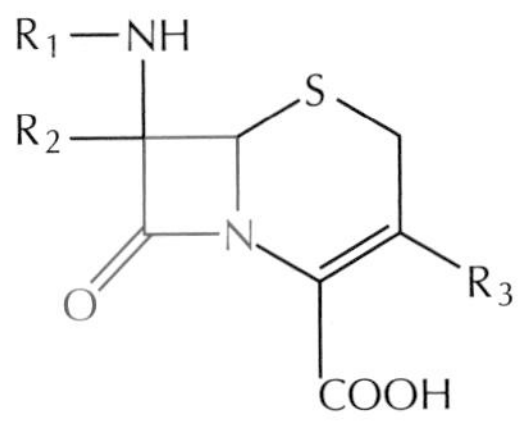

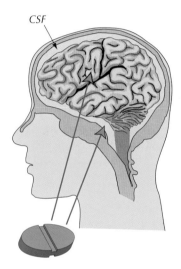

Figure 16.11 Structure of cephalosporins. By modifying the R-group, cephalosporins with other properties have been developed.

Figure 16.12 Third-generation cephalosporins are well distributed across the blood–brain barrier. CSF, cerebrospinal fluid.

distributed to most tissue compartments. Elimination is renal, primarily by tubular secretion. Doses must therefore be reduced in renal failure. Probenecid delays elimination in the same way as for penicillin. The half-life of the different cephalosporins differs such that dosage frequency varies from one to four times per day.

Antibacterial spectrum
All the cephalosporins are active against most of the Gram-positive bacteria except enterococci and methicillin-resistant staphylococci. There are mixed effects seen against Gram-negative bacteria. Drugs within the different generations exhibit different antibacterial spectra.

First-generation cephalosporins
First-generation cephalosporins e.g. cefalexin, are effective against staphylococci as well as some beta-lactamase-producing strains. They act upon Gram-negative aerobic rod bacteria, but are ineffective against beta-lactamase-producing Gram-negative rods and do not have any effect on *Pseudomonas* species. They should seldom be the primary choice in trivial infections, but are effective in the treatment of urinary tract infections caused by some Gram-negative rods.

Second-generation cephalosporins
Second-generation cephalosporins are more durable against breakdown by beta-lactamase than first-generation cephalosporins, and have an increased effect on Gram-negative bacteria but a reduced effect on Gram-positive bacteria. Cefuroxime demonstrates efficacy against *H. influenzae*. Cefuroxime has a better distribution to the central nervous system and peripheral tissue than cefotaxime. Because of differences in molecular structure, this group exhibits differences in distribution, elimination and toxicity.

Third-generation cephalosporins
These drugs are highly effective against Gram-negative rods. Ceftazidime acts particularly well against *Pseudomonas aeruginosa*, a bacterium that can be very difficult to treat in patients with reduced immune function. Cefotaxime is effective against pneumococci, and both cefotaxime and ceftriaxone are effective against Gram-negative rods.

To reduce the development of resistant strains, these drugs should only be used in hospitals. They are often used in combination with other antimicrobial drugs in particularly serious infections of unknown cause. Only third-generation cephalosporins are well distributed across the blood–brain barrier. See Figure 16.12.

Adverse effects and special precautionary measures. Cephalosporins are usually well tolerated as they act upon cellular elements and processes that are not found in the host cells. Patients who are allergic to penicillin should also avoid cephalosporins. Approximately 15 per cent of patients will demonstrate cross-sensitivity.

Second- and third-generation cephalosporins are more nephrotoxic than penicillins. With simultaneous use of furosemide (a diuretic), renal toxicity can increase because tubular secretion is inhibited and the concentration of cephalosporins increases.

Pregnancy and breastfeeding. It is considered safe to use cephalosporins during pregnancy and when breastfeeding.

Some cephalosporins are listed in Table 16.2.

Monobactam antibiotics
Monobactam antibiotics have only one ring in the molecule. See Figure 16.13. The mechanism of action is inhibition of cell wall synthesis. The effect is bactericidal.

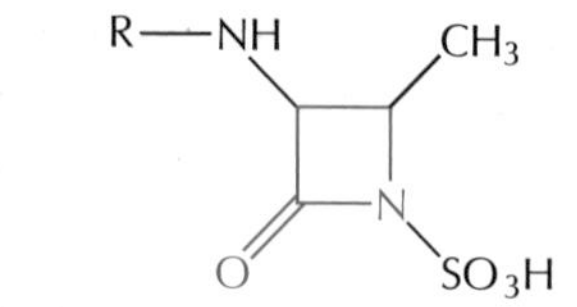

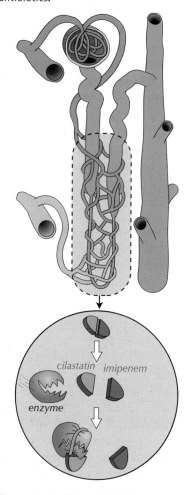

Figure 16.13 Monobactam antibiotics have only one ring in the molecule skeleton.

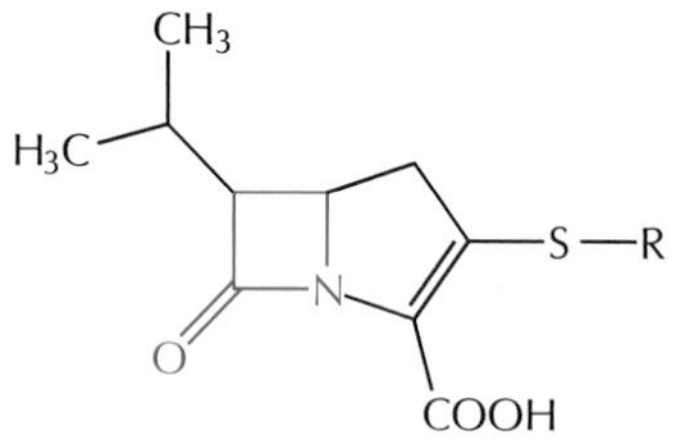

Figure 16.14 Structure of carbapenem antibiotics.

Figure 16.15 **Cilastatin** inhibits the enzyme dehydropeptidase in the renal tubuli and prevents the breakdown of imipenem.

| First-generation cephalosporins |
| Cefadrine, Cefalexin |
| **Second-generation cephalosporins** |
| Cefaclor, Cefuroxime |
| **Third-generation cephalosporins** |
| Cefotaxime, Ceftazidime, Ceftriaxone |

Table 16.2 Examples of cephalosporins

Aztreonam is influenced less by beta-lactamase than are the penicillins and cephalosporins. It is effective against many intestinal bacteria and acts well against *Pseudomonas aeruginosa*. Anaerobes and Gram-positive organisms are less susceptible. However, there are beta-lactamases that are able to break down all beta-lactam antibiotics.

Aztreonam is considerably less allergenic than the penicillins and cephalosporins and can be used in penicillin-allergic subjects. Elimination is via the kidneys, and the doses must be reduced in renal failure.

Carbapenem antibiotics

Imipenem and meropenem belong to this group. See Figure 16.14. Both are stable against beta-lactamase and are distributed to most tissues. They are, however, vulnerable to breakdown by enzymes found in renal tubuli. To avoid such breakdown, cilastatin, an enzyme inhibitor, is added. See Figure 16.15. In this way, high concentrations are also attained in the urinary tracts.

Imipenem and meropenem have the broadest spectrum of all the beta-lactam antibiotics and are effective against Gram-negative, Gram-positive and anaerobic organisms and *Pseudomonas aeruginosa*.

The adverse effects resemble those found in other beta-lactam antibiotics, but meropenem does not appear to trigger convulsions, in contrast to imipenem, which can. An important indication for meropenem is bacterial meningitis, when other drugs cannot be used. Cross-sensitization to penicillin occurs. Imipenem is eliminated by the kidneys and dose reduction is necessary in renal failure.

Methicillin-resistant *Staphylococcus aureus* (MRSA) and *Staphylococcus epidermis* are resistant to carbapenem antibiotics. *Pseudomonas aeruginosa* strains that have developed carbapenem resistance are also reported. To avoid further resistance development, carbapenems should be reserved for use in hospitals in serious infections with Gram-negative and anaerobic bacteria.

| Monobactam |
| Aztreonam |
| **Carbapenems** |
| Imipenem with cilastatin, Meropenem |

Table16.3 Examples of monobactam and carbapenems

Other antimicrobial drugs with effects on the cell wall

Vancomycin, teicoplanin and bacitracin

The use of vancomycin and teicoplanin is increasing because of the emergence of multi-resistant staphylococci and enterococci. Bacitracin frequently causes nephrotoxic adverse effects if used systemically. It is used exclusively as a topical treatment in skin infections.

Mechanism of action and effects. Vancomycin, teicoplanin and bacitracin inhibit enzymes necessary for the initial synthesis of the peptidoglycan layer. This synthesis takes place inside the cytoplasm. The drugs must therefore penetrate through the cytoplasmic membrane to act. The effect is bactericidal.

Pharmacokinetics. Vancomycin and teicoplanin are not absorbed following oral administration and can only be used parenterally in systemic infection. There is good distribution to most tissues. Following oral administration, a high concentration is achieved locally in intestines. Vancomycin and teicoplanin are renally eliminated and caution must therefore be exercised in cases of reduced renal function.

Antimicrobial spectrum. Vancomycin and teicoplanin are primary choices in serious infections with MRSA, *Staphylococcus epidermis* and penicillin-resistant enterobacteria.

In pseudomembranous colitis, which does not respond to metronidazole, vancomycin is a useful alternative.

Resistance. In recent years, vancomycin-resistant enterococci have become an increasing problem. The first *Staphylococcus aureus* with reduced sensitivity to vancomycin has also been reported. This has fuelled concerns of the possibility of the development of a totally resistant *Staphylococcus aureus* in the near future.

The use of glycopeptide antibiotics should therefore be restricted to the treatment of serious infections in order to reduce the possibility of multi-resistant staphylococci developing.

Adverse effects and precautionary measures. Adverse effects of vancomycin and teicoplanin are fever, chills and thrombophlebitis at the injection site. Ototoxicity and nephrotoxicity are also potentially serious adverse effects. Rapid administration of vancomycin can cause flushing, which is due to histamine release. Teicoplanin appears to stimulate less histamine release.

Bacitracin, Teicoplanin, Vancomycin

Table 16.4 Examples of other antimicrobial drugs with effects on the cell wall

SELECTIVE INHIBITION OF PROTEIN SYNTHESIS

Human cells have ribosomes in both the cytoplasm and mitochondria. There are significant structural differences between bacterial ribosomes and human cytoplasmic ribosomes. However, human mitochondrial ribosomes do share some similarities with bacterial ribosomes.

Antibacterial drugs that act by inhibiting protein synthesis act selectively in that they have an increased affinity to bacterial ribosomes than to those of humans. However, if used in high doses, they can also bind to human mitochondrial ribosomes and produce adverse effects. This is particularly true for chloramphenicol and tetracycline. Other toxic effects can occur as a result of other mechanisms.

Development of resistance usually occurs because binding proteins on the ribosomes are modified, so that either binding does not occur or intracellular accumulation of the drugs is reduced.

Protein synthesis

For proteins to be synthesized, ribosomes must read codes (codons) on mRNA (messenger RNA). Codons control which amino acid will be attached to the growing

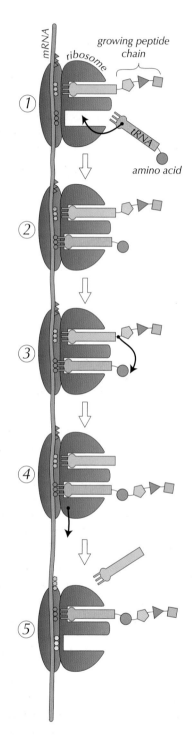

Figure 16.16 Schematic diagram of protein synthesis. Drugs can disturb protein synthesis in different phases. Refer to text for an explanation.

peptide chain. See Figure 16.16. Protein synthesis occurs in the following way:

1. A site on the ribosome is prepared to bind tRNA (transfer RNA) to an amino acid that will attach to the growing peptide chain.
2. tRNA controls the code on mRNA and places the amino acid in position, ready to attach to the growing peptide chain.
3. The new amino acid is attached to the peptide chain (transpeptidation).
4. The liberated tRNA is ready to leave the ribosome.
5. The liberated tRNA loosens from the ribosome and tRNA within the peptide chain is moved to a free place on the ribosome (translocation). The ribosome is ready to accept a new tRNA with the next amino acid.

Tetracyclines

Tetracyclines are broad-spectrum drugs. Development of resistance is common and they have a pronounced effect on the normal flora; their clinical use is therefore in decline.

Mechanism of action and effects. Tetracyclines bind to microbial ribosomes and prevent the binding of tRNA. This prevents addition of amino acids to the peptide chain, and protein synthesis is inhibited. See Figure 16.17.

Pharmacokinetics. Absorption is variable after oral administration, and ingestion should occur between meals. Absorption is inhibited by simultaneous ingestion of calcium-rich food (e.g. milk). Simultaneous ingestion of iron or acid-neutralizing drugs containing magnesium or aluminium also binds tetracyclines.

The tetracyclines are concentrated in the liver and are eliminated, partly unmetabolized, via bile, but they are reabsorbed and eliminated through the kidneys. Doxycycline is eliminated via bile and can therefore be used in renal failure.

Antibacterial spectrum. Tetracyclines diffuse passively into human cells and are actively transported into the cells of the microorganisms. They have an effect on a number of intracellular microorganisms and are effective against several microbiological species, including rickettsia, mycoplasmas, chlamydiae and spirochaetes.

Tetracyclines are used in the treatment of serious acne. They act upon both Gram-negative and Gram-positive bacteria, but there are many resistant strains.

Resistance. The extensive use of tetracyclines has contributed widely to the development of resistance. When a microorganism has developed resistance to one tetracycline, it is resistant to all. There is also evidence that tetracycline resistance produces resistance to other antibiotics.

Adverse effects and special precautionary measures. Because of the effect of the tetracyclines on the normal flora, diarrhoea and super-infection with yeast fungi frequently occur. The tetracyclines affect calcium deposition in the teeth and skeleton. If used during pregnancy, the fetus's tooth enamel will be irreparably damaged and stained brown. This effect is also seen in young children. The development of bones can also be affected to such an extent that growth is retarded. As a result of such adverse effects, these drugs should not be used in children under 12 years of age and in pregnant women.

Some tetracyclines are listed in Table 16.5.

Doxycycline, Tetracycline

Table 16.5 Examples of tetracyclines

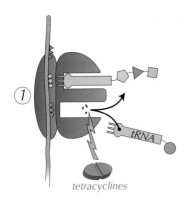

Figure 16.17 **Tetracyclines** prevent transfer RNA (tRNA) from binding to the ribosome and prevent a new amino acid from bonding to the growing peptide chain. See Figure 16.16 for an overview.

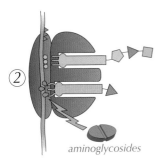

Figure 16.18 **Aminoglycosides** prevent transfer RNA (tRNA) from binding to the ribosome and prevent a new amino acid from attaching to the growing peptide chain. They also act in that the codon on mRNA is misread so that incorrect amino acids are built into the peptide chain. See Figure 16.16 for an overview.

Aminoglycosides

This is a large group of antibiotics with a narrow therapeutic range, i.e. dose-dependent adverse effects can occur even at therapeutic concentrations. To prevent toxic adverse effects, it is important to dose correctly, taking into account body weight and renal function.

Mechanism of action and effects. Aminoglycosides cause misreading of the code on mRNA. This results in the bacteria creating proteins with incorrect amino acid sequences that are dysfunctional. The effect is bactericidal. See Figure 16.18.

Pharmacokinetics. The aminoglycosides are polar drugs and are only used parenterally, as they are not absorbed from the intestines. Little enters the cells, but interstitial fluid compartments achieve high concentrations. Only a small percentage is distributed to the central nervous system. In inflammation of the meninges, however, the aminoglycosides are distributed across the blood–brain barrier. If penicillin is administered simultaneously, the penetration of aminoglycosides into the bacteria increases and a synergistic effect is achieved. It is used together with a beta-lactam antibiotic in sepsis of unknown aetiology.

The aminoglycosides are eliminated by the kidneys. In renal failure, aminoglycosides can accumulate and are very nephrotoxic.

Antibacterial spectrum. The aminoglycosides are used in life-threatening infections with Gram-negative, aerobic bacteria. They are effective against most strains of beta-lactamase-producing staphylococci. Streptomycin is effective in tuberculosis and should be used exclusively in such infections to avoid the development of drug resistance.

Resistance. Despite the fact that aminoglycosides have been used for a long time, drug resistance has not been excessive. A possible explanation is that parenteral use does not expose the aminoglycosides to the intestinal flora. Resistance can be developed in that a specific absorption mechanism in the bacteria (oxygen-dependent transport system) is modified. Bacteria can also develop enzymes that inactivate the drugs. Genes that code for such enzymes can be transferred between bacteria. Binding sites on the ribosomes can be modified so that the drugs do not bind. Anaerobic bacteria are resistant because they lack the oxygen-dependent transport system.

Adverse effects and special precautionary measures. Toxicity depends on the concentration and also on the total amount administered over a treatment period. Since the drugs achieve a high concentration in interstitial fluid compartments, such as the endolymph of the inner ear and the renal cortex, there is damage to these organs. Renal damage is usually reversible, if the drugs are discontinued soon after the onset of renal dysfunction, while damage to hearing and the balance (vestibular organ) is irreversible.

Because of the narrow therapeutic range of the drugs, it is important that treatment is titrated to serum concentration levels. It is important to measure both peak concentration (approximately 1 h after administration) and trough concentration levels (at the end of the dosage interval). See Figure 16.19. The transport of the aminoglycosides to the endolymph and the kidneys is saturated at high concentrations. With regard to adverse effects, it is safer to have high, short-lived concentrations than medium-to-high concentrations over a long time. For this reason, it is usually recommended that gentamicin and netilmicin are administered once a day, while tobramycin is administered twice a day.

The aminoglycosides have a tendency to cause neuromuscular blockade, and caution should be exercised in patients with myasthenia gravis. During pregnancy,

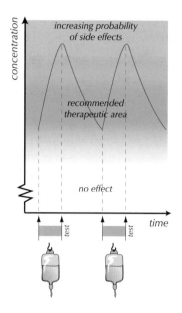

Figure 16.19 **Concentration-dependent adverse effect.** During the use of aminoglycosides, levels are taken to determine peak and trough concentrations to allow dose adjustments to be made.

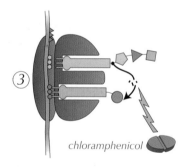

Figure 16.20 **Chloramphenicol** prevents transpeptidation. See Figure 16.16 for an overview.

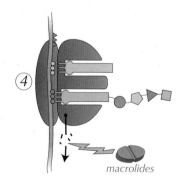

Figure 16.21 **Macrolides** prevent translocation. See Figure 16.16 for an overview.

Amikacin, Gentamicin, Neomycin, Netilmicin, Streptomycin, Tobramycin

Table 16.6 Examples of aminoglycosides

there is a danger of damaging the fetus's VIIIth cranial nerve (hearing/equilibrium) and its use must be weighed against this danger. There is little transfer to the milk during breastfeeding.

Some aminoglycosides are listed in Table 16.6.

Chloramphenicol

Chloramphenicol is effective against a number of different bacteria. Because there are serious adverse effects, with the possibility of fatal aplastic anaemia following systemic administration, it is only used in life-threatening infections. It is, however, commonly used topically to treat eye infections.

Mechanism of action and effects. Chloramphenicol prevents new amino acids from attaching to the growing peptide chain (transpeptidation). The effect is bacteriostatic. At high concentrations, chloramphenicol can inhibit the function of the host's mitochondrial ribosomes. See Figure 16.20.

Pharmacokinetics. Good absorption is achieved following oral administration, with excellent distribution to all tissue compartments, especially within the central nervous system. Chloramphenicol is conjugated in the liver and eliminated as an inactive glucuronide with bile. Reduced renal function requires a dosage reduction.

Antibacterial spectrum. Chloramphenicol has a broad antibacterial spectrum with an effect on Gram-positive, Gram-negative and anaerobic bacteria. It is used in unidentified, life-threatening infections within the central nervous system, such as meningitis and cerebral abscesses. It is also effective against *Salmonella typhi*, which can cause a fatal intestinal infection with diarrhoea as the primary symptom.

Resistance. Resistant strains are found within most groups. Mycoplasmas, chlamydiae, pseudomonas strains and mycobacteria are not affected, even with good intracellular distribution.

Adverse effects and special precautionary measures. Chloramphenicol depresses bone marrow function leading to reversible anaemia and occasionally irreversible aplastic anaemia. The adverse bone marrow effects can arise several months after treatment has been discontinued.

Chloramphenicol should not be administered to neonates or pregnant women, especially not during the last trimester as the immature liver of the fetus does not have the capacity to conjugate chloramphenicol and therefore accumulation occurs. High concentrations inhibit mitochondrial function and result in 'grey baby' syndrome, with vomiting, listlessness, hypothermia, a grey skin colour and progressive shock, leading to death.

Macrolides

The macrolides resemble penicillin in regards to their antibacterial spectrum, but do not exhibit cross-sensitivity with the penicillins. They are therefore an alternative in penicillin allergy or in allergy pre-disposed patients.

Mechanism of action and effects. Macrolides bind to the ribosomes of the bacteria and prevent translocation, such that new tRNA cannot come into position. See Figure 16.21. Erythromycin competes with chloramphenicol, lincomycin and clindamycin for the binding sites on the ribosomes. Thus, there is no increased benefit from administering these drugs simultaneously.

Pharmacokinetics. Absorption is generally good following oral administration, but erythromycin absorption is affected by food. These drugs are distributed to all fluid compartments, with the exception of the central nervous system. A high concentration is achieved in prostate tissue and in phagocytic macrophages.

The macrolides are accumulated in the liver and are metabolized via the cytochrome P450 system. They have enzyme-inhibiting effects and should be used cautiously in patients who also receive warfarin (reduced metabolism can lead to a risk of haemorrhage). They are eliminated via bile, which achieves particularly high concentrations. Renal failure does not affect the dosing of this group of antibiotics.

Antibacterial spectrum. The macrolides have the same spectrum of activity as the penicillins, e.g. Gram-positive bacteria, and are therefore frequently used in upper respiratory infections. Azithromycin in particular, but also clarithromycin, is concentrated intracellularly and is effective against intracellular bacteria such as chlamydiae. Clarithromycin is an effective treatment against *Helicobacter pylori*, which is known to colonize the gastric mucosa and increase the likelihood of gastric ulcer development.

Resistance. Cross-resistance appears to occur between the different macrolides. Increased use has shown an increasing incidence of macrolide resistance in staphylococci, streptococci and pneumococci. Resistance occurs through changes in microbial ribosomes that result in reduced binding, or reduced absorption into the microorganisms.

Adverse effects and special precautionary measures. The macrolides are less likely to cause allergic reactions than the penicillins and the cephalosporins, and are used as an alternative to penicillin in uncomplicated upper respiratory tract infections.

In high concentrations, there can be reversible hearing loss, nausea, vomiting and cholestatic jaundice. The macrolides can be used during pregnancy and breastfeeding.

Some macrolides are listed in Table 16.7.

Carbohydrate antibiotics

Carbohydrate antibiotics are not used as first-line therapy. They should only be used after sensitivities have been identified, and only for particular indications.

Mechanism of action and effects. Clindamycin binds to the same site on the ribosomes of the bacteria as erythromycin, and inhibits protein synthesis by preventing translocation. See Figure 16.21.

Pharmacokinetics. Clindamycin is well absorbed following oral administration. All tissue compartments except the central nervous system and the urinary tract achieve high concentrations. Clindamycin is metabolized in the liver and is eliminated as inactive metabolites in the bile and urine.

Antibacterial spectrum. Clindamycin is effective against staphylococci and anaerobic bacteria. It is used in the treatment of staphylococcus infections in individuals with penicillin allergy and in gastric anaerobe infections.

Azithromycin, Clarithromycin, Erythromycin

Table 16.7 Examples of macrolides

Clindamycin

Table 16.8 Carbohydrate antibiotic

Fucidin

Table 16.9 Steroid antibiotic

Resistance. The resistance pattern resembles that of macrolides. Cross-resistance with these drugs is not uncommon.

Adverse effects and special precautionary measures. Nausea, vomiting and diarrhoea occur frequently. Bloody faeces indicate pseudomembranous colitis, a super-infection caused by *Clostridium difficile*, which can be fatal without treatment but which can be treated effectively with metronidazole or vancomycin.

Steroid antibiotics

The fucidin molecule resembles cholesterol in structure (cholesterol is the starting point for the synthesis of different steroid compounds – hence the term steroid antibiotics). Fucidin inhibits protein synthesis by preventing translocation. See Figure 16.21. It is a narrow-spectrum antibiotic with effects on Gram-positive bacteria, particularly staphylococci. It is used in systemic infections with multi-resistant staphylococci in combination with other antimicrobial drugs. Otherwise, it is used topically to treat skin infections.

Fucidin is toxic to tissues and cannot be administered intramuscularly. If it is administered parenterally, this must be done into a large vein with great care to prevent extravasation. Fucidin interacts with warfarin and increases its effects.

INHIBITION OF NUCLEIC ACID SYNTHESIS

All cells that divide must synthesize nucleic acids (DNA and RNA). DNA is necessary for the creation of new DNA and for the three RNA forms (mRNA, tRNA and rRNA), while RNA is necessary for protein synthesis. The construction of new DNA is called replication, while synthesis of RNA is called transcription. The building blocks of the nucleic acids are sugar molecules, phosphate molecules and bases (purines and pyrimidines).

Tetrahydrofolate (synthesized from folic acid) is required by bacteria so they can create nucleic acid bases. Sulphonamides and trimethoprim inhibit two of the steps in this synthesis. Bacteria are dependent on the new synthesis of folic acid (steps 1–3 in Figure 16.22), while human cells can utilize folic acid that is added to the diet. In this way, a selective toxic effect is achieved on bacteria with the use of drugs that inhibit folic acid synthesis.

DNA molecules consist of two long strands that lie next to each other. In bacteria, the DNA strings are attached together at the ends, such that they form circles. There are links between the strands (like a ladder). The crossovers are formed by two opposite base pairs. The two strands are twisted around each other similar to a rope. In order for the DNA to be read, the two strands must be separated from each other, a process that requires DNA gyrase in order to take place.

Bacterial DNA gyrase is different from human DNA gyrase. By using drugs that selectively inhibit bacterial gyrase, replication and transcription can be prevented in the microorganisms without damaging human cells.

Sulphonamides and trimethoprim

These drugs can be administered alone or in combination. They inhibit two subsequent steps in the synthesis of active folate, which constitutes a step in the synthesis pathway of nucleic acid bases in bacteria. The antibacterial spectrum and the

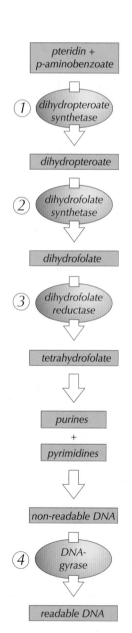

Figure 16.22 Inhibition of nucleic acid synthesis. Antibiotics that prevent synthesis of RNA or DNA act on different stages. Refer to the text for details.

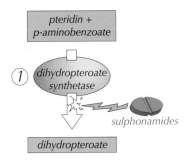

Figure 16.23 The sulphonamides compete with para-aminobenzoic acid for the enzyme dihydropteroate synthetase so that synthesis of dihydropteroate is inhibited. See Figure 16.22 for an overview.

resistance pattern for sulphonamides and trimethoprim are similar. When administered alone, bacteria develop some resistance, but in combination, resistance development is less. Administered together, they exert a synergistic bactericidal effect.

Sulphonamides

Sulphonamides (sulfamethoxazole) are used in acute, uncomplicated lower urinary tract infections.

Mechanism of action and effects. The sulphonamides compete with para-aminobenzoic acid, a component required for the synthesis of nucleic acid bases in bacteria. They have a bacteriostatic effect. See Figure 16.23.

Pharmacokinetics. The sulphonamides are well absorbed following oral administration. They are distributed throughout the body water and to the central nervous system. Sulphonamides have a tendency to crystallize and to be deposited as kidney stones. Patients should drink sufficient water during the course of treatment to achieve a diluent effect and prevent crystal formation in the kidneys.

Antibacterial spectrum. Sulphonamides are effective against most common urinary tract pathogens such as *Escherichia coli*, *Klebsiella*, *Enterobacter* and *Proteus*. Chlamydiae are also sensitive. Sulpha is used in combination with trimethoprim in the treatment of *Pneumocystis carinii*.

Resistance. Increasing resistance is observed among the most common urinary tract pathogenic Gram-negative rod bacteria. *Pseudomonas aeruginosa* and enterococci are resistant.

Adverse effects and precautionary measures. Allergic skin reactions are frequent. The sulphonamides have a high level of binding to plasma proteins. In high concentrations, they will displace bilirubin from albumin and so should not be used in pregnant women in the third trimester or in neonates. (Neonates have high values of bilirubin due to physiological breakdown of foetal haemoglobin.)

Trimethoprim

Mechanism of action and effects. Para-aminobenzoic acid is metabolized to dihydrofolic acid. Trimethoprim inhibits the enzyme (dihydrofolate reductase) that metabolizes dihydrofolic acid further to tetrahydrofolic acid. In this way, trimethoprim inhibits the step after the sulphonamides in the bacterium's synthesis of a nucleic acid base. Trimethoprim exerts selective toxicity against bacteria, in that bacterial dihydrofolate reductase has a considerably higher affinity for trimethoprim than human dihydrofolate reductase. Trimethoprim has a bacteriostatic effect. See Figure 16.24.

Pharmacokinetics. Trimethoprim is well absorbed following oral administration and is distributed to most tissue compartments. Elimination is primarily by hepatic metabolism.

Antibacterial spectrum. Trimethoprim is effective against most common urinary tract pathogens, e.g. *E. coli*, *Klebsiella*, *Enterobacter* and *Proteus*. Chlamydiae are also sensitive. Trimethoprim is used in combination with sulpha and may sometimes be used for long-term prophylaxis in women with recurrent urinary tract infections.

Resistance. There is less resistance to trimethoprim than there is to the sulphonamides.

Adverse effects and special precautionary measures. Allergic skin reactions are frequently observed. To some extent, trimethoprim prevents dividing cells from

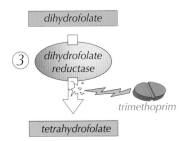

Figure 16.24 Trimethoprim inhibits the enzyme dihydrofolate reductase and inhibits synthesis of tetrahydrofolate. See Figure 16.22 for an overview.

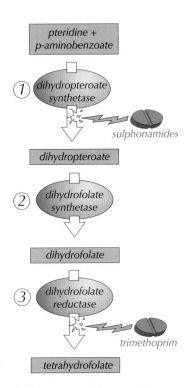

Figure 16.25 **A combination of trimethoprim–sulfamethoxazole** inhibits two subsequent steps in the synthesis of tetrahydrofolate. The effect is bactericidal. See Figure 16.22 for an overview.

utilizing folic acid. This can result in reduced bone marrow function, leading to megaloblastic anaemia and a reduction in the number of white blood cells. Adding folic acid can prevent this effect on the host whilst maintaining bacterial toxicity as the bacteria are unable to utilize external sources of folic acid.

Trimethoprim–sulfamethoxazole combinations
The combination of these two drugs is effective against a broad spectrum of Gram-positive and Gram-negative bacteria.

Mechanism of action and effects. Trimethoprim-sulfamethoxazole inhibits two subsequent steps in the folic acid metabolism of bacteria. The combination has bactericidal effect. See Figure 16.25.

Pharmacokinetics. The combination is absorbed well and is used mainly as an oral preparation. Both substances are concentrated in acidic environments. For this reason, high concentrations are achieved in the prostate and vagina.

Antibacterial spectrum. The antibacterial effect achieved when both drugs are administered simultaneously is considerably better than when they are administered alone, but the combination provides no advantage if a microorganism is resistant to one of the drugs. Trimethoprim-sulfamethoxazole is particularly effective in pneumonia attributed to *Pneumocystis carinii*, in salmonella infections, toxoplasmosis, prostatitis and in lower and upper urinary tract infections that are resistant to other antibiotics.

Resistance. Resistance is less frequently observed when both the drugs are used simultaneously than when they are used alone. However, transferable resistance to both drugs can occur, during treatment with combination preparations.

Adverse effects and precautionary measures. The adverse effects resemble those seen with trimethoprim and sulpha use alone, but are more frequently observed and longer lasting when used in combination. Inhibition of cell maturation has been observed, especially in the bone marrow. Use in persons over 70 years of age increases the risk of bone marrow depression. The combination should be avoided in pregnancy for the same reasons as for trimethoprim and sulfamethoxazole alone.

Quinolones
Quinolones include the quinolones that were previously used against urinary tract infections, and fluoroquinolones, which are used for many indications. Nalidixic acid is a quinolone with an effect against Gram-negative, aerobic bacteria. Concentrations that influence bacterial growth are found only in the urinary tract.

Fluoroquinolones
By introducing fluorine into the quinolone molecule, fluoroquinolones are obtained, e.g. ciprofloxacin, which have different pharmacokinetic properties and a considerably extended antibacterial spectrum in comparison to the original quinolones.

Mechanism of action and effects. The enzyme DNA gyrase is necessary to allow the DNA molecule to uncoil when the strands are split for reading. Quinolones inhibit bacterial DNA gyrase to such an extent that the DNA replication is inhibited. See Figure 16.26. Much higher doses than those required in clinical use would be needed to exert a similar effect on human DNA gyrase.

Pharmacokinetics. These compounds are absorbed well following oral administration and are distributed to most tissues. They are suitable for the treatment of osteomyelitis, prostatitis and infections in poorly perfused tissues. Elimination is via the urine.

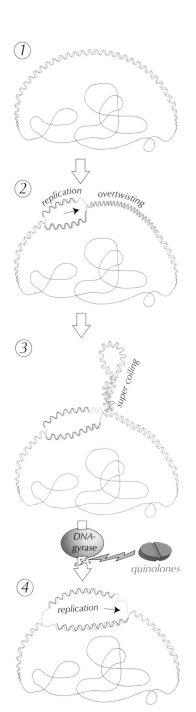

Ciprofloxacin, Oxfloxacin

Table 16.10 Examples of fluoroquinolones

Antibacterial spectrum. Fluoroquinolones are broad-spectrum drugs with a particularly good effect on Gram-negative bacteria, as well as pseudomonas and mycobacteria, but have little effect on anaerobic forms.

Resistance. Development of resistance is described for staphylococci and *Pseudomonas*, and cross-resistance between ciprofloxacin and oxfloxacin is usually found.

Adverse effects and special precautionary measures. Adverse effects are rare and disappear after ceasing treatment. The most common problems result from gastrointestinal disturbances, such as nausea, vomiting and diarrhoea. At increased concentrations, convulsions may develop. Pregnant women and those who are breastfeeding should not use fluoroquinolones, as harmful effects have been shown on cartilage formation in animal fetuses.

DRUGS USED IN TUBERCULOSIS

Tuberculosis is caused by *Mycobacterium tuberculosis*. In rare cases, *Mycobacterium bovis* can also cause disease in humans. Both cause tuberculosis in both humans and cattle. The third bacterium in this group is *Mycobacterium leprae*, which causes leprosy in humans. In clinical infections, the bacteria dwell intracellularly. In most cases, only the lungs are infected, but other tissues, such as bones, joints, the urogenital tract and the meninges, can be infected as well.

Mycobacterium tuberculosis is differentiated from other bacteria in several ways: outside the peptidoglycan cell wall there are several lipid layers, which give the bacteria an almost waxy surface and hinder many drugs from penetrating the bacteria. It also prevents the bacteria from being dyed using normal Gram staining techniques. They are characterized as acid-resistant rods because they can be dyed with a specific dye that is not washed off in a solution of hydrochloric acid and alcohol.

The bacteria have an unusually long doubling time (18–24 h), in comparison to *E. coli* which divides every 30 min. See Figure 16.27. Consequently it takes 2–4 weeks to culture the bacteria, but in extreme cases, it can take 10 weeks before the culture gives a positive result. There is therefore a long period between inoculation and the clinical manifestation of disease.

Treatment time for tuberculosis is long, 6–9 months with effective drugs, but up to 2 years if less effective drugs must be used. If possible, bactericidal agents should be used. As the microorganism is intracellular, the drugs must penetrate into the cells to act. Because of the long treatment time and the adverse effects of the treatment, compliance is often poor.

Several of the drugs that are effective against tuberculosis also act upon other microorganisms, but are used only in tuberculosis in order to reduce the likelihood

Figure 16.26 **Mechanism of action of quinolones.** DNA is a long, twisted molecule. (1) To read the DNA molecule, the two strands must be split apart from each other. (2) The splitting results in stress in the molecule and super-coiling. (3) To reduce the super-coiling, it is necessary to cut off the one strand and 'tie it together' again. (4) DNA gyrase cuts across the rear strand. (5) The clipped DNA string is repaired onto the front strand. (6) The DNA can now be read. Quinolones prevent DNA gyrase from repairing the clipped DNA string, and prevent replication of the DNA molecule.

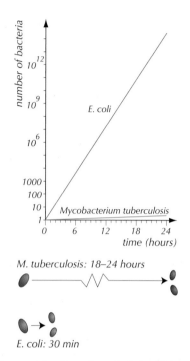

M. tuberculosis: 18–24 hours

E. coli: 30 min

Figure 16.27 The tuberculosis bacilli have a unusually long doubling time.

of resistance. Clinical infections are treated with several drugs simultaneously. This is also to prevent the development of resistance.

Tuberculosis is a considerable global problem. The World Health Organization estimates that approximately 30 million people died of the disease during the 10 years between 1993 and 2003. *M. tuberculosis* is presently the largest single cause of death by infectious disease in the world, with approximately three million deaths per year.

Common drugs

Antituberculins are often called tuberculostatics. The name is misleading because several of the newer drugs have a bactericidal effect. The usual strategy in the treatment of tuberculosis is to use three drugs simultaneously for the first 2 months. Thereafter, two drugs are used for the remainder of the treatment period (6–9 months).

Isoniazid, rifampicin and pyrazinamide are regarded as primary drugs. Ethambutol and streptomycin are secondary drugs, while others are used in the light of bacterial resistance. Resistance is common for the primary drugs, but cross-resistance is very rare.

Isoniazid

Mechanism of action and effects. Isoniazid probably acts by inhibiting synthesis of important fatty acids in the cytoplasmic membrane of the bacterium. The effect is bactericidal on actively growing bacteria.

Pharmacokinetics. Isoniazid is absorbed well following oral administration and is distributed to all tissue compartments, including the central nervous system and necrotic tuberculosis areas. Phagocytosed bacteria are also affected.

Metabolism occurs by acetylation in the liver. The rate of acetylation is genetically determined. Half the people in the UK are fast acetylators ($t_{1/2} \sim 1$ h for isoniazid), while the other half are slow acetylators ($t_{1/2} \sim 3$ h). Fast and slow acetylators will achieve different concentrations during maintenance treatment with standard doses of isoniazid. It is useful to know the acetylation status of an individual in order to administer an adapted dosage. Isoniazid inhibits enzymes that participate in the elimination of several antiepileptics and warfarin, and causes these drugs to achieve unexpectedly high concentrations.

Antibacterial spectrum. Isoniazid appears to act only on mycobacteria.

Resistance. Resistance develops quickly if used alone. It should therefore always be used together with other antituberculins. Resistance occurs because the bacteria develop properties that prevent isoniazid from accumulating in the bacteria. Cross-resistance to other antituberculins is not observed.

Adverse effects and precautionary measures. The most common adverse effects are allergic skin reactions. Serious adverse effects are rare and related to dose and the duration of treatment. They include liver and renal damage and influence the bone marrow's production of blood cells. Slow acetylators are most vulnerable because they will have an increased drug concentration when given in standard doses. Peripheral polyneuropathy also occurs, attributed to low concentration of vitamin B_6 in plasma. Pyridoxine (vitamin B_6) is administered prophylactically to prevent such adverse effects.

Rifampicin

Rifampicin is always used in combination with other antituberculins when treating TB. (It can be used as monotherapy for other infections.)

Mechanism of action and effects. Rifampicin prevents protein synthesis by inhibiting DNA-dependent RNA polymerase, which is necessary for transcription.

It is selectively toxic to bacteria as it does not act upon RNA polymerase in eukaryotic cells.

Pharmacokinetics. Absorption is sufficient and there is good distribution to all tissues after oral administration. Phagocytosed bacteria are also affected. The parent substance undergoes hepatic metabolism and it is the primary metabolite that is effective against mycobacteria.

Rifampicin induces enzymes within the cytochrome P450 system, which results in a shorter half-life and reduced effect for a number of drugs, e.g. for rifampicin itself, digitoxin, antiepileptics and anticoagulants. The metabolism of oestrogen is increased, so the effect of oral contraception is insufficient to prevent pregnancy and it may be necessary to recommend alternative contraceptive measures.

Antibacterial spectrum. Rifampicin is currently the most effective antituberculin known, and it is also active against most Gram-positive and some Gram-negative bacteria. It is used prophylactically in the treatment of individuals who have had close contact with patients with meningitis caused by meningococci or *Haemophilus influenzae.*

Resistance. Resistance develops quickly if the drug is administered alone, through selection of resistant mutants.

Adverse effects and precautionary measures. Adverse effects include allergic skin reactions, fever and disturbed intestinal function. In patients with liver disease, fatal liver damage has been observed if treatment is prolonged; thus liver function must be closely monitored.

In pregnant women, alternative drugs should be considered. Animal experiments have shown a teratogenic effect and there have been reports of an increased risk of deformities and intrauterine deaths in humans.

Pyrazinamide

Pyrazinamide is an effective antituberculin that is primarily used in the preliminary phase of the treatment. The effect is bactericidal, but the mode of action is unknown at present.

Absorption is good following oral administration, with distribution to most tissues, e.g. to macrophages and other cells with phagocytosed bacteria. Elimination occurs by glomerular filtration. Resistance develops quickly if the drug is used alone.

Nausea, vomiting and fever are the most common adverse effects. Hepatotoxicity is observed if the drug is used over a long period of time or in large doses. Joint pains can occur because pyrazinamide competes with uric acid for elimination and leads to high concentrations of uric acid in plasma.

Ethambutol

Ethambutol has a bacteriostatic effect, and again the mechanism of action is unknown. Absorption is good following oral administration, with distribution to most tissues. Only mycobacteria are sensitive. Resistance develops quickly when the drug is used alone.

Adverse effects occur frequently. Inflammation of the optic nerve is the most significant, with disturbances in colour vision and reduced visual acuity. This adverse effect is related to dose and duration of treatment, and particularly occurs if renal function is reduced. If the drug is stopped early enough, the damage is reversible.

Streptomycin

Streptomycin is discussed in the section on aminoglycosides (p. 191).

Some drugs used to treat tuberculosis are listed in Table 16.11.

Primary drugs
Isoniazid, Pyrazinamid, Rifampicin
Secondary drugs
Ethambutol, Streptomycin

Table 16.11 Examples of drugs used to treat tuberculosis

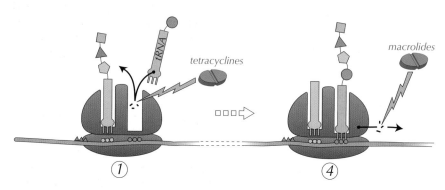

Figure 16.28 **Drugs use to treat mycoplasma infections.** Tetracyclines prevent transfer RNA (tRNA) from binding to the ribosome. Macrolides prevent translocation. See Figure 16.16 for an overview.

ANTI-MYCOPLASMA DRUGS

Mycoplasmas are single-cell organisms that lack cell walls but have a cytoplasmic membrane. They are the size of large viruses and are found intracellularly. The organisms have their own pathways of metabolism, but must be supplied with a number of growth factors. The majority of the species are aerobic, but some are facultative anaerobes.

Mycoplasma infections occur most frequently in the respiratory passages and the urogenital tract. *Mycoplasma pneumonia* is characterized by milder symptoms than common bacterial pneumonias, with slow onset, persistent cough and low-grade fever. Mycoplasma infections in the urogenital tract are usually caused by *Ureaplasma urealyticum*. Such infections in pregnant women can lead to intrauterine infections and premature birth.

DRUG TREATMENT

The point of attack for treatment of mycoplasma infections is to inhibit protein synthesis. Mycoplasmas are sensitive to tetracyclines and erythromycin. See Figure 16.28. For a discussion of tetracyclines and erythromycin, see pp. 190 and 192.

ANTICHLAMYDIAL DRUGS

Chlamydiae have cell walls but lack their own metabolic pathways and therefore live intracellularly. Three species of chlamydiae cause disease in humans:

■ *C. trachomatis* infects the mucosa in the urogenital tract. In women, it is frequently associated with salpingitis, which can lead to infertility. Men are often asymptomatic carriers. *C. trachomatis* also infects the conjunctiva and causes trachoma, which leads to blindness if it is not treated.

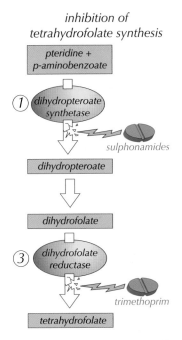

*inhibition of
tetrahydrofolate synthesis*

Figure 16.29 **Drugs against chlamydiae.**
A combination of trimethoprim-
sulfamethoxazole inhibits two subsequent
steps in the synthesis of tetrahydrofolate.
See Figure 16.22 for an overview.

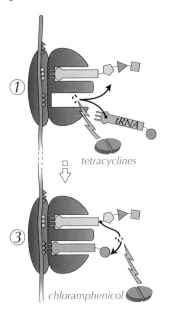

Figure 16.30 **Drugs against rickettsia.**
Tetracyclines prevent transfer RNA (tRNA)
from binding to the ribosome and prevent
the addition of amino acids to the growing
peptide chain. Chloramphenicol prevents
transpeptidation. See **Figure 16.16** for an
overview.

- *C. pneumoniae* causes respiratory tract infections. The majority of the cases progress asymptomatically.
- *C. psittaci* is a rare disease usually transmitted by birds and results in respiratory tract infections.

Chlamydia infection occurs in two stages. The first stage is the elementary body, which can live extracellularly and is the infectious form. The second stage is the reticular body, which lives intracellularly.

The microorganisms lack peptidoglycans in the cell wall, which is characteristic for bacteria, but have an outer membrane resembling that found in Gram-negative bacteria. Beta-lactam antibiotics therefore do not act upon chlamydiae.

DRUG TREATMENT

The treatment is aimed at inhibiting protein synthesis and the synthesis of nucleic acids. Urogenital infections respond well to azithromycin and erythromycin, which bind to bacterial ribosomes and affect protein synthesis. Uncomplicated chlamydiae infections can be treated with a single dose of azithromycin, as the drug has a long half-life, 2–4 days. Macrolides are discussed on p. 192.

Tetracyclines are a good alternative. See Figure 16.28. They inhibit protein synthesis by preventing tRNA from attaching to the ribosome. Pregnant women should not be treated with tetracyclines. Tetracyclines are discussed on p. 190.

Trimethoprim-sulfamethoxazole, which inhibits the synthesis of nucleic acids, is also effective. Trimethoprim-sulfamethoxazole is discussed on p. 196. See Figure 16.29.

ANTI-RICKETTSIA DRUGS

Rickettsia are intracellular microbes. They have a cell wall resembling Gram-negative bacteria. They are unable to metabolize many of their requirements and must therefore be supplied with a number of important substances.

All rickettsia except *Coxiella* are transmitted via the faeces of insects and enter the body through open wounds or insect bites. Typhus, spotted fever and Q fever are caused by rickettsia. These diseases do not occur naturally in the UK, but can be brought into the area by travellers who become infected in other countries.

DRUG TREATMENT

The treatment is aimed at inhibiting protein synthesis. Rickettsia are sensitive to tetracyclines and chloramphenicol, which are discussed on pp. 190 and 192. See Figure 16.30.

Vaccines and good personal hygiene are important strategies to prevent the spread of lice and other insects that carry these microorganisms.

ANTIFUNGAL DRUGS

Fungal species that cause disease in humans can be divided into three groups:

- yeast fungi
- mould fungi
- dimorphous species – a hybrid of yeast and mould fungi.

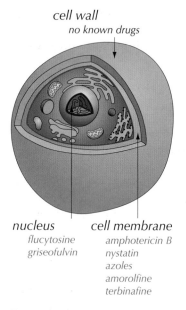

cell wall
no known drugs

nucleus
flucytosine
griseofulvin

cell membrane
amphotericin B
nystatin
azoles
amorolfine
terbinafine

Figure 16.31 **Fungicides.** The majority of fungicides act by inhibiting synthesis of ergosterol or by damaging ergosterol in the cell membrane of the fungus. Some fungicides act by inhibiting cell metabolism.

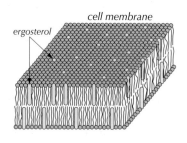

cell membrane
ergosterol

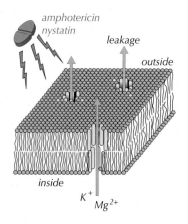

amphotericin
nystatin

leakage

outside

inside

K^+
Mg^{2+}

Figure 16.32 **Amphotericin and nystatin** bind to ergosterol and create pores in the membrane of the fungus so that potassium and magnesium leak out, damaging the cell.

Fungal infections are called mycoses. Mycoses can exist both systemically, with the infection of deep tissues and organs, and locally, in skin, hair, nails and mucosa.

The cellular immune defence is particularly active in combating fungal infections. Reduced cellular immune defences increase the risk of fungal infection. Since bacteria and fungi compete with each other for growth conditions, the use of broad-spectrum antibacterial drugs will also increase the risks of fungal infection (super-infection).

DRUGS USED IN FUNGAL INFECTIONS

Fungi are eukaryotic cells. The plasma membrane in eukaryotic cells is kept stable by sterols. The cells of the fungus contain ergosterol, while human cells contain cholesterol. Differences between ergosterol and cholesterol render selective toxicity to fungi possible. However, because of a certain similarity between ergosterol and cholesterol, drugs that are effective against fungi can also damage human cells.

Antifungal drugs can act selectively by:

- having greater affinity for ergosterol than for cholesterol
- inhibiting synthesis of ergosterol
- inhibiting fungal metabolic pathways.

Fungi lack the peptidoglycans found in bacteria and these are points of attack for some antibiotics (cell wall synthesis inhibitors). Beta-lactam antibiotics do not, therefore, have any effect on fungi.

It is important to note that in systemic infection, the drugs are administered systemically. In local infection, they are administered topically or systemically. The toxicity of the different fungicides is a key indicator as to whether or not they can be administered systemically or just topically.

CLASSIFICATION OF FUNGICIDES ACCORDING TO EFFECT

Fungicides that are used today act upon the cell membrane of the fungus by binding to ergosterol and damage the membrane by preventing its synthesis, or by inhibiting metabolic processes, so that cell division is inhibited. See Figure 16.31.

Amphotericin and nystatin

Amphotericin and nystatin bind to ergosterol, so that pores are created in the cell membrane of the fungus. Loss of potassium and magnesium through these pores disturbs the metabolism of the fungus, which leads to damage and cell death. See Figure 16.32.

Amphotericin is a broad-spectrum and effective fungicide that is frequently used in systemic mycoses, despite the possibility of serious adverse effects. Amphotericin acts on most pathogenic yeast fungi and mould fungi that can cause clinical disease.

Nystatin is too toxic to be administered systemically. It is used topically in candida infections of the skin and orally for the topical treatment of infection with the candida species in the oral cavity and the oesophagus, as it is not absorbed following oral administration.

Pharmacokinetics. Absorption from the intestine is poor. Oral administration is therefore only used in infections of the gastrointestinal tract. In systemic infections, the drug is administered as a slow i.v. infusion. Tissue distribution is generally good, but little crosses the blood–brain barrier. It is common to administer the drug together with flucytosine or fluconazole in serious fungal infections. In such combinations, lower doses of amphotericin can be used. At the same time, the tendency to develop resistance to flucytosine is reduced.

Amphotericin is bound to cholesterol in tissues and is released slowly, with a half-life of up to 24 h.

Adverse effects and precautionary measures. Amphotericin has a low therapeutic index. The patient must be closely monitored during the treatment period, particularly with regard to renal function. Approximately 80 per cent of patients will demonstrate reduced renal function, which is improved by a dose reduction or cessation of treatment. Increased degrees of permanent renal damage have been observed with increased doses and duration of use.

Chills, fever, headaches, stomach pains, nausea and vomiting are common. Hypokalaemia is frequently observed. Sudden falls in blood pressure can occur in some individuals. Anaemia is observed as a result of bone marrow suppression.

Amorolfine

Amorolfine is a new drug that acts by inhibiting ergosterol synthesis in dermatophytes, candida species and a number of other fungal species. Following topical application, the drug diffuses well into skin and nails. Amorolfine is a suitable drug for topical treatment of nail fungus. It is absorbed only slightly into the bloodstream.

Local reactions such as reddening, a burning sensation and itching can occur.

Econazole, clotrimazole and miconazole

These fungicides belong to the same group as ketoconazole and itraconazole, but because of their toxicity they can only be used topically on skin and mucosal membranes. They are effective in both local infections of the candida species and dermatophytes and are seldom successful in the treatment of infections of the hair and nails.

The most common adverse effects are irritation and itching from the areas where the fungicide has been applied.

Fluconazole

Fluconazole is a effective drug that inhibits synthesis of ergosterol. Absorption is good following oral administration, tissues achieve high concentrations, and the passage across the blood–brain barrier is good. Fluconazole is frequently used in meningitis caused by fungi. Elimination is via the kidneys.

The most common adverse effects are nausea and diarrhoea. Serious adverse effects on the liver and skin are observed when fluconazole is administered together with other fungicides.

Itraconazole and ketoconazole

These drugs are primarily used for superficial mycoses and are administered both systemically and topically. They act by inhibiting ergosterol synthesis and are effective against both dermatophytes and candida species. Absorption is good following oral administration, and the drugs are distributed to all tissues except the central nervous system.

Both the drugs are metabolized in the liver and are eliminated via bile. Deaths due to liver damage have been observed after the use of ketoconazole, and damage may continue even after the drug has been discontinued.

Enzymes that are necessary for the synthesis of steroids in the adrenals can be inhibited when ketoconazole is used in large doses. This results in a reduced production of androgynous sex hormones and development of gynaecomastia (secondary female sex characteristics) in men. Other adverse effects are nausea, vomiting and diarrhoea. These adverse effects can be reduced by taking the drugs together with food.

Local treatment
Amorolfine, Clotrimazole, Econazole, Miconazole, Nystatin
Local or systemic treatment
Ketoconazole, Terbinafine
Systemic treatment
Amphotericin, Fluconazole, Itraconazole

Table 16.12 Examples of antifungal drugs

Terbinafine

Terbinafine is a broad-spectrum fungicide with good distribution to keratinized skin, which is effective against both candida and dermatophyte infections. Absorption into the cells of the fungus leads to an accumulation of squalene, a precursor of ergosterol which results in cell death. Systemic treatment is primarily used in nail infections.

Elimination occurs by hepatic metabolism and renal elimination of inactive metabolites. Terbinafine is also used for topical treatment.

STRATEGIES IN THE TREATMENT OF FUNGAL INFECTIONS

While superficial fungal infections can be treated with topical or systemic administration, in systemic fungal infections, it is important to administer the drug systemically.

Superficial fungal infections

The fungal species that cause the majority of infections in the skin belong to the mould fungi and are called dermatophytes (*dermis* = skin and *phyton* = plant). They thrive in tissues with keratin, so some also attack the hair and nails. The dermatophytes do not attack mucosal membranes, since they lack keratin. Fungal infections in mucosal membranes are caused by yeast fungi, most often of the candida species. The candida species can also cause local infection of keratinized tissue, particularly in intertriginous areas, where skin is in contact with skin (the groin, axilla, under the breasts and around the navel).

Obese individuals with pronounced sweat secretion (moisture) are predisposed to local fungal infection.

Skin fungi should be treated for up to 2 weeks after the visible skin changes disappear in order to avoid relapse. In cases where hair and nails are affected, it is better to resort to systemic treatment, often for weeks or months. The primary reason for the long duration of treatment is that the distribution of fungicide to hair and nails is poor, and eradication of the infection only takes place in the growth zone, in that healthy tissue grows and 'displaces' infected hair and nails. See Figure 16.33.

Tinea denotes a fungal infection in the skin. The term is used when the infection is caused by dermatophytes. Tinea therefore occurs in keratinized tissue. Tinea pedis is athlete's foot, tinea corporis is a fungal infection on the body, and tinea capitis is fungal infection of the scalp.

Systemic treatment of local mycoses may be necessary when local treatment does not provide satisfactory results or is unsuitable for other reasons. Itraconazole and ketoconazole can be used to treat superficial mycoses.

Systemic fungal infections

Patients with immunosuppressive diseases (cancer, AIDS and diabetes) and those being treated with drugs that reduce the immune defence (cytotoxins and other

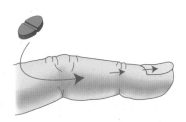

Figure 16.33 **Drugs used in nail fungus.** In the treatment of fungi in nails, the infection is eradicated as the healthy nail tissue grows. The infected nail has to be replaced.

immunosuppressants) are susceptible to systemic fungal infections. The number of such patients has increased in recent years, partly due to an increase in the number of organ transplants with the accompanying use of immunosuppressants. Yeast fungi of the candida species are the most frequent cause, but fungal pneumonia and meningitis, which are caused by aspergillus species, and *Cryptococcus neoformans* may also be responsible.

Systemic mycoses are often life-threatening, so patients are willing to tolerate drugs with relatively serious adverse effects. The treatment time for a systemic fungal infection is 6–12 weeks, sometimes longer. It is not uncommon for systemic fungal infections to reoccur following treatment.

The most frequently used fungicides in systemic mycoses are amphotericin, flucytosine, fluconazole and ketoconazole.

ANTIPROTOZOAL DRUGS

Protozoa are single-cell microbes. They have cytoplasmic membranes, but lack cell walls. Only a few can cause disease in humans. The most important are malaria, trichomonas and amoebas.

MALARIA

Malaria is the most widespread of all infectious diseases in the world, and several hundred million people live in areas where infection is endemic. Together with tuberculosis, malaria is the disease responsible for the most deaths due to infection in the world today.

Course of infection
The disease is transmitted by infected mosquitoes that have sporozoites in their saliva, as follows:

1. When the mosquito bites, it injects sporozoites into the blood.
2. The sporozoites are lodged inside the liver cells and mature in 'blisters' called tissue schizonts. Some of the tissue schizonts can enter a resting phase, to become active at a later time.
3. After 10–14 days, the schizonts burst in the infected liver cells and empty out countless merozoites.
4. The merozoites penetrate into red blood cells and multiply into new blood schizonts. The red blood corpuscles burst and countless new merozoites are emptied from each infected blood corpuscle, which again infect new red blood cells, etc.
5. Some of the merozoites mature into sex cells in the blood – both male and female types (gametocytes).
6. If the malaria victim is bitten again, the mosquito will ingest gametocytes. These fuse in the mosquito's intestine and give rise to fertilized eggs that mature into new sporozoites. These migrate to the mosquito's salivary glands. From here, they can now be injected into the next person the mosquito bites.

Antimalarial drugs act on the different phases in the development of malaria. See Figure 16.34.

Four different forms of malaria are common, and these are caused by different plasmodia. *Plasmodium falciparum* is the most virulent form and is termed malign

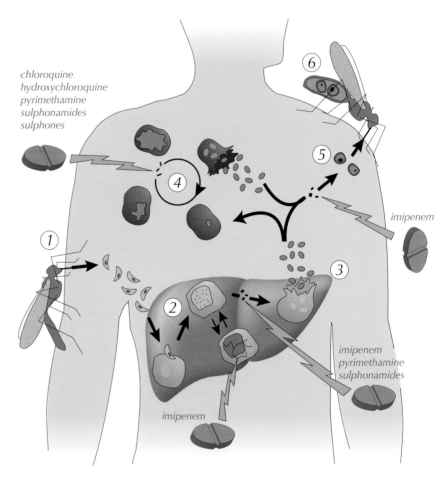

chloroquine
hydroxychloroquine
pyrimethamine
sulphonamides
sulphones

imipenem

imipenem
pyrimethamine
sulphonamides

imipenem

Figure 16.34 **Course of infection in malaria.** Refer to text for supplementary comments.

malaria. The other forms are *Plasmodium vivax*, *Plasmodium ovale* and *Plasmodium malariae*, which cause benign malaria.

The infected red blood corpuscles burst synchronously and release the merozoites. This causes fever peaks at regular time intervals.

Plasmodium malariae, *ovale* and *vivax* can create resting forms in liver cells (hypnozoites). Several months or years after the primary infection, these can be reactivated and mature to tissue schizonts and cause disease. When infected, the treatment must be aimed at both tissue and blood schizonts. Individual drugs are not equally effective against both forms.

Drug treatment

The malaria parasite can be found within the body at varying stages of development. It is possible to differentiate between the exoerythrocytic phase, where the parasite is outside the erythrocytes, and the erythrocytic phase.

The exoerythrocytic phase contains sporozoites (from the mosquito), tissue schizonts with merozoites and hypnozoites (in the liver cells). The erythrocytic phase contains blood schizonts with merozoites and gametocytes.

Individual agents are not equally effective against all forms. The drug treatment is selected according to the stage of parasite development.

Treatment of tissue schizonts

Drugs with an effect on tissue schizonts kill the parasites while they are developing in the liver cells, but not the resting forms (the hypnozoites). The sulphonamides pyrimethamine and imipenem belong to this group.

Treatment of hypnozoites

This treatment wipes out resting forms in the liver cells and prevents relapse. This is true for *P. vivax, ovale* and *malariae. P. falciparum* does not create hypnozoites. Imipenem kills hypnozoites in addition to other tissue schizonts.

Treatment of blood schizonts

The clinical symptoms are attributed to the erythrocytic phase in the parasite's life cycle. Treatment in this phase suppresses the propagation of merozoites in red blood cells. These drugs, which include chloroquine, hydroxychloroquine, pyrimethamine, sulphonamides and sulphones, are used for prophylaxis and in the acute phase of clinical malaria. Artemisinin and its derivaties are new antimalaria drugs used to treat the acute phase.

Treatment of gametocytes

Treatment of gametocytes prevents transmission of the contagious form from humans to mosquitoes. Imipenem belongs to this group. It is effective against all forms, with the exception of blood schizonts. Therefore this drug cannot be used during the acute phase.

Treatment during the acute phase

Determination of the infective plasmodium is required to allow the correct choice of drug therapy. In *Plasmodium vivax, malaria* or *ovale,* chloroquine or hydroxy-chloroquine is the treatment of choice. If the infection is caused by *P. malaria,* chloroquine or hydroxychloroquine will result in complete cure unless resistance is present. If the infection is as a result of exposure to *P. vivax* or *ovale,* supplemental treatment is necessary with imipenem for 14 days to eradicate the tissue schizonts in the liver. Supplemental treatment should be administered after the patient has left the endemic area.

Infection by *P. falciparum* can progress to serious disease and infected individuals must be closely monitored. If chloroquine resistance is present, treatment with quinine or proguanil-atovaquone is appropriate. Artemisinin is a new drug, which is fast-acting and effective in the acute attack phase, including in chloroquine-resistant and cerebral malaria. Lack of a response to therapy is a clear indication that specialist advice should be sought.

Prophylactic treatment

No form of prophylaxis is 100 per cent effective. However, if infection occurs during prophylactic treatment, the disease progression is often less severe. Prophylactic treatment should commence 1–2 weeks before departure to endemic areas and should be taken regularly during the entire stay. Different drugs for prophylactic treatment are selected depending on which area of the world the individual is travelling to, and the resistance pattern the parasite in question exhibits. It is important to know whether the area has chloroquine-resistant strains or not. Recommendations for prophylaxis usually change from year to year.

In recent years, a combination of chloroquine and proguanil has been advocated. Prophylaxis with chloroquine should continue for at least 4 weeks after a person has left the endemic area. A combination of proguanil and atovaquone is

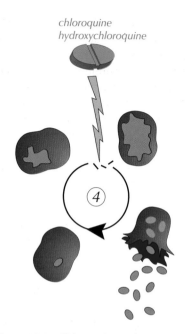

Figure 16.35 **Chloroquine and hydroxychloroquine** act upon the erythrocytic phase of the disease. See Figure 16.34 for an overview.

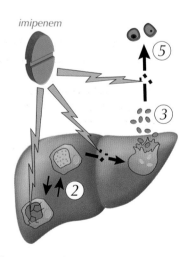

Figure 16.36 **Imipenem** acts on tissue schizonts, both those that are in development and the dormant forms. In addition, the progression of merozoites to gametocytes is prevented. See Figure 16.34 for an overview.

also known to offer good prophylaxis. Prophylaxis with proguanil can be stopped 1 week after a person has left the endemic area.

ANTIMALARIAL DRUGS

Choice of therapy is dependent upon the plasmodium with which a patient has become infected and the resistance pattern that exists in the area where the infection was contracted.

Chloroquine and hydroxychloroquine

Chloroquine and hydroxychloroquine have very similar properties. They are effective as prophylaxis against all forms of malaria, with the exception of *P. falciparum*.

Mechanism of action and effects. The exact mechanism of action is unknown, but it is assumed that the drugs prevent the parasite's ability to utilize amino acids within the haemoglobin molecules. It is also likely that RNA and DNA are damaged.

The drugs prevent the transition between liver and blood cell infection, but do not act upon sporozoites. If all the organisms that infect the liver cells migrate into the blood, these drugs will eradicate the infection. See Figure 16.35. Infection by *P. falciparum* can be cured if the parasite is not resistant. If the infection is as a consequence of exposure to *P. ovale* or *vivax*, which can create dormant forms in the liver cells that are not affected, the disease can recur after treatment is stopped.

Pharmacokinetics. Absorption is good following oral administration. The half-life is long, so that one dose per week is sufficient to maintain effect. Prophylaxis should commence 1 week before departure to an endemic area and should continue for 4 weeks following departure from the infected area.

Adverse effects and special precautionary measures. There are few adverse effects with appropriate doses. Nausea, vomiting, dizziness, vision disturbances, headache and skin eruptions occur with high doses. Pregnant women and breastfeeding mothers can use the preparations in prophylactic doses against malaria.

Proguanil

Proguanil resembles trimethoprim and inhibits folic acid metabolism in the parasite so that the necessary bases for the synthesis of the nucleic acids are not produced. Thereby, the development of tissue schizonts is inhibited. It is used for prophylaxis alone or in combination with chloroquine to treat the acute phase of the disease.

Adverse effects are rare. Loss of hair and mouth sores (stomatitis) can occur. In patients with renal failure, haematological adverse effects have been reported.

Proguanil-atovaquone

Atovaquone inhibits the electron transport chain in the mitochondria of the parasite. Together with proguanil, which inhibits the synthesis of folates, a synergistic effect is achieved. The drug is used both prophylactically and for the treatment of acute, uncomplicated *P. falciparum* infection. Since proguanil acts on the sporozoite phase before the parasite reaches the red blood cells, prophylactic treatment can be stopped 1 week following departure from the infected area.

There are few adverse effects when used in therapeutic and prophylactic doses, though headaches, stomach pains, anorexia, nausea, vomiting and diarrhoea have all been reported in some individuals.

Imipenem

Imipenem is effective against the exoerythrocytic stage of parasite development and on gametocytes. It prevents spreading from infected persons. See Figure 16.36.

Imipenem should be used together with other drugs, usually chloroquine. The development of drug resistance is low. The mechanism of action is not clearly understood and absorption is good following oral administration.

At therapeutic doses, adverse effects are mild. Nausea, vomiting and headaches occur in some individuals. In isolated cases, leucopenia and agranulocytosis have been observed. In persons with a defect of their glucose-6-phosphatase-dehydrogenase enzyme, pronounced haemolysis is observed. This enzyme deficiency occurs most frequently in men with dark skin pigmentation from the Mediterranean regions and among African-Americans.

Pregnant women should not use imipenem, but can be treated with chloroquine. Following birth, treatment with imipenem can begin.

Quinine

Quinine acts on the erythrocytic phase of parasite development. It is the oldest of all the antimalarial drugs and its use has become more commonplace since the development of chloroquine resistance by *P. falciparum*. The mechanism of action is somewhat uncertain, but nucleic acid synthesis is probably inhibited. Quinine is not used for prophylaxis, but for the treatment of the acute phase, especially if central nervous system involvement is suspected.

Tinnitus, dizziness, headaches, nausea and vomiting occur relatively frequently. In addition, hypoglycaemia, thrombocytopenia and haemolytic anaemia are observed at high doses. Quinine reduces the heart rate and can cause arrhythmias if high drug concentrations are achieved and should not be administered as a fast intravenous infusions or bolus injections.

Pyrimethamine-sulfadoxine

Pyrimethamine resembles trimethoprim and, in combination with sulfadoxine, resembles trimethoprim-sulfamethoxazole. The combination inhibits nucleic acid synthesis in the parasite. Toxic adverse effects limit prophylactic use. In acute treatment, the combination is used as a single dose, especially with chloroquine-resistant *P. falciparum*.

Artemisinin and derivatives

Artemisinin and its derivatives are used to treat the acute phase of malaria. There is no effect on liver hypnozoites. The drugs are concentrated in cells infected with parasites.

These drugs have few adverse effects and at present no resistance has been seen. Alone and in combination with other antimalarial drugs artemether (artemether with lumefantrine) is effective against multidrug-resistant malaria.

Artemisinin, Artesunate, Artemether with lumefantrene, Artether, Chloroquine, Hydroxychloroquine, Imipenem, Proguanil, Proguanil-atovaquone, Pyrimethamine–sulfadoxine, Quinine

---

Table 16.13 Examples of antimalarial drugs

INFECTION BY *TRICHOMONAS VAGINALIS*

Trichomonas vaginalis primarily causes infections within the vagina and the urinary tracts in both women and men. New studies indicate that aggressive infection with *T. vaginalis* increases the chances of becoming infected with HIV (human immunodeficiency virus) following exposure. *T. vaginalis* is effectively treated with nitroimidazoles.

INFECTION BY *ENTAMOEBA HISTOLYTICA*

Entamoeba histolytica is an amoeba that can cause serious diarrhoea, amoebic dysentery. The microorganism exists in two stages, a trophozoite form and a cyst form that colonizes the gastrointestinal tract, acting as a reservoir for the disease and allowing the transmission of infection via the faeces. An invasive form can cause abscess formation in both the gastrointestinal tract and liver.

The invasive form is treated first for approximately 10 days with nitroimidazole, and thereafter the cyst form is treated with diloxanide.

Nitroimidazoles

Cells with low oxygen tension and anaerobic microorganisms are dependent on specific proteins that accept electrons during metabolism. Metronidazole functions as a receiver molecule for such electrons. After receipt of such electrons, the molecule becomes reactive and exhibits a toxic effect on the cells by binding to cellular macromolecules such as proteins and DNA.

Oral absorption is good for these the drugs. Metronidazole undergoes hepatic metabolism.

These drugs are effective in treating *T. vaginalis* and the trophozoite form of *E. histolytica*, but not the cyst form. In addition, they produce a bactericidal effect against many anaerobic intestinal bacteria and *H. pylori* and, as such, are used prophylactically in abdominal surgery.

Ataxia and uncoordinated movements can occur as adverse effects, and combinations with alcohol can lead to severe nausea and vomiting. Bone marrow suppression can occur and its use potentiates the effects of warfarin. It is not recommended for use in pregnancy because it is teratogenic.

Diloxanide

Diloxanide is effective against the cyst form of *E. histolytica*. The mechanism of action is unknown. Its use is recommended after the invasive form has been treated with nitroimidazoles. It is also used to render healthy carriers of the cyst form non-infectious. Serious adverse effects are seldom reported.

ANTIVIRAL DRUGS

Viruses are not cells in their own right, but rather infectious particles that consist of genetic material (DNA or RNA) protected by a protein capsule. Some viruses also have an outer layer of lipoproteins and glycoproteins. See Figure 16.37. Structures within the capsule proteins and the glycoproteins in the outer layer make it possible for viruses to bind to sites on cell membranes and in this way penetrate cells and thus infect them.

Viruses do not have the genes that make it possible to produce the cellular components that are necessary for reproduction. They are therefore dependent on using the metabolic apparatus of the cells that they infect. Viruses therefore live and reproduce only inside the host cells.

The growing number of HIV infected people has led to a dramatic increase in the use of antiviral drugs.

VIRAL INFECTIONS OF HOST CELLS

Viruses penetrate host cells by first binding to the surface of the cell. The cell membrane then encloses the virus in a membranous 'cloak' and draws it into the

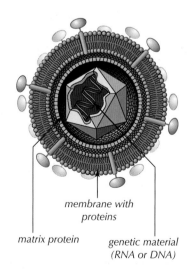

membrane with
proteins

matrix protein   genetic material
(RNA or DNA)

Figure 16.37 **Virus.** Common components of a virus.

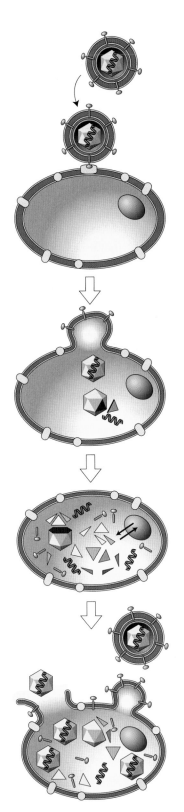

Figure 16.38 **Overview of viral multiplication.** The virus multiplies inside a cell.

cell. The membranous 'cloak' with the virus inside is released into the cell in the form of an endosome, within the cytosol of the cell (pinocytosis).

Finally, the genetic material within the virus is released (uncoating), and the formation of new virus particles begins. To replicate a virus, all elements (DNA, RNA and proteins) must be synthesized. See Figure 16.38 for an overview.

SPREAD OF VIRUSES IN THE BODY AND SYMPTOMS

Some viruses multiply rapidly and spread to different body tissues. This is especially true for influenza viruses. Symptoms therefore may be experienced as headache (viral meningitis), musculoskeletal pain (viral infection of muscles, ligaments and joints) nausea, vomiting and diarrhoea (infection of the gastrointestinal system).

With some viral infections, the number of virus particles often peaks before or close to the onset of clinical symptoms closely followed by the onset of the host immune response. Commencement of antiviral therapy at this point therefore will have little effect on the progression of the disease. This applies to influenza and herpes simplex infections. Treatment of influenza and herpes infections should therefore be started as early in the disease process as is possible to have any therapeutic effect.

Antiviral treatment is appropriate in chronic viral infections and also acute or recurring infections in patients with immunodeficiency attributed to disease; treatment is with cytotoxic drugs or other immunosuppressive drugs.

ANTIVIRAL DRUGS

The development of antiviral drugs has been slow when compared with the development of drugs to combat other microorganisms. This is mainly because viruses have few specific structural elements that can act as targets for drugs. Also since viruses use the metabolic apparatus of the cells that they infect, targeting the biological processes often will affect the host cells, even cells not infected by viruses. This often happens and is the main reason why many antiviral drugs are only used in serious diseases (when the positive drug effects may outweigh the adverse effects).

Antiviral drugs do not kill viruses, but inhibit the multiplication of the virus. Full recovery therefore depends on an intact immune system. That is why patients with a compromised immune system struggle to combat viral infections.

Since antiviral drugs often affect DNA synthesis, pregnant women should only use them when absolutely necessary and when the risks of not administering the drug outweigh the possible adverse effects.

During the last decade many new antiviral drugs have been developed, and more will follow as our understanding of the complicated interplay between viral multiplication and host cell function develops. Some examples of antiviral drugs are presented in Tables 16.14 and 16.15.

Antiviral drugs may act at various stages during the multiplication of viruses. The most important mechanisms (see below) are presented in Figure 16.38.

- Reduced attachment of the virus to the host cell membrane
  (Vaccines, immunglobulines and interferons)
- Reduced uncoating of the virus
  (Amantidine and rimantidine)
- Reduced synthesis of viral components e.g. DNA, RNA and proteins
  (Nucleoside analogues, inhibitors of reverse transcriptases and of viral proteases)
- Reduced penetration of the viruses through the cell membrane
  (Neuraminidase inhibitors).

The most serious adverse effect of antiviral drugs is bone marrow suppression, but other organ systems such as the gastrointestinal system and the CNS are frequently affected. Antiviral drugs that inhibit DNA synthesis can cause mutagenic damage during foetal development. Such drugs are not used during pregnancy.

Antiviral resistance occurs through mutation, and subsequent selection of resistant strains.

Reduced attachment of the virus to the cell membrane

It is difficult to treat viral infections after they have become established. Vaccines therefore have been developed that enhance the immune system's early response to specific viral infection. In addition to vaccines, the administration of immunoglobulins and interferons can contribute to an increased early immune response following viral infection. See step 1 of Figure 16.39.

Vaccines

Vaccines exert their effect by sensitizing the host's immune system to a particular virus or viral element. This then ensures an early and rapid response by the host immune system to a specific viral infection. As a result of this mechanism, most of the viruses are destroyed by cells of the immune system before they invade ordinary tissue cells. Several vaccines have been developed against bacterial disease but many exist to protect against viral infection. There are four main types of vaccines:

- *Toxoids* – toxins from microorganisms that have been treated so that their toxic effects have been lost or significantly diminished but their antigenic ability to stimulate the immune system is preserved
- *Killed microorganisms or components* – antigens from these components stimulate the immune system
- *Living, weakened strains of microorganisms (attenuated)* – these also act as antigens and stimulate the immune system
- *Recombinant produced antigens* – this is where the antigen component of the infective agent is reproduced utilizing recombinant DNA techniques in cell cultures.

The majority of adverse effects associated with vaccine use are mild and transitory. However, serious allergic reactions can arise with the use of parenterally administered vaccines. These reactions can be attributed to the active component within the vaccine, contamination or additives in the vaccine.

Precautionary measures

- Vaccination should be deferred in individuals with evidence of ongoing infectious disease
- Vaccines should not be administered to patients with serious systemic disease
- Patients treated with immunosuppressive drugs or cytotoxins should not be given live vaccines
- Patients who have previously had a serious allergic reaction to vaccine products should not receive the same product again
- Vaccines that are produced from egg cultures must not be administered to individuals with known egg allergies
- Pregnant women should not routinely be vaccinated with live vaccine preparations.

Many countries have established effective vaccination programmes. Vaccination of the majority of a population results in a 'herd immunity' and prevents the disease

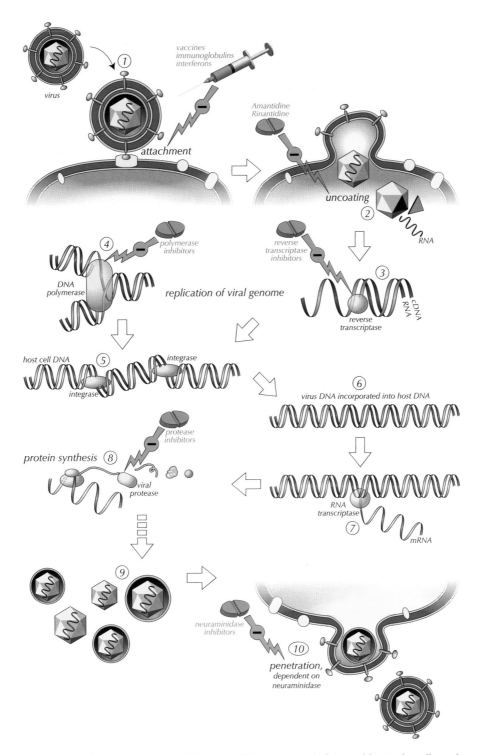

Figure 16.39 **Viral multiplication.** 1) A virus has reached the extracellular space ready for attaching to the cell membrane. The attachment may be inhibited by vaccines, immunglobulins and interferons. 2) Uncoating of the viral genetic material (here a RNA). Uncoating may be inhibited by amantidine or rimantidine. 3) Reverse transcriptase synthesises complementary DNA from viral RNA. Reverse transcriptase may be inhibited by reverse transcritpase inhibitors. 4) Viral DNA genomes are replicated by DNA polymerase. DNA polymerase may be inhibited by polymerase inhibitors. 5) Integrases assist in the incorporaton 6) of viral DNA into host DNA. 7) RNA transcriptase synthesizes viral RNA. 8) Synthesis of viral proteins cut to functional viral proteins by viral proteases. Viral protease may be inhibited by protease inhibitors. 9) Viral particles are made. 10) Penetration and spread of viruses from the infected cell. Penetration may be inhibited by neurominidase inhibitors.

from spreading. Herd immunity also protects the small number of individuals who are unable to receive the vaccine. The global eradication of smallpox was entirely due to an effective vaccination programme. In the UK childhood immunization programmes exist. All children are offered vaccination against diphtheria, tetanus, pertussis, measles, mumps, rubella, polio and TB. Specific vaccines against hepatitis A and B, influenza and pneumococcal infections are offered to certain at-risk groups, e.g. the influenza vaccine for the elderly.

Immunoglobulins

Immunoglobulin preparations contain antibodies against viruses. The antibodies bind to the capsule proteins of the virus and inhibit the virus attaching to the host cell. Immunoglobulins that bind to viruses stimulate antibody-producing B-lymphocytes and increase the efficiency of the immune system. Immunoglobulins are more effective prophylactically than therapeutically, because the antibodies present in the extracellular phase will bind to the invading virus and increase their destruction by the immune system before they penetrate the cells. Figures 12.3 and 12.4 (p. 117) gives some information of the complicated interplay between different immunocompetent cells. There are two main types of immunoglobulins: normal human immunoglobulin and specific immunoglobulin.

Normal human immunoglobulin – (also called pooled immunoglobulin) is produced by mixing plasma from several thousand blood donors. In this way, plasma is obtained that contains antibodies from individuals who have been exposed to all the most common viral diseases. These immunoglobulins are used prophylactically against measles, poliomyelitis and hepatitis A and after exposure to hepatitis B.

Specific immunoglobulin – is produced from the plasma of individuals with a particularly high content of specific antibodies. Such antibodies are used against hepatitis B, German measles (rubella), chickenpox, rabies and tetanus.

Immunoglobulins used in the treatment of viral infections can produce adverse effects in the form of allergic reactions.

Interferons

In patients with immunodeficiency, stimulation of the immune system may contribute to a more effective immune response when combating viral infections. Interferons are proteins (cytokines) that are synthesized and released from specific cells when exposed to a number of stimuli, e.g. viral antigens. They have several effects, including inhibiting the propagation of viruses. This is because interferons increases the synthesis of enzymes in host cells that degrade viral mRNA and prevent protein synthesis. In this way, synthesis of virus proteins and production of virus particles are significantly reduced.

Adverse effects of interferons include fever, lethargy, headache and myalgia. Disturbances of the cardiovascular, hepatic and thyroid function may occur as well as bone marrow depression.

Reduced uncoating of the virus

Uncoating of the virus is the release of the genetic material from the virus into the host cell cytoplasm. This step is essential for the virus DNA and RNA to reach the nucleus of the host cell, where the viral genetic material is replicated. The drugs amantadine and rimantadine inhibit the uncoating of the virus. They may be used in the treatment of influenza A. The mechanism of action is due to the inhibition of the proton transport within an ionic channel in the viral envelope which results in an inhibition in the transport of the viral genome out of the virus into the cell. The use of these drugs is restricted. See step 2 of Figure 16.39.

Reduced synthesis of viral components

The multiplication of viruses requires synthesis of viral nucleic acids (DNA or RNA), as well as viral proteins and other components that together create a complete virus particle. Viral multiplication can be reduced by the incorporation of modified components that terminate the viral DNA or RNA chain synthesis, or by the inhibition of important enzymes in the synthesis of viral nucleic acids or proteins.

Termination of nucleic acid synthesis

The principal elements of the nucleic acids are sugar molecules, bases and phosphates. The complex formed between a phosphate, a sugar molecule and a base makes up a *nucleotide* (a phosphorylated nucleoside). The nucleotide is the principal unit in nucleic acids. The complex between a sugar molecule and a base is termed a *nucleoside*.

Many antiviral drugs are nucleoside *analogues*. This means that the sugar molecule or the base of the nucleocide drug is similar to the endogenous nucleocide. With the help of enzymes, the nucleocides bind to energy-rich phosphate groups which are termed nucleotides. When this occurs in the presence of nucleocide drugs, false nucleotides are produced. Some viral enzymes are considerably more effective in the phosphorylation of the nucleocides than the enzymes of host cells. Cells that are infected with such viruses will therefore achieve high concentrations of phosphorylated nucleocide drugs, while virus-free cells do not achieve such high concentrations. The phosphorylated drugs (the false nucleotides) then compete with the native nucleotides available for synthesis of viral DNA. After a false nucleotide is linked to the growing DNA or RNA strand, synthesis is inhibited or terminated because connection of native nucleotides to the false nucleotides is prevented. See Figure 16.40.

Inhibition of enzymes

The nucleotides are connected to the growing DNA or RNA by a group of enzymes called polymerases. DNA-polymerases are necessary for synthesis of DNA. RNA-polymerases are necessary for synthesis of RNA. The false nucleotides to a different degree inhibit different polymerases. See step 4 in Figure 16.39.

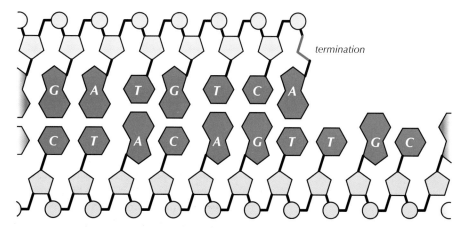

Figure 16.40 Termination of DNA chain elongation. When a false nucleoside analogue is phosphorylated and incorporated in the growing DNA chain, the synthesis of the viral DNA is terminated.

HIV-viruses are RNA-viruses. The RNA of the HIV-virus must be copied and a complementary DNA strand must be synthesized. This step is made possible by the enzyme *reverse transcriptase*, a specific DNA polymerase. This DNA is later integrated into the DNA of the host cell, where it is used as a template for the production of HIV RNA. Inhibitors of reverse transcriptase are used in the treatment of HIV-infection.

Proteases are enzymes that are important for modifying the peptide chain produced by the viral RNA to make up functional viral proteins. If viral proteases are inhibited, viral protein synthesis is disturbed. Inhibitors of viral proteases are used in the drug treatment of HIV-infection. See steps 3–8 of Figure 16.39.

Reduced penetration of viruses through the cell membrane

Neuraminidase is an enzyme that breaks down cellular barriers helping the virus to escape an infected cell and thereby increases the viral spread. Virus-infected cells produce neuraminidase. Inhibition of neuraminidase may reduce viral spread. See step 10 of Figure 16.39.

DRUGS USED IN THE TREATMENT OF IMPORTANT VIRAL INFECTIONS

Viral infections such as influenza, herpesvirus infections and cytomegalovirus infection, viral hepatitis and HIV infections may cause serious diseases.

Influenza

Influenza is transmitted almost exclusively by inhaled aerosol droplets. The virus, which over time constantly changes, predominantly infects the bronchial epithelium in the early phase of the disease. Zanamivir and oseltamivir inhibit neuraminidase. Amantadine and rimantadine reduce the viral multiplication and thus the viral spread by inhibiting viral uncoating.

Zanamivir and oseltamivir

Zanamivir and oseltamivir inhibit neuraminidase and prevent the virus from effectively infecting new cells. Zanamivir was the first antiviral drug shown to be effective against both influenza A and B. If it is administered early (within 48 hours of symptom onset) the length and severity of illness can be diminished. If the drug is taken late, it has no effect. The drug is inhaled to ensure high concentrations in the bronchial mucosa.

Bronchospasm and impaired pulmonary function can occur, particularly in patients with respiratory disease. In such cases, the drug is immediately discontinued.

Amantadine and rimantadine

Amantadine and rimantadine inhibit the uncoating of the virus and therefore multiplication in the early phase of the infection. The drugs are effective in the treatment of influenza A if started within 48 hours of the onset symptoms.

Herpesvirus and cytomegalovirus infection

Herpes simplex and *varicella-zoster* are the most important herpesvirus pathogens.

Herpes simplex serotype 1 often infects the mucous membranes of mouth and lips and sometimes the eye. Within the infected area painful blisters develop, leaving scabs after rupturing. After the primary (first) infection, the viruses infect and follow sensory nerves from the skin and are found in neural ganglia for the rest of the person's life. From this reservoir the virus may be activated and present as secondary infections many times. Immunocompromised patients may be infected in other areas of the skin. Herpesvirus serotype 2 is associated with infections of genitalia.

Mild infections in healthy individuals are usually treated with topical antiviral drugs. Severe infections and infections in immunocompromised patients are best treated with systemic antiviral drugs.

Varicella zoster cause chickenpox and herpes zoster (shingles) later in life. After the primary infection (chickenpox) the *Varicella zoster* virus lies dormant in neural ganglia like *Herpes simplex*. Usually chickenpox is mild, but in rare cases the infection can be life-threatening after infection of the lungs or the brain. Vaccines are used prophylactically to prevent chickenpox infections. Immunocompromised patients are treated with systemic antiviral drugs. Acicclovir, valaciclovir, famciclovir and idoxuridine are used to treat herpesvirus infections.

Following infection by cytomegalovirus the virus remains in the body for the rest of a person's life. Infection is usually asymptomatic but primary infection in a pregnant woman in the first trimester may harm the foetus. Immunocompromised patients may exhibit severe symptoms and may need systemic treatment. Ganciclovir, valaciclovir, valganciclovir, foscarnet and cidofovir are used to treat cytomegalovirus infections.

The drugs used to treat herpesvirus and cytomegalovirus infection all inhibit DNA polymerase.

Aciclovir and valaciclovir

Aciclovir is a nucleocide analogue that is particularly effective against the herpes virus. The herpes virus has an enzyme that is able to phosphorylate aciclovir, which then becomes active. Phosphorylated aciclovir inhibits viral DNA polymerase, which attaches the nucleotide to the growing DNA strand. The formation of new viral DNA is thus inhibited. In the herpes virus, the virus-specific enzyme is inhibited approximately 30 times more effectively than the human enzyme, so little effect is seen on the human host cells.

Aciclovir is used for the topical treatment of herpes infection of the cornea. Oral administration is used for infections of the skin and mucosa. In serious infections (herpes encephalitis) intravenous administration is required. It is important that the infusion does not extravasate outside the vein, as the solution is strongly alkaline and will cause serious tissue necrosis.

Usually aciclovir is well tolerated. Renal damage may occur at high doses and following rapid intravenous infusion, particularly in dehydrated patients. In renal failure the dose must be reduced. Nausea and headache are also reported.

Valaciclovir is a prodrug of aciclovir with considerably higher bioavailability than aciclovir. The drug can be given once a day.

Famciclovir and penciclovir

Famciclovir is a prodrug of penciclovir and is given orally. Penciclovir is a topical treatment formulated as a cream. It acts as an terminator of DNA chain enlongation and as an inhibitor of DNA polymerase in hepatitis B virus infection. The drugs are used in herpes genitalis and in herpes zoster.

Ganciclovir

Ganciclovir is phosphorylated in the same way as aciclovir by a virus-specific enzyme. The active drug prevents the formation of viral DNA by inhibiting viral DNA polymerase. It is considerably more effective than aciclovir against cytomegalovirus, which, in particular, causes clinical infections in patients with reduced immune defences, e.g. AIDS (acquired immune deficiency syndrome).

The effect on human cells is considerable. Bone marrow depression, adverse effects on liver and renal function, on the central nervous system and on male and female gametes are sufficiently severe to ensure that ganciclovir is used in only the most serious viral infections.

Cidofovir

Cidofovir competes with the native nucleotides to terminate the DNA strain and inhibit DNA polymerases. The drug is given once a week together with probeneid to reduce renal elimination so that the time in the body is prolonged.

Cidofovir is nephrotoxic and has a dose-limiting effect. Mutagenic, embryotoxic, teratogenic, carcinogenic and gonadotoxic effects are observed in animal studies.

Idoxuridine

Idoxuridine inhibits DNA synthesis by acting as a false nucleotide. The compound is phosphorylated not by virus-specific enzymes but by enzymes in the host cell. As a result the concentration of active drug will also be high in cells that are not infected. The effect on host cells is so significant that the drug is only used as a topical treatment.

It is used in oral herpes simplex, infection of the cornea and in serious herpes zoster (shingles) infection. Idoxuridine has shown a teratogenic effect in animal studies and is contraindicated in pregnancy.

Foscarnet

Foscarnet is a non-nucleotide that binds directly to DNA and RNA polymerase and inhibits nucleic acid synthesis. Viral polymerases are inhibited at lower concentrations than polymerases in the host cells. Foscarnet's main use is the treatment of cytomegalovirus in patients with HIV/AIDS who do not tolerate treatment with ganciclovir. There are frequent and serious nephrotoxic effects and adverse effects related to several other organ systems.

Viral hepatitis

Viral hepatitis constitutes the diseases hepatitis A, B and C.

Hepatitis A is transmitted by contaminated food or drinks, very often from faecal contamination. The disease course may be from mild to severe. At present there is no effective antiviral drug to treat hepatitis A, but immunoglobulins and vaccination may prevent the disease.

Hepatitis B is transmitted via blood or blood components. Intravenous drug abusers are at particular risk because of contaminated syringes. The course may be acute or chronic and infection may cause hepatic cancer. Hepatitis B may be treated with interferon alfa or lamivudine.

Hepatitis C is transmitted via blood or blood components. The course is usually mild during the acute phase, but may result in serious damage to the liver. Treatment can be with ribavirin or peginterferon alfa.

Interferon alfa

Interferon alfa is used in the treatment of hepatitis B (and in some forms of hepatic cancer). The drug is administered parenterally. The mechanism of action is the stimulation of immuncompetent cells to increase viral degradation and reduce viral multiplication. Adverse effects are influenza-like symptoms with fever, headaches, muscle pains and lethargy. Bone marrow depression and other effects are also described. It is contraindicated in patients receiving immunosuppressant treatment.

Ribavirin and peginterferon alfa

Ribavirin in combination with peginterferon alfa is used to treat chronic hepatitis C. The mechanism of action is uncertain, but ribavirin acts both as a nucleotide monophosphate and a nucleotidtriphosphate, by inhibiting the synthesis of viral nucleic acids, especially mRNA. For the treatment of hepatitis C ribavirin is given systemically (and by inhalation for the treatment of respiratory syncytial virus). Peginterferon alfa resembles interferon alfa, but is more effective than interferon alfa in treating hepatitis C in combination with ribavirin.

Inhibitors of DNA polymerase (nucleocide analogues)
Aciclovir, Cidofovir, Famciclovir, Ganciclovir, Idoxuridine, Penciclovir, Ribavirin, Valaciclovir

Inhibitor of DNA polymerase (non-nucleocide analogues)
Foscarnet

Interferons
Interferon alfa, Peginterferon alfa

Inhibitors of neuraminidase
Oseltamivir, Zanamivir

Inhibitors of viral uncoating
Amantadine, Rimantadine

Table 16.14 Examples of antiviral drugs (non HIV)

HIV infection and aids

The *Human immunodeficiency virus* (HIV) is a retrovirus with RNA as the genetic material. The infection is chronic and lifelong. Acquired immune deficiency syndrome (AIDS) is the clinical manifestation of HIV infection and can develop several years after HIV infection. Following the development of AIDS, the immune system is severely impaired, with T_4-lymphocyte function particularly affected.

Because of a significantly reduced immune defence, patients suffering from AIDS often develop opportunistic infections. Infection by *Pneumocystis carinii*, toxoplasmosis and cytomegalovirus occurs frequently. Tuberculosis is also more frequently observed in this patient group than in others, because the cellular immune defence is particularly important for combating such infections. This is the reason that this group of patients often has viral and fungal infections.

A fatal outcome is associated with AIDS, usually due to overwhelming infection associated with a failing immune system. Without treatment, fully developed AIDS has a current mortality rate of 80 per cent within 2 years and 100 per cent after 5 years.

Indication for use of anti-HIV drugs

Use of anti-HIV drugs is guided by laboratory tests that quantify the amount of HIV-RNA in plasma and the number of CD_4-positive T cells in peripheral blood, since there is a correlation between the amount of HIV-RNA (viral load) in plasma and the progression of the disease. Drug treatment should be started before the immune system is irreversibly damaged. Since anti-HIV drugs are associated with toxicity, the need for early treatment should be weighed up against this risk.

Drugs used to treat HIV infection and aids

Modern treatments for HIV and AIDS are inhibitors of reverse transcriptases or proteases. Most inhibitors of reverse transcriptases are nucleocide analogues that are phosphorylated to false nucleotides, but some are non-nucleocides. Mutation of the enzymes which the drugs act upon may lead to drug resistance. As HIV virus readily mutates, triple therapy is used: two nucleoside analogues in combination with a protease inhibitor.

Inhibitors of reverse transcriptases that are nucleocide analogues

Inhibitors of reverse transcriptases that are nucleocide analogues (phosphorylated to false nucleotides) have a selective toxicity for the HIV virus caused by a greater affinity for viral reverse transcriptases than for the cells' polymerases. All are able to terminate the growing DNA strand. They also inhibit the activity of reverse transcriptase. These drugs become less effective with change to the enzyme reverse transcriptase as a result of mutation. See Figure 16.40 (p. 215).

All drugs except didanosine are well absorbed following oral administration and are renally excreted (with the exception of abacavir).

As a class they have been associated with the development of fatty liver, neuropathy, myopathy, and pancreatitis. These adverse effects are thought to arise from the inhibition of mitochondrial DNA polymerases of the host cells which cause mitocondrial dysfunction. These adverse effects show that the 'selective toxicity' of this class is restricted. Zidovudine was the first drug to be developed in this group. Other drugs are presented in Table 16.15.

Inhibitors of reverse transcriptases that are non-nucleocide analogues

Inhibitors of reverse transcriptases that are non-nucleocide analogues do not require phosphorylation to be activated. Their selective toxicity is a result of their ability to deactivate reverse transcriptase. They do not share the effect of nucleocide analogues on cellular polymerases and therefore do not lead to mitocondrial dysfunction.

These drugs are well absorbed. Elimination is by the hepatic P-450 system. The drugs are therefore vulnerable to interactions with other drugs that share a similar metobolic pathway.

Maculopapular rashes are common adverse effects. Toxic hepatitis is associated with the use of nevirapine and the use of efavirenz is associated with neuropsychiatric effects. Tenofovir is a novel nucleotide analogue. The mechanism of action is similar to that of the nucleocide analogues. Since the phosphorylation step is not necessary, nucleotide analogues can incorporate into the viral DNA chain more rapidly than nucleocide analogues. More importantly, this will bypass emerging viral nucleocide resistance. Drugs of this type are presented in Table 16.15.

Inhibitors of proteases

HIV protease inhibitors are substrate analogues that prevent the enzyme from cutting long virus-produced proteins leading to the formation of functional proteins. In this way, 'immature' virus particles are created that cannot infect new cells. The HIV protease inhibitors have a selective affinity to HIV proteases and insignificant affinity to human proteases. The effect on viral multiplication is stronger than for the nucleotide analogues.

All drugs in this group are metabolized by the liver and are vulnerable to interactions with other drugs. The HIV virus can develop resistance to the protease inhibitors.

Gastrointestinal side effects with nausea and diarrhoea are the principal side effects. A syndrome of lipodystrophy, resembling the long-term use of glucocorticoids has been observed following extended use. See Table 16.15.

Inhibitors of reverse transcriptase (nucleocide analogues)
Abacavir, Didanosine, Lamivudine, Stavudine, Zalcitabine, Zidovudine

Inhibitors of reverse transcriptase (non-nucleocide analogues)
Delavirdine, Efavirenz, Nevirapine, Tenofovir

Inhibitors of HIV protease
Amprenavir, Indinavir, Nelfinavir, Ritonavir, Saquinavir

Table 16.15 Examples of drugs used to treat HIV-infections

SUMMARY

- Antimicrobial drugs exploit differences between microorganisms and animal cells to exert a selective toxicity. Aerobic and anaerobic microorganisms thrive in tissues with and without oxygen, respectively.

- Resistance is the ability of microorganisms to resist an external harmful influence. Some microorganisms have natural resistance; others can develop (acquire) resistance to antimicrobial drugs. There is a clear connection between the use of antimicrobial drugs and increased occurrence of resistant bacteria.

- Determinations of resistance are carried out to find an antimicrobial drug to which microorganisms are sensitive.

- When the disease-causing microbe is identified, a specific narrow-spectrum drug should be selected. In life-threatening infections without a known agent, a combination of antimicrobial drugs is used to treat the patient against the most probable microbes.

- Normal flora protects against disease-causing microorganisms. Patients with a reduced immune defence can succumb to infection with microorganisms that belong to the normal flora.

- Some antimicrobial drugs kill microbes, while others inhibit the growth so that the host's immune defence can overcome the infection.

- Adverse effects of antimicrobial drugs can occur in host cells that have similar properties to those of the microorganism and in tissues that achieve high concentrations of an antimicrobial drug.

- The important points of attack for antimicrobial drugs are inhibition of cell wall synthesis, protein synthesis, nucleic acid synthesis and functions within the cell membrane.

- Beta-lactam antibiotics damage the cell wall in bacteria. Synthetic penicillins have a broader spectrum than the natural penicillins. Some are resistant to beta-lactamase. The cephalosporins resemble the penicillins and often demonstrate cross-sensitivity.

- Sulphonamides, trimethoprim, quinolones, nitroimidazoles and rifampicin inhibit nucleic acid synthesis. Isoniazid disturbs the functions of the cytoplasmic membrane.

- Aminoglycosides inhibit protein synthesis in bacteria. The aminoglycosides can have toxic effects on the kidneys and hearing when used in high doses.

- Tetracyclines inhibit protein synthesis in bacteria. They have a broad spectrum and contribute to the development of resistance. Tetracyclines are not to be used for pregnant women or children because of discoloration of the tooth enamel and inhibition of bone growth.

- Macrolides inhibit protein synthesis in bacteria. The macrolides act upon virtually the same microorganisms as the natural penicillins, but have fewer tendencies to cause allergy.

- Chloramphenicol inhibits protein synthesis in bacteria and can cause toxic effects on the bone marrow up to several months after use. Neonates have a reduced ability for conjugation because of an immature liver and reduced ability to eliminate chloramphenicol.

- Use of clindamycin and lincomycin can cause adverse gastrointestinal effects due to pseudomembranous colitis, a super-infection in the colon.

- Sulphonamides and trimethoprim inhibit two subsequent steps in the synthesis of nucleic acid bases. They often cause allergic skin reactions.

- In the treatment of tuberculosis, two or three drugs are used simultaneously to prevent the development of resistant strains. The course of treatment is long because of the extended reproduction time seen in the causative organism.

- Patients with reduced immune defences are particularly susceptible to systemic fungal infections. The mould fungi thrive in tissues with keratin. Yeast fungi can grow in all tissues, but thrive in non-keratinized tissue. Fungal infections of the hair and nails require a prolonged period of treatment. The majority of fungicides act by inhibiting ergosterol synthesis or by damaging ergosterol in the membranes of the fungus.
- No antimalarial drugs are effective against both tissue and erythrocyte merozoites. Prophylactic treatment aims to prevent clinical malaria (the erythrocyte stage). After exposure, there is a short period of treatment with drugs against both tissue and blood schizonts to achieve eradication.
- Influenza, herpes virus infections, cytomegalovirus infection, vital hepatitis and HIV infections are important viral infections.
- Antiviral drugs act by reducing the attachment of the virus to the host cell, preventing the uncoating of the virus, reducing synthesis of viral components like DNA, RNA and proteins and reducing penetration of the viruses through the cell membrane. Antiviral drugs should not be used during pregnancy because of the danger of mutagenic damage to the fetus.
- Zanamivir was the first antiviral drug shown to be effective against both influenza A and B. It must be administered early in the diseases. Vaccination is the best prophylaxis against influenza.
- Drugs against HIV infection act by inhibiting HIV-specific reverse transcriptase or HIV-specific protease (protease inhibitors).

17 Drug used to treat diseases in the cardiovascular system

The cardiovascular system comprises a pump and pipe system for the transport of oxygen and nutrients to, and waste products from, all the cells in the body. In heart disease, the pump function will suffer. In vascular disease, the transport function will suffer. Since the tissues are dependent on this pump and pipe system, disease in the heart or vascular system can present as disease or malfunction in different organs, usually in several simultaneously.

In recent years, the role of the vascular system as both recipient and producer of endocrine substances has increased our understanding of how the physiology of the heart and vascular system is regulated. For example, the insides of blood vessels are lined by endothelial cells that have considerable endocrine function.

Patients with disease of the cardiovascular system often use drugs over a long period and often many drugs simultaneously, so it is important to consider potential drug interactions.

As several of the drug groups are used in different disorders, the diseases are examined first, followed by drug groups. Drugs used to treat coagulation disorders are covered in Chapter 20, Drugs used to treat diseases of the blood.

HYPERTENSION

Blood pressure is the pressure the blood exerts against the walls in a blood vessel. Generally, when we refer to blood pressure, we are referring to the pressure in the arteries of the systemic circulation. In large arteries, the blood pressure is related to the heart's pumping phase, and is highest closest to the heart. Blood pressure is usually measured indirectly with a sphygmomanometer and stethoscope – normally in the brachial artery of the upper arm. Blood pressure tends to rise with increased age. Therefore, the limits for what one perceives as elevated blood pressure vary with age. Blood pressure ≥140 mmHg systolic or ≥90 mmHg diastolic, at three separate measurements, is defined as high blood pressure, regardless of age. Hypertension is a persistent elevated systolic and/or diastolic blood pressure. Reduced salt intake, weight reduction, cessation of smoking and increased physical activity form the basis of all hypertension treatment. In the majority of cases, it is still uncertain what causes hypertension. It is considered multifactorial and touches on hereditary factors and lifestyle.

The decision concerning the use of drugs in the treatment of hypertension is based on the overall evaluation of several risk factors, of which the blood pressure is but one. In the case of concurrent diabetes or kidney disease, treatment at lower limits of hypertension is required than without such diseases.

PATHOPHYSIOLOGY OF HYPERTENSION

The blood circulates from the left atrium to the left ventricle, through arteries to the capillary network and through veins to the right atrium. This is the systemic circulation. From the right atrium, blood is delivered to the right ventricle and is pumped out into the pulmonary circulation. After gaseous exchange in the lungs, the blood is delivered back to the left atrium. See Figure 17.1.

When the ventricles contract (systole), blood is pumped simultaneously into both the systemic and pulmonary circulations. During this phase, blood pressure increases and reaches its peak value – systolic pressure. When the ventricles relax (diastole), the blood pressure drops, reaching its minimum value – diastolic pressure. The period of systole lasts for a shorter time than that of diastole. See Figure 17.2.

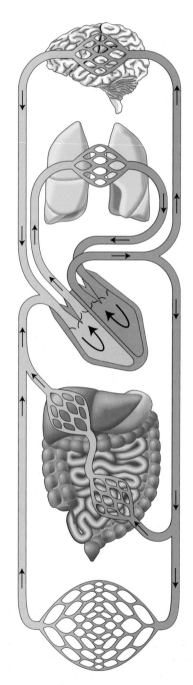

Figure 17.1 **Schematic diagram of the blood's circulation.** Notice that blood from the intestines passes through the liver before it flows back to the heart and is pumped out into the wider circulation. This is important for drugs with a high degree of first-pass metabolism in the liver, when they are taken by the enteral route.

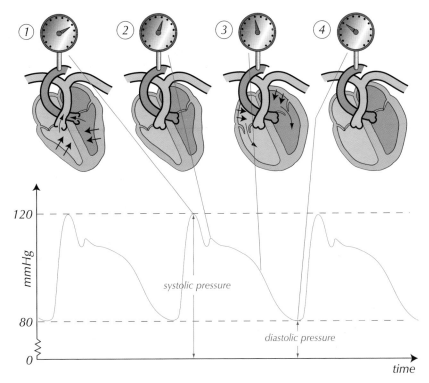

Figure 17.2 **The blood pressure varies through the heart's cycle.** (1) During systole, the heart's ventricles contract and pump blood out through the aorta (and the pulmonary artery). The systemic arterial pressure rises quickly to its highest value (systolic blood pressure). (2) When the contraction is over and the pressure in the ventricles drops, the aorta will have higher pressure than the ventricles for a short period. The blood will then tend to flow back, but is prevented because the valves in the aorta and the pulmonary artery close. The closing of the aortic valve results in a slight and brief increase in pressure. (3) During the heart's resting phase, there is a gradual pressure drop in the arteries because blood is carried outwards towards the capillary beds. However, the pressure is held above zero because of the elasticity of the veins. (4) The heart is ready for a new contraction. The pressure in the arteries is now at its lowest (diastolic blood pressure).

Regulation of the blood pressure

Imagine that you are going to blow air through a system of pipes of increasingly smaller diameter. As the diameter becomes smaller and smaller, so it becomes more difficult to blow air through them – more force is required. The larger the diameter of the pipe, the easier the air will circulate. The pressure of air in the pipe will be highest near where you blow in, and will decrease in the system gradually as the air passes through increasingly narrower passages. The pressure becomes greater if the resistance in the system and the circulating air quantity increase.

In the same way, the blood pressure is affected by the resistance against the narrow arterioles and by the circulating blood volume. The blood pressure (BP) can be expressed as:

$$BP = CO \times R$$

$$BP = SV \times f \times R$$

where CO is the cardiac output, R is the resistance (more correctly the total peripheral resistance) against the circulation, SV is the stroke volume (blood volume ejected with each heartbeat), and f is the frequency (number of heartbeats/min). The cardiac output is determined by the stroke volume and the frequency (CO = SV × f). From this, it can be seen that the value of the blood pressure increases when the cardiac output or the resistance increases.

Blood pressure is determined by the resistance against which the heart pumps and the volume that is ejected with each heartbeat. Hypertension can therefore occur when peripheral resistance increases (resistance hypertension) or when the circulating volume increases (volume-associated hypertension). The smallest arteries before the transition to capillaries, the arterioles, are the most important parts of the cardiovascular system for the regulation of blood pressure. The arterioles have smooth muscle orientated in a ring-like manner in their walls – so-called circular smooth muscle. If the muscles contract, the arteriole constricts (a process called vasoconstriction) and the resistance to blood flow increases. The heart must then pump harder to push the blood through the vessels, and the arterial blood pressure will rise. The blood vessels that form the transition from arterioles to the capillary vessels also have ring-shaped muscles, precapillary sphincters. These have the ability to contract and relax, and in doing so to regulate the blood flow into the capillary bed.

Regulation of blood pressure occurs mainly through two overlapping systems: the autonomic nervous system and the renin–angiotensin–aldosterone system. In people with hypertension, the pressure seems to be regulated to a 'higher level' than in people who are not hypertensive. This elevated pressure then becomes 'accepted' as their normal resting blood pressure.

The autonomic nervous system

In the large arteries near the heart (the aortic arch and right and left carotid arteries) and in the left ventricle there are pressure receptors (baroreceptors) that monitor blood pressure from moment to moment and are able to alter it via nervous regulation. For example, a rapid increase in the blood pressure will be sensed by the baroreceptors, as the artery and ventricular walls will be stretched to a greater extent. Action potentials will be transmitted to the cardiovascular centre in the medulla. In turn, this results in a decrease in heart rate, force of contraction and inhibition of vasoconstriction. By these effects, the blood pressure is returned to its normal value. The opposite occurs when blood pressure falls. This type of nervous regulation occurs quickly. See Figure 17.3.

The renin–angiotensin–aldosterone system

The kidneys contribute to regulation of blood pressure by influencing the degree of vasoconstriction and by changing the circulating blood volume. Baroreceptors in the arteries of the kidneys respond to changes in blood pressure. When the pressure drops, the hormone renin is released, which metabolizes angiotensinogen to angiotensin-I. In turn, angiotensin-I is metabolized to angiotensin-II in the presence of angiotensin-converting enzyme (ACE). Angiotensin-II is a very potent vasoconstrictor substance that results in an increase in blood pressure. In addition, angiotensin-II stimulates the adrenal glands to increase the release of aldosterone. Aldosterone increases the reabsorption of sodium from the urine to the blood. With sodium follows water. In this way, the circulating blood volume increases, which in turn produces a rise in blood pressure. See Figure 17.4.

Hypertension is a risk factor for disease

Hypertension is a pronounced risk factor for the development of cardiovascular disease because the high pressure acts as mechanical stress on both heart and

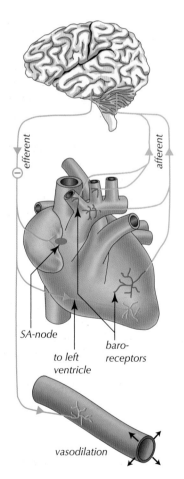

efferent

afferent

SA-node

to left ventricle

baro-receptors

vasodilation

Figure 17.3 Blood pressure regulation via baroreceptors and the autonomic nervous system. Refer to text for a more detailed explanation.

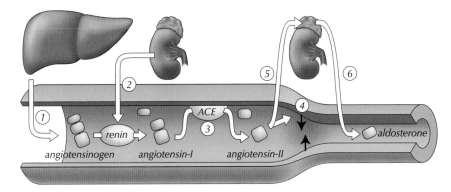

Figure 17.4 **Blood pressure regulation via the renin–angiotensin–aldosterone system.**
Angiotensinogen is synthesized in the liver (1). Renin is released by low arterial pressure in
the kidneys (2), which metabolizes angiotensinogen to angiotensin-I. Angiotensin-
converting enzyme (ACE) (3) metabolizes angiotensin-I to angiotensin-II, which has a
powerful vasoconstrictor effect (4) and stimulates the adrenal glands (5) to secrete
aldosterone (6). Aldosterone has sodium-retaining effect.

blood vessels. In the arteries, the circular smooth muscle is strengthened simultaneously, as hardening of the arteries (arteriosclerosis) develops more rapidly than
otherwise. In this process, the lumen of the vessels becomes smaller and the elasticity in the vessel walls is reduced (see Figure 17.5). The arterial wall can burst if a
high pressure persists over many years. An isolated moderate hypertension in itself
only involves a small increased risk if other risk factors do not exist simultaneously. Elevated blood pressure must therefore be seen in a wide context when drug
treatment is considered.

Arteriosclerosis often occurs in the large arteries; for example, it is pronounced
in the coronary arteries, the aorta, renal arteries and cranial arteries.

The increased pressure against which the heart pumps results in an increase in
the thickness of the heart muscles (hypertrophy). This puts the heart muscle's own
blood supply under further risk. The additional strain on the heart in hypertension makes the heart muscle extra sensitive to reduced blood supply, owing to
coronary artery arteriosclerosis.

Symptoms of hypertension

Symptoms of hypertension usually appear some considerable time after its initiation and first manifest themselves when there is already considerable damage to
blood vessels. Symptoms appear in organs most vulnerable to hypertension, e.g. the
heart, brain and kidneys. There can also be a poor peripheral circulation with cold
feet, and activity-related pain from muscles in the lower extremities (intermittent
claudication) is not uncommon.

Hypertension is a risk factor for the development of many serious diseases of
the cardiovascular system.

GOAL OF DRUG TREATMENT

The goal of treating people with hypertension is to reduce the development of
further serious disease in:

- the heart (angina pectoris, myocardial infarction, rhythm disturbances and
  cardiac failure)
- blood vessels (arteriosclerotic development)

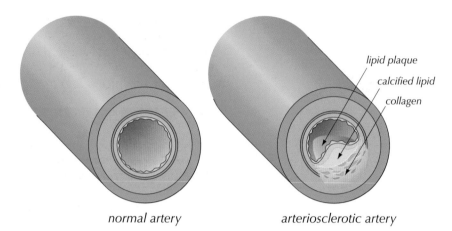

Figure 17.5 **Normal and arteriosclerotic arteries.** An arteriosclerotic artery has a reduced lumen diameter.

- the central nervous system (stroke with haemorrhage and thrombosis)
- the kidneys (renal failure).

Sustained elevated blood pressure must always be treated. Moderate increases in blood pressure with subsequent complications (angina pectoris, left ventricular hypertrophy, cerebral infarction and renal damage) must also be intensively treated. At the start of drug treatment, small doses of drugs should be used. Dose adjustment should wait until the full effect is achieved from the given dose. Large doses or rapid increases in dosage can cause a fall in blood pressure with undesirable effects (disturbed cerebral, coronary and renal blood flow).

All drugs used in hypertension achieve their effects via one or more of the following mechanisms:

- reduction of the cardiac output
- reduction of the resistance in the vascular system by causing the precapillary sphincters to dilate
- reduction of the circulating blood volume
- increase of the accumulation of blood on the venous side in the circuit (emergency treatment).

The choice of drug to treat hypertension is based on the cause of the hypertension, the degree of seriousness, how quickly it has progressed and the presence of other concurrent diseases.

Relevant drug groups
- Diuretics
- Beta-blockers
- ACE inhibitors
- Angiotensin-II-receptor antagonists
- Calcium-channel blockers.

ANGINA PECTORIS

Angina pectoris is chest pain attributable to a disparity between the heart's need for oxygen and the ability of the coronary arteries to supply the tissue with oxygen-rich blood. Hardening of the arteries constricts the coronary arteries and limits

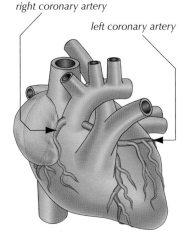

right coronary artery

left coronary artery

Figure 17.6 **Outlet of the coronary arteries.** The right and left coronary arteries have their origin in the aorta just above the aortic valve and supply the heart muscle with blood.

blood flow of the heart. The symptoms first present when sufferers exert themselves, e.g. exercise or increased work in exertion, but they can also be present during rest, in disease that has progressed. In angina pectoris, the pains are localized behind the sternum as a constricting feeling. The pains often radiate to the neck and left arm, and can be accompanied by dyspnoea.

PATHOPHYSIOLOGY OF ANGINA PECTORIS

The blood supply to the heart muscle is via the right and left coronary arteries, which have their outlet from the aorta, just above the aortic valve. See Figure 17.6. The coronary arteries each supply their own part of the heart and normally have few connections between them. The poor connectivity is exacerbated by the presence of end arteries. See Figure 17.7. Acute disturbances of blood flow in an area of the heart muscle can therefore only be slightly compensated by the increased blood flow in another, adjoining region. If the narrowing occurs gradually, adjacent arteries could take over some of the supply to such an area.

Circulation in the coronary arteries

In systole, when the heart contracts, the coronary arteries are partially squeezed together. There is therefore little coronary circulation in the wall of the left ventricle during the systole. During diastole, the heart muscle relaxes and the coronary circulation is re-established. The blood pressure in the aorta pushes the blood through the coronary arteries. This is why coronary circulation of blood occurs primarily in the diastole. See Figure 17.8. An increase in the heart rate shortens diastole and can therefore further reduce the coronary blood flow.

GOAL OF DRUG TREATMENT

The goal of the treatment is primarily to reduce pain, and to improve exercise tolerance, but also to reduce the chances for the development of serious rhythm disturbances and cardiac infarction. The treatment aims to make up for the disparity between the need for and supply of oxygen by improving the blood flow to the myocardium, or by reducing the heart's load such that the oxygen consumption is reduced. The latter can occur by reducing the heart's force of contraction, the

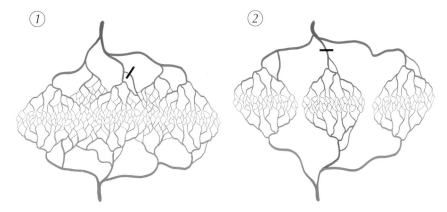

Figure 17.7 **Anastomosing arteries and end arteries.** If there is a blockage in an artery that has abundant anastomoses (1), the area will be supplied by adjacent arteries and the tissue damage in the area is minimal. If there is a blockage in the circulation in an end artery (2), the area that is supplied by the artery will lose its blood supply and die (grey area).

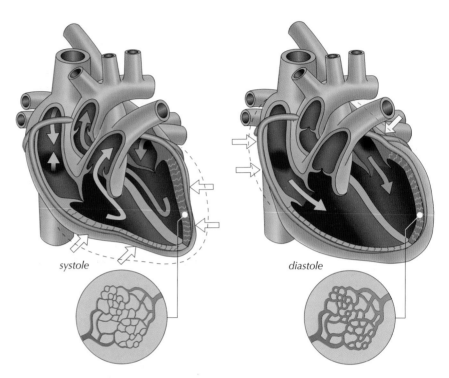

Figure 17.8 **Circulation in coronary arteries in systole and diastole.** The circulation in the wall of the left ventricle is reduced during systole because the blood vessels are compressed by the increased muscular force during contraction.

systole   *diastole*

blood pressure or the rate of contraction. Angina pectoris is a risk factor for development of myocardial infarction. To prevent myocardial infarction, the patients should be treated with low dose aspirin. Aspirin reduces blood platelet aggregation and platelet adhesion to the endothelial lining of arteries, thus reducing the risk of narrowing of the lumen and the development of arterial thromboses.

Relevant drug groups
- Organic nitrates
- Beta-blockers
- Calcium-channel blockers.

MYOCARDIAL INFARCTION

Myocardial infarction occurs when an area of the heart loses so much of the blood supply that the tissue dies from oxygen deficiency. The higher up in the coronary arteries the blockage occurs, the larger the area of the heart that will be affected.

PATHOPHYSIOLOGY OF MYOCARDIAL INFARCTION

A myocardial infarction can be a 'natural' consequence of progressive arteriosclerosis, but it can also appear without warning due to thrombosis in a coronary artery with only a modest degree of hardening of the arteries. The arteriosclerotic process is influenced by the plasma levels of cholesterol and other lipids. Smoking, a high intake of saturated fat, being overweight and taking little exercise further increase the formation of arteriosclerotic plaques in the arteries.

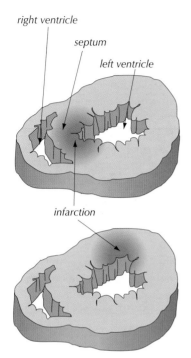

right ventricle

septum

left ventricle

infarction

Figure 17.9 **The localization of the infarction** is dependent on which coronary artery fails. The illustration shows infarction in the ventricle septum (damage of left coronary artery) and in the dorsal, left ventricle (damage of right coronary artery).

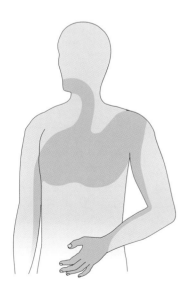

Figure 17.10 **Pain localization in myocardial infarction.** The distribution of pain in myocardial infarction is explained as 'referred pain'. See Figure 14.5 for further details (p. 151).

The immediate danger of an acute myocardial infarction is the development of arrhythmias and acute cardiac failure.

Size and localization of the infarct

If a person survives a myocardial infarction, the part of the myocardium that is damaged will be replaced by connective tissue. Connective tissue cannot contract. An infarction will therefore result in part of the myocardium losing its ability to contract. If the damage is great enough, cardiac failure can develop (post-infarction failure). If the infarction is in an area that is important for the transmission of cardiac action potentials (ventricular septum), it can lead to rhythm disturbance. If the heart's papillary muscles are affected by the infarction, the fibrous strands (chordae tendineae) that hold the valves in their correct position lose their attachment to the ventricular wall, such that the valves between the atria and ventricles fail. Such papillary muscle damage can cause life-threatening cardiac failure. See Figure 17.9.

Symptoms of myocardial infarction

Myocardial infarction presents with retrosternal, compression pains which radiate to the neck or jaws and/or to one or both arms. The pains resemble those seen in angina pectoris, but are usually stronger, last longer and are not relieved by rest. See Figure 17.10. Pain, anxiety, restlessness, nausea, rhythm disturbances, hypotension and cardiac failure are often seen in a myocardial infarction.

GOAL OF DRUG TREATMENT

In addition to suppressing the pain, the primary goal of drug treatment is to limit the size of the infarction and to reduce the risk of development of complications. The treatment is different between the acute phase and the phase after the infarction has occurred. Thrombus formation is present in all infarctions. If an ECG shows clear signs of infarction, thrombus-dissolving (thrombolytic) treatment is administered if no more than 8 h have passed since the symptoms presented.

It is important to treat the acute sequelae. Pain, anxiety, restlessness, nausea, rhythm disturbances, hypotension and cardiac failure exacerbate the situation and can increase the size of the infarction.

Analgesic drugs (usually morphine) also suppress anxiety and restlessness, but pure anxiolytic drugs may be administered. Nausea is treated with separate antiemetics. Rhythm disturbances, cardiac failure and hypotension are treated with drugs that are described elsewhere in this chapter.

Relevant drug groups

There are no distinct drugs used to treat myocardial infarction. The possible exception to this are drugs that dissolve fresh thrombotic masses, i.e. thrombolytics, and drugs that reduce activation of platelets, such as acetylsalicylic acid. Drugs that delay the arteriosclerotic process in the long term will reduce the risk of cardiac infarction. All other therapy is based on treatment of the sequelae of the myocardial infarction:

- Beta-blockers
- ACE inhibitors
- Diuretics
- Organic nitrates
- Calcium-channel blockers.

Thrombolytics, analgesics, anxiolytics and antiemetic drugs are discussed in other chapters.

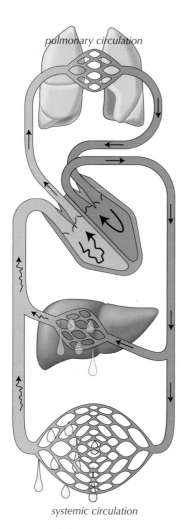

pulmonary circulation

systemic circulation

Figure 17.11 Failure in the right ventricle can cause congestion in the cardiovascular system, which presents itself as oedema in the lower extremities. In such a situation, there can also be congestion in internal organs, here symbolized by liver congestion.

CARDIAC FAILURE

Cardiac failure means failure in the heart's pumping function or in its relaxation. The main problem then, consists of either a failing systolic function (systolic failure) or disturbed relaxation (diastolic failure). Systolic failure is best characterized and easiest to treat. The most important causes of systolic failure are loss of muscle tissue after myocardial infarction and high blood pressure over many years. Damaged heart valves and rhythm disturbances can also lead to failure in the pump function.

Cardiac failure can develop gradually or occur acutely, and can affect the right, left or both ventricles. Because the right and left ventricles pump blood into the pulmonary and systemic circulations, respectively, the symptoms will be different depending on which ventricle fails.

PATHOPHYSIOLOGY OF CARDIAC FAILURE

The right ventricle receives blood from the right atrium which, in turn, receives the venous return. If the pump function of the right ventricle is reduced, the blood will be 'congested' in the veins in the same way as the amount of water will increase in a dammed-up river. Because of the congestion, the volume and the pressure in the ventricle will increase. The increase in pressure travels to the large veins and backwards to the capillary vessels, and plasma can thus leak from the bloodstream to the tissues. If the leakage from the blood to the tissue is greater than that drained back by the lymphatic vessels, oedema will develop. Because of gravity, right-sided cardiac failure will cause oedema in the lower extremities, but internal organs can also be affected. See Figure 17.11.

The left ventricle receives blood from the lungs. If the pump function of the left ventricle is inhibited, then blood will accumulate backwards towards the lungs. Depending on how pronounced the failure is, it can present as anything from mild dyspnoea to pronounced pulmonary oedema. See Figure 17.12.

The heart's ability to pump is controlled by the heart rate, the pressure in the ventricles when they are filled (preload), the resistance against which they pump (afterload) and the contractility in the heart muscle cells. Normally, the ventricles eject the same volume of blood with which they are filled. An increase in preload produces stretching of the heart muscle, which results in an increased ventricular volume and thereby a more favourable filling situation. In serious cardiac failure with loss of contractility, the ability to increase the pump function by stretching the heart muscle is fully utilized, and a continued increase in preload results in further increased congestion in supplying veins.

In cardiac failure, the body will redistribute the blood the heart manages to pump, so that blood supply to the vital organs is preserved. This occurs because arteries in some tissues vasoconstrict. The result is increased resistance to blood leaving the heart and a chronic increased load that stimulates hypertrophy of the heart muscle. In such a situation, the heart is strongly stimulated through sympathetic activation.

In the treatment of cardiac failure, it is necessary to reduce both preload and afterload. A high afterload is considerably more energy-demanding than a high preload, particularly when the heart's own blood supply is compromised.

Symptoms and findings in cardiac failure

Symptoms and findings in right-sided cardiac failure include a heavy feeling and swelling in the legs, weight increase and pressure below the right rib arch (liver congestion).

In left-sided cardiac failure, the symptoms are heavy breathing, coughing and gurgling respiration, depending on the degree of seriousness of the failure. The

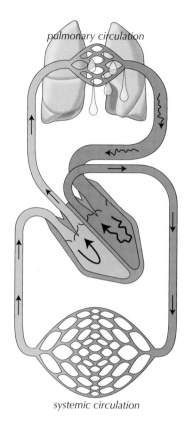

pulmonary circulation

systemic circulation

Figure 17.12 **Failure in the left ventricle** can cause congestion in the pulmonary circuit.

oedema will spread over the base of the lungs in a person who is upright, and throughout the lungs if the person is in a supine position. As left-sided cardiac failure develops, right-side cardiac failure will gradually develop.

In both right- and left-sided cardiac failure, fatigue and a low threshold for exhaustion are common.

Causes of cardiac failure
Acute cardiac failure can occur in association with myocardial infarction, valvular defects, rapid progressive hypertension and pulmonary embolism. Chronic cardiac failure is observed as a late result of minor infarctions, progressive valvular defect and hypertension.

All situations that put stress on the circulation, e.g. physical or mental stress, infection with pyrexia, anaemia or rhythm disturbances, can be triggering factors for failure and must be treated if the heart shows poor pump function.

GOAL OF DRUG TREATMENT

The goal of drug treatment is to improve the pump function of the heart thereby relieving symptoms, improving exercise tolerance, reducing the frequency of acute exacerbations and reducing mortality. This can be done by reducing the afterload, the resistance in the circulation (vasodilating drugs), the preload and circulating blood volume (diuretics), or by briefly strengthening the heart's force of contraction (positive inotropic drugs), which can be achieved by using one or a combination of the drugs listed below.

Relevant drug groups
- Diuretics (reduce the blood volume)
- ACE inhibitors or angiotensin-II-receptor inhibitors (vasodilation on the arterial side and reduction of the circulating blood volume)
- Glycerol nitrate/isosorbide mono- and dinitrate (vasodilation on the venous side)
- Cardiac glycosides (positive inotropic drugs)
- Others, e.g. aldosterone antagonists (reduce the blood volume)
- β-blockers (vasodilation on the arterial side by reduced activity in the sympathetic nervous system).

In the treatment of acute cardiac failure in hospital, other drugs are also used, e.g. dopamine, dobutamine and phosphodiesterase inhibitors. These drugs are used only briefly during intensive treatment since tolerance develops very quickly.

OVERVIEW OF DRUGS USED TO TREAT CARDIOVASCULAR DISEASES

Treatment of diseases of the cardiovascular system is complicated because the person who is being treated often has several diseases/conditions that interact with each other. A specific treatment can therefore improve one part of the disease complex while exacerbating another.

- Adrenergic receptor blockers (primarily β-blockers)
  - block receptors in the heart and arteries such that noradrenaline and adrenaline have reduced effect
  - suppress central nervous stimulation of the heart and arteries
  - suppress the activity in the renin–angiotensin–aldosterone system
- Calcium-channel blockers – inhibit influx of calcium ions in heart muscle and in vascular smooth muscle

- ACE inhibitors
  - inhibit the formation of angiotensin-II by inhibiting ACE
  - reduce the secretion of aldosterone
- Angiotensin-II-receptor antagonists – inhibit angiotensin-II by blocking angiotensin-II receptors
- Diuretics – increase urine elimination, thereby reducing the circulating blood volume and, indirectly, the fluid volume of the tissues
- Organic nitrates
  - primarily dilate veins, but also arteries, thereby causing a redistribution of the blood volume in the venous system
  - improve collateral blood flow in ischaemic tissue in the heart muscle
- Cardiac glycosides
  - increase the influx of calcium into heart muscle cells, thereby increasing the force of contraction
  - reduce the heart rate in supraventricular tachyarrhythmias
- Anti-atherogenic drugs
  - alter the ratio of atherogenic/anti-atherogenic substances in a favourable direction
  - can cause regression of previously formed arteriosclerotic masses
- Prostaglandin synthesis inhibitors – reduce the formation of thromboxanes (e.g. thromboxane A_2), thereby preventing platelet aggregation
- Methyldopa, clonidine and hydralazine – reduce central nervous stimulation of the heart and blood vessels and therefore lower the blood pressure.

ADRENERGIC BLOCKERS (ADRENOCEPTOR BLOCKERS)

Noradrenaline and adrenaline are naturally occurring substances that stimulate α- and β-adrenoceptors. These receptors are found in many of the body's tissues, in varying density and with varying ratios. Blockade of α- and β-adrenoceptors prevents noradrenaline and adrenaline from exerting their effects, and thereby has a primarily relaxing effect on muscles with such receptors.

The action of these drugs and further details of the autonomic nervous system can be found in Chapter 11, Structure and function of the nervous system.

Anatomy and physiology – receptors and effects

The adrenoceptors are divided into α_1-, α_2-, β_1- and β_2-receptors. The α-receptors are primarily found in the heart and large arteries, but also in smaller vessels. The β_1-receptors are found in cardiac muscle and in some vascular smooth muscle of small arteries. β_2-Receptors are predominantly in bronchial smooth muscle and uterine smooth muscle, but are also found in arteries in the skeletal muscle. See Figure 17.13.

Noradrenaline and adrenaline stimulate both α- and β-receptors. α_1-Receptors are located postsynaptically. Their stimulation causes contraction of muscle with such receptors. Blockade of these receptors causes reduced contraction. α_2-Receptors are located presynaptically. Stimulating these receptors inhibits the release of noradrenaline from the presynaptic terminal, while blockade causes increased release of noradrenaline. Blockade of the α_2-receptors is therefore undesirable in situations where it is necessary to reduce adrenergic stimulation.

Stimulation of β_1-receptors causes an increase in heart rate and force of contraction. Blockade of these receptors produces the opposite effect. Stimulation of β_2-receptors causes dilation of some smooth muscles – bronchial and uterine.

The ratio of α- and β-receptors in smooth muscle in different areas of a vascular bed vary and difference in the affinity of these receptors for different drugs account for the characteristic effects seen when such drugs are used.

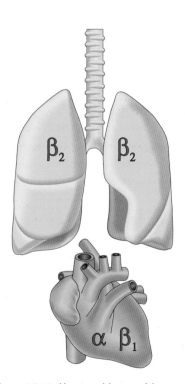

Figure 17.13 **Heart and lungs with receptor types.** The heart has primarily α- and β_1-receptors. The lungs have primarily β_2-receptors.

Non–selective and selective blockers

Drugs with a blocking effect on either α- or β-adrenoceptors can be useful in different cardiovascular diseases. Those that act on both β_1- and β_2-adrenoceptors are called non-selective blockers. Those that primarily act on α_1-receptors are called selective α_1-blockers. Those that primarily act on β_1-receptors are called selective β_1-blockers.

Blockade of a particular receptor type can result in reflex or adaptive compensation measures in other physiological processes. The adaptive compensation can occur either quickly or gradually.

The α–receptor blockers (α–blockers)

In non-selective blockade of the α-receptors, the α_1-receptors and the α_2-receptors are blocked. Blockade of α_2-receptors results in increased influx of calcium in the presynaptic neuron and thereby causes an increased release of noradrenaline. The effect of released noradrenaline on the α_1-receptors is blocked, but noradrenaline can cause tachycardia by stimulation of the β_1-receptors. See Figure 17.14. In clinical use, only drugs with α_1-blocking and combined α_1- and non-selective β-blocking properties are used.

Blockade of α_1-receptors causes dilation of large and small arteries. Peripheral resistance is reduced, so that the blood pressure falls. As the β-receptors are not blocked, there can be a mild reflex increase in the heart rate. By combining α_1-blockers with β-blockers, it is possible to prevent the reflex increase in heart rate.

Adverse effects. If the dosage is high, there is a hypotensive effect and reduced cardiac output. This is particularly pronounced after the first dose.

Because of the effect on α-receptors in other tissues of the body, it is also possible to experience other adverse effects such as contraction of the ciliary muscle of the eye, congestion of the nose due to swollen mucosa, and peripheral oedema due to vasodilation.

Indications for use

The primary use of α_1-receptor blockers is in the treatment of resistant hypertension. α_1-receptor blockers do not affect the bronchial muscle, and are therefore well suited for asthmatics with hypertension. The favourable long-term effects of reduced cardiovascular morbidity (seen when using β-blockers) are not seen when using α_1-receptor blockers. α_1-receptor blockers are also used to improve micturition in benign prostatic hypertrophy, in that the muscles in the neck of the bladder and the prostate gland are dilated by blockade of α_1-receptors.

The β–receptor blockers (β–blockers)

Different β-blockers have different properties. The most important properties are selectivity and water/lipid solubility. These properties partly determine the choice of drug, based on expected effect, adverse effects and concurrent diseases, especially cardiac failure, obstructive lung diseases, renal failure and diabetes mellitus.

Selectivity in the effect of β-receptor blockers

Non-selective β-blockers have effects on both β_1- and β_2-receptors. Large doses of selective β_1-blockers also cause blockade of the β_2-receptors. Peripheral vascular effects, e.g. cold hands and feet, are least pronounced with the use of selective β_1-blockers. The selectivity is relative and not equally pronounced in all patients.

Pharmacokinetics. Absorption after oral administration is good, but lipid-soluble drugs have varying biological availability in different users. This is probably associated with individual differences in metabolism.

Lipid solubility and metabolism. Some β-blockers are more lipid-soluble than others and easily cross the blood–brain barrier. The concentration in the central

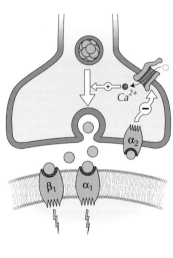

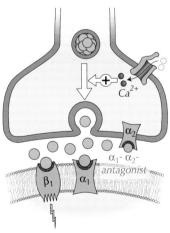

Figure 17.14 Blockade of α_1- and α_2-receptors. Blockade of α_2-receptors increases the release of noradrenaline, which stimulates the β_1-receptors.

	LS	↓RD
Non-selective β-blockers		
Nadolol	No	Yes
Oxprenolol	Yes	No
Pindolol	Mod	Mod
Propanolol	Yes	No
Sotalol	No	Yes
Timolol	Mod	Mod
Selective β$_1$-blockers		
Acebutolol	Yes	No
Atenolol	No	Yes
Bisoprolol	Mod	Mod
Celiprolol	No	Yes
Esmolol	Yes	No
Metoprolol	Mod	Mod
Nebivolol	Yes	No

Table 17.1 Overview of some β-blockers

LS, lipid solubility; ↓RD, reduced dose in renal failure; Mod, moderate.

nervous system increases and central nervous system adverse effects such as nightmares and hallucinations are more pronounced with these than with the more water-soluble ones. Lipid-soluble drugs are largely metabolized in the liver, while water-soluble drugs are eliminated unmetabolized in the urine. This influences the choice of drug in patients with renal failure and those who suffer adverse effects from the central nervous system (see Table 17.1).

Effects. The load of the heart and its metabolism are lowered by a reduction in both its force and rate of contraction. In turn, the heart's requirements for oxygen are lowered. Initially, an increase in peripheral vessel resistance is often observed, which can contribute to maintenance of the elevated blood pressure, but the peripheral resistance is gradually reduced to its original value and blood pressure drops.

Adverse effects. The adverse effects are moderate with normal dosing. When the dose is too high, and therefore the effect is too strong, cardiac failure can be triggered with reduced cardiac output, hypotension, dizziness and other adverse effects as consequences. Reduced peripheral circulation, with cold hands and feet, is common. Rhythm disturbances, particularly in the form of atrioventricular blockages and symptomatic bradycardia, can be a result of their inhibitory effect on the heart's conduction system.

Other observed adverse effects include effects on the central nervous system, such as listlessness, sleep disturbances, nightmares, hallucinations and depression. Gastrointestinal adverse effects, such as nausea, vomiting and diarrhoea, cause some people to stop taking these drugs.

During hypoglycaemia, β$_2$-receptors in the liver are stimulated, resulting in an increased release of glucose. Use of β-blockers can reduce the release of glucose and mask hypoglycaemic symptoms such as tremor and tachycardia. These drugs must therefore be used with caution in diabetics.

Prolonged use of β-blockers has adverse effects on blood lipids, resulting in an increase in triglycerides and a reduction in high-density lipoprotein (HDL) cholesterol. However, the clinical significance of these alterations is overshadowed by the favourable effects of the drugs in the treatment of hypertension and arrhythmia.

Pregnancy and breastfeeding. Generally, β-blockers are suitable for pregnant women when it is necessary to treat hypertension, e.g. at the end of the pregnancy. Caution should be exercised, however, when using them over a longer period, since growth retardation in fetuses has been reported. The transfer of water-soluble β-blockers into breast milk is less than that of lipid-soluble β-blockers.

Indications for use

Adrenergic blockers are particularly useful in the treatment of hypertension, angina pectoris, myocardial infarction and rhythm disturbances.

Hypertension. β-blockers are useful in the treatment of hypertension, and are particularly well suited if there is concurrent angina pectoris and/or a rapid heart rate. Even though their mechanisms of action are not completely understood, it is assumed that their effects are due to a combination of direct blockade of catecholamines, reduced sympathetic activity and reduced activity in the renin–angiotensin–aldosterone system. All these effects contribute to a lowering of blood pressure. If blood pressure is not lowered with a β-blocker alone, a supplement of diuretics or a calcium antagonist can be useful.

Important clinical studies have shown that β-blockers have a primary preventive effect on the harmful consequences of hypertension.

Angina pectoris. The beneficial effect in the treatment of angina pectoris is due to reduced load of the heart because the force of contraction is reduced. When the heart's load decreases, the requirements of the heart, which are met by the coronary circulation are reduced. Because the rate of contraction is lowered, the length of the diastole increases, i.e. the period when blood flow through the coronary circulation is greatest. Gradual reduction of β-blockers is advised as sudden withdrawal may exacerbate angina.

Myocardial infarction. Extensive studies have shown that use of both selective and non-selective β-blockers increases survival in patients who have suffered myocardial infarction. β-Blockers administered within 12 h from the onset of symptoms can reduce both the size of the infarction and the tendency to develop arrhythmias. β-blockers administered later after an infarction can reduce the chance of a new infarction and the one-year mortality rate by approximately 25 per cent. Using β-blockers following myocardial infarction is unsuitable for patients with obstructive airway disease, uncontrolled cardiac failure, hypertension and bradycardia.

Cardiac failure. Beta-blockers have a beneficial effect in cardiac failure. Because they have a negative inotropic effect on the heart, there has long been scepticism about the use of β-blockers in this disorder. However, several studies have shown that selective β_1-blockers and combined α_1-blockers and non-selective β-blockers reduce both symptoms and mortality in moderate to serious cardiac failure with reduced systolic function.

Rhythm disturbances. By delaying the conduction rate of cardiac action potentials, β-blockers will reduce the ventricular rate in atrial triggered flutter and fibrillation. Extra ventricular beats are reduced in cases where high sympathetic activity contributes to increased impulse traffic. However, when used in those with a tendency for atrioventricular blockage, they can exacerbate the blockage.

Other uses of β-blockers. Beta-blockers are also used in the treatment of glaucoma, migraine and as preliminary treatment before surgery of the thyroid in hyperthyroidism.

α₁–selective blockers
Doxazosin, Indoramin, Prazosin, Terazosin

Combined α₁–selective and and non–selective β–blockers
Labetalol, Carvedilol

β–blockers, nonselective
Nadolol, Oxprenolol, Pindolol, Propanolol, Sotalol, Timolol

β₁–selective blockers
Acebutolol, Atenolol, Bisoprolol, Celiprolol, Esmolol, Metoprolol, Nebivolol

Table 17.2 Adrenoceptor blocking drugs

Some adrenergic blockers are listed in Table 17.2.

CALCIUM-CHANNEL BLOCKERS

Calcium is necessary for the muscle filaments to interact with each other and therefore contract. This is true in both vascular and cardiac muscle. In addition, impulses that control the heart rate and the conduction rate of cardiac action potentials in the heart's conduction system will be inhibited by low calcium levels in the cells. Thus, the blood pressure and both the heart's force of contraction and rate of contraction are decreased by a reduction in the calcium concentration.

Selectivity in the effect on different types of muscle
There are several types of calcium channel, therefore an individual calcium-channel blocker may have different effects in cardiac muscle from those it has in vascular smooth muscle. Equally, differing concentrations of a drug may produce different effects in the same tissue. Skeletal muscles are largely unaffected by calcium-channel blockers. The calcium channels have binding sites to which the different calcium-channel blockers can bind. Likewise, just as it is possible to exploit the differences in the β-blockers, it is possible to exploit the differences between the calcium-channel blockers with choice of drug.

Calcium-channel blockers with the greatest effect on blood vessels
Calcium-channel blockers that have the greatest effect on vascular smooth muscle in arterioles will produce a decrease in peripheral resistance. Their use is favoured in disease with poor peripheral resistance, e.g. diabetes, and in treating hypertension in asthmatics. See Figure 17.15.

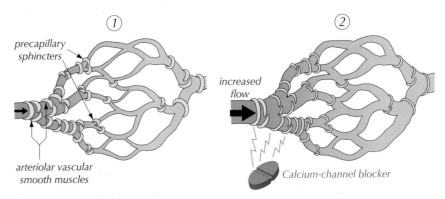

Figure 17.15 **Calcium-channel blockers** with an effect on vascular smooth muscle in small arteries cause a reduction in resistance by dilating arterioles.

Nimodipine has been shown to have particular effects on blood vessels in the cerebral circulation, and produces reduced vascular spasms and improved blood flow after subarachnoid haemorrhage.

Calcium-channel blockers with the greatest effect on the heart

Verapamil and diltiazem have a more pronounced inhibitory effect on the contractile force of heart muscle and on the heart's conduction of cardiac action potentials than do other calcium-channel blockers. The uses of these are for hypertension without poor peripheral blood flow with a simultaneous high heart rate and in supraventricular tachycardias. See Figure 17.16.

Mechanism of action and effects. The calcium content of muscle cells is regulated with the help of calcium channels and is determined by the extent to which the channels are open. By blocking calcium channels, it is possible to reduce the calcium content in the cells. See Figure 17.17.

Pharmacokinetics. The calcium-channel blockers are absorbed well after oral administration. They undergo metabolism in the liver and are eliminated largely as inactive metabolites through the kidneys. All are highly protein-bound. The half-life varies from 3 to 50 h. The time to achieve their effect varies, as does the time required to clear a toxic dose.

Adverse effects. Calcium-channel blockers which have the greatest effect on the heart's force of contraction and conduction of action potentials can cause too large a reduction in blood pressure and an increased tendency to the development of cardiac failure. Likewise, blockage of the impulse conduction in the atrioventricular node can be pronounced. See Figure 17.16. Verapamil and diltiazem should therefore not be combined with β-blockers in conduction disturbances, or where there is a tendency for cardiac failure.

Calcium-channel blockers which have the greatest effect on the smooth muscle of blood vessels have less serious dose-dependent adverse effects than the other group.

Other rare adverse effects are flushing, dizziness, peripheral oedemas, nausea and constipation.

Pregnancy and breastfeeding. Calcium antagonists should not be administered to pregnant women as there have been reports of embryo toxicity. There is little documentation regarding breastfeeding and harmful effects.

Indications for use

Calcium-channel blockers are useful in hypertension, angina pectoris and rhythm disturbances.

Hypertension. Calcium-channel blockers are used in the treatment of hypertension. Favourable effects can be achieved in conditions where there is also a poor peripheral circulation, as in angina pectoris, diabetes mellitus, and hypertension in asthmatics where the contraction of bronchial smooth muscle should be avoided. If treatment with calcium-channel blockers alone is ineffective, a supplement of a β-blocker or a diuretic can be useful. It is has not been shown that calcium-channel blockers have the same favourable preventive effects against the consequences of hypertension as do diuretics, β-blockers or ACE inhibitors.

Angina pectoris. The beneficial effect of calcium-channel blockers in the treatment of angina is assumed to arise from reduced load of the heart due to a reduced force of contraction and reduced need for coronary circulation. Reduced peripheral resistance will also reduce afterload. When the heart rate is lowered and the time

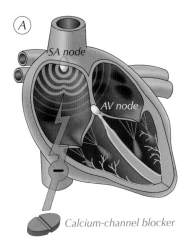

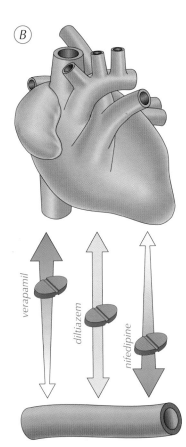

Figure 17.16 Calcium-channel blockers can cause blockade of action potential conduction when they are used in large doses. Calcium-channel blockers have selectivity. Some calcium-channel blockers have a greater effect on action potential generation and conduction than others that have their primary effect on vascular smooth muscle in small arteries.

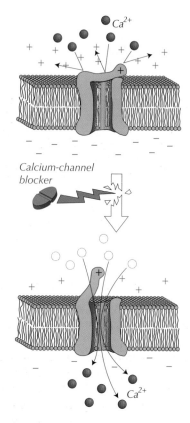

Figure 17.17 Calcium–channel blockers inhibit the opening of calcium channels and thereby reduce the influx of calcium ions in muscle cells in the heart and arteries.

Calcium–channel blockers with the greatest effect on blood vessels
Amlodipine, Felodipine, Isradipine, Lacidipine, Lercandipine, Nicardipine, Nifedipine, Nimodipine, Nisoldipine

Calcium–channel blockers with the greatest effect on the heart
Diltiazem, Verapamil

Table 17.3 Calcium–channel blockers

spent in diastole increases, so blood flow through the coronary circulation increases.

Rhythm disturbances. By delaying the conduction of cardiac action potentials, calcium-channel blockers will reduce the ventricular rate in supraventricular flutter and fibrillation. Atrioventricular blockage can be exacerbated by the simultaneous use of β-blockers and verapamil or diltiazem. These combinations are contraindicated in patients with a tendency to develop blockage of the impulse conduction in the heart.

Other uses of calcium-channel blockers. Reduced vasoconstriction of cerebral vessels and improved cerebral blood flow after subarachnoid haemorrhage have given nimodipine a place in treating the condition. The use of calcium antagonists in some patients suffering from migraine and Raynaud's disease (vascular spasms) has been shown to be beneficial.

Some calcium-channel blockers are listed in Table 17.3.

ACE INHIBITORS

Angiotensin-converting enzyme inhibitors are drugs that prevent the formation of angiotensin-II. Therefore, a direct vasoconstrictor effect on small arteries is prevented, and stimulation of aldosterone secretion from the adrenals is reduced. In addition, the breakdown of bradykinin, a peptide that is mainly created in inflamed tissue and that has vasodilatory effect on small arteries, is reduced. The result is reduced peripheral resistance (i.e. reduced afterload).

Mechanism of action and effects. Renin is an enzyme produced in the juxtaglomerular apparatus (JGA) of the nephron. Renin diffuses to the blood and converts a peptide, angiotensinogen, which is synthesized in the liver, to angiotensin-I. When angiotensin-I reaches the lungs, ACE will metabolize (convert) angiotensin-I to angiotensin-II, which:

- is one of the body's most potent vasoconstrictor substances
- contributes to central nervous system signals which result in vasoconstriction
- is important for the autoregulation of blood pressure in the kidneys and therefore glomerular filtration
- stimulates the release of aldosterone from the adrenal cortex; aldosterone increases the absorption of sodium, and therefore circulating blood volume
- increases the feeling of thirst.

Use of ACE inhibitors reduces a number of stimuli that contribute directly and indirectly to increased peripheral resistance and increased blood volume. See Figures 17.4 (p. 227) and 17.18. Both preload and afterload are thereby reduced, and the load of the heart is decreased.

Pharmacokinetics. Absorption of ACE inhibitors is generally good after oral administration, although the absorption of captopril is delayed by food intake.

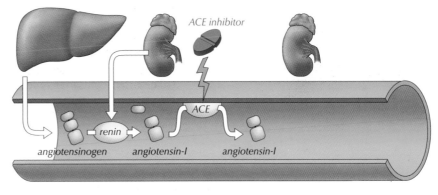

Figure 17.18 **ACE inhibitors** prevent the angiotensin-converting enzyme (ACE) from converting angiotensin-I to angiotensin-II. The vasoconstrictor effect and secretion of aldosterone from the adrenal cortex are reduced.

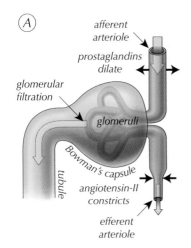

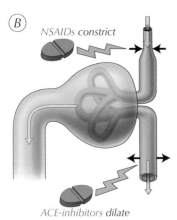

Figure 17.19 **Effect of ACE inhibitors and NSAIDs on glomerular blood flow.** Angiotensin-II contracts efferent arterioles from glomeruli, as shown in (A). ACE inhibitors reduce the formation of angiotensin-II and thereby dilate efferent glomerular arterioles (B). This results in a drop in the arterial pressure in glomeruli, and less plasma is filtered across to the proximal tubuli, which reduces the renal function. Combining ACE inhibitors may further reduce the glomerular blood flow, and should be avoided.

Elimination is primarily renal, so patients with renal failure should have a reduced dosage.

Adverse effects. Patients who are hypovolaemic from the use of diuretics, salt restriction or other volume loss can experience serious hypotension with the use of ACE inhibitors. This occurs due to a reduced aldosterone secretion and further loss of sodium, and thereby reduced circulating blood volume. The dose should therefore be evaluated in all situations where there is the possibility of a large drop in blood pressure. Since reduced aldosterone secretion results in increased plasma potassium concentration, hyperkalaemia can occur in patients who are using potassium-sparing diuretics simultaneously.

In patients with renal artery stenosis and poor renal blood flow, angiotensin-II is important for the physiological contraction of efferent arterioles arising from glomeruli, such that the pressure in Bowman's capsule, and thereby glomerular filtration, are maintained. Glomerular filtration is necessary for urine production and for elimination of substances that are removed by this mechanism. Use of ACE inhibitors in this patient group can compromise renal function. It is helpful to follow up patients with measurements of creatinine in serum. See Figure 17.19.

Coughing due to reduced breakdown of bradykinin (which stimulates coughing) can be so troublesome that the drug must be discontinued. A reduced sense of taste, nausea, headaches, skin eruptions, fever and increases in liver enzymes may occur.

Pregnancy and breastfeeding. Pregnant women should not use ACE inhibitors, especially in the last two trimesters, because of the possibility of low blood pressure and reduced urine production in the fetus, deformities and death.

Indications for use

The ACE inhibitors are used in hypertension and cardiac failure, especially in patients with concurrent diabetes.

Hypertension. Angiotensin-converting enzyme inhibitors are valuable in the treatment of hypertension, especially in patients with concurrent cardiac failure and poor peripheral circulation, as peripheral resistance is lowered. In hypertension with increased heart rate, ACE inhibitors can be combined with β-blockers. The use of ACE inhibitors has been shown to reduce cardiovascular morbidity and mortality.

ACE inhibitors
Captopril, Cilazapril, Enalapril, Fosinopril, Imidapril, Lisinopril,
Moexipril, Perindopril, Quinapril, Ramipril, Trandolapril

Angiotensin-II-receptor antagonists
Candesartan, Eprosartan, Irbesartan, Losartan, Olmesartan, Telmisartan,
Valsartan

Table 17.4 ACE inhibitors and angiotensin-II-receptor antagonists

Cardiac failure. Angiotensin-converting enzyme inhibitors are the primary drugs of choice in both symptomatic and asymptomatic cardiac failure. Their effects are potentiated by adding a small dose of a diuretic.

Angina pectoris. Angiotensin-converting enzyme inhibitors are not used alone in the treatment of angina pectoris. However, patients with hypertension and concurrent angina pectoris will benefit from the use of these drugs in that the reduction in blood pressure reduces cardiac workload and the need for oxygen.

ANGIOTENSIN-II-RECEPTOR ANTAGONISTS

Losartan is an example of an angiotensin-II-receptor antagonist. These drugs achieve a similar purpose to ACE inhibitors but they act by preventing angiotensin-II from binding to its receptors. Most of the effects of angiotensin-II are inhibited, but aldosterone secretion is only slightly inhibited. Coughing is less pronounced than with the ACE inhibitors. These drugs are used in the treatment of hypertension and cardiac failure.

Some ACE inhibitors and angiotensin-II-receptor antagonists are listed in Table 17.4.

DIURETICS

In adults, approximately 180 L of plasma per day are filtered through the glomeruli of the kidneys and into the nephrons – this is the glomerular filtrate or preurine. During the transport along the nephrons, approximately 99 per cent of the glomerular filtrate is reabsorbed back to the blood. The final urine volume is some 1–2 L. Varying amounts of dissolved substances that are found in the glomerular filtrate are also reabsorbed. See Figure 17.20.

Diuretics are drugs that increase the volume of urine produced by the kidneys. This occurs because the 'normal' reabsorption of electrolytes, especially sodium, from the glomerular filtrate back to the blood, is inhibited. In this way electrolytes (and therefore water) are retained in the urine, which then has a greater volume. This leads to a decrease in the circulating blood volume, since the urine is produced from the blood. When the circulating blood volume is decreased, fluid is drawn from the tissues into the bloodstream. The overall effect achieved is that fluid moves from the tissues to the blood, and from the blood to the urine, whereby it is excreted. In this way, tissue oedema can be reduced.

The most important indications for the use of diuretics are hypertension and cardiac failure with concurrent oedema. However, it is important to be aware of the disturbances in electrolytes, especially when using diuretics.

Diuretics vary in their site of action in the nephron, their efficacy, their duration of action, and how the absorption of electrolytes is affected.

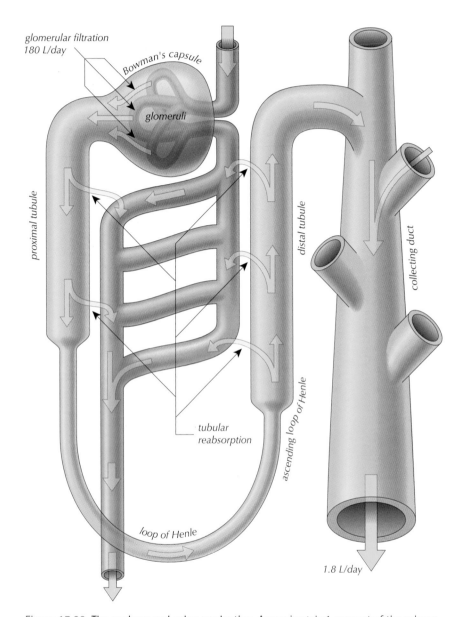

Figure 17.20 **The nephron and urine production.** Approximately 1 per cent of the volume of plasma that reaches the proximal tubules by glomerular filtration leaves the body in the form of urine. Ninety-nine per cent is reabsorbed to the blood at different places along the nephron. The reabsorption occurs because electrolytes in the glomerular filtrate are actively reabsorbed, while water follows passively along.

Regulation of the fluid and electrolyte balance and site of action for diuretics

A nephron is the functional unit of the kidneys. Three processes in the nephron influence the final quantity and composition of the urine:

- *Glomerular filtration* – filtration of plasma in glomeruli, which creates the glomerular filtrate. The glomerular filtrate has the same content of dissolved substances as plasma, but larger particles such as blood corpuscles and proteins are retained in the plasma.

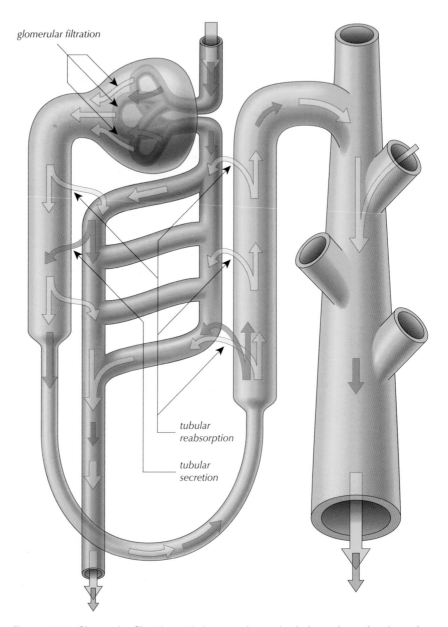

glomerular filtration

tubular reabsorption

tubular secretion

Figure 17.21 **Glomerular filtration, tubular secretion and tubular reabsorption** determine how much of a drug is eliminated via the kidneys. Tubular reabsorption and secretion take place in different parts of the nephron for different substances.

■ *Tubular reabsorption* – this process takes place along the entire length of the nephron, where small molecules are reabsorbed from the glomerular filtrate and back into the bloodstream. Reabsorption of water is linked to this process.
■ *Tubular secretion* – this process takes place in the proximal and distal convoluted tubules, where substances are actively transported from the blood to the glomerular filtrate.

The sum of glomerular filtration, tubular reabsorption and tubular secretion determines the volume of urine and which substances are eliminated via the urine. See Figure 17.21.

Proximal tubules

Approximately 70 per cent of the glomerular filtrate that is formed in the glomeruli is reabsorbed back into the blood in the proximal tubules by tubular reabsorption. In this region, glucose, bicarbonate and amino acids are also reabsorbed. Organic acids (e.g. uric acid) and bases, some antibiotics and a few diuretics themselves are eliminated by tubular secretion in this part of the tubule. The tubular secretion of organic acids (uric acids) can be saturated. Such saturation occurs more easily if diuretics are used at the same time, since these drugs are also eliminated from the blood by the transport system for organic acids. This explains why there can be a decrease in uric acid secretion with use of some diuretics, leading to an acute attack of gout. Cimetidine is a base that is removed by tubular secretion.

The loop of Henle

The U-shaped medullary portion of the nephron between the proximal and distal tubule is the loop of Henle. When the glomerular filtrate has passed through the loop of Henle, approximately 80 per cent of the urine volume and 90 per cent of the sodium have been reabsorbed back to the blood.

Diuretics that act in this part of the nephron (loop diuretics, e.g. bumetanide, furosemide and ethacrynic acid) inhibit the absorption of sodium, potassium and chloride in the ascending limb of the loop of Henle. Loop diuretics are the most potent diuretics for pharmacokinetic reasons and have the most rapid onset of action.

The distal tubule and collecting duct

The distal tubule is the portion of the nephron between the loop of Henle and the collecting duct. Sodium is reabsorbed actively in this part; water and chloride follow passively along. Potassium in the glomerular filtrate is usually reabsorbed effectively in the proximal tubule and in the loop of Henle. In the collecting ducts, a fine adjustment of the urine's potassium content takes place as a result of the action of angiotensin-II and aldosterone.

The distal tubule connects to the collecting ducts where antidiuretic hormone (ADH) increases the absorption of water from the glomerular filtrate. When this fluid, which has now become urine, leaves the collecting ducts, approximately 99 per cent of the volume and 99.5 per cent of sodium in the original glomerular filtrate have been reabsorbed back into the blood.

Diuretics that act in the distal tubules inhibit the absorption of sodium and chloride, and thereby of water.

Contribution of the kidneys to development of oedema in cardiac failure

In cardiac failure, arteries in the kidneys will 'experience' low blood pressure, possibly due to a reduced circulating blood volume. The secretion of renin and aldosterone increases to maintain sodium and water levels in the blood. The increased blood volume results in congestion, development of oedema and exacerbation of cardiac failure. In the following sections, diuretics are discussed in the order according to the location in the nephron where they act.

Diuretics that act in the loop of Henle: loop diuretics

It is common to refer to diuretics that act in the loop of Henle as 'loop diuretics'. They act in the thick segment of the ascending loop.

Mechanism of action and effects. Loop diuretics increase the renal blood flow and thereby cause increased glomerular filtration. In addition, the reabsorption of sodium, potassium and chloride from the glomerular filtrate to the blood is

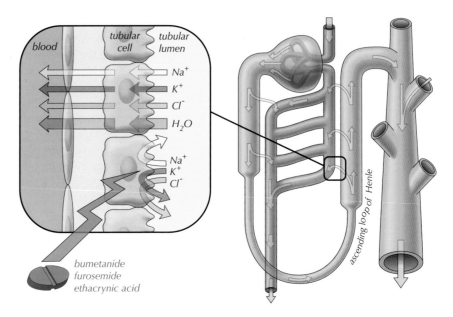

Figure 17.22 **Loop diuretics** act in the ascending limb of the loop of Henle by inhibiting active reabsorption of sodium, potassium and chloride, and thereby the passive absorption of water.

inhibited in the ascending limb of the loop of Henle. See Figure 17.22. Because these substances are held in the lumen of the nephron, and so is water, increased volumes of urine are excreted. Magnesium is also lost with the use of loop diuretics. In addition to the diuretic effect, loop diuretics have a vasodilating effect.

Given by oral administration, the diuretic effect lasts approximately 4–6 h. Loop diuretics should be administered in the morning (and afternoon if necessary) but not in the evening so as to avoid nocturnal diuresis.

Adverse effects. The most important adverse effects are potassium loss leading to hypokalaemia and therefore an effect on the excitability of the heart's conduction system and on cardiac muscle, leading to a tendency to develop arrhythmias. With use over a longer period of time, it is therefore often necessary to give potassium as a supplement or to add potassium sparing diuretics if the effect of loop diuretics is insufficient. When loop diuretics are combined with cardiac glycosides, patients are at high risk arrhythmias if plasma potassium is low. At particularly low plasma potassium concentrations, hydrogen ions are eliminated in the urine in exchange for potassium, simultaneously as bicarbonate is formed. In this way, loop diuretics can contribute to metabolic alkalosis with concurrent acid urine (paradoxical aciduria).

Gout can be triggered when the tubular secretion of uric acids is saturated by elimination of the loop diuretics. Patients with gout should therefore take great care when using these drugs for prolonged periods of time.

High doses can cause volume loss with hypotension and development of shock, especially with the simultaneous use of ACE inhibitors, which inhibit the aldosterone secretion and cause further sodium and volume loss. The elderly are at particular risk from side effects so lower initial doses should be used. In renal failure doses should be reduced.

Pregnancy and breastfeeding. Generally, diuretics should be avoided in pregnancy and breastfeeding. Loop diuretics are however the primary choice if diuretics must be used during pregnancy.

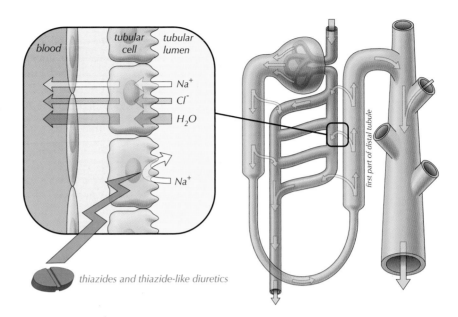

Figure 17.23 **Thiazides and thiazide-like diuretics** act by inhibiting active reabsorption of sodium and the passive accompanying reabsorption of chloride and water in the first section of the distal tubules.

Indication for use
Oedema of cardiac (pulmonary or ankle oedema), renal (global oedema or hypertension) or hepatic (acites) origin is the most important indication for the use of loop diuretics. The vasodilating effect on large veins appears immediately after absorption and is faster than the diuretic effect. Vessel dilatation and the reduction in circulating blood volume reduce venous return and therefore the load of the heart (preload decreases). This effect is particularly valuable in the treatment of acute left-sided cardiac failure with congestion in the pulmonary circulation. Right-sided cardiac failure with congestion in the systemic circulation is also treated with loop diuretics. Acute hypercalcaemia can be treated with an infusion of glucose or saline solution containing loop diuretics, which will promote excretion of the excess calcium. If the oedema is caused by a decrease in renal function, loop diuretics will increase the volume of urine produced, leading to reduced tissue oedema. Oedema of hepatic origin is most often due to decreased synthesis of albumin and therefore a loss of osmotic potential in the blood. Loop diuretics are effective in reducing tissue oedema caused by hepatic failure.

Diuretics with a site of action in the first portion of the distal tubule: thiazides
This group of diuretics is known as the thiazides and thiazide-like diuretics.

Mechanism of action and effects. Thiazides inhibit the active absorption of sodium and the passive accompanying absorption of chloride in the first section of the distal tubule. By doing so, elimination of sodium, chloride and water also increases. See Figure 17.23. The glomerular filtrate will have an increased concentration of sodium when it reaches the distal tubules, where it will have a tendency to be drawn into the tubule cells. This results in an increased negative charge in the lumen of the collecting duct. Potassium is therefore drawn out of the cells and into the lumen, and is lost with the urine. This potassium loss makes it relevant to add potassium to these drugs. Several of these drugs are often combined with potassium.

The elimination of bicarbonate is less than the corresponding sodium elimination, to the extent that a metabolic alkalosis develops with long-term use of thiazides. The blood pressure-reducing effect is initially associated with volume loss, but with long-term use, the reduction in blood pressure is maintained by the vasodilatatory effect of the thiazides. In comparison with loop diuretics, the diuretic effect of the thiazides is decreased in renal failure.

Adverse effects. With the use of thiazides, potassium is exchanged for sodium. A small dose of thiazides produces a maximal or close to maximal lowering effect on blood pressure compared to a higher dose. Higher doses may result in marked disturbances of plasma electrolytes, especially hypokalemia. Supplements of potassium are often necessary if a thiazide with a potassium supplement is not used.

Gout can be triggered because the tubular secretion of organic acids is saturated by elimination of the thiazides themselves.

Thiazide diuretics render the β cells in the pancreas less sensitive to high glucose concentration in the blood (increased glucose tolerance), such that the secretion of insulin decreases. In this way, a higher plasma glucose concentration is tolerated. This can provoke latent diabetes.

Thiazides reduce the elimination of lithium. It is necessary to monitor lithium levels in those patients who use the drugs simultaneously.

Pregnancy and breastfeeding. Thiazides are not recommended for pregnant women and women who are breastfeeding. Use during pregnancy causes reduced placental blood flow. Electrolyte disturbances can occur in both mother and fetus and reduced milk production is seen in breastfeeding mothers.

Indication for use
These drugs have a moderate blood pressure-reducing effect and are used to treat hypertension and heart failure. Thiazides are often the first choice of drugs used in the treatment of moderate hypertension and can be used as supplements to most other antihypertensive drugs.

Diuretics with a site of action in the last section of the distal tubule: potassium-sparing diuretics

Aldosterone antagonists and potassium-sparing drugs without aldosterone-inhibiting effects belong to this group.

Mechanism of action and effects. The aldosterone antagonists prevent the action of aldosterone in the distal tubule. As aldosterone increases the absorption of sodium and the secretion of potassium, the use of aldosterone antagonists results in loss of sodium and retention of potassium.

Amiloride inhibits the absorption of sodium in the last section of the distal tubule, and the elimination of sodium, chloride and water increases. The secretion of potassium and magnesium is inhibited. See Figure 17.24.

Adverse effects. Hyperkalaemia is the greatest danger, and potassium supplements should not be administered together with these drugs. Gynaecomastia and impotence are observed in male users, and hirsutism and menstrual disturbances in females. The explanation for this is that the aldosterone antagonists can stimulate steroid receptors that influence the synthesis of sex hormones.

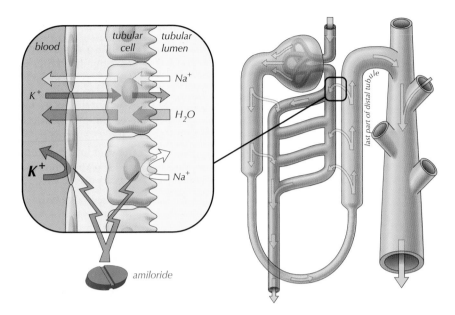

Figure 17.24 **Potassium-sparing diuretics.** Sodium is reabsorbed against potassium in the last section of the distal tubule. Diuretics that act in this part of the nephron increase the elimination of sodium and water, and cause increased concentration of potassium in the blood.

Pregnancy and breastfeeding. These drugs should not be used by pregnant women or women who are breastfeeding because of possible growth retardation (reduced placental circulation) and reduced milk production.

Indications for use
Used alone, these drugs have a weak to moderate diuretic effect. Aldosterone antagonists are used in situations where high plasma concentrations of aldosterone exist, such as in cirrhosis of the liver, right-sided cardiac failure and in tumours in the adrenal cortex, where aldosterone is synthesized.

Potassium-sparing diuretics are therefore often used together with a thiazide or a loop diuretic, especially in cardiac failure with oedema. Therefore, it is possible to avoid dangerous cardiac arrhythmias that can occur with low potassium concentrations. It is also possible to utilize a potassium-sparing diuretic together with digitalis in cardiac failure, if the patient does not receive other potassium supplements.

Some diuretics are listed in Table 17.5.

Loop diuretics
Furosemide, Bumetanide, Torasemide

Thiazide diuretics
Bendroflumethiazide, Chlortalidone, Cyclopenthiazide, Indapamide, Metolazone, Xipamide

Potassium sparing diuretics
Amiloride, Triamterene

Aldosterone antagonists
Spironolactone, Epleronone

Table 17.5 Diuretics

ORGANIC NITRATES

Organic nitrates have two somewhat different primary indications for use, angina pectoris and acute congestive heart failure. They include drugs such as glyceryl trinitrate and isosorbide mononitrate and dinitrate.

Mechanism of action and effects. Organic nitrates act by releasing nitric oxide (NO), which causes smooth muscle to relax. In small doses, the nitrates have a relaxing effect on the veins in muscles, reducing venous return to the heart. The volume load (preload) is lowered, and the pressures in both the pulmonary circulation and the systemic circulation are reduced. This improves circulatory function in patients with congestive heart failure.

With increasing doses, both veins and arteries are dilated, so the pressure in the systemic circulation, and therefore the afterload, is reduced; thus, the heart's workload and need for oxygen are lowered. In addition, the blood is redistributed to ischaemic areas of the heart by increased collateral circulation. See Figure 17.25.

Pharmacokinetics. Glyceryl trinitrate (nitroglycerine), which is used in tablets that are placed under the tongue or as a mouth spray, is absorbed quickly across the oral mucosa and provides pain relief after approximately 1 min. It is used to suppress acute attacks of chest pain and as a short-lasting prophylactic. The tablets are not effective if they are swallowed because they undergo rapid first-pass metabolism. Glyceryl trinitrate is absorbed well through the skin, and several preparations are available as patches with and without a depot effect.

The isosorbide dinitrates and mononitrates are used as tablets that provide a longer effect because they have less first-pass metabolism and a longer half-life.

Because of the reduced effect with continuous use (i.e. tolerance develops), it is necessary to include an 8–10 h period during the day when patients know by experience they are least troubled by angina pains and are unlikely to need the drug.

Adverse effects. Other than hypotension, which is observed particularly in the upright position and at high doses, there are no serious adverse effects with the use of plasters or enteral formulations when they are taken in the recommended doses.

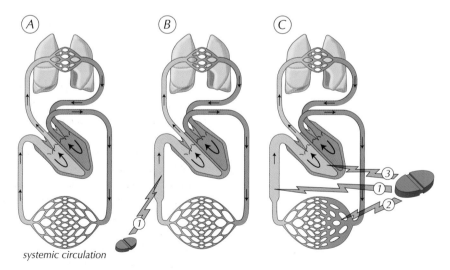

systemic circulation

Figure 17.25 **Organic nitrates.** (A) Normal situation. (B) In small doses, organic nitrates cause dilation of veins, particularly capacitance vessels (1). (C) Larger doses also dilate arterioles (2), and collateral blood flow in the heart improves (3).

Organic nitrates
Glyceryl trinitrate, Isosorbide dinitrate, Isosorbide mononitrate

---

Table 17.6 Organic nitrates

However, throbbing headaches, flushing and nausea can occur. Following high-dose intravenous administration, these effects can be pronounced.

Indications for use

Sublingual forms are suitable for treating and preventing attacks of angina pectoris in that the therapeutic effect is quickly achieved and they have few systemic adverse effects. Also during an acute phase of myocardial infarction sublingual or intravenous forms are used to dilate big veins (capacitance vessels) thereby reducing the heart's load. For prophylactic use, it is better to choose tablets or patches that provide a reasonably consistent plasma concentration over a longer period of time. Intravenous forms are used in unstable angina pectoris and in acute congestive heart failure.

Some organic nitrates are listed in Table 17.6.

CARDIAC GLYCOSIDES

The two most important cardiac glycosides are digoxin and digitoxin. These drugs produce an increased force of contraction of the heart and are used to supplement treatment of congestive heart failure and in rapid supraventricular arrhythmias. Digitalis reduces morbidity in congestive heart failure.

Mechanism of action and effects. The cardiac glycosides inhibit an energy-requiring transport system, the Na^+/K^+-ATPase (sodium–potassium pump) in the membrane of cardiac muscle cells. The inhibition of Na^+/K^+-ATPase causes an increase in intracellular sodium concentration. In turn this inhibits a sodium (in)/calcium (out) transporter which results in an increase in intracellular calcium concentration. See Figure 17.26. Increased intracellular calcium causes an increase in calcium in the sarcoplasmic reticulum. Thus, a larger amount of calcium is released when an action potential is triggered and a stronger contractile response is triggered. Corresponding inhibition of Na^+/K^+-ATPase also occurs in the baroreceptors. In doing so, these seem to regain their function, which is reduced in untreated cardiac failure.

The cardiac glycosides also exert beneficial effects via the autonomic nervous system via increased vagal tone, which possibly contributes even more to a positive inotropic effect than does the increased calcium concentration in the cardiac muscle cells. With an increase in the force of contraction, blood is pumped more efficiently out of the heart. There is an increase in renal blood flow which helps to reduce oedema, often seen in cardiac failure.

Digitalis also results in inhibition of conduction with reduced ventricular rate, with a risk of increased activity in ectopic pacemakers by shortening phase IV in ventricular myocardial cells. A reduced heart rate is possible due to a direct stimulation of the vagus (parasympathetic nerve). The cardiac glycosides compete with potassium for the binding site on Na^+/K^+-ATPase. If the plasma potassium concentration is low, the degree of glycoside binding will increase. Low potassium concentration therefore produces an increased effect of a given concentration of digitalis. As this effect increases, the danger for arrhythmia also increases. Digitalis preparations have mild diuretic and vasoconstrictor effect.

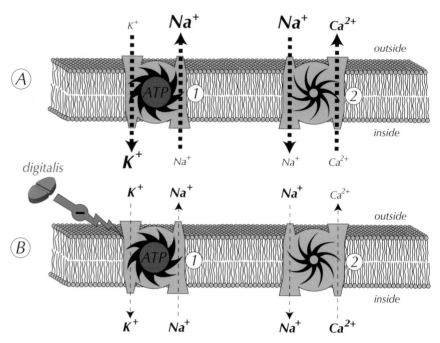

Figure 17.26 **The mechanism of action of digitalis.** (A) During depolarization, sodium flows in and potassium flows out of the cardiac muscle cells. Sodium–potassium-ATPase pumps a large amount of sodium out of the cell (1). The sodium–calcium exchange (2) pumps out calcium and helps to maintain the concentration of intracellular sodium at its normal level. (B) shows the result when digitalis inhibits sodium–potassium-ATPase. This will result in such a high concentration of intracellular sodium that the sodium–calcium exchange is inhibited and the cell's concentration of intracellular calcium will increase.

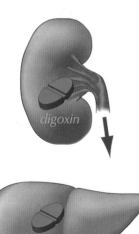

Figure 17.27 **Elimination of digitoxin and digoxin.** Digitoxin is metabolized in the liver. Digoxin is eliminated unmetabolized across the kidneys.

Pharmacokinetics. Digoxin and digitoxin differ from each other in absorption, elimination and duration of action. Absorption after oral administration is satisfactory for both, but better for digitoxin. Both are largely distributed to tissues outside the bloodstream and have a large apparent volume of distribution.

Digitoxin is metabolized in the liver before elimination via the bile. The metabolites are inactive. The half-life is longest for digitoxin (5–7 days). Digoxin is eliminated via the kidneys with a half-life of approximately 1.5 days. See Figure 17.27. In renal failure doses must be reduced.

A long half-life means that it takes a long time before a steady state concentration is established. It is therefore common to administer loading doses of digoxin or digitoxin if these drugs are to be used in the treatment of acute cardiac failure.

From these differences in pharmacokinetics, it is possible to conclude that in the case of overdose, it takes longer before the plasma concentrations are reduced to therapeutic level for digitoxin than it does for digoxin. Digitoxin is better suited for use in renal failure than digoxin.

Adverse effects. Digitalis has a narrow therapeutic range and overdose can occur. Adequate monitoring of plasma levels is necessary. Most adverse effects occurring at a normal dosage are mainly gastrointestinal, e.g. anorexia, nausea and vomiting. Cloudy vision, altered colour vision (yellow vision, or xanthopsia) and cardiac arrhythmias are signs of overdosing. The adverse effects associated with overdoses are more pronounced if the plasma potassium level is low.

Cardiac glycosides
Digitoxin, Digoxin

Table 17.7 Cardiac glycosides

Pregnancy and breastfeeding. Digitalis is regarded as safe to use during pregnancy and breastfeeding.

Indications for use
The primary indications for use of digitalis are chronic heart failure and rapid supraventricular arrhythmias. In recent years, it has become more common to try ACE inhibitors in cardiac failure. Digitalis is now used, especially if the patient presents with symptoms despite optimal treatment with ACE inhibitors and diuretics.

Cardiac glycosides are listed in Table 17.7.

CENTRALLY ACTING ANTIHYPERTENSIVE DRUGS

Methyldopa, clonidine and moxonidine are centrally acting antihypertensive drugs. They are seldom used alone, but rather in combination with other blood pressure-reducing drugs. Methyldopa can be used by pregnant women.

These drugs reduce blood pressure by inhibiting sympathetic activity at both central and peripheral sites. Moxonidine is used for mild to moderate essential hypertension when other antihypertensives are not appropriate.

Methyldopa, Clonidine, Moxonidine

Table 17.8 Centrally acting antihypertensive drugs

CARDIAC ARRHYTHMIAS

The heart muscle contracts in a rhythmic, synchronous manner. In serious cardiac arrhythmias, the pump function is reduced, because the contractions become too disorganized, the filling time becomes too short, or there is too much time between each heartbeat.

PATHOPHYSIOLOGY OF CARDIAC ARRHYTHMIAS

The impulses resulting in heartbeats are spontaneous electrical signals that are created in the heart. They are normally triggered from the sinus node and reach the ventricular muscles via the atrioventricular (AV) node, the bundle of His and the Purkinje fibres. This is the heart's conduction system, which can be compared with nerve fibres elsewhere in the body. See Figure 17.28. The impulses generated from the sinus node produce sinus rhythm. Any other rhythms generated are termed arrhythmias.

Spontaneous electrical impulses can occur elsewhere in cardiac muscle. The heart, however, has a hierarchical arrangement with the fastest spontaneous impulse rate in the sinus node. The rate of contraction is also influenced by impulses from the central nervous system and stress hormones.

In heart disease, this hierarchical arrangement can be disturbed and the conduction system damaged. This increases the risk of arrhythmias. Ischaemia in cardiac

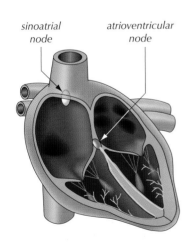

sinoatrial node   *atrioventricular node*

Figure 17.28 **Anatomical localization of the heart's conduction system.** A myocardial infarction in the ventricle septum can damage the impulse diffusion.

muscle, cardiac failure, febrile illness, physical and mental exertions and electrolyte disturbances are examples of conditions that can trigger arrhythmia. Use of drugs and excessive use of coffee, alcohol and tobacco can also cause rhythm disturbances.

Description of heart rhythms

To describe a heart rhythm, it is necessary to consider both the origin of the electrical impulse initiating the heartbeat and the rate at which it originates.

Origin of heart rhythms

If the impulse originates in the sinus node, sinus rhythm is generated. If it starts elsewhere in the atria, an atrial rhythm is generated. An origin in the AV node causes an atrioventricular rhythm, and an origin in the ventricles causes a ventricular rhythm. Rhythms that have their origin in the sinus node, atria or the AV node are called supraventricular rhythms (above the ventricles), as distinguished from ventricular rhythms.

Frequency of the heart rhythm

If the frequency is below 50 beats/min, it is described as bradycardia (slow rhythm). If the rate is above 100 beats/min, it is described as tachycardia (fast rhythm). In atrial flutter, the impulses occur chaotically at different places in the atrial muscles, while in ventricular flutter, the impulses occur chaotically at different places in the ventricles.

Normal heart rhythm

The normal heart rhythm at rest is the sinus rhythm, where the rate varies between 50 and 80 beats/min (with severe exertion in young, healthy persons, the rate can reach 200–225 beats/min). In sinus rhythm, an impulse starts in the sinus node and spreads across the atrial muscles. This impulse causes the atrial muscles to contract and pump blood down into the ventricles. The impulse proceeds to the AV node and is conducted further in the bundle of His to the Purkinje fibres. The ventricles contract when the impulse reaches the Purkinje fibres. Because the signal is delayed through the AV node, the atria will contract before the ventricles – this produces an optimal pump function.

Interaction between atria and ventricles – blockage

If every impulse that is generated in the atria is conducted across to the ventricles, the atria and ventricles will beat synchronously and with the same rate. If the rate is more than 200 beats/min, the AV node will have problems conducting all the impulses further, and some impulses are blocked. The block can be even, e.g. every other impulse is blocked (2:1 block) or every third impulse is blocked (3:1 block), or uneven, as in atrial flutter and fibrillation. In total block, the atria and ventricles beat asynchronously and with different rates, as there is dissociation between them.

Severity of cardiac arrhythmias

Rhythms that are generated in the ventricles cause a poorer coordinated contraction than a sinus node-triggered contraction, and cause poorer pump function. Low and high rates of beating are more dangerous the closer they are to the extreme points, because the cardiac output is lowered. In bradycardia, the cardiac output will be low because of only a few beats per minute. The extreme point here is asystole – no impulse, and thus no contraction.

In ventricular tachycardia or ventricular flutter or fibrillation, the muscles will contract so frequently that blood cannot reach the ventricle between the contractions.

Ventricular fibrillation is the extreme situation and results in an immediate circulatory arrest. Ventricular arrhythmias always require treatment if they persist. Ectopic beats appearing spontaneously with normal heart beats rarely require drug treatment.

Symptoms of cardiac arrhythmias

A person who is suffering from an arrhythmia will notice different symptoms that are due to a reduced cardiac output, hypotension and reduced cerebral blood flow. The most common are dyspnoea, chest pains, dizziness and disturbances of consciousness. The seriousness of symptoms depends on how much the cardiac output is reduced.

GOAL OF DRUG TREATMENT

By using antiarrhythmic drugs, the aim of treatment is to prevent abnormal rhythms, prevent new attacks of rhythm disturbance and restore the normal ventricular rate. However, it is a paradox that in only a few forms of arrhythmia has it been shown that treatment with antiarrhythmics can result in increased survival. This may be due to the fact that almost all of the drugs used to treat arrhythmias have, in themselves, arrhythmogenic properties, i.e. they can cause arrhythmias.

In most cases, patients with arrhythmias requiring treatment have other heart disease as a cause of the arrhythmia. It is therefore important to identify such disease before the arrhythmia is treated. Drugs that influence the transmission and rate of impulse conduction always affect the heart's pumping function. In choosing a drug, it is necessary to consider the risk of triggering cardiac failure.

In some forms of arrhythmia, it is possible to physically destroy conduction bundles in the heart that allow arrhythmias to be maintained. Such arrhythmia treatment can result in permanent recovery and is today an important alternative to drug treatment in re-entry arrhythmias. In re-entry arrhythmias, the impulses are normally conducted in an extra conduction bundle between the atria and ventricles.

Grouping of antiarrhythmics

There are several ways of classifying antiarrhythmic drugs. One of these is to classify drugs according to where in the heart they have their primary effect. Another way is to group the drugs according to which phase of the action potential they act upon when a cell is depolarized. It is customary to group them according to this latter method, which is known as the Vaughan Williams method.

Depolarization and repolarization of a cell

In all living cells, a potential difference can be measured across the cell membrane. The cells are negatively charged on the inside and positively charged on the outside. In some cells, such as nerve cells and heart muscle cells, this membrane potential can be altered because ions flow quickly across the membrane through ion channels. When the potential difference between the inside and the outside moves towards zero, the cell is said to be depolarized. As it returns back to its resting value, the cell is said to be repolarizing. Antiarrhythmic drugs act by influencing the ionic currents and thereby the tendency for depolarization and repolarization to occur.

Phases of depolarization and repolarization

The cells in the heart's conduction system are characterized by the tendency for spontaneous depolarization. In disease and with other biochemical changes in the heart, the tendency for spontaneous impulse generation from places other than the conduction system increases. Depolarization and repolarization are divided into five phases. The transition between the phases is continual. See Figure 17.29.

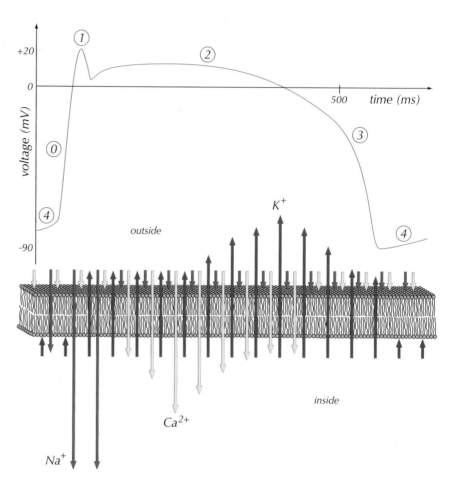

Figure 17.29 **The voltage change between the inside and outside of a cell during the depolarization and repolarization.** The illustration shows the values recorded from the heart's conduction system (Purkinje fibres, where all the phases can be recorded). The voltage change is indicated by the red line. The ionic currents across the cell membrane are indicated corresponding the different phases, from 0 to 4. If the voltage changes occurring due to depolarization/repolarization are recorded in the sinoatrial (SA) node, phase 4 will have faster rising than phase 4 in the Purkinje fibres. This causes the sinus node to reach the threshold value where phase 0 begins earlier, and depolarization takes place. Thus, the sinus node normally governs the impulse generation. In arrhythmia, these conditions are altered.

Phase 0: fast depolarization phase. The voltage is changed in a short time from negative (approximately $-85\,mV$) to positive (approximately $+20\,mV$). This happens because positive sodium ions flow quickly into the cell through sodium channels, but then quickly stop. The sodium channels shut and do not open until some time later in phase 3. The period when the sodium channels do not open is called the cell's refractory period. During the refractory period, the cell cannot generate a new action potential.

Phase 1: partial repolarization. In this phase, the flow of sodium into the cell stops. Simultaneously, a slow efflux of positive potassium ions begins.

Phase 2: plateau phase. The potential difference remains stable for a relatively long time. Potassium flows slowly out of the cell, and calcium flows slowly into it.

Phase 3: repolarization phase. The potential difference drops quite quickly to a value below the starting point before the depolarization. The calcium influx ceases and the potassium efflux increases until, just as quickly, it ceases at the end of this phase. The membrane potential is then restored.

Phase 4: resting phase – quiet depolarization. In this phase, there are few ionic currents. The phase is characterized by the cell's potential difference drifting towards the threshold value when a new action potential will be generated. In phase 4, the slow depolarization of the cells is probably associated with a slow influx of potassium ions.

Vaughan Williams classification method
Antiarrhythmics are divided into four classes, even if there are 5 phases, 0–4, according to this classification. The problem with this formulation is that not all drugs used in antiarrhythmic treatment fit into the classes. It is necessary to be aware that the different drugs used as antiarrhythmics have different abilities to affect arrhythmias, depending on whether the origin is in the atria or in the ventricles. Some antiarrhythmics affect the ionic currents in several of the phases.

Class I antiarrhythmics: sodium channel blockers. These drugs block the influx of sodium ions through sodium channels in the cell membrane. They act primarily in phases 0 and 1, but to a certain extent also in phase 3. Lidocaine, mexiletine, disopyramide and procainamide belong to class 1 antiarrhythmics. They are used less frequently now than in the past.

Class II antiarrhythmics: β-blockers. These drugs are discussed elsewhere in this chapter (p. 235). The heart rate is lowered in that phase 4 is extended. The rate of conduction in the heart's conduction system is lowered. β-Blockers are used to treat attacks of rapid supraventricular arrhythmias associated with a high sympathetic drive and also as prophylactic treatment of supraventricular tachycardias.

Class III antiarrhythmics: drugs that extend the refractory period. This group has its primary effect in delaying the efflux of potassium, such that the plateau phase is extended. Amiodarone is regarded as part of this group, even though the drug also has properties that apply to other classes of antiarrhythmic drugs. Amiodarone extends the duration of the action potential and the refractory period in all parts of the myocardium, and causes a unique antiarrhythmic effect in both supraventricular and ventricular rhythm disturbances.

Because of serious adverse effects (pulmonary fibrosis is the most significant), amiodarone must be used with caution. Sensitivity to light with a blue coloration of sun-exposed skin develops in many of the users. These problems can be reduced with the use of suntan lotions with a high degree of protection. Amiodarone has iodine in the molecule. Some users can therefore develop hypo- or hyperthyroidism. The frequency of adverse effects is clearly dose-dependent, so low doses are seldom associated with serious adverse effects. Because of its unique antiarrhythmic effect the use of amiodarone has increased in the last few years.

The β-blocker sotalol also has a class III effect on the conduction system, in addition to its class II effect.

Class IV antiarrhythmics: calcium-channel blockers. Calcium-channel blockers inhibit the influx of calcium into myocardial cells. These drugs also extend the refractory period in the same way as the class III group. They are used in conjunction

Class I antiarrhythmics
Quinidine, Lidocaine, Flecainide, Procainamide

Class II antiarrhythmics
β-blockers (see Table 17.2, p. 238)

Class III antiarrhythmics
Amiodarone, Sotalol (also class II)

Class IV antiarrhythmics
Verapamil, Diltiazem

Table 17.9 Antiarrhythmics

with β-blockers in rapid supraventricular arrhythmias and in re-entry arrhythmias, but seldom in ventricular tachycardias. In re-entry arrhythmias, the impulses are normally conducted in an extra conduction bundle between the atria and ventricles.

Indications for use
Antiarrhythmics are used for several indications, and the choice between the different groups is determined based on arrhythmia type and presence of other diseases. Today, the drugs used as pure antiarrhythmics are mainly those of classes II and III.
   Some antiarrhythmics are listed in Table 17.9.

HYPERLIPIDAEMIAS

Hyperlipidaemia means persistently high concentrations of a number of different fatty compounds (lipids) in the blood. Cholesterol and triglycerides are examples of such fatty compounds. The amount of cholesterol in the circulation is affected by the fat content in the diet and the body's biosynthesis of cholesterol. Hyperlipidaemia, and particularly a high level of cholesterol, is associated with an increased tendency for arteriosclerosis and diseases associated with arteriosclerosis. The most important element in the treatment of hyperlipidaemias is a change in lifestyle that every individual can undertake. Weight reduction, increased physical activity, stopping smoking and a diet with reduced amounts of saturated fat form the basis of the treatment.

PATHOPHYSIOLOGY OF HYPERLIPIDAEMIAS

The lipids circulate in the blood bound to proteins. Different combinations of lipids and proteins are called lipoproteins. The lipoproteins consist of an external 'sheath' of phospholipids and proteins and an internal 'core' of lipids (triglycerides and cholesterol). They are spherical particles that are classified according to the relative distribution between lipids and proteins. Large lipoproteins contain lipids with a high proportion of triglycerides and are of low density. Small lipoproteins have fewer lipids, but a high proportion of cholesterol and are of higher density. The lipoproteins can be divided into four main classes:

- Chylomicrons are the largest lipoproteins. They are created in the mucosal cells of the intestines from lipids in the diet and are emptied into the blood via the lymph.
- Very low-density lipoproteins (VLDLs) are created in the hepatocytes and are released to the blood.
- Low-density lipoproteins (LDLs) are created in the circulation from VLDLs.
- High-density lipoproteins (HDLs) are created in the liver and are released to the blood.

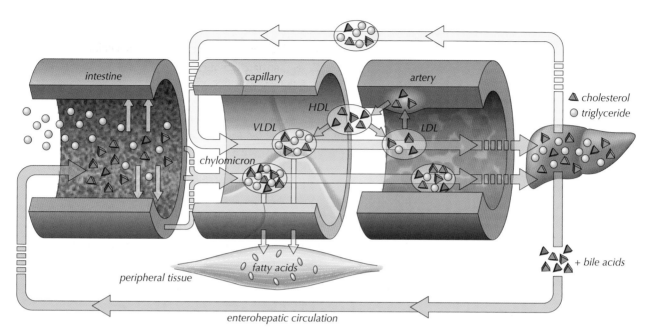

Figure 17.30 **Lipid metabolism.** Triglycerides and cholesterol from the diet are absorbed via the mucosal cells of the intestines and are packed in large lipoprotein particles or chylomicrons. Chylomicrons release free fatty acids (FFAs) from triglycerides to adipose and muscle tissue (peripheral tissue) and are then absorbed in the liver. Very low-density lipoproteins (VLDLs) are created in the liver and are released to the blood. Here, VLDLs are metabolized to low-density lipoproteins (LDLs) after metabolism of triglycerides and release of free fatty acids. LDLs transport cholesterol to peripheral tissue, but the majority are absorbed by the hepatocytes because they bind to LDL receptors. High-density lipoproteins (HDLs) are formed in the liver. They draw on cholesterol from peripheral tissue and transmit it to LDLs and VLDLs.

Contribution of diet to lipoproteins and cholesterol

After ingesting fat, triglycerides and cholesterol are absorbed across the mucosal cells of the intestines. Here, the lipids are 'packed' in large lipoprotein particles, chylomicrons, which have an external sheath of phospholipids and proteins. Chylomicrons are absorbed into lymph and are then emptied into the venous circulation. When the chylomicron particles circulate in the capillary beds in adipose and muscle tissue, the lipids are attacked by lipoprotein lipases, enzymes that break down the triglycerides, while cholesterol is largely untouched. Free fatty acids from the triglycerides are absorbed to adipose and muscle cells, where they are stored or used for energy production. The chylomicron remnants (with cholesterol) are absorbed and metabolized by the hepatocytes when they reach the liver. Cholesterol is released and can be stored, form part of the VLDL particles or be metabolized to bile acids. The bile acids are created from cholesterol and are necessary for absorption of fat. They recirculate in the enterohepatic circuit. See Figure 17.30.

Biosynthesis of lipoproteins and cholesterol

Cholesterol is synthesized in the liver with the help of the enzyme HMG-CoA reductase. See Figure 17.31. Self-synthesized cholesterol and triglycerides are packed together with cholesterol and triglycerides from the chylomicron remnants and are released to the blood in the form of VLDL particles. Lipoprotein lipases in the capillary beds of fat and muscle tissue release triglycerides in VLDLs in the same way as in chylomicrons. In this way, the remnants of VLDLs create LDLs, which are rich in cholesterol. The LDL particles have surface antigens that are recognized by receptors on the cell surfaces of hepatocytes, smooth muscle cells in the arterial wall and macrophages. Most of the LDLs are bound via this mechanism and are

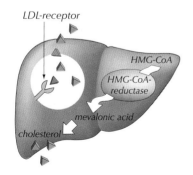

Figure 17.31 **The liver's cholesterol synthesis.** Most of the cholesterol in the body is synthesized in the liver with the help of the enzyme HMG-CoA reductase.

absorbed in the liver cells. In this way, cholesterol is removed from the circulation. Because some LDLs are bound to other cells and are absorbed by them, they increase their cholesterol content. In this way, LDLs transport cholesterol to the body's cells. Smooth muscle cells and macrophages in the arterial wall with high cholesterol content contribute largely to the arteriosclerotic process. See Figure 17.30.

HDL particles have the ability to absorb cholesterol from cells and transfer it to VLDL and LDL particles. Because a number of LDLs are absorbed by the liver cells, HDLs will, in this way, help to remove cholesterol from the cells. When a large amount of cholesterol is transported back to the liver cells, the liver's biosynthesis of cholesterol is reduced. The liver's biosynthesis of cholesterol contributes considerably more to the total cholesterol concentration in plasma than does cholesterol from the diet.

Effect of lipid profile on the arteriosclerotic process

Chylomicrons primarily contain triglycerides that are metabolized and which release free fatty acids to adipose tissue and muscle tissue, where they are stored or used as a source of energy. VLDLs are also carriers of triglycerides, elevated levels of which are a moderate risk factor for arteriosclerotic disease. LDLs contain considerable amounts of cholesterol and are strongly associated with development of arteriosclerotic disease. HDLs also contain a large amount of cholesterol. Since HDLs transport cholesterol from the cells, a high value of HDLs is associated with reduced development of arteriosclerosis.

GOAL OF DRUG TREATMENT

The goal of drug treatment is to reduce the arteriosclerotic process and partially remove previously formed arteriosclerotic material. In this way, it is possible to reduce the risk of the development of serious diseases such as hypertension, angina pectoris, myocardial infarction, kidney failure and stroke. Drug treatment attempts to alter the distribution of the lipoproteins in a favourable direction. It is especially desirable to lower the total cholesterol.

In the light of many clinical studies that have been conducted with lipid-lowering drugs in relation to cardiovascular diseases, there is agreement about the need for secondary prophylaxis in such diseases. Lipid-lowering treatment is being considered for all patients with myocardial infarction. The benefit of primary prophylaxis is somewhat less certain, but the use of effective lipid-lowering drugs is recommended for everyone with total cholesterol above certain values, and especially to people with familial hypercholesterolaemia.

Four different drug groups are useful in the treatment of hyperlipidaemias.

Statins

Statins inhibit HMG-CoA reductase, an enzyme (mainly located in the liver cells) responsible for the synthesis of cholesterol. In addition, there is an increase in the creation of new LDL receptors, especially in the liver, which bind and break down LDL cholesterol. In this way, the level of LDL cholesterol is lowered, while HDL cholesterol increases and the lipid profile improves. See Figure 17.32. Extensive studies have shown reduced numbers of myocardial infarctions, reduced arteriosclerosis and improved survival in people with moderately elevated cholesterol who receive HMG-CoA reductase inhibitors. There are few adverse effects with the use of statins, but rhabdomyolysis (muscle lysis) is a serious adverse effect that has received considerable attention. It has been shown that rhabdomyolysis occurs more frequently with use of one of the statins (cerivastatin) compared with the others. This adverse effect can occur at any time during treatment and the risk

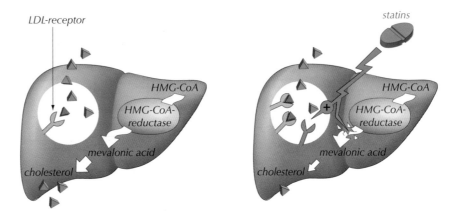

Figure 17.32 Inhibition of HMG–CoA reductase. Statins inhibit a critical step in the synthesis of cholesterol in the liver. In addition, the number of low-density lipoprotein (LDL) receptors on the liver cells increases, such that more LDL cholesterol is removed from the circulation.

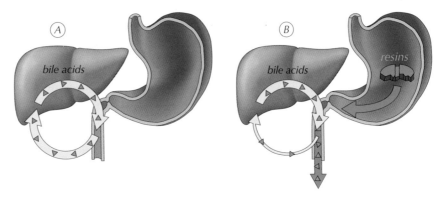

Figure 17.33 Resins bind bile acids in the intestines and prevent them from recirculating in the enterohepatic circuit. Thereby, cholesterol is utilized.

increases with simultaneous use of erythromycin (antibiotic) or gemfibrozil (lipid-lowering).

Resins

Bile acids are synthesized by cholesterol and are necessary for the absorption of lipids in the small intestine. Resins are drugs that bind bile acids in the intestines. Because the bile acids that are bound are removed with the faeces, cholesterol is 'utilized'. The absorption of cholesterol from the intestines is simultaneously lowered. Low blood cholesterol increases the amount of LDL receptors in the liver, which remove LDLs from the circulation. Resins are therefore particularly effective in patients with high LDL cholesterol. See Figure 17.33. Use of these drugs for secondary prophylaxis has reduced the number of patients suffering myocardial infarctions.

The resins are not absorbed so there are few systemic adverse effects, but constipation, stomach pains, nausea, vomiting and diarrhoea are common.

A number of drugs bind to resins in the intestines, and must be taken at least 1 h before or 4 h after ingestion of resins.

Fibrates

Fibrates increase the activity of lipoprotein lipase, which breaks down lipoproteins, so the blood's concentrations of triglycerides and VLDLs are reduced.

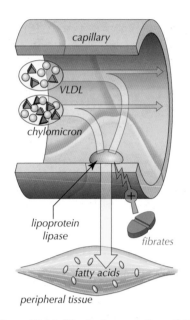

Figure 17.34 Fibrates increase the activity of lipoprotein lipase. In this way, the numbers of chylomicron remnants and very low-density lipoproteins (VLDLs) that return to the liver are reduced.

Statins
Atorvastatin, Fluvastatin, Pravastatin, Rosuvastatin, Simvastatin
Resins
Colestyramine, Colestipol
Fibrates
Benzafibrate, Ciprofibrate, Fenofibrate, Gemfibrozil
Fish oils
Omega-3-acid ethyl esters, Omega-3-marine triglycerides

Table 17.10 Lipid-regulating drugs

See Figure 17.34. The fibrates also reduce the liver's synthesis of cholesterol and increase the secretion of cholesterol with bile. The LDL concentration drops while the HDL concentration increases.

Fish oil concentrates
Fish oil concentrates contain omega-3 fatty acids. The main effect is that the concentration of HDL cholesterol increases and the triglycerides are reduced, thus improving the lipid profile.

Indications for use
If there is an inappropriate lipid profile with symptoms of coronary heart disease and dietary treatment does not provide sufficient effect, statins should be recommended. Fibrates are relevant in cases of persistent high triglycerides. Omega-3 fatty acids are recommended if HDLs are low or if other treatment is not satisfactory.

Drugs used to treat hyperlipidaemias are listed in Table 17.10.

SUMMARY

- The most important elements in regulating blood pressure are the baroreceptors, the autonomic nervous system and the renin–angiotensin–aldosterone system.
- Hypertension increases the arteriosclerotic process and increases the risk of development of all serious diseases in the cardiovascular system. Drug treatment attempts to reduce systolic and diastolic pressure, to lower the risk of associated diseases.
- Angina pectoris is associated with poor circulation in the heart muscle and is exacerbated by situations that require increased cardiac load. Drug treatment attempts to improve the blood flow to the myocardium and/or reduce the load of the heart. Thereby, pain and the risk for further disease are reduced.
- Myocardial infarction occurs when a part of the myocardium dies from insufficient blood supply. It is caused by thromboembolic events clogging a coronary artery. Drug treatment attempts to reduce the size of the infarct, to lower the risk of rhythm disturbances, the development of acute and chronic cardiac failure and the development of new thromboembolic events.
- Cardiac failure is due to failing pump function (systolic failure) in the right, left or both ventricles, or reduced compliance in cardiac muscle (diastolic failure). Right-sided failure causes congestion in the systemic circulation and internal organs. Left-sided cardiac failure causes congestion in the pulmonary circulation. The most frequent cause of failure is myocardial infarction. Drug treatment attempts to improve systolic and diastolic function.

- Adrenergic neuron blocking drugs block receptors in the heart and arteries, such that noradrenaline and adrenaline have a reduced effect. They also reduce the release of noradrenaline and adrenaline. In addition, central nervous stimulation of the heart and arteries is inhibited and the activity in the renin–angiotensin–aldosterone system is reduced. The most important indications for use are hypertension, angina pectoris, myocardial infarction and arrhythmias. The most frequent dose-related adverse effects are hypotension, cardiac failure, atrioventricular block and cold hands and feet. Bronchoconstriction can occur in predisposed asthmatic individuals. Selective β_1-blockers can be used to avoid affecting β_2-receptors.

- Calcium-channel blockers inhibit influx of calcium ions into cardiac muscle cells and vascular smooth muscle. The most important indications for their use are hypertension, angina pectoris and arrhythmias. The most frequent dose-related adverse effects are hypotension, cardiac failure, blockage of the impulse conduction in the AV node and reduced peripheral circulation.

- ACE inhibitors inhibit the formation of angiotensin-II by inhibiting angiotensin-converting enzyme. The most important indications for use are dry cough, hypertension and cardiac failure. The most frequent dose-related adverse effects are dry cough, hypotension, cardiac failure and, in some cases, hyperkalaemia.

- Angiotensin-II-receptor antagonists prevent angiotensin-II from binding to angiotensin-II receptors. The important indications for their use are hypertension and heart failure. There are fewer adverse effects than with ACE inhibitors.

- Diuretics increase urine volume and reduce the circulating blood volume and tissue oedema. They act in different sections of the nephron. The most important indications for their use are hypertension and the treatment of oedema, particularly with concurrent congestion. The most frequent dose-related adverse effects are hypotension and electrolyte disturbances. Serious hyperkalaemia can occur with potassium-sparing diuretics.

- Organic nitrates dilate both veins and arteries and cause a redistribution of the blood volume in the venous system. Collateral blood flow improves in ischaemic tissue in cardiac muscle. Extremely useful drugs in the treatment of angina pectoris, organic nitrates can also be used to treat congestive heart failure. The most frequent dose-related adverse effects are hypotension and throbbing headaches.

- Cardiac glycosides increase the concentration of calcium in heart muscle cells, thereby increasing the heart's force of contraction. Heart rate in supraventricular tachyarrhythmias is reduced. The most important indications for their use are heart failure and supraventricular tachycardias. The most frequent dose-related adverse effects are gastrointestinal problems and a tendency for arrhythmias. Altered colour vision and cloudy vision occur at high concentrations.

- All cardiac arrhythmias result in reduced pump function compared with that seen in normal sinus rhythm. Ventricular arrhythmias are more dangerous than supraventricular arrhythmias, and always require treatment if they persist. Drug treatment attempts to prevent abnormal rhythms, prevent new attacks of rhythm disturbance and restore the normal ventricular rate.

- Almost all antiarrhythmic drugs have properties that can contribute to arrhythmia, particularly if they are used in high doses. In the treatment of arrhythmia, it is equally important to treat underlying diseases as it is to administer drugs against the arrhythmia.

- Methyldopa, clonidine and moxonidine reduce central nervous stimulation to the heart and blood vessels. Their most important use is in the treatment of hypertension, but they are not the primary choice, except in pregnancy.

■ Hyperlipidaemia is persistently high concentrations of lipids in the blood, leading to arteriosclerosis. Drug treatment attempts to reduce the progression of arteriosclerosis and thereby to lower the risk of associated diseases.

■ Anti-atherogenic drugs alter the ratio of atherogenic and anti-atherogenic substances in a favourable direction and can dissolve previously formed arteriosclerotic masses. The most important indication for their use is total cholesterol and high fraction of LDL. Other important drugs in the treatment of hyperlipidaemias are statins, resins, fibrates and fish oil concentrates.

18 Drugs used to treat diseases of the pulmonary system

The primary function of the pulmonary system is to enable gaseous exchange between the blood and the atmosphere, where oxygen diffuses to the blood and carbon dioxide diffuses from the blood. Diseases that disturb gaseous exchange affect oxygen saturation in blood and tissues and contribute to acid–base disturbances. Since the lungs and airways are in direct contact with the atmosphere, they are exposed to a number of harmful agents which may cause disease. The most frequent diseases of the pulmonary system are acute infections, allergies and inflammation, which contribute to obstructive lung diseases which may lead to lower alveolor ventilation and reduced gas exchange.

Drugs acting on the pulmonary system can be administered locally via inhalation. By using local administration lower doses compared with systemic administration are needed, thereby reducing unwanted systemic effects and adverse effects. This chapter deals with drugs used to treat coughing, obstructive pulmonary diseases, bronchiectasis and cystic fibrosis.

COUGHING

Coughing is a physiological reflex (the so-called tussive reflex) which acts to clear the airways leading to cough. The reflex starts in the bronchial wall where afferent nerves transmit signals to the cough reflex center in the brain stem. In turn, the brain stem relays impulses back to the muscles of the lanynx and to the ventilatory muscles. Simultaneously, the larynx occludes the airways and the ventilatory muscles start a fast and forced contraction, preparing for a powerful expiratory breath. Suddenly the larynx opens and the air is expelled at a high speed. In this way cough helps to clear the airways of mucus and particles at the bronchial surface which initiated the cough.

PATHOPHYSIOLOGY

Hypersensitivity of the bronchial wall will increase the generation and the transmission of impulses leading to cough. Inflammation of the bronchial wall (bronchitis) and inhaled particles increase the sensitivity of the bronchial wall. Inflammation of the bronchial wall is most often caused by viral or bacterial infections or by different allergens. Acute and chronic bronchitis and asthma are diseases in which bronchial inflammation often is pronounced. Left ventricular failure leads to oedema of the bronchial mucosa and increased sensitivity. Pulmonary tumours and foreign bodies in the airways may induce coughing induced by local inflammation of the bronchial wall.

Classification
Coughs may be described as either non-productive (dry cough) or productive. In non-productive cough there is not production of excessive volumes of mucus. A productive cough is one in which there is an increased mucus secretion from the airway mucosa. It is helpful to examine this hypersecretion to differentiate between purulent (yellow/green mucus) and non-purulent (greyish/white or non-coloured mucus) secretions, since this indicates what sort of treatment is appropriate.

Bacterial infections often result in a productive cough which is usually purulent, whilst increased secretions seen in allergic reactions and asthma are generally non-purulent. Viral infections and infections with, for example, Chlamydia or Mycoplasma often produce a dry cough or a cough with low volume, greyish secretion.

Exercise-induced coughing and constant recurrent cough in children are characteristic of asthma. Exertion-triggered coughing in the elderly may be a symptom of right ventricular failure.

DRUGS USED TO TREAT HYPERSECRETION AND COUGH

In the evaluation of coughing, it is important to consider the possibility of serious underlying diseases that require treatment, e.g. infections, asthma, chronic bronchitis, cardiac failure or pulmonary tumours. The most important part of the treatment of a cough is that any underlying disease should be treated rather than just the symptom.

Dry cough may be treated with cough suppressants. Productive cough should not principally be treated by antitussive drugs, since this will inhibit the cough reflex and prevent the removal of excessive mucus. This may in turn lead to plugging of the airways with mucus. If the mucus that plugs the airways is purulent there is an increased risk of spreading infection distal to the plugging and development of pulmonary infection. Plugging may also prevent distribution of inhaled air to alveoli distal to the plug, thus leading to oxygen deficiency in this part of the lung. If the excessive amount of mucus is viscous, mucolytics may be used. If the mucus is purulent or there is suspicion of bronchial infection, antibiotics should be considered.

Expectorants
It is claimed that expectorants facilitate the mucociliary transport of bronchial secretions. None of the expectorants has proved to be effective, but they may be useful as an 'effective' placebo.

Centrally acting cough suppressants
The most effective antitussive drugs are the opioids. These drugs suppress the cough reflex via an action in the central nervous system which results in inhibition

Expectorants
Ammonia and Ipecacuanha, Simple linctus
Centrally acting cough suppressants
Codeine, Dextromethorphan, Pholcodine

Table18.1 Expectorants and cough suppressants

of efferent impulses to the muscles that are activated during coughing. They have an effect on both dry and productive coughs. All the drugs, except pholcodine and noscapine, have narcotic properties. They cause drowsiness and there is a danger of dependence with long-term use. Large doses of opioids may cause nausea and there is a tendency for the development of constipation.

The addition of ephedrine to opioid-containing cough mixtures has a relaxing effect on the bronchial muscles. The opioids are more thoroughly discussed in Chapter 14, Drugs with central and peripheral analgesic effect.

Other cough suppressants

Other compounds, e.g. diphenhydramine (an antihistamine), are used in some preparations as an antitussive agent. The efficacy of such compounds is questionable.

Drugs used to treat coughing are listed in Table 18.1.

OBSTRUCTIVE LUNG DISEASES

Obstructive lung diseases prevent the normal flow of air into, but particularly out of the lungs. Chronic bronchitis and emphysema are chronic obstructive lung diseases where there is variable airflow obstruction that may or may not be reversible. Bronchial asthma is a chronic disease that is periodically obstructive. Distinguishing between different obstructive diseases may be difficult as they share a number of common presenting symptoms, e.g. cough and airflow obstruction. In many instances, the symptoms and problems associated with a particular disease vary considerably.

PATHOPHYSIOLOGY

The majority of lung tissue consists of bronchi and alveoli. The bronchi branch to produce increasingly narrower airway tubes before they terminate in alveoli. Gaseous exchange occurs in the alveoli, so alveolar ventilation is of primary importance in determining its efficiency. In serious obstructive lung diseases, airflow to the alveoli may be compromised to such an extent that gaseous exchange is severely impaired and the tissue needs for oxygen delivery and carbon dioxide removal may not be met.

The obstruction to the airflow may be caused by several components, like muscular contraction, increased mucus production, oedema of the bronchial wall and increased filling of the capillaries in the bronchial mucosa (see Figure 18.1):

- The airways consist of a number of dichotomously branching 'tubes' which originate from the trachea. The initial segments of the airways are called bronchi. Larger bronchi (i.e. those nearer to the trachea) have C-shaped structures of cartilage in their walls. As the larger bronchi divide, the C-shapes are replaced by irregular and random plates of cartilage. The bronchi also contain circular smooth muscle in their walls. Contraction of this muscle will

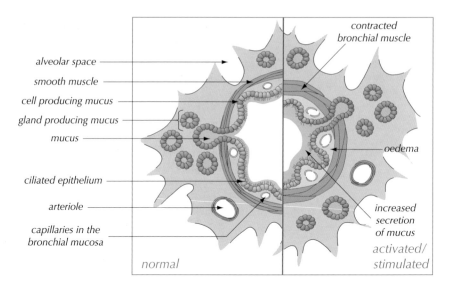

alveolar space

smooth muscle

cell producing mucus

gland producing mucus

mucus

ciliated epithelium

arteriole

capillaries in the
bronchial mucosa

contracted
bronchial muscle

oedema

increased
secretion
of mucus

activated/
stimulated

normal

Figure 18.1 **Cross-section through normal and pathological bronchioles.** Contraction of bronchial muscles results in reduction of the lumen diameter. Increased mucus secretion, increased mucosal oedema and increased filling of capillaries in the bronchial mucosa obstruct the lumen.

have a minimal effect in obstructing the lumen due to the presence of cartilage. Obstruction in this region of the airways is primarily due to the increased production of mucus, tumours or foreign bodies. Those airways which lack cartilage are called bronchioles. Contraction of circular smooth muscle in bronchioles has a significant effect in obstructing the lumen. This is an important component in asthma attacks.

■ The airways are lined with mucosal epithelium which secretes a thin mucus layer. The mucus traps inhaled particles and transports them towards the pharynx, where they are swallowed or expectorated. Reduced mucus transport and/or increased mucus production can result in accumulation of secretions, which obstructs the lumen, thus reducing airflow. This is a particularly important component in chronic bronchitis, but also occurs in asthma.

■ Inflammation in the mucosa can cause fluid to leak from blood vessels (particularly venules) and cause significant mucosal oedema. Together with the mucosal oedema, increased filling of the venules in the mucosa during inflammation will contribute to occlude the lumen of the airways which results in airflow obstruction. This is an important component in asthma attacks, chronic bronchitis and also acute exacerbation of chronic bronchitis. Inflammation also causes contraction of the circular muscles of the bronchioles, reducing the diameter of the airways.

■ The elasticity in the lung tissue holds the fine branches of the airways open to allow a smooth airflow to and from the alveoli. Loss of elastic tissue can cause the bronchioles to collapse and prevent airflow. This is an important component in emphysema.

Asthma

Asthma is an inflammatory disease of the airways characterized by episodic obstruction of small respiratory passages. Sufferers of this disease form IgE antibodies to common allergens, which embed themselves in the membrane of mast cells. Upon subsequent exposure to the allergen, the allergen binds to the IgE antibodies which results in disruption of the mast cell membrane and the release of a number of pro-inflammatory mediators, e.g. histamine. These inflammatory mediators initiate the pathophysiological consequences of an asthma attack, i.e. bronchoconstriction, mucosal oedema and the recruitment and activation of other inflammatory cells. Asthma attacks can also be triggered by infections, tobacco smoke, physical exertion, cold air, psychological stress and drugs (e.g. aspirin). Drug treatment of asthma should particularly take into account the local inflammatory process and the bronchial constriction. The treatment is approached step by step, each step either increasing the dose or altering the means of administration of the drug, or adding a new drug.

Chronic bronchitis

Chronic bronchitis is characterized by increased mucus production and retention of mucus that severely limits airflow in the respiratory airways. Mucosal oedema may occur as well as inflammation of the airway mucosa. Coughing and bacterial respiratory infections frequently occur in periods of active disease. The criterion required for diagnosis of chronic bronchitis is the presence of a productive cough for the majority of days over a period of 3 months per year for more than 1 year. The disease is strongly associated with long-term smoking and often coexists with emphysema. Drug treatment of chronic bronchitis should particularly take into account the local inflammatory process and the increased mucus secretion.

Emphysema

Emphysema is tissue degeneration with the loss of both alveolar tissue (septa) inside the alveolar acinus and of capillary vessels embedded in the alveolar septa. This leads to reduced elasticity of the lung tissue and collapse of small airways and thereby to compromised ventilation. In addition, there is reduced gaseous exchange because of the loss of alveolar area and capillary vessels. Emphysema is strongly associated with long-term smoking. In plain emphysema no drugs can improve the respiratory failure and the reduced gaseous exchange. Improvement of the oxygen deficit can only be compensated for with a small increase in the oxygen content of the inhaled air. Since emphysema most often coexists with chronic bronchitis, drug therapy should address the treatment of this disease.

DRUGS USED TO TREAT OBSTRUCTIVE LUNG DISEASES

For adequate drug therapy in obstructive lung diseases, the challenge is to identify the current pathophysiological change or changes that contribute to the reduced ventilation, since different pathophysiological changes may often present with the same symptoms. In addition, the same patient may have components of asthma, chronic bronchitis and emphysema simultaneously, and these components may change over time. It is therefore difficult to know which is the primary contributing factor to the reduced ventilation.

In treating obstructive lung diseases there may be some benefit in combining drugs with different effects, e.g. reversing bronchoconstriction, suppressing inflammatory responses, reducing mucus secretion and mucosal oedema. See Figure 18.2.

Drugs used to treat obstructive lung diseases include glucocorticoids, β_2-agonists, cromoglicate, anticholinergics, leukotriene antagonists and theophylline. With the exception of theophylline, all the drugs can be administered locally via inhalation. The advantage of local administration is that the dose can be reduced considerably

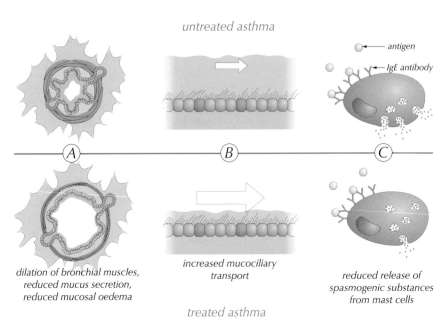

untreated asthma

antigen

IgE antibody

(A) (B) (C)

dilation of bronchial muscles,
reduced mucus secretion,
reduced mucosal oedema

increased mucociliary
transport

reduced release of
spasmogenic substances
from mast cells

treated asthma

Figure 18.2 **Site of action for drugs used in obstructive lung disease.** (A) Dilation of bronchial muscles, reduced mucus secretion and reduced mucosal oedema. (B) Increased ciliary transport. (C) Reduced release of inflammatory and bronchoconstrictor substances.

in comparison with that which would need to be given by systemic administration. Additionally, the time for the drug to exert its effects is reduced when administered locally. However, when administered by inhalation, only 10–25 per cent of the administered dose will reach the small airways. The remainder is deposited on the mucosa of the oral cavity, larynx and large airways, where it has no effect. See Figure 18.3. To get the optimal effect of local administration, a good inhalation technique must be learned.

Inhaled glucocorticoids

The use of inhaled glucocorticoids (e.g. budesonide, fluticasone, beclomethasone) has increased since the acceptance of asthma as an inflammatory airway disease. Their use is now a major therapy for the treatment of asthma and is recommended as standard treatment if the need for β_2-agonists is greater than two doses three days per week. In some cases of severe asthma, the use of systematic glucocorticoids may be necessary. However, this is only appropriate when other drug treatments have failed to control the disease.

Mechanism of action and effects. Glucocorticoids have significant anti-inflammatory effects expressed by a decrease in the production of inflammatory substances and an increase in the production of anti-inflammatory substances. These effects are mediated by altering gene transcription in the cells which they target i.e. they have the ability to turn on and turn off a variety of genes. They also reduce the number of eosinophils and other inflammatory cells that migrate to the tissue during inflammatory disorders. Since they inhibit the production of pro-inflammatory mediators and prevent the recruitment and activation of inflammatory cells, their effects include a reduction in venule permeability and hence a reduction in oedema formation. They also produce a reduction in

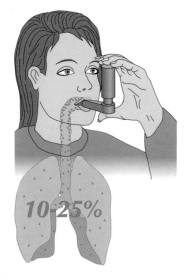

10–25%

Figure 18.3 **Drug administration by inhalation.** Only a small portion of the dose reaches the site of action by local administration.

viscosity of bronchial secretions. Glucocorticoids do not have a direct relaxant effect on bronchoconstriction, nor do they inhibit the effect of released histamine from mast cells.

Given their mechanism of action, i.e. the alteration of gene activity, glucocorticoids are not fast-acting drugs. Their role is in preventing the development of asthma attacks rather than providing symptomatic relief of the immediate effects of an asthma attack.

Pharmacokinetics. Seventy-five to ninety per cent of an inhaled dose attaches to the mucosa of the oral cavity, pharynx and larynx. A large portion of that which is swallowed undergoes first-pass metabolism in the liver. In this way, systemic effects and adverse effects are minimized.

Adverse effects. Glucocorticoids administered by inhalation have considerably fewer adverse effects than those resulting from systemic administration, because considerably smaller doses can be administered by inhalation than with the use of tablets. Fungal infections of the oral mucosa can occur, but they can be prevented by rinsing out the mouth after inhalation and by good oral hygiene.

In adults who are treated with inhaled glucocorticoids, systemic effects can be observed with inhaled daily doses of budesonide $>1200\,\mu g/day$, and of beclometasone $>1000\,\mu g/day$.

Glucocorticoids are more thoroughly described in Chapter 21, Drugs used to treat endocrinological disorders.

β_2-receptor agonists

Drugs that stimulate β_2-receptors are termed β_2-agonists. β_2-receptors are found predominantly in airway smooth muscle, but also in uterine and vascular smooth muscle. Stimulation of the β_2-receptors results in relaxation of smooth muscle. Activation of these receptors is therefore beneficial in the treatment of asthma attacks, where bronchial muscular contraction is pronounced (and also in the treatment of premature contractions in pregnant women). If there is a need to use β_2-agonists more than three times per week, it is recommended that treatment is changed to inhaled glucocorticoids as standard treatment. In the step by step increase in the use of anti-asthmatic drugs, β_2-agonists are the first drugs to be added to inhaled glucocorticoids in severe asthma. Systemic β_2-agonists may be added to inhaled glucocorticoids and β_2-agonists when these alone fail to control asthmatic symptoms.

Mechanism of action and effects. The primary effect of β_2-agonists in the respiratory tract is the dilation of the airway by relaxing the smooth muscle. For this reason they are used to provide immediate symptomatic relief of an asthmatic attack. They also increase the rate of ciliary transport of mucus and decrease the release of mediators which, for example, result in the formation of oedema. See Figure 18.4. All three of the effects will improve ventilation during an asthma attack. β_2-agonists possess no anti-inflammatory effects.

β_2-agonists may be classified as either short-acting or long-acting. Short-acting β_2-agonists relieve the immediate effects of a mild asthma attack and may be used in anticipation that an attack is about to occur. Long-acting β_2-agonists are used to prevent asthma rather than providing symptomatic relief from an acute attack. They are often used together with inhaled glucocorticoids. See Table 18.2.

Pharmacokinetics. β_2-agonists are most frequently administered by inhalation, although they can be administered orally. With inhalation, it is possible to use

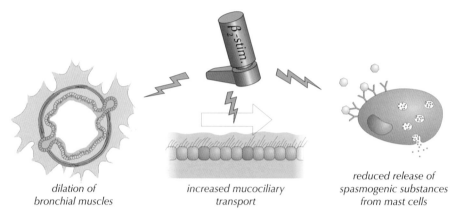

dilation of
bronchial muscles

increased mucociliary
transport

reduced release of
spasmogenic substances
from mast cells

Figure 18.4 **β₂-agonists.** The primary effect of β₂-agonists is dilation of airways by relaxing the smooth muscle. In addition, they increase ciliary transport and reduce degranulation of mast cells.

Drug name	Time to effect	Duration of effect
Fast acting β₂-receptor agonists		
Salbutamol	minutes	4–6 hours
Fenoterol	minutes	6–8 hours
Slow acting β₂-receptor agonists		
Bambuterol (Terbutalin)		
Terbutalin	minutes	6–8 hours
Formoterol	minutes	circa 12 hours
Salmeterol	10–20 minutes	12–16 hours

Table18.2 β₂-receptor agonists, time to effect and duration

lower doses than would be used with systemic administration. Elimination is primarily by metabolism to inactive metabolites.

Adverse effects. With moderate use, adverse effects will be minimized. However, with several subsequent doses or with the use of oral forms of drugs (i.e. larger doses), patients can experience palpitations, tremor and peripheral vasodilation with a mild drop in blood pressure. Palpitations are associated with stimulation of β₁-receptors in the heart whilst the vasodilation is due to activation of β₂-receptors in peripheral blood vessels. Tremors are associated with central nervous stimulation.

Since these drugs can stimulate the heart, they must be used with caution in patients with hypertension or ischaemic heart disease.

Theophylline

The main effect of theophylline is bronchodilation. It may be added to inhaled glucocorticoids and β₂-agonists when these alone fail to control asthmatic symptoms. It can be administered as tablets on a regular basis or intravenously as aminophylline in the treatment of acute, severe asthma attacks.

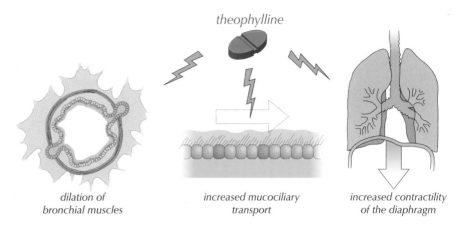

theophylline

dilation of
bronchial muscles

increased mucociliary
transport

increased contractility
of the diaphragm

Figure 18.5 **Theophylline.** The primary effect of theophylline is bronchodilation. In addition, it increases mucociliary transport and contractility of the diaphragm, which improves ventilation.

Mechanism of action and effects. The mechanism of action of theophylline is not well understood. The principal effect is bronchodilation by relaxation of smooth muscles. In addition to causing bronchodilation, theophylline increases mucociliary transport, stimulates the contractility of the diaphragm and increases the sensitivity of the medullary respiratory centre for CO_2, especially in premature children. It has a weak diuretic effect and enhances the effect of β_2-agonists. It may also prevent the release of mediators associated with the development of inflammation. See Figure 18.5.

Pharmacokinetics. Theophylline is well absorbed after oral administration, and peak plasma concentration is achieved 1–2 h after ingestion. Elimination is primarily by hepatic metabolism. However, there are large individual differences in the half-life of the drug. Cardiac failure, reduced renal function, acute viral respiratory infections and chronic obstructive lung disease appear to increase the half-life, so that the concentration in plasma increases. In smokers, the drug appears to have a shorter half-life and so there is a need to increase the dose. Patients treated with theophylline need regular monitoring of plasma concentrations in order to optimize their treatment. The use of depot preparations provides the possibility of a reduced number of administrations and a more stable plasma concentration.

Adverse effects. Theophylline has a narrow therapeutic range. Adverse effects within the normal therapeutic plasma concentrations include increased wakefulness, headaches, nausea and diarrhoea. Tachycardia and vasodilation with a drop in blood pressure are frequently experienced. High plasma concentrations may induce cramps. Large doses and high plasma concentrations should be avoided in pregnant women, as the drug easily crosses the placenta and can cause tachycardia, irritability and gastrointestinal problems in the fetus.

Leukotriene antagonists

The use of leukotriene antagonists (e.g. montelukast, zafirlukast) represents another line of treatment of obstructive lung diseases. The rationale is that

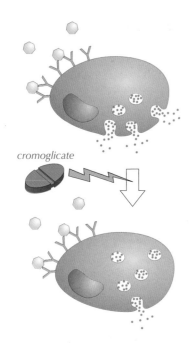

cromoglicate

Figure 18.6 **Cromoglicate.** Cromoglicate reduces the release of histamine and other spasmogenic substances.

leukotrienes are released from different cells during the inflammation. They both maintain and stimulate further the inflammatory process by stimulating different receptors, which lead to increased bronchial constriction, increased mucosal secretion and oedema and increased bronchial reactivity. By blocking the receptors to which leukotrienes bind, these effects are reduced. Leukotriene antagonists are administered orally.

The drugs take some time to produce clinical effects, although not as long as the glucocorticoids, so they are not effective in the immediate treatment of an acute asthma attack. Leukotriene antagonists may be added to inhaled glucocorticoids and β_2-agonists (instead of theophylline) when these alone fail to control asthmatic symptoms.

The most common adverse effects are fatigue, stomach pains, dizziness, headache and insomnia. In rare cases, there are serious allergic reactions to the drugs.

Cromoglicate

Cromoglicate is used prophylactically in exercise-induced and allergic asthma. The drug appears to be less effective than local administration of glucocorticoids and it has no effect in suppressing an acute attack once it has started.

Mechanism of action and effects. Cromoglicate inhibits immediate and delayed antigen-triggered release of histamine and other pro-inflammatory mediators from mast cells in lung tissue. See Figure 18.6. Chronic treatment with cromoglicate will provide the airways with some protection against the harmful effects of these mediators.

Pharmacokinetics. There is insignificant absorption of the drug if it is administered orally, so cromoglicate is only administered locally by inhalation. The majority of the dose administered is eliminated unmetabolized by mucociliary transport out of the lungs.

Adverse effects. With the exception of local irritation and a feeling of dryness in the throat, there are few adverse effects. However, the use of cromoglicate has been reduced in recent years primarily due to the efficacy of inhaled glucocorticoids.

Ipratropium

Ipratropium possess anticholinergic activity and can inhibit the bronchoconstriction evoked during an allergic asthma attack.

Mechanism of action and effects. Ipratropium is an antagonist at muscarinic cholinergic receptors in the parasympathetic autonomic nervous system. By blocking the effect of acetylcholine on muscarinic receptors in the bronchial mucosa, the parasympathetic activity is inhibited. This results in reduced contraction of the airway smooth muscle and also a reduction in mucus secretion. See Figure 18.7. Ipratropium is used in the treatment of chronic bronchitis, when mucus secretion can be considerable.

Pharmacokinetics. Ipratropium is administered locally as an aerosol. It is poorly absorbed and consequently will not have significant actions at muscarinic cholinergic receptors other than those located in the airways.

Adverse effects. When administered by inhalation, there are a few, mild anticholinergic adverse effects, e.g. dry mouth, constipation etc. Failure to fully inhale a dose results in deposition of the drug in the oral cavity and further dryness of the mouth.

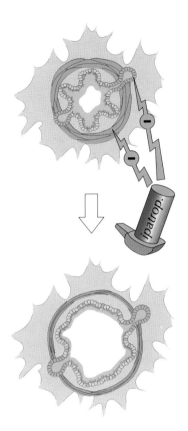

Figure 18.7 **Ipatropium bromide** relaxes bronchial constriction and reduces bronchial secretion without inhibiting the mucociliary transport.

MANAGEMENT OF CHRONIC ASTHMA IN ADULTS AND SCHOOL CHILDREN

In chronic asthma a step by step increase in medication is advised. The progression could be as follows:

Step 1
Inhale short-acting β_2-agonists to relieve acute attacks.
   If needed more than two times a day more than three days a week or
   if night symptoms appear more than once a week or
   if exacerbation during the last two years requiring systemic corticosteroids or nebulized bronchodilator,
   move to step 2.

Step 2
Add to Step 1 regular standard-dose of inhaled glucocorticoids.
   If symptoms are not controlled move to step 3.

Step 3
Add to Step 2 regular standard doses of inhaled long-acting β_2-agonists.
   If symptoms are not controlled, discontinue inhalation of long-acting β_2-agonists and increase doses of inhaled glucocorticoids to upper range.
   If symptoms are not controlled, add a
         leukotriene antagonist or
         slow-release theophylline formulation or
         oral β_2-agonist.
   If symptoms are not controlled move to step 4.

Step 4
Add to Step 3 the second or/and the third of the reminding alternatives in step 3.
If symptoms are not controlled move to step 5.

Step 5
Add to Step 4 a single dose of prednisolone tablets.
   If symptoms are not controlled the patient should be referred to an asthmatic clinic.

Review treatment every three months. Step down prednisolone doses carefully to the lowest dose that controls the symptoms. Step further down if possible. Educate patient in self-management of medication.

PATIENT EDUCATION AND SELF-MANAGEMENT OF OBSTRUCTIVE LUNG DISEASES

There is a policy to establish good self-treatment protocols in patients with chronic obstructive lung disease. This involves patients in becoming familiar with their disease and making changes in the basic medication according to their own needs. Obstructive lung diseases display seasonal variability in many patients. Drug treatment should vary with the severity of the disease.
   Drugs used to treat obstructive lung disease are listed in Table 18.3.

Inhaled glucocorticoids
Beclometasone, Budesonide, Fluticasone, Mometasone

β2-agonists
Bambuterol, Fenoterol, Formoterol, Salbutamol, Salmeterol, Terbutaline

Theophylline
Theophylline, Aminophylline

Leukotriene antagonists
Montelukast, Zafirlukast

Chromglicate
Cromoglicate

Anticholinergics
Ipratropium, Tiotropium

Table18.3 Drugs used to treat obstructive lung diseases

BRONCHIECTASIS AND CYSTIC FIBROSIS

Bronchiectasis is a pathological dilation of the bronchi. The bronchial wall is inflamed and thickened with a reduced mucociliary transport. The disease presents with coughing and production of considerable amounts of mucus, which is often infected. The cause of the disease is uncertain, but repeated respiratory infections probably play a considerable role. Viscous mucus may be treated with mucolytics.

Some patients are helped by the use of a bronchodilator, but drug treatment consists primarily of antibiotic therapy.

Cystic fibrosis is an autosomal recessive disease affecting the exocrine glands in the body that disrupts mucus production, resulting in a viscous mucus with a reduced water and sodium chloride content. The symptoms from the respiratory tract are obstruction of small airways and an increased tendency for respiratory infections, often triggered by the bacteria *Staphylococcus aureus* or *Pseudomonas aeruginosa*. Such infections require intensive antibiotic therapy. Viscous secretion may be treated with mucolytics.

Mucolytics

Airway mucus contains varying amounts of polysaccharides, glycoproteins, albumin and DNA from necrotic cells, all of which contribute to its viscosity. Mucolytics (e.g. mecysteine hydrochloride) act by making the mucus less viscous, thereby increasing the ciliary transport of mucus out of the airways to the mouth. The effectiveness of these drugs has been questioned.

Dornase alfa is an enzyme (deoxyribonuclease) that breaks down free extracellular DNA which is found in the increased amounts of infected mucus in the respiratory passages. This makes the mucus less viscous. It is used prophylactically to prevent the accumulation of DNA in the mucus thereby limiting airway complications.

Drugs used as mucolytics are listed in Table 18.4.

Mucolytics
Carbocisteine, Dornase alfa, Meycysteine

Table18.4 Mucolytics

SUMMARY

- Coughing is a symptom of underlying disease and a physiological reflex that can be triggered by irritation of the mucosa in the respiratory passages. Dry cough can be treated with cough suppressants, and productive coughs can be treated with expectorants. With purulent expectorations, underlying infections should be treated with antibiotics.
- Obstructive lung disease results in reduced ventilation and reduced gas exchange and may be due to asthma, chronic bronchitis or emphysema. In asthma and chronic bronchitis, the airways are hyperactive and respond to a variety of different agents by contraction of bronchial smooth muscle and the development of inflammation, hypersecretion and oedema. In emphysema, there is degeneration of alveolar tissue and capillaries, leading to reduced elasticity of the lung tissue with bronchiolar collapse and reduced gaseous exchange.
- In these diseases, drugs are used that inhibit bronchoconstriction, inflammation, oedema and mucus secretion.
- Glucocorticoids have strong anti-inflammatory effect because they inhibit the production and release of pro-inflammatory mediators and increase the synthesis of anti-inflammatory substances. Local use (inhalation) produces effects at doses lower than those necessary for systemic administration. They are used increasingly as the drug of choice in patients whose asthma cannot be controlled with β_2-agonists.
- β_2-agonists are usually administered locally. The drugs produce a bronchodilation primarily, but also increase mucociliary transport and inhibit the release of some of the mediators that contribute to the development of inflammation in the airway mucosa.
- Theophylline is administered systemically. It produces a bronchodilation, increased mucociliary transport and increased contractility of the diaphragm. In newborns, the medullary respiratory centre is sensitized to CO_2.
- Leukotriene antagonists inhibit the binding of leukotrienes to their receptors and in doing so inhibit the effects of these inflammatory mediators.
- Cromoglicate is used prophylactically. It inhibits the immediate and delayed release of histamine and other pro-inflammatory mediators.
- Ipratropium exerts an anticholinergic effect on muscarinic receptors in the airways when it is administered via inhalation, resulting in reduced airway secretions and inhibition of bronchoconstriction.
- Viscous secretion in cystic fibrosis may be treated with Dornase alfa.

19 Drugs used to treat gastrointestinal diseases

The gastrointestinal tract is a muscular hollow organ leading from the mouth to the anus. Peristaltic movements facilitate the transport of the intestinal contents from the oral cavity towards the rectum. Throughout its length, different glands in the gastrointestinal tract produce and secrete enzymes that contribute to breaking down the food into small molecules that are absorbed by the small intestine. Fluids and electrolytes are reabsorbed in the large intestine, so the intestinal contents gradually become firmer before the intestinal contents reach the rectum, from which it is emptied. In addition, the composition of the intestinal contents is crucial for local hormonal and nervous reflexes that influence the activity of the intestinal tract. There are several disorders that can affect the gastrointestinal tract. Different structure and functions in different parts of the intestinal tract can give rise to different regional disorders.

GASTRO-OESOPHAGEAL REFLUX

Gastro-oesophageal reflux means that contents from the stomach are pushed upwards (i.e. refluxed) into the oesophagus.

PATHOPHYSIOLOGY OF GASTRO-OESOPHAGEAL REFLUX

When food is not being moved through the oesophagus, it is kept closed by a two muscular sphincters at its top and bottom as well as by muscular tone along its entire length. Under normal conditions, the stomach contents will not be pushed up into the oesophagus as the lower (gastro-oesophageal) sphincter remains closed unless food is being passed into the stomach.

In some individuals, closing of this sphincter is incomplete due to periodic relaxation of the muscles or increased upward pressure of the gastric contents, so that some of the contents move back up through the sphincter (this may occur in hiatus hernia). This can cause gastro-oesophageal reflux disease (GORD) where reflux of acidic stomach contents leads to irritation and inflammation of the mucosa in the oesophagus. See Figure 19.1.

Symptoms

Acid reflux causes burning pains in the throat. Bending over forwards, lifting heavy objects and enjoying large meals with fatty, fried and heavily spiced foods exacerbate the problem. The symptoms can sometimes be difficult to distinguish from those seen in coronary disease.

Long-term inflammation of the oesophageal mucosa can lead to the development of stenosis in the sphincter between the oesophagus and the stomach. Changes in the mucosa of the oesophagus can increase the risk of developing cancer.

Gastro-oesophageal reflux can be reduced by avoiding large meals, particularly just before bedtime. Excessive intake of caffeine should be reduced. Similarly, consumption of tobacco, alcohol and foods that provoke the problem should also be reduced. It is important to lose excess weight.

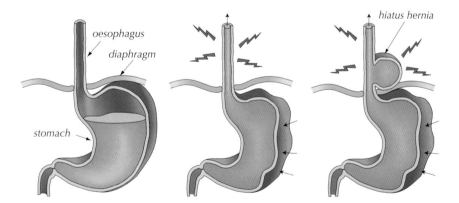

Figure 19.1 **Gastro-oesophageal reflux.** The stomach contents are moved upwards into the oesophagus. The acidic stomach contents damage the mucosa in the oesophagus and cause a burning sensation (dyspepsia). Hiatus hernias increase the possibility of this problem.

DRUGS USED TO TREAT GASTRO–OESOPHAGEAL REFLUX

Drug treatment is aimed at:

- increasing tone in the gastro-oesophageal sphincter and improving gastrointestinal motility
- protecting the oesophageal mucosa
- using acid-neutralizing drugs
- inhibiting acid secretion in the stomach
- relieving pain and discomfort.

The three last items are discussed in the section on ulcers (below).

Drugs inducing increased tone in the gastro-oesophageal sphincter and improved gastrointestinal motility

By increasing the tone of the gastro-oesophageal sphincter the gastric contents will be kept in the stomach. By increasing the gastrointestinal motility, the gastric contents will be more easily propelled along the intestinal route. Both processes result in reduced gastro-oesophageal reflux. Metoclopramide improves the muscle tone in the intestinal tract.

Metoclopramide

Mechanism of action and effects. Metoclopramide causes an increased release of acetylcholine locally in the intestinal tract, and thereby increased tone in the lower part of the oesophagus. Gastrointestinal motility is simultaneously stimulated, which improves the emptying of the stomach and duodenum. The effect is increased emptying of the stomach and reduced gastro-oesophageal reflux.

Adverse effects, precautionary measures and elimination. Sedation and extrapyramidal effects, drowsiness, restlessness and diarrhoea are seen in some patients. Metoclopramide is mainly eliminated by renal excretion. Patients with a reduced renal function should start with a reduced dose.

Protection of the oesophageal mucosa

The oesophageal mucosa may be protected by covering the gastric content with foamy gel. Alginates prevent the stomach contents from being moved up into the oesophagus.

Alignates

Mechanism of action and effects. These preparations are a combination of alginate and antacids in the form of alkaline aluminium, magnesium and/or sodium carbonate or hydroxide. When alginate with added carbonate is stirred in water, a foam is created that will lie like a gel uppermost in the stomach, preventing reflux. See Figure 19.2. Aluminium or magnesium compounds contribute to a more favourable environment, as they provide an almost neutral pH.

Adverse effects and precautionary measures. There can be increased sodium absorption in the form of sodium bicarbonate. Increased sodium absorption will ultimately lead to an increase in blood volume. In patients with cardiac failure, increased sodium absorption can therefore lead to exacerbation of the failure.

PEPTIC ULCERS

Ulcers may occur in the stomach or duodenum at sites where the mucosal epithelium is exposed to pepsin and acid. This condition is associated with inflammatory

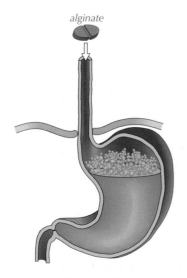

alginate

Figure 19.2 **Alginate** lies like a protective 'cover' over the stomach contents and prevents reflux.

damage to the mucosa and underlying structures. Epigastric burning pain is the major symptom of peptic ulcers. The pain of stomach ulcers most often arises during meals, while the pain associated with duodenal ulcers typically arises some time after meals, very often during the night. The pain is reduced by a reduction in gastric acid secretion or by antacids. Dyspepsia is a term often used to describe symptoms of peptic ulcers, which covers epigastrial pain, fullness, early satiety, bloating and nausea.

PATHOPHYSIOLOGY OF PEPTIC ULCERS

The stomach mucosa comprises several different cells:

- mucus-producing cells – the mucus forms a protective layer over the stomach's internal surface
- parietal cells – these produce hydrochloric acid; histamine stimulates the parietal cells to increase hydrochloric acid production
- chief cells – these produce pepsinogen, which is converted to pepsin in the acidic environment
- gastrin-producing cells – these cells produce gastrin which stimulates increased acid production. Hydrochloric acid and pepsin can contribute to ulceration of the mucosa of the stomach surface. See Figure 19.3.

Peptic ulcers are caused by the effects of pepsin and hydrochloric acid at the epithelial surface. The bacterium *Helicobacter pylori* is present in the edge of the ulcer of the mucosa in almost every subject with duodenal ulcers and in most with gastric ulcers, which contributes to local inflammation. Treatment that eradicates the bacterium is very effective in healing ulcers.

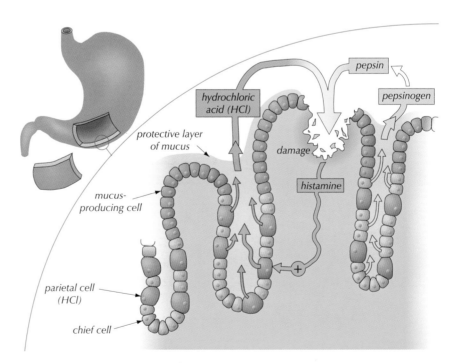

Figure 19.3 **Mucosal damage in peptic ulcers.** Tissue damage leads to a release of histamine. Hydrochloric acid and pepsin stimulate the histamine release, which in turn leads to increased secretion of hydrochloric acid. A peptic ulcer can penetrate considerably more deeply than shown in the figure.

Alcohol and smoking will exacerbate gastric problems in many cases. Non-steroidal anti-inflammatory drugs (NSAIDs) exacerbate ulcer problems and are contraindicated in this condition. These drugs are discussed in Chapter 14, Drugs with central and peripheral analgesic effects.

In the past, many patients underwent surgical removal of a part of the stomach or had the fibres of the vagus nerve cut (which stimulates acid secretion). Since the development of drugs that reduce acid secretion, surgical treatment has been considerably reduced.

Control of acid secretion

Gastrin, histamine and acetylcholine stimulate the secretion of hydrochloric acid by activating protein kinase. Protein kinase then stimulates a proton pump, which pumps H^+ ions into the lumen of the stomach. Prostaglandin I_2 and E_2 inhibit parietal cell acid secretion by inhibiting adenylyl cyclase, which in turn results in decreased protein kinase activity. Control of acid secretion is shown in Figure 19.4.

DRUGS USED TO TREAT PEPTIC ULCERS

The aim of drug treatment is to reduce the risk of complications of excessive acid secretion. Haemorrhage occurs because ulcers have exposed blood vessels which are damaged and bleed. Perforation of the stomach wall can occur, causing the contents to seep out into the abdominal cavity, resulting in peritonitis. Scar formation and fibrosis can lead to obstruction of gastric outflow.

Drug treatment is aimed at:

- reducing acid secretion
- increasing mucosal protection
- neutralizing the hydrochloric acid

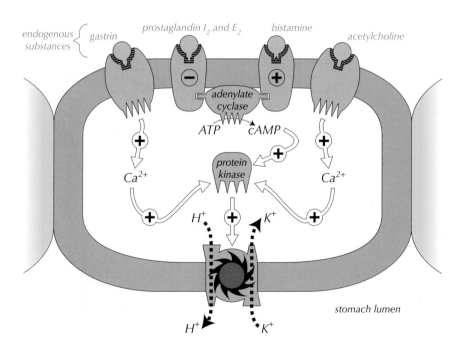

Figure 19.4 **Effect of endogenous substances.** Gastrin, histamine and acetylcholine stimulate receptors on the parietal cells leading to increased acid production. Prostaglandin I_2 and E_2 have an inhibitory effect on acid production.

■ eradication of *Helicobacter pylori*
■ relieving pain (in practice, the pain is relieved when the acid secretion is reduced or when the ulcer development and the inflammation cease).

Drugs that reduce the acid secretion

By inhibiting the acid secretion, the pH at the surface of the mucosa is increased (i.e. the stomach contents become less acidic). Histamine H_2-receptor antagonists, prostaglandins and proton pump inhibitors all act differently to reduce the acid secretion.

Histamine H_2-receptor antagonists

Histamine H_2-receptor antagonists reduce both basal and stimulated acid secretion from the gastric mucosa.

Mechanism of action and effects. By blocking the histamine H_2 receptors, the intracellular concentration of cAMP is reduced, protein kinase activity is reduced and hence proton pump activity is decreased, resulting in decreased acid secretion into the stomach.

These drugs accelerate the healing of the ulcers and improve gastric problems. Many individuals notice relief of symptoms a short time after commencing therapy. For patients who experience a relapse after they stop taking the drugs, a small daily dose can be of help and may prevent the development of new ulcers. The histamine H_2-receptor antagonists also provide relief in many patients with gastro-oesophageal reflux. See Figure 19.5.

Adverse effects, precautionary measures and elimination. Used in recommended doses, there are few adverse effects of these drugs. Cimetidine inhibits

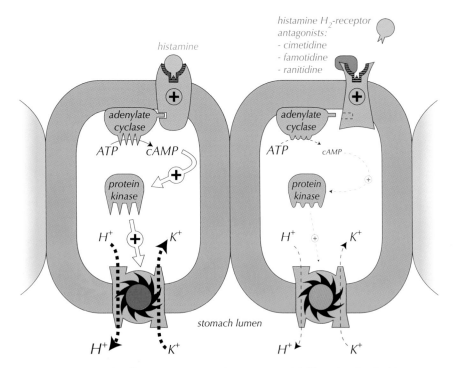

Figure 19.5 Histamine H_2-receptor antagonists compete with histamine for the H_2-receptors. This prevents the activation of adenylyl cyclase. The result is reduced acid secretion.

cytochrome P450 and can thereby contribute to slower metabolism of other drugs, such that the concentration of these drugs will be increased. Long-term treatment with large doses of cimetidine can cause gynaecomastia in some patients. Ranitidine does not produce this effect in therapeutic doses.

Approximately 70 per cent is eliminated unchanged across the kidneys; the remainder undergoes hepatic metabolism. For pregnant women with acid reflux requiring treatment, acid-neutralizing drugs may be more appropriate.

Proton pump inhibitors

At present, proton pump inhibitors are probably the most effective inhibitors of acid secretion.

Mechanism of action and effects. Omeprazole inhibits the enzyme hydrogen/potassium ATPase (H^+/K^+-ATPase), which acts as a proton pump. This is the last step in the secretion of hydrochloric acid into the lumen of the stomach. Inhibition of the pump lowers the acidity of gastric juices. The effect is achieved approximately 2 h after ingestion. Used prophylactically, the full effect is observed after 3–5 days. See Figure 19.6.

Adverse effects, precautionary measures and elimination. There are few adverse effects with the use of therapeutic doses of these drugs. Headaches, nausea, diarrhoea and flatulence are the most common.

Omeprazole can reduce the elimination of drugs metabolized by cytochrome P450 in the liver. Lansoprazole has a higher bioavailability than omeprazole.

Prostaglandins

Prostaglandins E_1 and I_2, which are synthesized in gastric mucosa cells, inhibit adenylyl cyclase so that less cAMP is created, and consequently the proton pump receives a reduced stimulus for acid secretion.

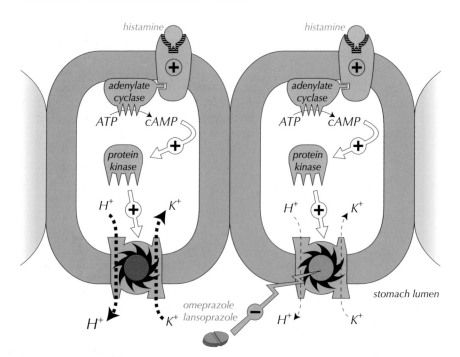

Figure 19.6 **Proton pump inhibitors** inhibit hydrogen/potassium ATPase and inhibit acid secretion. See Figure 19.4 for an overview.

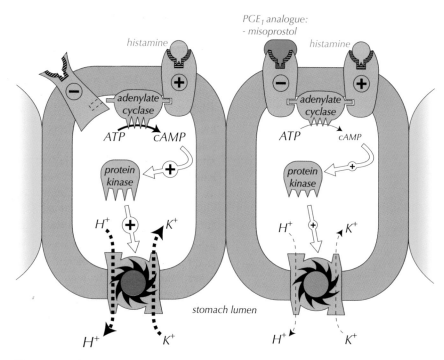

Figure 19.7 Prostaglandin E$_1$ agonists increase the inhibition of adenylyl cyclase. The result is less acid secretion. See Figure 9.4 for an overview.

Mechanism of action and effects. Misoprostol is a prostaglandin E$_1$ analogue that stimulates prostaglandin receptors in the gastric mucosa and inhibits adenylyl cyclase, thereby lowering the acid production. See Figure 19.7. In addition, secretion of mucus and bicarbonate is stimulated, so that the gastric surface is protected. Misoprostol can be used to prevent gastric ulcers in patients receiving treatment with NSAIDs.

Adverse effects, precautionary measures and elimination. Dose-dependent diarrhoea occurs, but is reduced if ingestion is in association with meals. Some prostaglandins can stimulate the uterus. Misoprostol is therefore contraindicated in pregnant women.

Drugs that increase mucosal resistance
The mucosal resistance can be increased by the use of drugs that bind to the ulcer surface and prevent hydrochloric acid and pepsin from eroding further into the mucosa. Sucralfate is such a drug.

Sucralfate
Sucralfate protects the ulcer surface by covering it.

Mechanism of action and effects. Sucralfate binds to proteins on the surface of a gastric ulcer and functions as a protective barrier against hydrochloric acid and pepsin. In addition, mucus secretion is stimulated. See Figure 19.8.

Adverse effects, precautionary measures and elimination. Sucralfate is hardly absorbed in the small intestine and thus there are few adverse effects of the drug. Some individuals may become constipated.

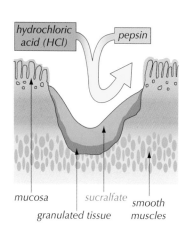

Figure 19.8 Sucralfate binds to the ulcer surface and protects against hydrochloric acid and pepsin.

Drugs that neutralize hydrochloric acid

Substances that neutralize the gastric acid will indirectly protect the epithelial cells of the stomach and duodenum from the effect of the hydrochloric acid and pepsin.

Antacids

Antacids are drugs that react with hydrochloric acid and form water-soluble salts. There are a number of different antacids.

Mechanism of action and effects. Antacids neutralize hydrochloric acid. The drugs contain aluminium or magnesium and/or sodium carbonate or hydroxide. As aluminium and magnesium salts are relatively insoluble, they remain in the stomach for a long time. Because the pH increases, conditions will be less favourable for pepsin activity. Antacids that contain aluminium also bind bile salts and exert a protective effect on the gastric mucosa. Symptoms arising from high gastric acidity can be relieved by antacids, but relatively large doses are required after each meal and at bedtime.

Adverse effects, precautionary measures and elimination. Protracted use can lead to disturbances in calcium phosphate metabolism, leading to demineralization of the skeleton. In reduced renal function, magnesium or aluminium can accumulate and cause symptoms of poisoning. Antacids can bind a number of drugs, e.g. digoxin, iron, tetracyclines and histamine H_2-receptor antagonists. Aluminium and magnesium are combined in several of the preparations used. Aluminium has a tendency to cause constipation, while magnesium can cause diarrhoea. Antacids containing sodium may exacerbate cardiac failure because sodium retains water, thereby increasing the circulating blood volume. The use of antacids has been reduced in recent years.

Antidepressants and anticholinergics

Antidepressants and anticholinergics have a limited effect on gastric ulcers. Because of their adverse effects, they are considered a poor alternative to newer drugs, and are used less and less for this purpose.

Eradication of H. pylori

The treatment usually combines inhibition of the acid secretion with antibiotics (and bismuth). The most common treatment is to use proton pump inhibitors, but histamine H_2-receptor antagonists are also used together with two different antibiotics and bismuth. Choice of antibiotics, dosage and dosage frequency vary in different treatment regimens.

Drugs used in the treatment of gastro-oesophageal reflux and peptic ulcers are listed in Table 19.1.

CHRONIC INFLAMMATORY BOWEL DISEASE: ULCERATIVE COLITIS AND CROHN'S DISEASE

Ulcerative colitis and Crohn's disease are chronic inflammatory diseases that can cause ulceration in the intestine. The primary cause is not well known, but may be due to changes in the sufferer's immune system, probably influenced by genetics and the environment. Often active disease periods are accompanied by skin, eye, joint, liver and kidney problems.

Ulcerative colitis causes ulceration in the colon. Patients show symptoms of bloody diarrhoea, fever and weight loss. The disease has several degrees of severity, and a pattern of relapse and remission is often observed. In the long term there is an increased chance of developing cancer of the large intestine.

Reduction of gastro-oesophageal reflux
Metoclopramide

Alginates with antacids
Alginic acid with aluminium hydroxide-magnesium carbonate

Histamine H$_2$-receptor antagonists
Cimetidine, Famotidine, Nizatidine, Ranitidine

Proton pump inhibitors
Esomeprazole, Lansprazole, Omeprazole, Pantoprazole, Rabeprazole

Prostaglandin analogues
Misoprostol

Drugs binding to ulcer surface
Bismuth, Sucralfate

Neutralization of acid
Antacids

Antibiotics to treat *Helicobacter pylori*
Amoxicillin, Claritromycin, Metronidazole

Table 19.1 Drugs used to treat gastro-oesophageal reflux and peptic ulcers

Crohn's disease can occur in both the small and large intestines. Refractory patients with this disease eventually require surgery to remove affected parts of the intestine. When large sections of the small intestine are removed, the length of the intestine is reduced, resulting in a reduced ability to absorb nutrients. Following surgery, relapse can occur in the remaining part of the intestines. Surgical treatment is not necessarily curative in the long term, as it is in ulcerative colitis.

DRUGS USED TO TREAT CHRONIC INFLAMMATORY BOWEL DISEASE

The purpose of drug treatment is to:

- alleviate acute attacks
- suppress the immunological and inflammatory activity
- prevent new attacks
- counteract complications.

Drug treatment is by use of aminosalisylates and corticosteroids. Local applications are used to treat disease affecting the rectum or the recto-sigmoid part of the large intestine.

Immune modulating drugs like cyclosporin, azathioprine, mercaptopurine or methothrexate may be used by specialists in severed inflammatory bowel disease. Infliximab is licensed to treat severe Crohn's disease when the disease has not responded to conventional immunosuppressants. These drugs are dealt with in Chapter 22, Drugs used in allergy, for immune suppression and in cancer treatment.

Aminosalisylates
These drugs form the primary medication used to maintain remission in ulcerative colitis and Crohn's disease. Sulfasalazine is the primary choice.

Mechanism of action and effects. Sulfasalazine is a compound made up of 5-aminosalicylic acid (5-ASA) and sulfapyridine. Olsalazine is a coupling together of two molecules of 5-aminosalicylic acid. Both sulfasalazine and osalazine are broken down in the intestine by intestinal bacteria. The active compound is 5-aminosalicylic acid.

| **Aminosalicylates** |
| Balsalazide, Mesalazine, Olsalazine, Sulfasaline |
| **Corticosteroids** |
| Budesonide, Hydrocortisone, Prednisolone |
| **Other drugs used to treat chronic inflammatory bowel disease** |
| Azathioprine, cyclosporin, mercaptopurine, methothrexate, infliximab |

Table 19.2 Drugs used to treat chronic inflammatory bowel disease

Their mode of action is unknown but these drugs may cause inhibition of leucocyte chemotaxis. The substances possibly have both anti-inflammatory and immunosuppressive effects. They suppress disease activity and reduce the number of relapses. The treatment period is long, and termination of treatment is not recommended until at least 2 years after the patient has been symptom-free.

Adverse effects, precautionary measures and elimination. The most common adverse effects are nausea, loss of appetite, headaches, dizziness, vomiting and tinnitus. In some cases, there is blood dyscrasia. Use in men results in a reduced sperm count, which is restored when drug treatment is concluded. Most adverse effects are dose-dependent.

Elimination shows genetic differences. Some individuals eliminate the drugs more slowly than others and are the most vulnerable group to adverse effects.

Glucocorticoids

As ulcerative colitis and Crohn's disease are considered to be disorders of immunological origin, it may be of value to use glucocorticoids, which suppress activity in the immune system. These drugs are used both locally and systemically.

Systemic administration of glucocorticoids is often the first choice for drug treatment of Crohn's disease, particularly when the small intestine is affected or when ulcerative colitis is also present. Initially, relatively high doses are used, but it is important to reduce the dose to the lowest possible maintenance treatment. The basis of treatment with glucocorticoids is their anti-inflammatory activity.

Glucocorticoids are discussed in Chapter 21, Drugs used to treat endocrinological disorders.

Drugs used in the treatment of chronic inflammatory bowel disease are listed in Table 19.2.

NAUSEA AND VOMITING

Nausea can be triggered by disease, by stimulation of certain senses (e.g. unpleasant sights) and by different substances in the intestinal tract that directly or indirectly activate the vomiting centres in the lateral reticular formation of the medulla. See Figure 19.9.

PATHOPHYSIOLOGY OF NAUSEA AND VOMITING

The vomiting centres lie in the lateral reticular formation of the medulla oblongata and can only be affected by substances that have crossed the blood–brain barrier. There is, however, an area, the chemoreceptor trigger zone, in the floor of the fourth ventricle where the blood–brain barrier is not intact. Water-soluble drugs and toxins can be distributed to this area and can activate chemoreceptors which communicate signals to the vomiting centre and trigger the vomiting reflex. In this way, nausea and vomiting are closely associated. See Figure 19.10. The chemoreceptors in the chemoreceptor trigger zone are associated with dopamine and

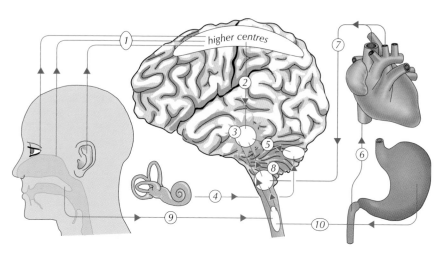

Figure 19.9 Mechanisms for triggering nausea and vomiting. Sensory stimuli from visual impressions, smell, taste or sounds (1) can be processed in higher centres and stimulate (2) the vomiting centres (3). Such sensory stimuli can be enhanced by previous experience. Stimuli from the vestibular disturbances in the inner ear are conducted (4) via the cerebellum and from there (5) to the vomiting centre. Toxins from the intestinal tract are absorbed into the blood (6) and are carried with the blood (7) to the chemoreceptor trigger zone in the floor of the fourth ventricle of the brain (8). The vomiting centres are stimulated from the chemoreceptor trigger zone (see also Figure 19.10). Impulses from local stimulation of the oesophageal wall (9) and the intestinal tract (10) are conducted via afferent nerve paths to areas in the medulla oblongata. From here, there are stimulation routes to both the chemoreceptor trigger zone and the vomiting centre.

5-hydroxytryptamine receptors. Renal failure and liver failure cause increased amounts of endogenous and exogenous breakdown products that are likely to stimulate the vomiting centre via this mechanism. The same is true with several drugs. Infections with viruses and other microbes can trigger nausea.

The vomiting centre can also be activated by visual or aural experiences, by smell, before certain events, such as examinations or going into combat, and by certain movement patterns (motion sickness). In addition, increased cerebral pressure, cardiac infarction and obstruction in the intestinal tract are associated with nausea.

DRUGS USED TO TREAT NAUSEA AND VOMITING

The most effective antiemetics block dopamine and 5-hydroxytryptamine receptors in the chemoreceptor trigger zone. See Figure 19.10. Granisetron, ondansetron and tropisetron selectively inhibit the 5-HT$_3$ receptor. These drugs are particularly effective in treating cytotoxic drug- and radiation-induced nausea.

Metoclopramide blocks dopamine receptors in low doses and 5-hydroxytryptamine receptors at high doses. In addition, gastric emptying and intestinal motility are stimulated. High doses are effective in cytotoxin- and radiation-induced nausea. Metoclopramide is often used in opiate-induced nausea following treatment for myocardial infarction. If combined with antipsychotics, extrapyramidal adverse effects can be pronounced. High doses cause sedation.

Antipsychotic drugs can have an antiemetic effect because they block the dopamine receptors in the chemoreceptor trigger zone. Apart from motion sickness, they are effective in most other forms of vomiting. Prolonged use can cause irreversible damage with uncontrolled muscular twitches (tardive dyskenesias).

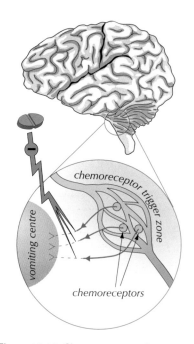

Figure 19.10 Chemoreceptor trigger zone. Drugs used to treat nausea and vomiting inhibit 5-hydroxytryptamine and dopamine receptors in the chemoreceptor trigger zone so that the vomiting centre does not receive stimulating signals from the chemoreceptor trigger zone.

5-HT₃ receptor antagonists
Granisetron, Ondansetrol, Tropisetron

Dopamine antagonists
Domperidone, Metoclopramide

Antipsychotics
Chlorpromaxine, Haloperidol, Levomepromazine,
Perphenazine, Prochlorperazine, Trifluoperazine

Antihistamines
Cinnarizine, Cyclizine, Meclozine, Promethazine

Table 19.3 Drugs used to treat nausea and vomiting

Antipsychotic drugs are discussed in more detail in Chapter 13, Drugs used to treat psychiatric disorders.

Older generation antihistamines have varying degrees of effect on 5-hydroxytryptamine receptors and muscarinic receptors that probably contribute to reducing nausea. They are used extensively in travel sickness and, to some extent, to treat vomiting in pregnancy. These antihistamines also have different degrees of sedative effect. Antihistamines are discussed further in Chapter 22, Drugs used in allergy, for immune suppression and cancer treatment.

Drugs used in the treatment of nausea and vomiting are listed in Table 19.3.

DIARRHOEA

Substances that bind water in the intestines, inflammation of the intestinal mucosa, toxins from microorganisms and altered intestinal flora can trigger diarrhoea.

Sudden diarrhoea occurs frequently, usually lasts a short time and normally does not require treatment. Diarrhoea that lasts more than 1 week should be investigated. Prolonged diarrhoea, where the patient cannot maintain sufficient fluid intake, together with clinical symptoms such as fever and poor general condition, may require hospital treatment.

The main goal of treatment of diarrhoea is to prevent dehydration and loss of electrolytes and to avoid unnecessarily frequent emptying. By inhibiting intestinal motility and increasing fluid and electrolyte absorption in the large intestine, the degree of diarrhoea can be modified. In many cases, however, such treatment is not necessarily desirable, as diarrhoea also removes toxins and causative microorganisms from the intestine.

DRUGS THAT COUNTERACT DIARRHOEA

Opiates reduce the intestinal motility considerably and were in considerable use at one time. Because of the risk of abuse, their use has been reduced to a minimum.

Loperamide is a synthetic opioid that probably exerts a local effect in the intestines. Intestinal motility is reduced and the passage of the intestinal contents is slowed, so that the time for absorption of fluid and electrolytes is increased. In addition, secretion to the intestinal lumen is reduced while the absorption is increased.

Loperamide does not cross the blood–brain barrier and does not have the opioids' potential for abuse. In recommended doses, there are few adverse effects, although large doses can lead to constipation and stomach pains. The pharmacological effect is increased by adding loperamide as a prodrug in the form of loperamide oxide.

FUNCTIONAL INTESTINAL DISEASE

Functional intestinal disease is the term used to describe long-term irregularities of faecal excretion. There are alternating periods of sluggish and loose bowel movements, flatus and stomach pains, but there is no established organic explanation for the problems which some individuals experience periodically.

IRRITABLE COLON: IRRITABLE BOWEL SYNDROME

Irritable colon is a condition characterized by frequent production of loose stools mixed with mucus, interrupted by periods with harder or lumpy stools. No drugs have a well documented success rate in this condition, although opioids and 5-hydroxytryptamine antagonists have met with varying degrees of success. It is important that the patient receives a thorough clinical (and sometimes X-ray/ endoscopic) examination. Regular meals are important and, allied to a diet rich in fibre and exercise to stimulate the intestinal motility, can have a favourable effect.

CONSTIPATION

Intestinal contents are transported down the intestinal lumen by spontaneous peristaltic movements. Increased volume in the intestines and increased secretion to the intestinal lumen increase the peristaltic movements and expel the intestinal contents more rapidly.

Constipation is a subjective feeling of not defecating frequently enough, with sufficient ease or in sufficient amounts. Neuroleptic drugs and antidepressant drugs have anticholinergic effects and can reduce secretion and motility in the intestines and thereby lead to constipation. Opiates also have an inhibitory effect on the intestinal motility. Diseases that prevent passage of the intestinal contents can cause constipation.

DRUGS USED TO TREAT FUNCTIONAL INTESTINAL DISEASE

Chronic use of laxatives often results in the user developing a type of 'dependence' on the drugs. This happens because the neuro-muscular reflexes that lead to the emptying function become so poor that the use of the laxative has to be maintained. Regular meals, exercise and fibre-rich diets are useful in regulating intestinal emptying in a natural way. Laxatives act by local stimulation so that intestinal motility is increased or by increasing secretion, or by softening the intestinal contents.

These drugs can be grouped into bulk-forming laxatives, osmotic laxatives, faecal softening laxatives and stimulant laxatives.

Bulk-forming laxatives

Bulk-forming laxatives consist of long-chain polysaccharides and salts, both of which bind water and increase the volume of the intestinal contents. The increase in volume causes the intestinal wall to stretch which stimulates the emptying reflex. See Figure 19.11. Bulk forming laxatives are useful in treating patients with colostomy, ileostomy, haemorrhoids, anal fissure and irritable bowel syndrome. Sufficient fluid intake is important to soften the intestinal content and avoid intestinal obstruction.

Bran is an example of a polysaccharide that is not broken down or absorbed in the intestines of humans, but binds water and increases the volume of the intestinal contents. The effect first appears after a few days of use. There are few adverse effects. These drugs are recommended when laxatives 'must' be used.

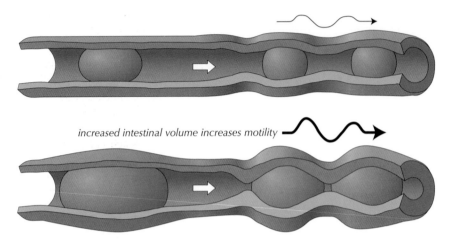

Figure 19.11 **Bulk-forming laxatives** cause increased peristalsis and push the intestinal contents out of the intestines.

Osmotic laxatives

Saline laxatives (magnesium or sodium salts) bind water in the intestines. Absorption of salt can be a problem. Magnesium salts can cause hypermagnesaemia in renal failure. Sodium salts can cause fluid retention and exacerbation of heart failure. Lactulose is a disaccharide that is broken down by bacteria in the colon and is metabolized to lactic acid and acetic acid with a water-binding effect.

Softening laxatives

Liquid paraffin is a mineral oil that is only slightly absorbed but which lubricates and softens the intestinal contents. However, paraffin binds lipid-soluble vitamins and regular use can cause hypocalcaemia associated with vitamin D deficiency and coagulation disturbances associated with vitamin K deficiency.

Stimulant laxatives

Stimulant laxatives, such as senna, increase the secretion and stimulate peristaltic movements. See Figure 19.12. The drugs are not recommended for use in chronic constipation, but are well suited to emptying the intestines before an internal

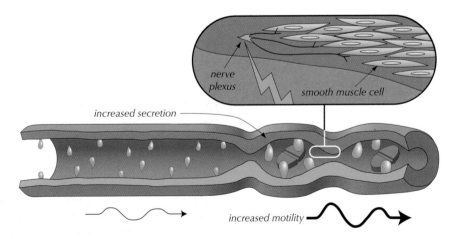

Figure 19.12 **Stimulant laxatives** increase secretion and peristaltic movements so that the emptying function improves.

Diarrhoea
Kaolin, Loperamide

Bulk-forming laxatives
Ispaghula husk, Methylcellulose, Sterculia

Osmotic laxatives
Lactulose, Macrogols, Magnesium salts

Softening laxatives
Arachis oil, liquid paraffin

Stimulant laxatives
Bisacodyl, Dantron, Docusate, Glycerol, Senna

Table 19.4 Drugs used to treat diarrhoea and constipation

examination. In long-term use, increased secretion from the intestinal mucosa can lead to a loss of electrolytes, particularly potassium.

Drugs used in the treatment of diarrhoea and constipation are listed in Table 19.4.

ITCHING AROUND THE ANUS (PRURITUS)

Many individuals experience itching around the anus. There are several possible causes, such as perianal eczema, secretion from the anal mucosa, anal fistulas, fungal infection, anal incontinence and increased perspiration due to warm clothing.

Mechanical stimulation in the form of scratching exacerbates the situation. When washing, rubbing should be avoided. Exaggerated washing with soap tends to exacerbate the problem.

DRUGS USED TO TREAT ITCHING AROUND THE ANUS

Excessive use of common soap should be avoided and soap with a low pH should be used. The skin can be lubricated with a water-repellent salve that can be washed off in the evening. Thereafter, cream or salve containing glucocorticoids might be applied. Glucocorticoids have a good antipruritic effect and suppress the inflammation and eczema. If there is fungal infection, this should be treated separately with an antifungal agent.

HAEMORRHOIDS

The causes of haemorrhoids are unknown, but the condition often arises or is exacerbated as a result of increased intra-abdominal pressure. An increase in abdominal pressure results in partly compressed inferior vena cava and inhibition of venous flow. This in turn leads to an increase in the venous pressure distal to the venous obstruction, spreading to the veins around the anus, leading to enlargement and prolapse of these veins. In women, haemorrhoids can occur during pregnancy because of the increased intra-abdominal pressure caused by the growing uterus. With haemorrhoids, it is therefore important not to increase abdominal pressure, i.e. cause increased pressure in the abdomen by straining the abdominal muscles, such as with heavy lifting, or performing a Valsalva manoeuvre to encourage defecation.

Soothing haemorrhoidal preparations Different preparations on sale to the public
Local corticosteroids Hydrocortisone, other haemorrhoidal preparations with corticosteroids
Local sclerosants Ethanolamine oleate, Sodium tetradecyl sulphate

Table 19.5 Drugs used to treat itching around the anus and haemorrhoids

Common symptoms are small haemorrhages. Pain occurs with thrombosis of enlarged veins. Because of difficulty in keeping the area clean, itching and burning occur relatively frequently.

Prevention of constipation is important. Surgical treatment of internal haemorrhoids is by use of elastic band ligation. External haemorrhoids can be surgically removed.

DRUGS USED TO TREAT HAEMORRHOIDS

Drugs with an astringent and anti-inflammatory effect can be used. Astringent drugs act locally by irritating the mucosa in the rectum and producing a vessel-contracting effect. After a while, they will reach the fibrosis in the mucosa and possibly in the vascular wall. In this way, there is a 'strengthening' of the tissue, which can prevent the tendency for varicose veins and prolapse.

Glucocorticoids act as anti-inflammatory agents. They are most effective in acute haemorrhoids. Suppositories and creams can be used several times a day initially; thereafter, the frequency of the application is reduced.

Many individuals are helped by short-term treatment of 5–10 days' duration, although prolonged use of glucocorticoids can cause mucosal atrophy.

OBESITY

The connection between obesity and diseases such as hypertension, other cardiovascular diseases and diabetes has encouraged research into new treatment regimes for obesity. Changing an unhealthy diet and increased activity are probably the most important elements in weight reduction. However, for overweight individuals who do not achieve results from a change in their lifestyle, some drugs are available, but their effectiveness is yet to be fully established.

DRUGS USED TO TREAT OBESITY

Drug treatment of obesity should be given in combination with other weight-reducing programmes.

Orlistat

Orlistat acts by inhibiting intestinal lipases from breaking down fat in the diet to absorbable triglycerides and free fatty acids. Thus approximately 30 per cent of the fat passes through intestine without being absorbed. With such a high fat content in the faeces, many individuals experience diarrhoea, a problem that can be minimized by reducing the fat intake.

The drug may be chosen for patients with a high fat intake.

Inhibition of intestinal lipases
Orlistat

Apetite suppressant
Sibutramine

Table 19.6 Drugs used to treat obesity

Sibutramine
Sibutramine is an amphetamine like centrally acting appetite suppressant that acts by inhibiting the re-uptake of serotonin and noradrenaline. The drug might be chosen for patients who can not control eating. Increased blood pressure is seen in many users, which increases the risk of cardiovascular diseases.

SUMMARY

- Gastro-oesophageal reflux exists when gastric contents pass back up the oesophagus. Drug treatment aims to increase the tone in the oesophagus (metoclopramide); prevent reflux (alginate); reduce acid secretion (histamine H_2-receptor antagonists and proton pump inhibitors); and neutralize hydrochloric acid (antacids).
- Ulcers in the stomach or duodenum develop when the mucosa does not protect against the harmful effects of hydrochloric acid, pepsin and the bacterium *Helicobacter pylori*. Drug treatment aims to reduce acid secretion (H_2-receptor antagonists and proton pump inhibitors), protect the mucosa (sucralfate), neutralize the hydrochloric acid and eradicate bacterial infection (antibiotics).
- Ulcerative colitis and Crohn's disease are autoimmune, inflammatory intestinal diseases in the colon and the entire intestine, respectively. Drug treatment aims to alleviate acute attacks, suppress the inflammatory activity and prevent new attacks. Aminosalicylic acid compounds and local administration of glucocorticoids form the primary medication, but in particularly active periods, systematic glucocorticoids are also used.
- Nausea and vomiting are triggered by direct or indirect influences on the vomiting centres in the medulla oblongata. Antiemetics act by blocking 5-hydroxytryptamine and dopamine receptors.
- Diarrhoea is the consequence of increased secretion of fluid and electrolytes to the intestinal lumen and reduced absorption in the colon. Diarrhoea may be treated with drugs that reduce intestinal motility (loperamide).
- Functional intestinal diseases such as irritable bowel syndrome and constipation often result in unnecessarily large consumption of laxatives that reduce the intestine's physiological emptying function. If drugs are necessary, bulk-forming, osmotic, softening or stimulant laxatives can be used.
- Itching around the anus and haemorrhoids can be treated locally with anti-inflammatory drugs, drugs with an astringent effect, or antifungal agents.
- Treatment of obesity best involves a change in lifestyle as its basis. Drugs that reduce the fat absorption in the intestines can be tried in those individuals who do not achieve satisfactory results with the former approach. Drugs that suppress appetite may be effective.

20 Drugs used to treat diseases of the blood

Blood consists of cells and plasma. Blood cells are formed in the bone marrow and comprise red and white cells and platelets. The primary components of plasma are water, proteins, salts, lipids, carbohydrates and gases. See Figure 20.1.

A normal number of functioning red blood cells (erythrocytes) is important for the transport of oxygen and carbon dioxide to and from the tissues. White cells are necessary for a functioning immune system. Platelets and plasma proteins (coagulation factors) are important for stopping haemorrhages and for normal coagulation.

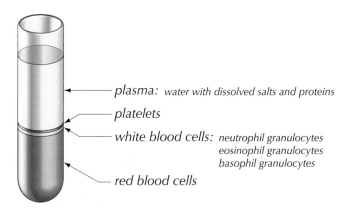

plasma: water with dissolved salts and proteins

platelets

white blood cells: neutrophil granulocytes
eosinophil granulocytes
basophil granulocytes

red blood cells

Figure 20.1 **The blood's components:** plasma, platelets, white blood cells and red blood cells.

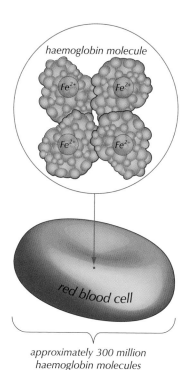

approximately 300 million haemoglobin molecules

Figure 20.2 **Red blood cells.** Each cell contains many haemoglobin molecules.

THE ANAEMIAS

Red blood cells contain haemoglobin, which carries oxygen from the lungs to the tissues. When the amount of haemoglobin drops, the blood's ability to transport oxygen is reduced. Haemoglobin concentration below certain limits is characterized as anaemia, and it is usually an indication of underlying disease.

PATHOPHYSIOLOGY OF ANAEMIAS

Production of red blood cells (erythrocytes) is called erythropoiesis and takes place in the bone marrow. Erythropoiesis is stimulated by the hormone erythropoietin, which is released from the kidneys in response to low oxygen saturations in the tissues. Each red blood cell contains approximately 300 million haemoglobin molecules. Haemoglobin consists of four protein molecules with a central haem molecule in each. Each haem molecule consists of a pyrrol ring with divalent iron in the centre. See Figure 20.2. Normal erythropoiesis requires supplies of iron, vitamin B_{12} and folic acid. A deficiency of one or more of these components results in reduced erythropoiesis, low haemoglobin and the gradual development of anaemia.

Haemoglobin concentration changes during life

The concentration of haemoglobin in the blood varies throughout the different stages of life. It is highest at birth and drops gradually to its lowest value at the age of 3 months. The rapid drop is due to the breakdown of fetal haemoglobin after the child is born. From then, the haemoglobin concentration rises gradually towards puberty, when it reaches its adult value. See Figure 20.3. At adult age, men have a somewhat higher haemoglobin value than women. The criteria that define anaemia are therefore related to age and gender. Anaemia is diagnosed if the haemoglobin concentration in adult males is lower than 13.0 g/dL, and in adult females is lower than 12.0 g/dL.

The symptoms of anaemia are associated with oxygen deficiency in the tissues. They are related to the severity of the anaemia and how quickly it develops. The general symptoms of anaemia are as follows:

■ listlessness and increased tiredness as a result of poor oxygen supply to the tissues
■ pallor due to the low haemoglobin value of the blood that circulates in skin and mucous membranes – an assessment of the colour of the mucosal membranes can therefore give a crude indicator of the likelihood of anaemia

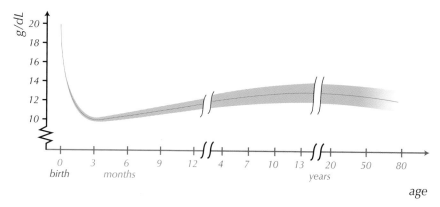

Figure 20.3 **Haemoglobin concentration.** The haemoglobin concentration varies with age. After birth, it drops quickly because fetal haemoglobin is broken down.

■ shortness of breath and palpitations – indicators that the tissues are receiving too little oxygen; this leads to increased stimuli to the respiratory muscles to increase ventilation, and to the heart to increase cardiac output to maximize oxygen delivery to the tissues

■ dizziness and a tendency to faint – again, these are the result of poor oxygen supply to the brain. Additional symptoms can also exist, depending on the cause of the anaemia.

■ angina pectoris (chest pain) or exacerbation of cardiac failure in the elderly with coronary artery disease.

Classification of anaemias

In this text, anaemias are classified according to cause (aetiological classification). The most common anaemias result from a deficiency of iron, folic acid or vitamin B_{12}. Haemolytic anaemia is often associated with hereditary defects in the red blood cells, while aplastic anaemia is often the result of adverse drug effects. See Figure 20.4. Another way of classifying anaemias is according to the shape and size of red blood cells (morphological classification).

IRON DEFICIENCY ANAEMIA

Iron deficiency anaemia develops as a result of a low iron content in the diet, low iron absorption or chronic haemorrhage, where the body continuously loses iron. Morphologically, iron deficiency anaemia is characterized by small erythrocytes (microcytic anaemia) with low haemoglobin content (hypochromic anaemia).

Vulnerable groups are premature children, women with heavy menstrual bleeding and individuals with an iron-poor diet. Patients who have had a part of the gastric mucosa surgically removed can also have iron deficiency anaemia because they have reduced production of hydrochloric acid, which is necessary for ionization of the iron before absorption.

The diagnosis is confirmed by various blood tests:

■ low serum iron (iron in serum that is not associated with haemoglobin)

■ high TIBC (total iron binding capacity) because the availability of transferrin (transport protein for iron) increases in iron deficiency

■ low ferritin – ferritin is a storage form of iron that 'leaks' into the plasma and reflects the body's iron storage. Ferritin can be normal or high in severe infections as it is also an acute-phase protein

■ lack of haemosiderin (storage form of iron) in bone marrow preparations.

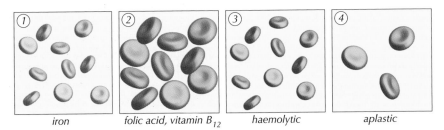

iron *folic acid, vitamin B_{12}* *haemolytic* *aplastic*

Figure 20.4 **Different forms of anaemia.** (1) Iron deficiency anaemia produces small erythrocytes. (2) A deficiency of folic acid or vitamin B_{12} produces large immature erythrocytes. (3) Haemolytic anaemia produces small erythrocytes. (4) Aplastic anaemia produces few erythrocytes with normal appearance.

Drugs used to treat iron deficiency anaemia

Iron deficiency can usually be corrected by iron supplements; the administration of divalent iron/ferrous salts (Fe^{2+}) orally is common but trivalent iron/ferric salts (Fe^{3+}) are also used.

Mechanism of action and effects. Divalent iron is essential for the haemoglobin molecule to bind oxygen. Trivalent iron (Fe^{3+}) must be reduced to divalent iron (Fe^{2+}) before it is absorbed. The effects of iron supplementation are increased haemoglobin synthesis and increased ability to transport oxygen.

Pharmacokinetics. In the acidic environment of the stomach, iron binds to proteins that keep it in solution within the small intestine and available for absorption. In iron deficiency, absorption of iron from the small intestine is increased. Ascorbic acid (vitamin C) increases absorption of iron by reducing trivalent to divalent iron. Absorption occurs because iron binds to a transport protein in the mucosal cell and is transferred to transferrin in plasma or to ferritin, a storage protein in the mucosal cell. The iron is transported to the bone marrow, bound to transferrin. Immature red blood cells bind transferrin and release the protein when the iron is absorbed.

Iron absorption is inhibited by tea and by the simultaneous use of antacids or tetracycline, which binds iron and other divalent metals. When there is deficient iron absorption, parenteral administration of iron may be necessary.

Adverse effects and precautionary measures. Constipation, diarrhoea, nausea and stomach pains are the most common adverse effects. Starting with low-dose supplementation can minimize the chances of adverse effects. Different individuals react differently to the different iron preparations available. It is often worthwhile changing the iron preparation if the adverse effects are severe.

ANAEMIAS ATTRIBUTED TO DEFICIENCY OF FOLIC ACID OR VITAMIN B_{12}

Folic acid and vitamin B_{12} are essential co-factors for the synthesis of DNA and are necessary for cell division. Deficiency particularly affects the production of blood cells in the bone marrow and generally first manifests itself in the form of anaemia because the synthesis of erythrocytes is inhibited. Anaemias attributed to deficiency of folic acid or vitamin B_{12} are also called megaloblastic anaemias. They derive their name from the appearance of the red blood cells in the bone marrow (*mega* = large, *blast* = spire). Blood films (the microscopic examination of the blood cells) taken from the bone marrow are therefore characterized by large, red blood cells that appear young, evaluated on the basis of colour and the ratio between the size of the nucleus and the cytoplasm. A deficiency of folic acid or vitamin B_{12} can also cause reduced cell division in the mucosal cells, particularly within the intestinal tract.

The body has considerably smaller stores of folic acid than of vitamin B_{12}. In individuals who suffer from malabsorption or who have an unbalanced diet, anaemia appears as a result of folic acid deficiency earlier than is the case with vitamin B_{12} deficiency. Anaemia attributed to vitamin B_{12} deficiency nonetheless occurs more frequently than anaemia attributed to folic acid deficiency.

Chronic alcoholics often have a diet with insufficient content of folic acid and vitamin B_{12}. Other risk groups are patients who have had a part of the gastric mucosa removed and who exhibit a reduced production of intrinsic factor (necessary for the absorption of vitamin B_{12}), and patients who have undergone long-term treatment with proton pump inhibitors. The risk is also increased in diabetes and thyroid disease, as the immunological mechanism that lies behind these diseases can also cause atrophic gastritis with reduced production of intrinsic factor.

Drugs used to treat anaemias due to deficiency in folic acid or vitamin B_{12}
Deficiency in vitamin B_{12} or folic acid should be compensated for by supplements.

Folic acid
The most important cause of folic acid deficiency is reduced absorption due to malabsorption in the small intestine. There is an increased need for folic acid in thyrotoxicosis, haemolytic anaemia and pregnancy. In malignant disease, folic acid supplements should not be administered, in order to avoid the proliferation of malignant cells.

Pharmacokinetics. Folic acid is usually administered orally and is absorbed in the duodenum. Only small amounts are stored in the body. In the light of inadequate intake of folic acid, anaemia develops within the course of a few months. Anaemia associated with folic acid deficiency is quickly corrected by folic acid supplements, usually within 1–2 months.

Vitamin B_{12} supplements
Vitamin B_{12} cannot be synthesized in the body and must be supplied from the diet. In a normal diet, the tissue depots will be sufficient for 2–5 years. Deficiency diseases as a result of reduced supply are therefore rare.

In addition to anaemia, vitamin B_{12} deficiency can cause damage to nerves in the spinal cord, which transmit stimuli from the peripheral nerves. This probably occurs because non-functional fatty acids are synthesized. In this way, the sense of vibration and proprioception (stimuli that indicate body position) can be affected and result in diminished balance and disorders of gait. When neurogenic symptoms are present, treatment must be started quickly to avoid irreversible nerve damage.

Where there is a suspicion of anaemia associated with folic acid or vitamin B_{12} deficiency, both should be administered simultaneously. This is because the anaemia is corrected by supplements of folic acid even if vitamin B_{12} remains deficient, but the risk of neurogenic damage is unchanged.

Pharmacokinetics. Vitamin B_{12} is absorbed in the duodenum. Absorption is dependent on a carrier molecule, intrinsic factor, which is secreted by parietal cells in the stomach. Pernicious anaemia is an autoimmune disease in which antibodies are created against parietal cells, and atrophic gastritis develops. In atrophic gastritis or following surgical removal of parts of the stomach, the secretion of intrinsic factor is diminished and leads to a reduction in the absorption of vitamin B_{12}.

In patients with reduced intrinsic factor, supplements of vitamin B_{12} must be administered parenterally. Oral maintenance treatment can be used in some patients, since large doses of vitamin B_{12} provide sufficient absorption without intrinsic factor. Vitamin B_{12} is carried to the cells by a protein that can be saturated. In large doses, the majority is therefore eliminated. Hydroxycobalamin is a form of vitamin B_{12} that provides long-lasting absorption, such that dosing is only necessary every 2–3 months.

Treatment with vitamin B_{12} is generally required for life. Parenteral treatment usually normalizes the blood profile after 6 weeks.

Anaemia associated with a folic acid or vitamin B_{12} deficiency responds quickly following treatment with a large increase in the number of red blood cells in the circulation. This results in a rapid increase of haematocrit (concentration of haemoglobin in the blood). Under such conditions, patients with cardiac failure can experience circulation problems due to increased viscosity of the blood.

HAEMOLYTIC ANAEMIA

Haemolytic anaemia is a disease in which the body destroys red blood cells (haemolysis) prematurely. If production cannot keep pace with destruction, anaemia develops. Drugs are not used to treat haemolytic anaemia.

APLASTIC ANAEMIA

In aplastic anaemia, there is a failure in the bone marrow's production of red blood cells. Normally, all the cell lines are affected, such that the numbers of red cells, white cells and platelets (thrombocytes) are reduced. The disease can develop without a known cause or be associated with external influences such as drugs, radiation or viral infection.

Drug-induced aplastic anaemia is usually caused by cytotoxic drugs, antirheumatics (gold salts and penicillamine) and chloramphenicol. NSAIDs, sulphonamides, antiepileptics, psychopharmaceuticals and oral hypoglycaemics can also cause aplastic anaemia. If the cause can be removed, the production of blood cells will usually recover.

Glucocorticoids, ciclosporin and anabolic steroids are used to treat aplastic anaemia. If the disease does not improve, bone marrow transplantation can be attempted. Otherwise, supportive treatment is required in the form of blood transfusions and antibiotic therapy (increased risk of infection due a reduction in the number of white blood cells).

POLYCYTHAEMIA

Polycythaemia is an abnormal increase in the number of circulating red blood cells. Polycythaemia is often secondary to diseases that result in poor oxygenation of the red blood cells (hypoxic heart/lung disease). In these conditions, the body will try to compensate for the hypoxia by synthesizing more red blood cells, which in turn transport more oxygen. The increased production of red blood cells will lead to a high haematocrit value, which can trigger cardiac failure due to the increased viscosity of the blood.

In polycythaemia, there can also be increased numbers of white blood cells and platelets. The disease is then called polycythaemia vera. It is considered to be a less aggressive form of bone marrow cancer (myeloproliferative disease).

Cytotoxic drugs are used in the treatment of polycythaemia vera.

Ferrous salts – oral formulations
Ferrous fumarate, Ferrous gluconate, Ferrous sulphate

Ferric salts – parenteral formulations
Iron dextran, Iron sucrose

Vitamin B$_{12}$
Cyanocobolamin, Hydroxocobolamin

Folates
Folic acid, Folinic acid

Table 20.1 Drugs used to treat anaemias

DYSFUNCTION OF WHITE BLOOD CELLS

Dysfunction of white blood cells primarily includes reduced formation in the bone marrow or increased production of immature, non-functioning cells, as is the case

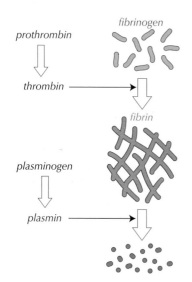

prothrombin

fibrinogen

thrombin

fibrin

plasminogen

plasmin

Figure 20.5 **The coagulation process – the last part.** Thrombin converts fibrinogen to fibrin. Plasmin breaks down the fibrin molecules.

in the leukaemias. Drugs that can influence white blood cells are discussed in Chapter 22, Drugs used in allergy, for immune suppression and in cancer treatment.

THROMBOEMBOLIC DISEASES

Under normal conditions, the blood circulates without platelets forming aggregates with each other or adhering to the vascular wall, and without the blood coagulating. Thrombosis is a process whereby the blood forms solid elements, thrombi, which bind to the vascular wall. If a thrombus mass detaches and is moved along with the circulation, the solid mass is called an embolus. Thromboses vary according to their size and whether they are formed in the arterial or venous circulation.

PATHOPHYSIOLOGY OF THROMBOEMBOLIC DISEASES

The fluidity of the blood is determined by factors contributing to coagulation and factors counteracting coagulation. Coagulation factors and platelets initiate the coagulation process, while endothelial cells and plasmin inhibit it. Coagulation factors are found in the blood in an inactive form. When the process starts, one factor activates the next (cascade). The last part of the coagulation occurs when prothrombin is activated to thrombin, which activates fibrinogen to fibrin. Fibrin is required for the formation of both arterial and venous thrombi, and makes the thrombus mass difficult to dissolve.

The blood also contains plasminogen, which can be activated to plasmin. Activated plasmin has the ability to decompose fibrin and dissolve a thrombus mass. This process is called fibrinolysis. The last part of the coagulation process and fibrinolysis are shown in Figure 20.5.

Arterial thrombi are initiated by activated platelets, primarily through damage to the vascular wall. Such damage can occur slowly over several decades (arteriosclerosis) or over a matter of hours as a result of acute damage to the vascular wall. Thrombus formation can develop over a short time. Arterial thrombus masses consist of a large number of platelets, but also of leucocytes and a fibrin network.

Venous thrombi develop mainly through activation of the coagulation factors, over a short time and often after damage to the vascular wall. In addition to fibrin, the thrombus mass consists of a number of platelets and leucocytes. The process of thrombus formation is shown in Figure 20.6.

When a piece of the thrombus mass loosens, the size of the embolus and where it lodges will be crucial in determining the extent of damage caused. The damage is associated with insufficient supply of oxygen and nutrients to the tissue (ischaemia) and an increase in the amount of waste products produced as a result of anaerobic cell metabolism in the tissue distal to the thrombus. Thrombi that are formed over a short time are easier to dissolve using drugs than those that are formed over a long period.

DRUGS USED TO TREAT THROMBOEMBOLIC DISEASES

Drugs used to treat thromboembolic disease are directed at preventing thrombosis formation or dissolving formed thrombus masses. There are three points of attack for such treatment:

■ anticoagulants – reduce the blood's ability to coagulate
■ platelet inhibitors – reduce platelet activation and platelet adhesion
■ fibrinolytics – increase the breakdown of fibrin and dissolve arterial and venous thrombi.

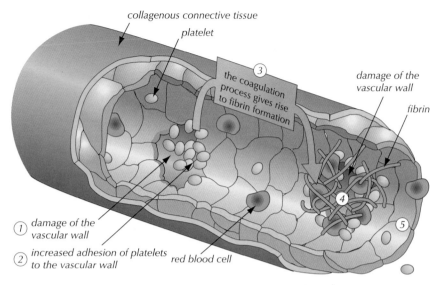

Figure 20.6 Thrombus formation. (1) Following damage to the vascular wall, collagenous connective tissue will activate platelets, which form aggregates with each other (2) and exhibit increased adhesion to the vascular wall. (3) Substances from activated platelets stimulate the coagulation process. (4) Aggregates of platelets and fibrin form the thrombus mass that grows on the arterial wall (5).

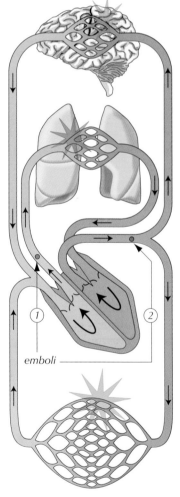

Figure 20.7 **Embolization.** (1) Venous embolisms lodge in the arteries of the pulmonary circulation. (2) Arterial emboli lodge in the arteries of the systemic circulation.

Prevention of thromboses

Thrombi on the arterial side of the circulatory system are prevented by the use of platelet inhibitors. If an arterial thrombus mass loosens, it will lodge in a smaller artery in the circulatory system. Atrial flutter poses a high risk for the development of atrial thrombi, particularly with simultaneous cardiac infarction, mitral valve failure or enlarged atrium. This is due to turbulent blood flow within the atria which is more prone to clot. Thrombi on the venous side are prevented by the use of anticoagulants. If a venous thrombus loosens and follows the blood flow, it will lodge in a pulmonary artery leading to a pulmonary embolus. See Figure 20.7.

Arterial thrombi

Thrombus masses from the left atrium can detach and be carried with the arterial blood flow to vital organs such as the brain, kidneys and abdominal arteries. Thrombus masses in the heart's atrium are treated primarily with anticoagulants. Arterial emboli must be treated quickly to prevent devastating ischaemia distal to the clot. Fibrinolytic treatment or surgical removal is often indicated.

Venous thrombi

Superficial thrombi are relatively harmless and do not require drug treatment. On the other hand, deep thrombi in large vessels require special treatment. It is important to prevent detachment and the development of pulmonary embolisms and post-thrombotic syndrome, which damage the venous valves and the veins with the further development of varices, oedema and an increased tendency for chronic leg eczema and ulceration. Thrombi located below the knee do not lead to post-thrombotic syndrome.

In the case of pelvic vein thrombus, deep femoral vein thrombus and, particularly, in massive pulmonary embolisms, fibrinolytic treatment must be considered.

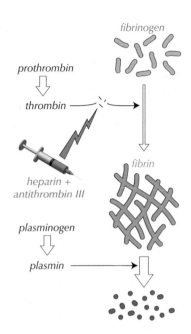

fibrinogen

prothrombin

thrombin

fibrin

heparin +
antithrombin III

plasminogen

plasmin

Figure 20.8 Heparin binds to antithrombin III and increases the inhibitory effect it has on the synthesis of fibrin.

Likewise, venous thrombi in the vital organs, such as the liver, kidneys and mesentery, also require urgent treatment with fibrinolytics.

It is important to be aware that both anticoagulants and fibrinolytics lead to an increased tendency to haemorrhage.

Anticoagulants

Anticoagulants can be divided into the two groups: heparins and vitamin K antagonists. They have different mechanisms of action and consequently different applications.

Heparins

Heparin is a sugar compound, a glucose amino glycan that occurs in mast cells, endothelial cells and plasma. It is a large molecule with varying molecular weight depending on the composition but is usually around 40 000 daltons (Da). Low-molecular-weight heparins are fragments of heparin with a molecular weight of 4000–15 000 which also have anticoagulant properties.

Mechanism of action and effects. Heparin acts primarily by binding to naturally occurring antithrombin III and enhancing its ability to inactivate thrombin, reducing the conversion of fibrinogen to fibrin. In addition, platelet aggregation is somewhat inhibited. See Figure 20.8. Prolonged use of heparin appears to reduce the production of antithrombin III, which in the long run increases the risk of venous thrombus formation. Low-molecular-weight heparins do not appear to have this property.

Because heparin prevents the formation of fibrin, thrombus formation or further growth of a thrombus is avoided. It is used prophylactically when there is an acute need for an anticoagulant effect, and in deep vein thromboses until an effect with other anticoagulants is achieved. Pregnant women should always use heparin when there is need for anticoagulation.

Pharmacokinetics. Heparin must be injected subcutaneously or intravenously. Intramuscular injections must be avoided because they can result in haemorrhage within the muscle. Heparin is removed from the circulation by the reticulo-endothelial system, where endothelial cells and macrophages are active. The half-life is relatively short, around 40–90 min.

Adverse effects. The most important adverse effect is haemorrhage, which occurs with too high a dose. It is important to test the blood's ability to coagulate and to titrate heparin therapy accordingly. Use of heparin can affect platelet formation and lead to the development of platelet antibodies (heparin-induced thrombocytopenia). In such cases, other anticoagulant agents must be used.

Protamine sulphate is an antidote for heparin and reduces/cancels the effect by creating an inactive complex with the heparin molecule.

Vitamin K antagonists

Warfarin, a vitamin K antagonist, is used when there is a long-term need for anticoagulant therapy.

Mechanism of action and effects. Synthesis of the coagulation factors II, VII, IX and X (proteins) takes place in the liver and is dependent on vitamin K. See Figure 20.9. Warfarin inhibits vitamin K from exerting its effect as a co-factor and results in reduced production of coagulation factors and also a reduction in proteins C and S, which have an anticoagulant effect. Because the production of coagulation factors is reduced, it takes a while before the effects are seen. Coagulation factors that are synthesized before commencing the drugs must be consumed

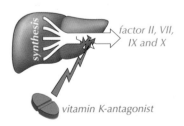

synthesis

factor II, VII, IX and X

vitamin K-antagonist

Figure 20.9 Vitamin K antagonists inhibit synthesis in the liver of the coagulation factors that are dependent on vitamin K.

before the full effect sets in. The time taken is dependent on the half-life of the coagulation factors. Full therapeutic effect is achieved after 5–7 days.

Since the synthesis of proteins C and S is inhibited after a shorter time (5–7 h) than the coagulation factors, there is an increased risk of thrombus formation immediately after commencing warfarin therapy. It is customary for patients to start heparin simultaneously with warfarin, and for the heparin to be continued for 2–3 days while a sufficient effect of warfarin is achieved. By administering warfarin, new thrombus formation is prevented.

Pharmacokinetics. Warfarin is well absorbed following oral administration. Elimination is by liver metabolism. A number of drugs are known to affect the metabolism of warfarin. It is therefore important to monitor the effects of warfarin by measuring the clotting profile frequently when a patient ceases or starts treatment with drugs that are known to affect its metabolism.

Adverse effects and precautionary measures. There is an increased tendency of haemorrhage from the nose, gums, stomach/intestines, urinary tract and skin. Serious haemorrhages occur in 2–5 per cent of users, including brain haemorrhage. The effect of warfarin is measured using the international normalized ratio (INR), a marker of clotting. Optimal therapeutic drug doses should produce an INR value of 2.0–3.5, depending on the indication for its use.

Experience shows that serious haemorrhage complications develop most frequently in elderly patients. It is therefore important to make certain that the patients understand the dosing regime and can cooperate precisely regarding treatment. Combinations with drugs that inhibit platelet function (NSAIDs) increase the risk of haemorrhage and must only be used in certain conditions.

Commencement of warfarin therapy must be closely monitored, especially if the patient has recently suffered tissue damage or has undergone any surgical intervention. In planned surgery, the dosage should be reduced to achieve a lower INR value. Women who breastfeed can use warfarin, but pregnant women must not use it as there is a possibility of fetal damage.

Haemorrhages are treated with vitamin K (antidote) or fresh plasma.

Platelet inhibitors

A number of substances affect the adhesiveness and function of platelets. Healthy vascular endothelium produces prostacyclin, which inhibits platelet activation and adhesion. Damaged endothelial cells activate the platelets such that they aggregate and attach to the vascular wall. Activated platelets release thromboxane, which increases platelet aggregation.

Acetylsalicylic acid

The most important platelet inhibitor is acetylsalicylic acid (ASA). ASA is used prophylactically to reduce the tendency for thrombus formation by patients with unstable angina pectoris and after myocardial infarction. Also ASA is used to

---

Standard heparin
Heparin

Low molecular heparins
Dalteparin, Enoxaparin, Tinzaparin

Vitamin K–antagonist
Warfarin

Table 20.2 Anticoagulants

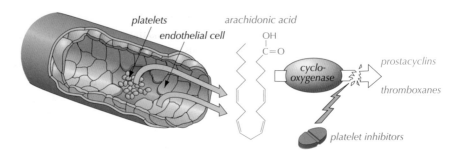

Figure 20.10 **Platelet inhibitors** reduce the synthesis of thromboxanes in platelets and prostacyclins from endothelial cells.

reduce the tendency for thrombus formation in implanted grafts after coronary artery bypass operations and after stenting thrombosed coronary arteries.

Platelet inhibitors inactivate cyclooxygenase by irreversibly acetylating the active enzyme. This reduces thromboxane synthesis in platelets and the prostacyclin synthesis in endothelial cells. Endothelial cells can, however, synthesize new enzyme, but a platelet that contains inhibited inactivated cyclooxygenase remains inhibited for the remainder of the platelet's lifetime. It takes 7–10 days to regain a population of unaffected platelets after a dose of acetylsalicylic acid. Because cyclooxygenase in endothelial cells requires a higher concentration of acetylsalicylic acid, selective effects on thromboxane synthesis in the platelets can be achieved with low-dose administration. See Figure 20.10.

By reducing the platelet activation, the risk of arterial thrombi is reduced. Acetylsalicylic acid is discussed further in Chapter 14, Drugs with central and peripheral analgesic effect.

Dipyridamole

This is used in combination with anticoagulants in patients with artificial heart valves and those who do not achieve a satisfactory effect from oral anticoagulation treatment. Production of thromboxane is reduced. Combination with acetylsalicylic acid enhances the platelet-inhibiting effect.

Clopidogrel

Clopidogrel irreversibly inhibits the binding of adenosine diphosphate (ADP) to thrombocyte receptors and so inhibits ADP-induced platelet aggregation. The drug is used for the same indications as acetylsalicylic acid, but is not a first choice because of its high cost when compared with other effective agents.

Glycoprotein IIb/IIIa inhibitors

Fibrinogen receptors (glycoprotein IIb/IIIa receptors) are located on platelets. Drugs that bind to these receptors inhibit fibrinogen from binding and thereby reduce platelet aggregation. These drugs are used as an adjunct to heparin and aspirin to reduce the risk of ischaemic complications in high-risk patients undergoing percutaneous transluminal coronary angioplasty (PTCA) or to prevent myocardial infarction in patients with unstable angina pectoris.

Antiplatelet drugs
Aspirin, Dipyridamole (cyclooxygenase inhibitors)
Clopidogrel (ADP inhibitor)
Abciximab, Eptifibatide, Triofiban (glycoprotein IIb/IIIa inhibitors)

Table 20.3 Platelet inhibitors

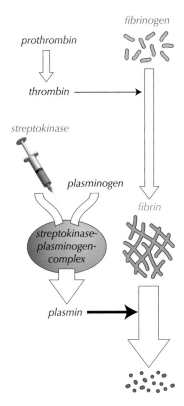

Figure 20.11 **Streptokinase** forms a complex with circulating plasminogen, which increases the metabolism of plasminogen to plasmin. Plasmin decomposes fibrin.

Fibrinolytics

Fibrinolysis is the breakdown of fibrin in thrombi. Drugs used to increase the fibrinolysis are known as fibrinolytics. The process is activated by plasmin, which is metabolized from the inactive form, plasminogen, under the effect of a plasminogen activator. Plasminogen circulates in the blood but is also found bound to the fibrin fibres in a thrombus. The circulating plasminogen activators bind to plasminogen and split the molecule at a specific site, leading to increased release of plasmin. Plasmin decomposes fibrin, fibrinogen and some other coagulation factors. The decomposition of fibrin creates fibrinogen degradation products (FDPs). Increased FDP values are seen as a result of increased fibrinolysis.

The treatment is effective for dissolving fibrin in formed thrombus masses. Large doses of fibrinolytics increase the risk for haemorrhage.

Streptokinase

Streptokinase is a protein (produced in β-haemolytic streptococci) which forms a stable complex with plasminogen – both plasminogen that is found in the circulation and that which is bound to thrombus material. The complex formation results in the creation of plasmin. The plasmin decomposes fibrin and in this way has a thrombolytic effect. See Figure 20.11. Because streptokinase is a foreign protein, and as such can act antigenically, its use may result in anaphylactic reactions.

Alteplase and reteplase

Alteplase and reteplase are naturally occurring activators of plasminogen that are produced using recombinant DNA technology. They might be thought of as target-guided rockets, since they only bind to plasminogen when it is bound to fibrin thrombus masses. Alteplase rarely causes allergic reactions, but its use is limited by its high cost.

Use of fibrinolytics

Fibrinolytics are very beneficial in the treatment of acute cardiac infarction. When treatment is administered early after occlusion of the coronary arteries, reperfusion occurs in approximately 70 per cent of cases. The mortality associated with cardiac infarction is reduced by approximately 25 per cent if such treatment is started within 6 h after the onset of infarction. Later treatment has also demonstrated some benefits if there are clinical or ECG-related signs of ischaemia.

Fibrinolytics are used, in some cases, to treat venous thrombi in the large veins.

The following patient groups should not be treated with fibrinolytics:

- patients with previous cerebral insult (haemorrhage)
- hypertension that requires treatment or is poorly controlled
- cerebral tumours
- recent puncture of a large artery
- surgical intervention during the past 10 days
- gastrointestinal haemorrhage during the past 2 months
- known increased risk for haemorrhage
- polytraumas.

Some fibrinolytics are listed in Table 20.4.

Fibrinolytics
Alteplase, Reteplase, Streptokinase

Table 20.4 Fibrinolytics

SUMMARY

■ Anaemia exists when the haemoglobin value is below defined, age-related limits for women and men. The symptoms are the result of poor tissue oxygenation.

■ Iron deficiency anaemia is the most frequently occurring form, but deficiency of vitamin B_{12} and folic acid can also give rise to reduced haemoglobin synthesis. In deficiency anaemias, the deficient substances must be supplied.

■ Iron is part of the haemoglobin molecule as divalent Fe^{2+}. Folic acid and vitamin B_{12} are essential for the maturation of all cells. Where there is intrinsic factor deficiency, vitamin B_{12} must be supplied parenterally. Maintenance treatment can often be by oral administration of vitamin B_{12}.

■ Aplastic anaemia is the result of reduced production of red blood cells in the bone marrow. This form of anaemia can be caused by bone marrow suppression as the result of some drug therapies.

■ Thromboembolic disease results in blockage of blood vessels and may be followed by the detachment of thrombus masses to produce free-floating emboli. Emboli from thrombus masses in veins lodge in the pulmonary arteries; those from thrombus masses in the left atrium and arteries lodge in the systemic arteries.

■ Anticoagulants reduce thrombus formation mainly on the venous side. Heparins enhance the effect of antithrombin III. Vitamin K antagonists reduce the production of coagulation factors in the liver. Both substances are effective in reducing thrombus formation by inhibiting various steps in the coagulation process.

■ Platelet inhibitors reduce thrombosis formation on the arterial side. They reduce activation of platelets by reducing the production of thromboxanes or by inhibiting ADP-induced platelet aggregation.

■ Fibrinolytics break down thrombus masses on both the venous and the arterial sides. Streptokinase, alteplase and reteplase increase the breakdown of fibrin and dissolve arterial and venous thrombus masses by the breakdown of fibrin.

■ All drugs that are used in thromboembolic disease lead to an increased risk of haemorrhage.

21 Drugs used to treat endocrinological disorders

In multicellular organisms, physiological functions are regulated by both the nervous system and the endocrine system. Endocrine glands synthesize and release physiologically active substances – hormones. These hormones are generally released into the vascular system whereupon they are transported to their target tissue where they produce their physiological effects. The target tissue may be a further endocrine gland or it may be a non-endocrine structure. In some instances, e.g. in the case of so-called local hormones, endocrine tissue secretes hormones but this secretion is not into the vascular system. Instead, the released hormone diffuses in interstitial fluid to an adjacent tissue where it produces its physiological effect – hence the term local hormone.

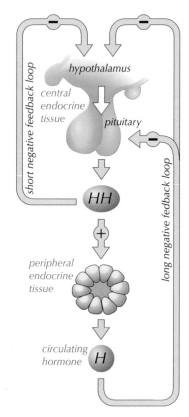

Figure 21.1 Organization of the hypothalamo–pituitary axis.

Disease in endocrine tissue can result in either an increased or decreased release of hormones. The use of drugs in endocrine disorders aims to restore the normal physiological concentration of the hormone concerned, and thus reduce the symptoms associated with its hyper- or hypo-secretion. In other instances, where there is an absolute lack of a particular hormone, replacement therapy may be used, e.g. hormone replacement therapy (HRT) in postmenopausal women or insulin in diabetics. There are also certain diseases or disorders that are hormone-dependent; in these cases, 'anti-hormone' therapy is employed, e.g. the use of hormone antagonists in the treatment of prostate and breast cancer.

HYPOTHALAMUS AND PITUITARY GLAND

The hypothalamus and pituitary gland, the latter of which is divided into a posterior lobe and an anterior lobe, are considered to be the major controlling influences over the remainder of the endocrine system. In turn they are subject to influences from higher regions of the central nervous system. The secretions of the anterior and posterior pituitary glands are considered later in this chapter.

The hypothalamus releases a variety of hormones, so-called release hormones or release-inhibiting hormones, which result in an increase or decrease, respectively, in the secretion of hormones from the anterior pituitary gland. Secretions from the posterior pituitary gland are not under this control.

The secretions of the anterior pituitary gland themselves are hormones whose targets are endocrine glands elsewhere in the body – peripheral endocrine organs. In turn, these endocrine glands secrete hormones which have a physiological effect in target organs elsewhere in the body. The hypothalamo-pituitary axis controls and coordinates the endocrine activity of the body via this hierarchical system.

The maintenance of appropriate levels of hormones is controlled by negative feedback loops. The hormone secretions of the peripheral endocrine organs may inhibit the secretions of the hypothalamus and posterior pituitary gland if their plasma levels rise too high. Equally, the hormones of the posterior pituitary gland may inhibit secretions of release and release-inhibiting hormones of the hypothalamus if their concentration levels are too high. These negative feedback loops are known as long and short feedback loops, respectively. See Figure 21.1.

PITUITARY HORMONES AND DISEASES

The most common diseases involving disrupted secretion of pituitary hormones are tumours, either in the pituitary gland itself or in surrounding tissue. Such tumours may result in an increased secretion of pituitary hormones that stimulate peripheral endocrine organs. This is an important cause of increased hormone secretion. Tumours in or near the pituitary can also reduce the release of pituitary hormones. If the release of hormones from the pituitary fails, peripheral endocrine organs will fail to synthesize and release their hormones. This is an important cause of failing hormone production.

It is common to divide the pituitary into the anterior pituitary gland (adenohypophysis) and the posterior pituitary gland part (neurohypophysis). The different areas of the pituitary secrete different hormones. See Figure 21.2.

Secretions from the anterior pituitary

The anterior pituitary secretes several hormones that act on peripheral endocrine glands. One of these, growth hormone (GH, somatotrophin), affects general growth

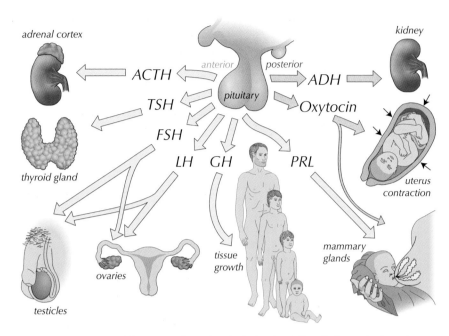

Figure 21.2 Release of hormones from the pituitary gland. The pituitary gland regulates the activity of peripheral endocrine glands by the secretion of trophic hormones. In addition growth hormone and prolactin are secreted from this part of the pituitary gland. The posterior pituitary gland secretes oxytocin and ADH. Adrenocorticotrophic hormone (ACTH), thyroid-stimulating hormone (TSH), follicle-stimulating hormone (FSH), luteinizing hormone (LH), growth hormone (GH) and prolactin (PRL), antidiuretic hormone (ADH).

and development and also the metabolism of proteins, fat and carbohydrates. In the past, a deficiency of GH was treated by the administration of GH obtained from cadavers. However, genetic engineering now makes it possible to produce a substance that is identical to GH, known as somatotrophin. A surplus of GH release results in gigantism in children and acromegaly in adults, while a deficiency of GH results in pituitary dwarfism.

Sermorelin is a synthetic analogue of growth hormone-releasing hormone (GHRH, released from the hypothalamus), which acts by releasing GH from the anterior pituitary gland. It is used diagnostically to determine the pituitary's ability to release GH in situations where GH levels are reduced. Pegvisomant is a genetically modified analogue of human growth hormone. It is a highly selective growth hormone receptor antagonist licensed for the treatment of acromegaly in patients with inadequate response to surgery or radiation.

The release of prolactin from the anterior pituitary gland stimulates the mammary glands to produce milk. Release of prolactin is inhibited by dopamine (prolactin release-inhibiting hormone, from the hypothalamus) and by high plasma levels of oestrogen and progesterone. However, the growth of mammary tissue is dependent upon oestrogen and progesterone. During pregnancy, the production of oestrogen and progesterone increases, such that the mammary gland development increases. After birth, there is a reduction in the plasma concentrations of oestrogen and progesterone, and the release of prolactin increases, which promotes the production of milk. Prolactin inhibits the release of hormones that are necessary for ovulation, and therefore represents a natural contraceptive mechanism in breastfeeding mothers. Maintenance of prolactin synthesis depends on

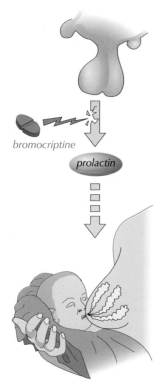

Figure 21.3 **Inhibition of prolactin release.** Dopamine agonists, e.g. bromocriptine, inhibit the release of prolactin and prevent the mammary glands from producing milk.

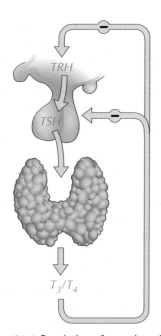

Figure 21.4 **Regulation of secretion of** T_3 **and** T_4. The released hormones have negative feedback effects on the pituitary and hypothalamus.

Growth hormone analogues
Somatropin
Growth hormone antagonists
Pegvisomant, Sermorelin
Prolactin release inhibitors
Bromocriptine, Cabergoline, Quinagolide
Posterior pituitary hormones – ADH
Vasopressin, Desmopressin, Terlipressin
Posterior pituitary hormones – Oxytocin
Oxytocin

Table 21.1 Drugs used to treat hypothalamic/pituitary disorders

maintenance of breastfeeding. It is thought that breastfeeding results in the hypothalamus releasing a prolactin-releasing hormone which promotes the release of prolactin from the anterior pituitary.

Bromocriptine and cabergoline are drugs with a similar effect as dopamine, i.e. they act as dopamine agonists at dopamine receptors. Dopamine, released from the hypothalamus, acts as a prolactin release-inhibiting hormone. These drugs inhibit the release of prolactin and thus prevent lactation. See Figure 21.3. Bromocriptine has other therapeutic uses. For example, it also inhibits the release of GH and is sometimes used in the treatment of acromegaly. It is used in the treatment of Parkinson's disease, which is discussed more thoroughly in Chapter 12, Drugs used to treat neurological disorders.

Secretions from the posterior pituitary

The posterior pituitary gland releases two hormones: antidiuretic hormone (ADH, or arginine vasopressin) and oxytocin. They are both released (into the vascular system) from the axonal endings of neurons whose cell bodies are located in the hypothalamus, and are both examples of neurohormones.

Oxytocin stimulates expulsion of milk from the milk ducts of the mammary gland and contraction of uterine smooth muscle during childbirth. ADH acts on the distal tubule and collecting duct of the nephron to increase the reabsorption of water, so that a smaller volume of urine is produced. In pharmacological doses, it also has a vasoconstrictor effect on vascular smooth muscle.

Desmopressin is an analogue of ADH and is used in the treatment of diabetes insipidus, a condition characterized by diminished secretion of ADH, which, in the worst case, can lead to death due to loss of large volumes of fluid. Desmopressin may also be used in the treatment of nocturnal enuresis in children. It increases the level of coagulation factor VIII and von Willebrand's factor, and can be used in haemophiliacs as a prophylactic treatment prior to dental extractions. It is also used in the treatment of bleeding oesophageal varices. These uses are due to its vasoconstrictive properties.

The adverse effects of desmopressin are also related to its vasoconstrictive properties, and it must be used with caution in patients with a poor peripheral circulation, particularly elderly patients with angina pectoris.

Drugs used to treat hypothalamic/pituitary disorders are listed in Table 21.1.

THYROID GLAND AND METABOLIC DISORDERS

The hormones tri-iodothyronine (T_3) and thyroxine (T_4), which are known as thyroid hormones, are produced in follicle cells of the thyroid gland, which is located in front of and on the sides of the trachea, just under the larynx. The follicle cells have the ability to concentrate iodine, which forms part of T_3 and T_4. The thyroid hormones regulate the metabolism of the body's cells. A deficiency of thyroid hormones in infants causes cretinism.

REGULATION OF THYROID HORMONES

The production of T_3 and T_4 is regulated by thyrotrophin-releasing hormone (TRH) from the hypothalamus, which in turn stimulates the anterior pituitary gland to secrete thyroid-stimulating hormone (TSH), in turn stimulating the thyroid gland to release T_3 and T_4. Plasma levels of these hormones are regulated by negative feedback mechanisms. See Figures 21.1 and 21.4.

The synthesis of the thyroid hormones begins in the follicle cells of the thyroid gland with synthesis of the protein thyroglobulin, which contains several residues of the amino acid tyrosine. The tyrosine residues then bind one or two iodine atoms, forming mono- or di-iodothyronine (MIT and DIT), respectively. Coupling of these molecules in the appropriate ratios results in the formation of T_3 and T_4. The hormones are secreted to the blood because the thyroglobulin molecule is hydrolysed and releases the iodinated tyrosine residues, i.e. T_3 and T_4. See Figure 21.5. Additionally, MIT and DIT are also released. The iodine is removed from these molecules and recycled. Excess iodine in the follicle cells inhibits the binding of iodine to the amino acid tyrosine.

IMBALANCE IN SECRETION OF METABOLIC HORMONES

Hyperthyroidism (thyrotoxicosis) occurs when there is an elevated plasma concentration of thyroid hormones. There are several types of thyrotoxicosis, including Graves' disease which is an autoimmune disease of TSH receptors. Another common cause is the development of benign tumours of the thyroid gland. The most pronounced effects of excess thyroid hormones are manifested in the cardiovascular system by accelerated heart rate, in the neuromuscular system by hyperactive reflexes and fine tremor of the muscles. Generally there is an acceleration of all bodily metabolic functions leading to weight loss despite increased food intake, heat intolerance and nervousness.

Hypothyroidism occurs when there is a reduced plasma concentration of thyroid hormones. The condition may be the result of an autoimmune disease of the thyroid gland, insufficient thyroid tissue after treatment with radioiodine or surgery, or a lack of stimulation of the thyroid due to low release of TSH from the anterior pituitary gland. The symptoms of hypothyroidism include a low heart rate, constipation, dry skin, cold intolerance and mental slowness that is often mistaken for depression. Hyper- and hypothyroidism can occur with either a normal or an enlarged thyroid gland. The latter is known as goitre. When goitre is present, therefore, there may be either an increase or a decrease in the secretion of thyroid hormones.

DRUGS USED TO TREAT HYPERTHYROIDISM (THYROTOXICOSIS)

The activity of the thyroid gland can be reduced by drugs that inhibit the incorporation of iodine into tyrosine residues (thyrostatics), by administration of large doses of iodine, which inhibits secretion of the thyroid hormones, or by radioactive iodine, which irradiates and damages the tissue where thyroglobulin is synthesized. In some cases, thyroid tissue is surgically removed. The aim of both drug treatment and surgical removal of tissue is that sufficient tissue remains for normal hormone production.

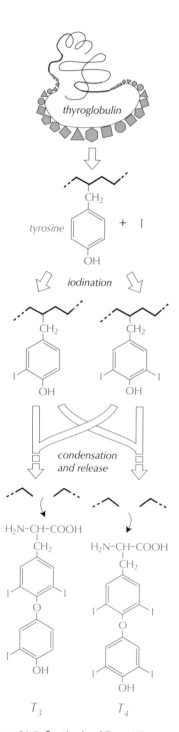

Figure 21.5 Synthesis of T_3 and T_4. Hydrolysis of thyroglobulin and release of T_3 and T_4 are stimulated by thyroid-stimulating hormone (TSH). Refer to the text for a detailed explanation.

Administration of iodine in large doses blocks the iodination of tyrosine residues in thyroglobulin and also reduces the release of the hormones. The effect appears quickly, within 1–2 days, and is used in thyrotoxic crisis and as a pre-treatment before surgical removal of thyroid tissue, i.e. to reduce the vascularization of tissues. The treatment should not be used for long periods, as the antithyroid effect decreases after some 10–15 days.

Radioiodine is used in the treatment of elderly patients and in the treatment of toxic adenomas (benign tumours of the thyroid gland). Radioactive iodine is concentrated in the thyroid tissue and damages it, so that hormone production is reduced. Large doses of radioiodine lead to hypothyroidism, which must be treated with substitution therapy.

Surgical treatment is used on large goitres, which, if left untreated, may grow to such a size that they put pressure on, and may partially occlude, the trachea. Surgery can lead to paralysis of the vocal cords because of the possibility of damage to the recurrent laryngeal nerve during the procedure.

Thyrostatics

Thyrostatics, e.g. carbimazole and propylthiouracil, are substances that inhibit the production of thyroid hormones. This is the treatment of choice in children and young adults. Both drugs are administered orally. Carbimazole is itself inactive, but is metabolized to metimazol, which is an active metabolite.

Mechanism of action and effects. Carbimazole and propylthiouracil are concentrated in the follicle cells in the thyroid and inhibit the iodination of tyrosine residues in thyroglobulin. In addition, they seem to inhibit the condensation of MIT and DIT, so that production of T_3 and T_4 is reduced. See Figure 21.6. In the target cells of the thyroid hormones, T_4 must be deiodinated to T_3 for it to have maximal effects. This process is inhibited by propylthiouracil. However, the drugs have no effect on pre-formed (at the start of therapy) thyroid hormones. It takes some 3–4 weeks of treatment to see a return to normality; this corresponds to the use of pre-formed hormones.

Adverse effects. The most serious adverse effect of thyrostatics is bone marrow suppression with agranulocytosis and thrombocytopenia, which appears in about 0.5 per cent of users within 3–6 weeks, and which is reversed when the treatment is stopped. A small reduction in leucocyte numbers may occur but this is no reason to stop treatment, though it requires careful monitoring. Rashes, headaches, joint pains and hepatitis are also reported adverse effects.

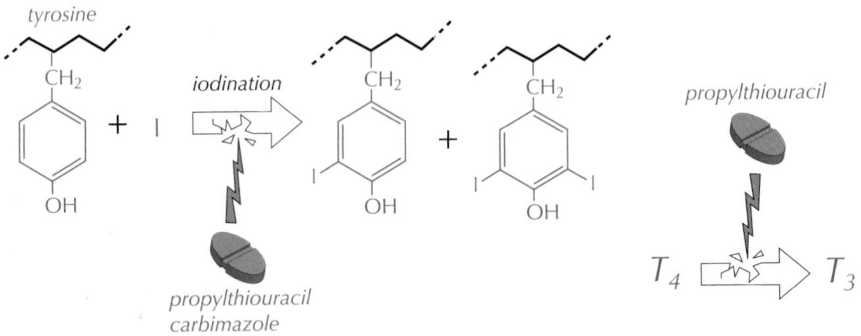

Figure 21.6 **Propylthiouracil and carbimazole** inhibit the iodination of tyrosine. In addition, the metabolism of T_4 to T_3 is inhibited by propylthiouracil.

In comparison to carbimazole, propylthiouracil is less likely to cross the blood–placenta barrier or enter breast milk. These drugs must be used with caution in pregnant women and should not be used in lactating women.

Beta-blockers

Several of the symptoms of hyperthyroidism can be reduced by the use of β-blockers, which inhibit the increased adrenergic activity that occurs in hyperthyroidism. β-Blockers are discussed in more detail in Chapter 17, Drug used to treat diseases in the cardiovascular system.

DRUGS USED TO TREAT HYPOTHYROIDISM

Hypothyroidism is associated with a reduction in the plasma concentration of thyroid hormones. Because of the general reduction in metabolism associated with hypothyroidism, similarly there is a reduction in the metabolism of drugs. It is usually appropriate to assess the need for dose reduction of a drug taken by patients with hypothyroidism. The treatment of hypothyroidism is via substitution of thyroid hormones.

Substitution with metabolic hormones

The aim of substitution therapy is to make the patient normothyroid (euthyroid) and to reduce the problems associated with a low metabolic rate. Substitution treatment in hypothyroidism is achieved with the administration of synthetic T_3 (liothyronine) and T_4 (levothyroxine). Both are absorbed well after oral administration. The time to effect is quicker for T_3 than for T_4, but its effects are less long-lasting. It is more common to use the T_4 form, as this gives the least fluctuation in plasma concentration and only requires one dose per day. The full effect is achieved after 4–6 weeks. T_3 and T_4 are highly protein-bound and so the dose required is controlled by measuring the concentration of free T_4 and TSH in the plasma and the clinical effect produced. T_4 is metabolized to T_3 in the cells. Both substances undergo hepatic metabolism.

Mechanism of action and effects. The metabolic hormones regulate metabolism in all the body's cells primarily by increased synthesis of proteins that are necessary for optimal cellular metabolism. They cause an increase in the number of mitochondria in the cells, which in turn causes an increase in energy metabolism and increased oxygen consumption. T_3 stimulates growth, especially bone tissue, and is essential for the normal differentiation of cells in the central nervous system in fetal life and in early childhood.

Adverse effects. Following an overdose, symptoms of hyperthyroidism can occur. Caution is required during the initial dosing period. This is particularly the case in patients with underlying cardiovascular disease where there is a risk of precipitating angina, arrhythmias or cardiac failure.

Drugs used to treat thyroid disease are listed in Table 21.2.

Hyperthyroidism
Carbimazole, Iodine/Iodide, Propylthiouracil, Propanalol (an example of a β-blocker)

Hypothyroidism
Levothyroxine, Liothyronine

Table 21.2 Drugs used to treat thyroid disease

CALCIUM METABOLISM

Calcium is required for the formation of the skeleton, maintaining excitability in neuromuscular tissue and for the maintenance of normal blood coagulation. The skeleton gradually becomes decalcified with increasing age. This process is pronounced in postmenopausal women. Both hypercalcaemia and hypocalcaemia result in adverse effects.

PHYSIOLOGICAL EFFECTS OF CALCIUM

Approximately 99 per cent of the amount of calcium in the body resides in the bone tissue, which acts as a depot for calcium. In bone, osteoclasts and osteoblasts are found, which are cells with bone-modulating effect. Stimulation of the osteoclasts results in the reabsorption of bone mass, increased release of calcium and a rise in plasma calcium levels. Stimulation of the osteoblasts results in a bone-building effect and helps to incorporate calcium into the bone substance, resulting in a lower plasma calcium concentration. Chronic loss of calcium or reduced absorption results in demineralization of the bone substance and increased risk of fractures. The plasma calcium concentration affects excitability in nerve tissue by regulating the release of neurotransmitter substances and the contractility of muscle tissue, by regulating the binding between the contractile elements in muscles. A low plasma concentration of calcium increases the risk of convulsions and development of tetany, while an increased plasma concentration of calcium leads to diminished neuromuscular excitability and generalized muscular weakness. It also increases the risk of cardiac arrhythmias and the deposition of calcium salts in the soft tissues, especially in the kidneys.

REGULATION OF CALCIUM METABOLISM

To maintain normal mineralization of the bone mass and optimal excitability of neuromuscular tissue, the plasma concentration is maintained within narrow limits (2.2–2.6 mmol/L). This regulation is controlled by the hormones parathyroid hormone (PTH), vitamin D hormone and calcitonin, which influence:

- the release of calcium from bone tissue
- the absorption of calcium from the small intestine
- the elimination of calcium via the kidneys.

Parathyroid hormone is released from the parathyroid glands, four small glands that lie posterior to the thyroid gland. PTH stimulates the osteoclasts to release calcium from bone tissue, to increase the absorption of calcium from the small intestine and to reduce the renal loss of calcium. The release of PTH is controlled by the plasma calcium concentration via a negative feedback loop. See Figure 21.7.

Vitamin D (calcitriol). Vitamin D is a collective term for several hormones. Vitamin D_3 (cholecalciferol) is the natural form in humans and is formed by the action of ultraviolet light on steroid precursors. Vitamin D_2 (ergocalciferol) is obtained from dietary sources. It is absorbed in the small intestine and metabolized to vitamin D_3. Vitamin D_3 is metabolized in the liver, and thereafter in the kidneys, to calcitriol (1,25-dihydroxycholecalciferol), the most potent form of vitamin D. See Figure 21.8. When there is a low plasma calcium concentration, PTH stimulates the synthesis of calcitriol. Calcitriol increases the plasma concentration of calcium by increasing its absorption in the small intestine, reducing its loss via the kidneys and mobilizing calcium from the skeleton.

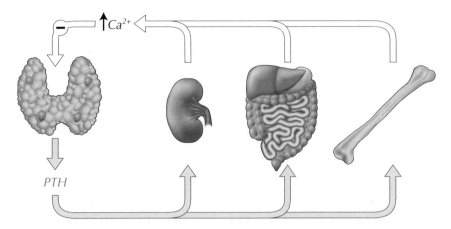

Figure 21.7 **Regulation of plasma calcium concentration.** Parathyroid hormone (PTH) stimulates the increased reabsorption of calcium in the kidneys, increased absorption from the intestines and increased osteoclast activity in bone tissue.

Calcitonin is produced in cells that lie throughout the thyroid gland. The secretion of calcitonin is regulated by the concentration of calcium in plasma. Calcitonin reduces the plasma calcium concentration by inhibiting the activity of osteoclasts in bone tissue.

HYPERCALCAEMIA

A high plasma calcium concentration is associated with an increased secretion of PTH from parathyroid tissue (primary hyperparathyroidism) caused by benign or malignant tumours originating in parathyroid tissue. Malignant tumours from other tissue sometimes release a parathyroid-like substance (PTHrP, parathyroid hormone-related peptide), which stimulates the osteoclasts and results in increased plasma calcium concentration in the terminal phase of disease. Hypercalcaemia can also be caused by a high consumption of vitamin D, by the use of thiazide diuretics which inhibit calcium excretion in the kidneys (loop diuretics increase the elimination of calcium), or by a large consumption of milk (milk-alkali syndrome).

A plasma calcium concentration above 3 mmol/L can be life-threatening (hypercalcaemic crisis). Symptoms of hypercalcaemia include nausea and vomiting, confusion and restlessness. Additionally, renal failure, serious cardiac arrhythmias, cerebral disturbances and coma can also occur.

Osteoporosis

Demineralization of the skeleton is a physiological process that gradually increases after the age of 40, in both men and women. Demineralization leads to hypercalcaemia. The loss of calcium from the skeleton happens more quickly in postmenopausal women than in men. The increased demineralization is associated with reduced oestrogen levels postmenopausally.

Osteoporosis is a systemic skeletal disease that is characterized by a reduced bone density together with altered microarchitecture resulting in reduced bone strength and an increased risk of fractures. The most frequent fractures occur in the dorsal vertebrae, the neck of the femur and the forearm.

HYPOCALCAEMIA

Hypocalcaemia occurs less frequently than hypercalcaemia and is usually caused by removal of parathyroid tissue during surgery on the thyroid or after radioiodine

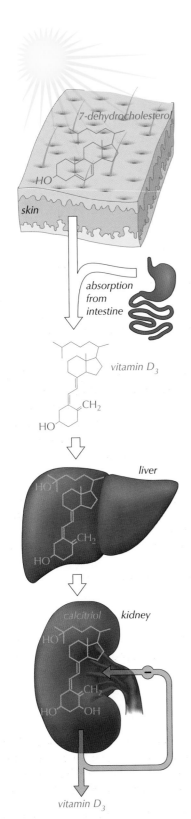

Figure 21.8 **Synthesis of vitamin D₃.** Refer to the text for a detailed explanation.

treatment. However, renal failure (resulting in reduced synthesis of vitamin D), deficient diet or reduced UV radiation of the skin can also cause hypocalcaemia. Hypocalcaemia that causes a deficiency in the bone structure in children is called rickets; in adults it is called osteomalacia.

A low plasma calcium concentration causes increased excitability of neuro-muscular tissue. This means that nerve and muscle tissues are 'unstable', so that impulses are more easily triggered, which can result in tonic convulsions. The symptoms of hypocalcaemia are most pronounced if the reduction in the plasma calcium concentration takes places over a short time.

Drug treatment consists of administration of calcium or vitamin D, both of which increase the calcium concentration.

DRUGS USED TO TREAT HYPERCALCAEMIA

In hypercalcaemia, drug treatment aims to normalize the plasma calcium concentration, avoid acute neuromuscular disturbances, prevent deposition of calcium salts in soft tissues and prevent demineralization of the skeleton.

Calcitonin

Calcitonin is used when there is a need for rapid reduction of the plasma calcium concentration. The drug is destroyed by proteases in the gastrointestinal tract and therefore is administered subcutaneously, intramuscularly or as a nasal spray.

Mechanism of action and effects. Calcitonin inhibits osteoclast activity by binding to receptors on the osteoclasts, and in so doing inhibits the release of calcium from the skeleton. In addition, the reabsorption of calcium in the kidneys is reduced. The effect is a reduction in plasma calcium concentration. This is seen soon after administration, but the response is short-lived, probably due to downregulation of the receptors to which the calcitonin binds.

Adverse effects. Nausea, vomiting, diarrhoea and periodic feelings of warmth occur. No reliable information is available regarding the effects in pregnant and lactating women.

Bisphosphonates

Bisphosphonates, e.g. clodronate and pamidronate, are used to reduce the plasma calcium concentration in malign hypercalcaemia and pronounced osteoporosis where there is an increased risk of fractures (e.g. alendronate and etidronate).

Mechanism of action and effects. Bisphosphonates bind to the crystalline elements of bone and reduce its breakdown by inhibiting the regeneration and function of osteoclasts, i.e. they inhibit the release of calcium from bone. The reduction in plasma calcium concentration takes several days to appear. The drugs are useful when there is persistent release of calcium from the skeleton, as with malignant tumours. It has also been shown that prolonged use of alendronate and etidronate reduces demineralization and increases bone density in postmenopausal women; the frequency of fractures is also reduced in this group. Absorption of bisphosphonates is impaired by the presence of food in the stomach, so they must be taken before eating.

Adverse effects. Nausea and diarrhoea occur, especially following oral administration. With prolonged use, localized demineralization with an increased risk of bone fracture can occur. About 50 per cent of each dose is eliminated unmetabolized via the kidneys. With reduced renal function, the dose must be reduced so as to avoid too pronounced an effect, i.e. hypocalcaemia.

Calcitonin
Calcitonin

Bisphosphonates
Alendronic acid, Etidronate, Clodronate, Ibandronic acid, Pamidronate, Risedronate, Strontium ranelate, Tiludronic acid, Zoledronic acid

Calcimimetic
Cinacalcet

PTH-analogue (synthetic form of parathyroid hormone)
Teriparatide

Table 21.3 Drugs used to treat hypercalcaemia

Calcimimetics

Calcimimetics are drugs that target the calcium-sensing receptor and lower parathyroid hormone levels without increasing calcium and phosphorus levels. Cinacalcet is a calcimimetic used to treat hypercalcemia in patients with secondary hyperparathyroidism (elevated levels of parathyroid hormone) and concomitant chronic kidney disease, in patients receiving dialysis and in patients with parathyroid carcinoma. The most commonly reported side effects are nausea and vomiting.

PTH-analouge

Teriparatide is a synthetic form of parathyroid hormone (PTH) given by subcutaneous injection for the treatment of osteoporosis in men and post-menopausal women who are at high risk of a fracture. The drug stimulates osteoblasts to induce new bone growth and improve bone density. Synthetic PTH may have the potential to replace depleted bone stores. Side effects include headache, asthenia, hypotension, angina pectoris, syncope, nausea, dizziness and depression.

Glucocorticoids

Glucocorticoids are hormones that are produced in the adrenal cortex. They reduce the absorption of calcium in the small intestine and increase its excretion by the kidneys. They have a rapid effect in the treatment of hypercalcaemia due to excessive consumption of calcium or vitamin D hormone. Glucocorticoids are dealt with later in this chapter (see p. 320).

Drugs used to treat hypercalcaemia are listed in Table 21.3.

DRUGS USED TO TREAT HYPOCALCAEMIA

In hypocalcaemia, it is necessary to reduce the renal excretion of calcium or to promote its intestinal absorption. Alternatively, it is possible to administer calcium supplements.

Vitamin D and vitamin D-like preparations
These drugs affect both the absorption and elimination of calcium.

Mechanism of action and effects. Calcitriol increases the absorption of calcium in the small intestine and also its reabsorption in the kidneys. In addition, the osteoblasts are stimulated, resulting in incorporation of calcium in the bone tissue. In rickets and osteomalacia, calcitriol can contribute to mineralization of the bone mass.

Adverse effects. Large doses can cause hypercalcaemia, with nausea, vomiting, fatigue and headaches. The kidneys have a reduced ability to concentrate the urine, which results in polyuria and thirst.

Vitamin D and vitamin D analogues
Alfacalcidol, Calcitrol, Colecalciferol, Ergocalciferol

Table 21.4 Drugs used to treat hypocalcaemia

Ergocalciferol or alfacalcidol must be metabolized to calcitriol in the kidneys before they exert their effects. Since calcitriol may disturb the normal negative feedback mechanism that controls plasma calcium levels, plasma concentrations of calcium must be carefully monitored.

Calcium preparations

Administration of calcium is intended to increase the absorption and thereby the concentration of calcium in plasma. By administering vitamin D hormone simultaneously, calcium absorption is maximized whilst the secretion of PTH is inhibited. Consequently, osteoclast activity is inhibited and bone breakdown is reduced, while the bone-building effect of the osteoblasts increases.

There is a risk of hypercalcaemia and deposits in the form of kidney stones with continuous use. The risk is increased in patients suffering from renal failure.

Drugs used to treat hypocalcaemia are listed in Table 21.4.

ADRENOCORTICOSTEROIDS

The adrenal glands are located superior to the upper surface of the kidneys. They consist of an outer layer (the cortex) and an inner layer (the medulla). The cortex is divided into three functional zones, each of which produces a variety of hormones derived ultimately from cholesterol:

- In the *outer layer*, mineralocorticoids are produced. They are important for regulation of water and electrolyte balance in the body, especially in relation to the secretion of sodium and potassium via the kidneys. Aldosterone is an example of such a mineralocorticoid.
- In the *middle layer*, glucocorticoids are produced. These hormones have different effects on different tissue. They are important in regulating the metabolism of carbohydrates, proteins and fat, and have an immunomodulating effect and an anti-inflammatory effect. Cortisol is an example of a glucocorticoid.
- In the *inner layer*, androgens are produced. These are hormones with both anabolic and masculinizing effects. However, the main site of production of androgens is the testes in men.

These hormones are discussed later in the chapter.

The adrenocorticosteroid hormones are not stored in the adrenal cortex, but are synthesized and released as needed. The signal for synthesis of these hormones is adrenocorticotrophic hormone (ACTH), which is released from the anterior pituitary gland. Figure 21.9 shows that the release of ACTH is regulated by a factor (corticotrophin-releasing factor, CRF) released from the hypothalamus.

Preganglionic neurons of the sympathetic nervous system form synapses within the adrenal medulla. When there is increased activity in the sympathetic nervous system, the adrenal medulla responds by releasing adrenaline, although a small amount of noradrenaline is also released.

Glucocorticoids

With a range of different effects in different tissue, glucocorticoids are used in a number of allergic, inflammatory and autoimmune diseases and in the treatment of

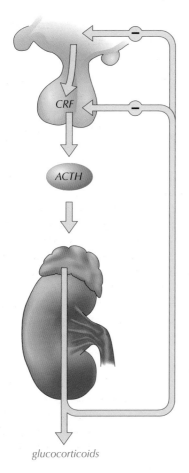

glucocorticoids

Figure 21.9 **Regulation of the glucocorticoid synthesis.** ACTH, adrenocorticotrophic hormone; CRF, corticotrophin-releasing factor.

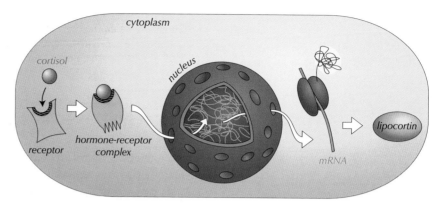

Figure 21.10 **Steroid hormones.** The steroid hormones bind to a cytoplasmic receptor and influence the production of mRNA and, subsequently, protein synthesis. The illustration shows how cortisol increases the synthesis of lipocortin.

anaphylactic shock. They are used to prevent organ rejection after transplantation and also in the treatment of malignant diseases in combination with cytotoxic drugs.

Cortisol is an example of a glucocorticoid. The production of cortisol varies throughout the day, and subsequently its plasma concentration fluctuates from about 110 nmol/L at 4am to approximately 450 nmol/L at 8am. Synthetic glucocorticoids include prednisolone, dexamethasone and budesonide.

Mechanism of action and effects. The glucocorticoids bind to cytoplasmic receptors in the target cell. The receptor– glucocorticoid complex is then transferred to the nucleus where it binds to DNA. Here, it modifies gene transcription by turning genes 'on' or 'off' – this is dependent on the tissue it is acting upon. Since the majority of the effects are mediated via altered protein synthesis, it takes a considerable time before the effects of these drugs are observed. See Figure 21.10.

Glucocorticoids increase gluconeogenesis (synthesis of glucose) and the production of glycogen in the liver. Simultaneously, metabolism in muscle and fatty tissue shifts from consumption of carbohydrates to consumption of amino acids and fat. In this way, they contribute to an increased plasma glucose concentration. In muscle, a catabolic status is initiated, with decomposition of proteins resulting in a reduction in muscle mass. In fatty tissue, lipolytic activity increases, and there is a redistribution of fat within the body. With long term use of glucocorticoids, the result is a change of body appearance, as is seen in Cushing's syndrome.

The anti-inflammatory and immunosuppressive effects are complex. The anti-inflammatory effect is mediated by an increase in lipocortin production. Lipocortin inhibits phospholipase A_2 so that the release of arachidonic acid from cell membranes is reduced, and the production of leukotrienes and prostaglandins that cause inflammation is inhibited (see Figure 15.2, p. 166). This results in reduced vasodilation and oedema in inflamed areas. In acute inflammation, the number and activity of leucocytes are reduced, and in chronic inflammation, there is a reduced activity of mononuclear cells, reduced proliferation of new blood vessels and less fibrosis. An important effect is the reduced proliferation of T- and B-lymphocytes in lymphatic tissue and subsequently a reduction in the production of T-cell-mediated cytokines. Fewer complement factors are produced in the blood.

When there is a reduced number of leucocytes and lymphocytes, both the immune response and the inflammatory response that are initiated by release of pro-inflammatory mediators from these cells are also inhibited. The release of histamine from mast cells is inhibited.

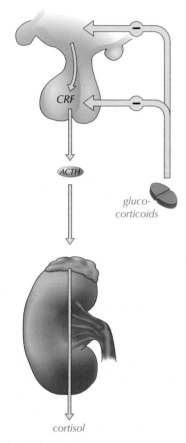

CRF

ACTH

*gluco-
corticoids*

cortisol

Figure 21.11 Atrophy of the adrenal cortex. Large doses of glucocorticoids inhibit the secretion of adrenocorticotrophic hormone (ACTH) from the pituitary. With that, the adrenal cortex loses its trigger to release cortisol and atrophies.

Glucocorticoids
Betamethasone, Cortisone, Deflazacort, Dexamethasone, Hydrocortisone, Methylprednisolone, Prednisolone, Triamcinolone
Mineralocorticoids
Fludrocortisone

Table 21.5 Corticosteroids

Pharmacokinetics. Glucocorticoids are used in many different dosage forms. Elimination occurs by conjugation in the liver and secretion with bile. The glucocorticoids have a pronounced negative feedback effect on ACTH release from the anterior pituitary gland. Prolonged use of glucocorticoids will suppress adrenal gland activity to such an extent that it may atrophy. This means that endogenous production of glucocorticoids is significantly reduced. It is important to remember that patients on long-term treatment with glucocorticoids do not have a functional pituitary/adrenal cortex axis. Sudden cessation of glucocorticoid administration will lead to acute failure to produce cortisol, as a result of an atrophied adrenal cortex. See Figure 21.11.

Adverse effects. Every treatment with corticosteroids is associated with predictable, dose-dependent adverse effects that arise after prolonged use of high doses. Single doses or treatments of less than 14 days do not produce any noticeable adverse effects. It is unnecessary to withdraw treatment gradually after such short treatments. After long term, high dose treatments, withdrawal should follow strict guidelines. Users should carry a 'Steroid Treatment Card' to inform health professionals about their use, since sudden discontinuation may be life threatening. The most important adverse effects are reduced defence against infection, catabolic protein metabolism that causes reduced muscle mass and reduced healing of sores due to reduced formation of connective tissue, a suppression of endogenous glucocorticoid synthesis, metabolic influences such as in Cushing's syndrome and demineralization of bones. Diabetogenic effects arise when there is reduced peripheral utilization of glucose and increased production of glucose in the liver. Secretion of hydrochloric acid and pepsin in the stomach increases and can result in damage to the mucous membrane.

Mineralocorticoids
Mineralocorticoids, e.g. aldosterone and fludrocortisone, increase the reabsorption of sodium in the distal renal tubules, simultaneously as it increases the secretion of K^+ and H^+ ions. Mineralocorticoids are used only as substitution therapy when there is insufficient endogenous synthesis to regulate the sodium and potassium secretion.

Aldosterone antagonists, e.g. spironolactone, are used in the treatment of hypertension and act by inhibiting the sodium-retaining ability of aldosterone. In so doing they produce a diuretic effect.

Some corticosteriod drugs are listed in Table 21.5.

DIABETES MELLITUS

Diabetes mellitus, also called diabetes, is defined as chronic hyperglycaemia along with other metabolic disturbances that are due to an absolute or relative insulin deficiency, often together with a reduced insulin effect (so-called insulin resistance).

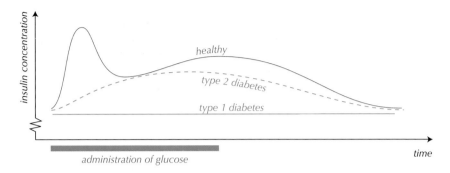

Figure 21.12 **Change in insulin concentration.** When glucose is administered, the insulin response shows a biphasic response in healthy individuals. Type 1 diabetics are individuals who lack insulin production. Type 2 diabetics have reduced insulin response.

Insulin

Insulin is a hormone produced in the islets of Langerhans in the pancreas. It consists of two peptide chains bound together by a disulphide bridge. It is released by β cells in the islets of Langerhans of the pancreas. The hormone is released directly into the blood in an inactive form (pro-insulin). In the blood, a small segment of peptide splits off, and active insulin is formed.

Mechanism of action and effects. As a response to an increased plasma glucose concentration, the absolute secretion and the rate of secretion of insulin are increased. The insulin response to glucose has two phases: first, there is an initial rapid response, which represents the release of pre-formed and stored insulin; the second phase is a slower, longer-lasting phase that represents both the synthesis and release of 'new' insulin. In diabetics, this response is abnormal. See Figure 21.12. Insulin exerts its effects on target cells (liver, muscle and fat) via insulin receptors, which results in an increased uptake of glucose from the plasma into the target cells. However, there are also some long term effects of insulin which are mediated via effects on DNA and RNA function.

Insulin can be considered as a fuel-storing hormone. It also influences cell growth and differentiation. The primary effect, however, is on glucose metabolism. The plasma concentration of glucose is reduced because insulin increases the glucose uptake from blood to muscle, liver and fat, and because glycogen synthesis in the liver increases while gluconeogenesis and glycogen breakdown are reduced.

Insulin also has significant effects on fat metabolism. The importance of this is seen in some of the symptoms of diabetes, i.e. incomplete fat metabolism and the production of ketoacids during insulin deficiency. This may result in diabetic ketoacidosis and development of coma. A long term insulin deficiency results in protein breakdown with listlessness and emaciation, often seen in diabetes in young people before the disease is recognized.

Other substances with an effect on glucose metabolism

Alpha cells in the pancreas secrete glucagon, which has the opposite effect of insulin on glucose metabolism. Glucagon can be considered a fuel-mobilizing hormone that stimulates gluconeogenesis, glycogenolysis and lipolysis. It increases the plasma concentration of glucose.

Glucocorticoids increase gluconeogenesis and reduce glucose uptake and utilization. Adrenaline and noradrenaline influence plasma glucose levels by increasing glycogenolysis and reducing glucose uptake. Both lead to increased plasma glucose concentration as a response to hypoglycaemia.

CLASSIFICATION OF DIABETES

There is a clinical difference between insulin-dependent diabetes mellitus (IDDM, type 1 diabetes) and non-insulin-dependent diabetes mellitus (NIDDM, type 2 diabetes). Type 1 diabetes presents before the age of 40, usually in childhood or adolescence. In this form, the insulin deficiency is due to autoimmune destruction of the β cells in the islets of Langerhans in the pancreas. Type 2 diabetes usually presents after the age of 40. In this form, there is both insufficient insulin production and insulin resistance. It is often associated with obesity, hypertension and disturbances in lipoprotein metabolism. People suffering from diabetes have an increased rate of development of atherosclerosis, which again increases the risk of development of cardiovascular diseases. This unfortunate effect is further increased if the plasma glucose concentration remains high in the long term. Diabetes can occur secondary to other diseases, such as inflammation of the pancreas. Drugs such as thiazide diuretics and glucocorticosteroids can trigger a diabetic state by reducing insulin secretion, reducing the peripheral glucose uptake and increasing the production of glucose in the liver.

DRUGS USED TO TREAT DIABETES MELLITUS

The goal of the treatment of diabetes is to achieve freedom from symptoms, a good quality of life, normal plasma glucose concentration and reduction in the risk of developing complicating diseases of diabetes. There are a number of drugs which can be used to treat diabetes: insulin and oral antidiabetics, including the sulphonylureas, biguanides, alpha-glucosidase inhibitors, glinitides and glitazones.

Insulin

Insulin may be extracted from either bovine or porcine pancreas or it may be produced by recombinant DNA technology. It is possible to modify porcine insulin to make it more human-like.

Pharmacokinetics. Because insulin has a very short half-life (~10 min), so maintenance of normal plasma levels of glucose depends on a constant production from the pancreas. In the treatment of diabetes mellitus by administration of insulin, the dose to be administered must be titrated against the amount of carbohydrate consumed. Time to action and insulin elimination may be modified by adding different substances that insulin adheres to, affecting the release of insulin from its injection site.

By adding different substances to insulin, the drug is divided into four 'types', depending on the time to effect after the dose is given by subcutaneous injection and the duration of the effect. See Figure 21.13. Note that the insulin molecule is the same in all formulations.

- *Short-acting insulin* produces an effect after 10–30 min depending on which short-acting insulin is used, the site of injection (fastest via the abdomen) and the degree of physical activity. Maximum effect occurs some 1–3 h after injection and is complete after 8 h. This form of insulin is pure dissolved insulin.
- *Intermediate long-acting insulin* produces an effect about 1–1.5 h after administration. The maximum effect is some 4–12 h after administration and is complete after 24 h. This form of insulin is a suspension where insulin is bound to protamine.
- *Very long-acting insulin* produces an effect 4 h after administration. The maximum effect occurs 8–24 h after administration and is complete after about 28 h. This form of insulin is a suspension where insulin is bound to crystalline zinc.
- *Combinations of short- and intermediate long-acting insulin* are available in varying ratios. The combinations produce an effect 30 min after administration. The

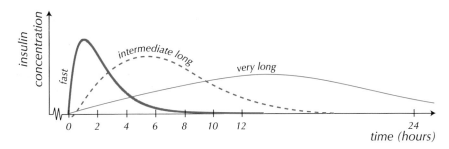

Figure 21.13 **Insulin concentration.** Different types of insulin have different times of action. Refer to the text for a more detailed explanation.

maximum effect is seen 4–8 hours after administration and is complete after about 24 h. The drug is a suspension of dissolved insulin plus insulin bound to protamine. Short-acting insulins are injected subcutaneously, intramuscularly and intravenously, while slow-acting insulins must not be injected intravenously because of the addition of protamine and zinc.

Insulin analogues (e.g. insulin lispro) are gene-modified human insulin products, produced by switching a lysine and proline residue in the polypeptide chain. The insulin effect is the same as in natural insulin, but the release from subcutaneous fat is faster and it tends to act for a shorter time. Insulin analogues can therefore be injected shortly before meals – 15 min before eating.

The primary indication for the use of insulin is in the treatment of type 1 diabetes. However, it is also used in intercurrent disease, e.g. infections, and in surgical intervention in type 2 diabetics. Pregnant women with diabetes should always use insulin if there is need for drug treatment.

Adverse effects. A major adverse effect of insulin injections is lipdystrophy, i.e. the atrophy or hypertrophy of fat in the skin at the site of injection. This tends to be less of a problem with newer insulins and the problem can be minimized by altering the site of injection. Probably the most common, and serious, adverse effect is the development of hypoglycaemia which results from an imbalance between glucose intake, glucose utilization and dose of insulin.

Oral hypoglycaemics

The plasma concentration of glucose can be influenced by stimulating the release of insulin from the β cells of the islets of Langerhans, by reducing hepatic synthesis of glucose and by altering the absorption of glucose from the intestine.

Glibenclamide, glimepiride, glipizide and chlorpropamide are examples sulphonylurea derivatives. They are synthetic compounds that stimulate the β cells in the pancreas to increase insulin release, especially in the initial phase, i.e. the release of pre-formed insulin. See Figure 21.14. Use of these preparations assumes that there is still some functional capacity of the pancreas to produce insulin. This is only true for type 2 diabetes patients. The adverse effects of these drugs include a late appearing hypoglycaemia, which, particularly in elderly individuals, can be long-lasting. Additionally, there are occasional allergic reactions, e.g. in the skin.

Metformin is a biguanide which acts by reducing the synthesis of glucose in the liver and thereby causes a reduced secretion of glucose into the plasma. It also reduces glucose absorption from the intestine. Metformin does not cause hypoglycaemia. It should be the drug of choice in overweight type 2 diabetes patients since this patient group is largely insulin-resistant and metformin has the additional

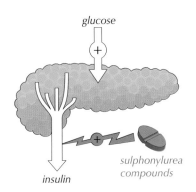

Figure 21.14 **Increased insulin release.** Sulphonylurea compounds stimulate the pancreas cells to increase the release of insulin when the glucose concentration rises.

Insulins – short-acting
Insulin aspart, Insulin lispro, Soluble insulin

Insulins – intermediate and long-acting
Insulin determir, Insulin glargine, Isophane insulin, Protamine zinc insulin

Insulins – very long-acting
Insulin zinc suspension

Insulins – combinations
Biphasic isophane insulins, Biphasic insulin aspart, Biphasic insulin lispro

Sulfonylureas
Chlorpropramide, Glibenclamide, Gliclazide, Glimepride, Glipizide, Gliquidone, Tolbutamide

Biguanides
Metformin

Other antidiabetics
Acarbose, Nataglinide, Pioglitazone, Rosiglitazone

Drugs used to treat hypoglycaemia
Glucagon, Glucose

Table 21.6 Drugs used to treat diabetes

advantage of lowering plasma triglyceride levels. It has a better protective effect than do the sulphonylurea derivatives against the complications of diabetes despite the fact that the blood sugar-lowering effect is no better. Patients with reduced renal function, alcoholism, poor general condition and uncompensated cardiac failure should not use metformin. This is because these patients are at increased risk of developing serious lactic acidosis, which may prove to be fatal.

Acarbose acts by inhibiting the enzyme glucosidase, which breaks down disaccharides, oligosaccharides and polysaccharides in the intestine. Since carbohydrates are absorbed as monosaccharides, the absorption of glucose is therefore reduced. Consequently, the rise in plasma glucose concentration seen after eating a meal is reduced.

Rosiglitazone and pioglitazone are glitazones (thiazolidinediones). These drugs reduce insulin resistance in fat, muscle and liver cells. The plasma glucose-lowering effect takes up to 8 weeks to develop after therapy has been started. Although they can be used in isolation, they can also be used in combination with metformin or the sulphonylureas. Patients with uncompensated cardiac failure should not use these drugs as they have a tendency to cause fluid retention and exacerbate the cardiac failure. There is also the possibility that they may cause liver damage, and so regular liver function tests are recommended.

Drugs used to treat diabetes are listed in Table 21.6.

DRUGS USED TO TREAT ACUTE HYPOGLYCAEMIA

Acute hypoglycaemia is best treated by drinking milk or drinks containing glucose, if the patient is conscious. Hypoglycaemia which causes unconsciousness is an emergency which may be treated by injection or infusion of glucose in unconscious patients. Injection of glucagon, a hormone produced by the pancreatic α-cells in the islets of Langerhans, is an alternative to glucose. Glucagon rapidly mobilizes glucose from glycogen stored in the liver. Side effects are nausea, vomiting, abdominal pain, hypokalemia and hypotension.

SEX HORMONES

Sex hormones (sex steroids) include androgens, oestrogens and progestogens. Androgens are male sex hormones; testosterone is the main endogenous androgen. Oestrogens are female sex hormones; the most potent endogenous oestrogen is oestradiol. Progestogens are also female sex hormones, the main one being progesterone.

MALE SEX HORMONES

Testosterone is mainly produced in the testicles under stimulation of luteinizing hormone (LH) from the anterior pituitary gland. It is also produced in small quantities in the ovaries and in the adrenal cortex in both men and women. Testosterone is responsible for the development of secondary sex characteristics in men. Follicle-stimulating hormone (FSH), released from the anterior pituitary gland in men, is responsible for spermatogenesis. In women, it has been suggested that testosterone aids the libido and the ability to reach orgasm. At high plasma concentrations, it has a masculinizing effect in women.

Testosterone is a steroid that acts in exactly the same way as the glucocorticoids described earlier in this chapter, i.e. it influences gene activity. Testosterone is used as substitute treatment in testicular dysfunction, e.g. hypogonadism or hypopituitarism, where there is inadequate stimulation of the testicles by anterior pituitary gland hormones.

Anabolic steroids are often abused in sports. They increase the muscle strength and are included in the list of illegal preparations. These steroids have considerable adverse effects in the form of increased aggressiveness and violence. Large doses inhibit pituitary function and lead to sterility because they suppress the release of FSH, which is necessary for sperm production. There is also an increased risk of liver damage following prolonged use.

Male sex hormones are listed in Table 21.7.

Androgens
Testosterone, Mesterolone
Anabolic steroid
Nandrolone

Table 21.7 Male sex hormones and anabolic steroid

FEMALE SEX HORMONES

Oestrogens and progesterone are the female sex hormones, which coordinate the physiology and developmental activity of female genitalia and mammary glands. The hormones have important pharmacological applications as contraceptives (birth control pills) and in prevention of postmenopausal problems, such as vaginal dryness and osteoporosis. The risk of taking oestrogen and progesterone supplements is that hormone sensitive tissue e.g. breast and endometrium may undergo changes and become cancerous. Also there is an increased risk of developing thromboembolic diseases like deep vein thrombosis, heart disease and strokes.

Oestrogens

Oestrogens are produced in the ovaries. They stimulate the development of secondary sex characteristics in women. Natural oestrogen occurs in three forms, oestrone, oestradiol and oestriol, the most potent of which is oestradiol.

Oestrogens have a mild anabolic effect; they contribute to the elasticity of the skin and to mineralization of bones. They also increase the ratio of high-density lipoprotein (HDL) to low-density lipoprotein (LDL). In young women this is advantageous since it affords some protection against the development of atherosclerosis and cardiovascular disease. However, the synthesis of some of the coagulation factors is increased, which increases the risk of thromboembolic disease.

After the menopause, there is a significant decline in oestrogen levels resulting in gradual atrophy of the breasts and vagina. The skin, especially the mucous membranes, becomes dryer and less elastic. This may cause sexual dysfunction in some women and can lead to an increased incidence of urinary tract infections because the secretion of antibacterial substances in the vagina and urethra is reduced. The decline in oestrogen levels also leads to demineralization of the skeleton, with an increased risk of fractures. Additionally, there is also increased risk of the development of cardiovascular problems, regardless of age.

The primary use of oestrogen supplements is for chemical contraception and in postmenopausal substitution therapy. Contraception is achieved by disturbing the normal physiological oestrogen secretion. Substitution therapy after the menopause reduces the demineralization of bones and maintains the elasticity of the epithelial mucosa. Additionally, problems with thermoregulation (hot flushes) and emotional instability are also reduced.

Pharmacological doses of oestrogen increase the blood's ability to coagulate through the influence of different coagulation factors. This is also the reason for the increased risk of thromboembolic disease in women taking some forms of the contraceptive pill. Oestrogen supplements also lead to retention of salt and water, tenderness in the breasts, nausea, vomiting and anorexia. Some women also experience weight gain. Postmenopausal substitution of oestrogen can result in menstrual-like bleeding and endometrial hyperplasia.

Progesterone

Progesterone is produced by the corpus luteum – the remainder of the follicle after ovulation has occurred. If the egg is not fertilized, however, the corpus luteum disintegrates, and the plasma levels of progesterone drop rapidly. As with oestrogens, progesterone binds to cytoplasmic receptors and influences the transcription of DNA.

The primary use of progesterone is in contraceptive pills. To understand its (and oestrogen's) role in contraception, it is necessary to understand the regulation of a normal menstrual cycle.

REGULATION OF THE MENSTRUAL CYCLE

The menstrual cycle begins on day one of the period, when menses (bleeding) begins. The menstrual cycle is regulated by close interactions between the hypothalamus, the anterior pituitary gland and the ovaries. The hypothalamus secretes gonadotrophin-releasing hormone (GnRH) in pulses, which stimulates the pituitary to release follicle-stimulating hormone (FSH) and luteinizing hormone (LH), as shown in Figure 21.2. FSH stimulates the development of a number of follicles in the ovaries. One of the follicles develops into a Graafian follicle, which will later release a mature egg (ovulation).

Follicle cells produce oestrogens in response to stimulation by FSH. The oestrogens promote endometrial proliferation in the first half of the menstrual cycle and in this way prepare it for the possible implantation of a fertilized egg. In addition, oestrogens sensitize cells in the anterior pituitary gland to increase the release of LH. This LH surge comes approximately midway through the menstrual cycle, i.e.

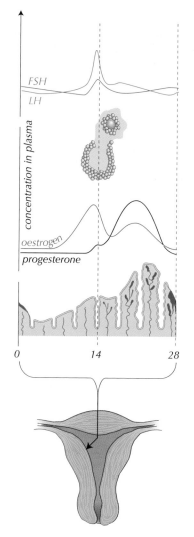

Figure 21.15 **Regulation of the menstrual cycle.**

on about day 14 of the cycle. The follicle ruptures in response to the increased levels of LH and the egg within it is released (ovulation). After ovulation, the oestrogens, by a negative feedback effect, cause a reduced release of FSH and GnRH. LH continues to influence the ruptured follicle, so that the cells within it proliferate and the follicle, now called the corpus luteum, secretes progesterone. Progesterone stimulates the endometrium to further develop in anticipation of a fertilized egg. If the egg is not fertilized and consequently fails to implant, the release of progesterone from the corpus luteum stops. The sudden drop in progesterone production results in a contraction of arteries in the endometrial membrane, which thereby receives insufficient blood supply. The endometrium is shed and a new menstrual cycle starts with the onset of menses. See Figure 21.15.

CONTRACEPTIVE (BIRTH CONTROL) PILLS

Birth control pills prevent pregnancy by preventing ovulation, reducing oestrogen-induced proliferation of the endometrium and changing the viscosity of the mucus in the cervix. This prevents the sperm from reaching the egg and makes the endometrium less receptive for a fertilized egg.

There are two types of birth control pills: combination pills and minipills. Combination pills contain both oestrogen and progesterone. This type of pill can be divided into two subgroups: one has a fixed quantity of oestrogen (monophasic preparations) while the other has varying quantities of oestrogen (sequence preparations or three-phase pills). Sequence preparations give a lower total dose of supplied hormones than the monophasic preparations. The pill is taken once a day for 3 weeks followed by a pill-free week. In some preparations, the pill-free week is replaced with a week of placebo tablets. In the placebo or pill-free week, there is menstrual-like bleeding. The effectiveness of the combination pill in preventing pregnancy is almost 100 per cent if the pills are taken as prescribed. See Figure 21.16.

Minipills contain progesterone only. They are taken daily throughout the entire cycle, including during the bleeding phase. They are not as effective as the combination pill in preventing pregnancy.

Mechanism of action and effects. By consuming combination pills, the body is supplied with oestrogen and progesterone in concentrations that suppresses FSH production (oestrogen) and LH production (progesterone). Follicle development is inhibited and ovulation is suppressed. Equally, the endometrium is hostile to the

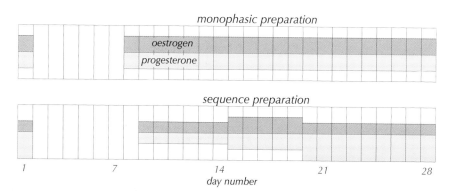

Figure 21.16 **Birth control pills.** The oestrogen and progesterone content of monophasic preparations and sequence preparations. The red colour shows the oestrogen content, while the blue colour shows the progesterone content.

Combined hormonal contraceptives – low strength
Ethinylestradiol with norethisterone, Ethinylestradiol with desogestrel,
Ethinylestradiol with gestodene

Combined hormonal contraceptives – standard strength
Ethinylestradiol with: levonorgestrel, norethisterone, norgestimate, desogestrel,
drospirenone, gestodene, cyproterone acetate

Progestogen-only contraceptives (oral, parenteral and intra-uterine forms are
available)
Desogestrel, Etynodiol diacetate, Levonorgestrel, Norethisterone

Also be aware of the intra-uterine contraceptive devices

Table 21.8 Contraceptives

implantation of a fertilized egg. Progesterone in minipills makes the mucus in the cervix more viscous, so that the sperm have difficulty in reaching the egg and fertilizing it. It also hinders the normal development of the endometrium.

Adverse effects. The adverse effects of low-dose combination pills include trace bleeding throughout the cycle, nausea, weight gain and skin pigmentation. Some women experience a reduced libido and no bleeding. Studies have shown an increased risk for developing venous thrombosis with subsequent pulmonary embolism, cardiac infarction and stroke. The most vulnerable are women with other risk factors like obesity, smoking, hyperlipidemia, hypertension, diabetes mellitus, age over 35 years or a family history of myocardial infarction. It is suggested that the oral contraceptive pill should be used with caution if there is one risk factor for arterial disease, but avoided if there are two or more. Birth control pills should be stopped at least 14 days before planned surgical intervention because of the risk of developing a thromboembolic disorder. The use of the combination pill protects against ovarian and endometrial cancer. There is a possible connection between the pill and the development of breast and endometrial cancer.

Contraceptives are listed in Table 21.8.

HORMONE REPLACEMENT THERAPY

When ovulation stops, the cyclic production of oestrogen and progesterone stops. This is assumed to be the cause of many problems in postmenopausal women. Early problems include hot flushes, insomnia, emotional instability and concentration difficulties. Some notice problems with dry and sore mucous membranes in the vagina, resulting in stinging pain when urinating, stress incontinence and recurring cystitis. This is a consequence of a reduced mucus secretion and a reduced synthesis of collagen and elastic connective tissue in the mucous membrane. Longer-term changes include a gradual demineralization of the skeleton, an increase in LDL cholesterol and a reduction in HDL cholesterol, with the increased risk of development of cardiovascular disease. Postmenopausal substitution therapy with oestrogen delays the demineralization of bones.

Both oestrogen and a combination of oestrogen and progesterone are used as substitution therapy. For postmenopausal use, the dose of oestrogen that is administered is less than that which is used in the contraceptive pill.

Because of the physiological changes associated with the reduced hormone secretion at menopause, hormone replacement therapy (HRT) has been questioned. For many years it was considered that maintaining appropriate hormone levels was beneficial. However, there is increasing evidence that the risks associated

---

Oestrogens for hormone replacement therapy
Oestrogen conjugated only, Oestrogens conjugated with progestogen, Estradiol only, Estradiol with progestogen, Estriol, Estrone, Ethinylestradiol
Others
Tibolone, Raloxifene

Table 21.9 Drugs used in hormone replacement therapy

with HRT may outweigh the benefits, since the risk of developing breast cancer, endometrial cancer, venous thromboembolism and strokes have all been shown to be increased. When needed, the minimum effective dose of HRT therefore should be used for the shortest possible duration.

The increased risk of breast cancer, caused by all types of HRT, is related to duration of use. Women with a family history of breast cancer are specifically at risk. The risk of developing a venous thromboembolism is also specifically elevated during the first year of use. Predisposing factors are a personal or family history of deep vein thrombosis or pulmonary embolism, smoking, obesity, major trauma, prolonged bed-rest and severe varicose veins. Major surgery under general anaesthesia involves an increased risk for the development of venous thromboembolism. It is therefore advisable to stop HRT 4–6 weeks before surgery. It is now no longer believed that HRT protects against the development of coronary heart disease.

Women with natural early or surgical menopause are at a high risk of developing osteoporosis. HRT therefore may be advised in these women until the approximate age of natural menopause.

If a woman has an intact uterus an oestrogen with cyclical progesterone for the last half of the cycle may be used. In women without a uterus an oestrogen alone is advisable. Topical HRT may be applied for a short time to improve the vaginal mucous membrane in menopausal athropic vaginitis. Modified-release vaginal tablets and an impregnated vaginal ring are available.

Drugs used in hormone replacement therapy are listed in Table 21.9.

SUMMARY

- Endocrine disturbances can lead to both over- and underproduction of hormones. The hypothalamus and pituitary gland exercise the highest level of endocrinological control. Their hormones control the release of hormones from peripheral endocrine glands. Hormone levels are regulated by negative feedback. Deficiency in pituitary function can lead to an array of hormone disturbances.
- Release of the thyroid hormones T_3 and T_4 occurs from the thyroid gland. Hyperthyroidism is an elevated concentration of thyroid hormones in the plasma. It can be treated by the use of radioactive iodine that is concentrated in the thyroid gland and destroys the tissue. It may also be treated by the use of thyrostatics – drugs that inhibit the production of thyroid hormones. Bone marrow suppression is a serious but often reversible adverse effect that occurs in a minority of the users. Hypothyroidism is low plasma concentration of thyroid hormones. In hypothyroidism, substitute therapy must be used.
- The calcium concentration in plasma is regulated by parathyroid hormone, vitamin D hormone and calcitonin. Chronic loss of calcium results in demineralization of the skeleton. In hypercalcaemia, drugs are used that both reduce the release and

increase the incorporation of calcium in the bone mass. Calcitonin and bisphosphonates have such an effect. Hypocalcaemia causes increased excitability of neuromuscular tissue and can trigger convulsions. Vitamin D increases the absorption of calcium from the intestines and the reabsorption of calcium in the kidneys.

■ The adrenal cortex secretes mineralocorticoids, glucocorticoids and androgens. Administration of glucocorticoids is used in inflammatory disorders and to suppress activity in the immune system in immunological disorders. The drugs have different effects in different tissues. There are many serious dose-dependent adverse effects: reduced immune function, reduced protein synthesis, reduced formation of connective tissue, demineralization of the skeleton and increased secretion of hydrochloric acid and pepsin. Aldosterone antagonists are used to treat hypertension to reduce the retention of sodium.

■ Release of insulin is stimulated by a high plasma glucose concentration. Diabetics have a deficient release of insulin into the plasma. In type 1 diabetes (IDDM), the ability to release insulin is lost and insulin substitution is necessary. There are four types of insulin: short-acting, intermediate long-acting, very long-acting and combinations of short- and intermediate long-acting preparations. The insulin is the same but is bound to different additives so that the time it takes to produce an effect varies. In type 2 diabetes (NIDDM), the response to an elevated plasma glucose concentration is reduced. These patients can use drugs that increase the release of insulin.

■ Oestrogens and progestogens are used as drugs to prevent pregnancy, prevent post-menopausal problems and reduce demineralization of the skeleton in women. Birth control pills are available in monophasic preparations with fixed hormone content and in sequence preparations with varying hormone content of oestrogen and progesterone. Minipills contain progesterone only and are less reliable than combination pills. Birth control pills prevent pregnancy by disturbing the natural release of oestrogen and progesterone, such that ovulation does not take place. Because the viscosity in the mucus in the cervix increases, the chance for an egg to become fertilized and implanted in the endometrium is reduced. Use of birth control pills seems to reduce the risk of cancer in ovaries and the endometrium, but possibly increases the risk of breast cancer. In menopausal difficulties, less potent oestrogens are used than those that are found in birth control pills. Substitution with oestrogens causes an increased risk of breast cancer, endometrial cancer and thromboembolic disease.

22 Drugs used in allergy, for immune suppression and in cancer treatment

The immune system protects the body against infection and removes damaged, diseased and dead cells. To perform this task without damaging the individual's own tissue, the immune system must differentiate between its own and foreign tissue. This ability is developed in fetal life and is usually maintained throughout life. Differences in membrane protein structures primarily characterize tissue. If the ability to differentiate between one's own and foreign tissue is lost, the immune system 'attacks' the person's own tissue and autoimmune disorders arise.

Structures that activate the immune system are called antigens. When antigens activate the immune system in an inappropriate way, the response is called hypersensitivity. Hay fever, asthma, autoimmune disorders or rejection of transplanted tissue are examples of hypersensitivity reactions. It may be necessary to suppress such reactions with drugs.

In cancer, several of a cell's normal properties change. They lose normal control of growth and grow in an uninhibited manner by steady cell division. There are also changes to cellular structures. The immune system normally removes such cells. In some cases, however, the difference between cancer cells and normal cells is insufficient for the body's immune system to be activated and remove them.

Drugs used to treat cancer try to exploit differences between healthy and diseased cells, and between cells in the stationary phase and the division phase of the cell cycle. Since the differences can be small, the drugs are often inadequately selective towards the cancer cells and attack both diseased and healthy cells. Inadequate selectivity is part of the explanation for the serious adverse effects of these drugs.

Since the immune system has as its central task the fighting off of infections, the use of immunosuppressive drugs and cytotoxics, which suppress activity in the immune system, increase the risk of infection.

THE IMMUNE SYSTEM

The immune system is complex in function and consists of many different components. It is often divided into a specific or acquired system and a non-specific or natural system. Antigens trigger activity in both systems. The non-specific system is activated by many different antigens and is active from first exposure. The specific immune system requires contact with an antigen to develop. Both systems act cooperatively to the extent that the division seems artificial. To understand the immunological reactions that are activated by hypersensitivity reactions, autoimmune diseases and rejection of transplanted tissue, it is important to understand the most important components of the immune system.

FIRST-, SECOND- AND THIRD-LINE DEFENCE

In addition to the immune system, the body has mechanical barriers that protect against disease and damage from microorganisms and chemical and organic material. The mechanical barriers consist of the outer layer of skin (epidermis), mucous membranes with dissolved enzymes, and the normal microbial flora. Mechanical barriers can be considered as first-line defence, the non-specific immune system as the second-line defence, and the specific immune system as the third-line defence. See Figure 22.1.

Non-specific immune system
Neutrophil granulocytes, monocytes and macrophages are all components of the non-specific immune system and have the ability to phagocytose many different antigens. These antigens can be microorganisms or products of microorganisms. They do not need specific receptors to bind to antigens and form the basis of the non-specific immune system. They are active in both the blood and tissue outside the bloodstream. Neutrophil granulocytes and monocytes are active in the bloodstream. When monocytes migrate out of the bloodstream to tissue, they are called macrophages.

Specific immune system
Lymphocytes are immunological active cells that are produced in the bone marrow. They are divided into B-lymphocytes and T-lymphocytes. The B-lymphocytes are produced and developed in the bone marrow, while the T-lymphocytes are produced in the bone marrow but develop in the thymus. The lymphocytes have protein structures in the outer membrane which only react with specific antigens. This property is the origin of the term 'the specific immune system'.

When B-lymphocytes are exposed to antigens, they will multiply and produce plasma cells, which secrete large amounts of antibodies (immunoglobulins) that circulate in the bloodstream and bind to the antigens that initially stimulated the B-lymphocytes. The immunoglobulins are divided into five different classes (IgA, IgE, IgD, IgG and IgM) that have different functions. Antigens bound to antibodies are more effectively intercepted by the immune system than antigens without antibodies. Simultaneously as plasma cells are produced, B cells will be produced that 'remember' the antigen (memory B cells). On subsequent stimulation from the same (specific) antigen, these cells will remember the antigen and quickly contribute to the formation of large quantities of antibodies directed against it. The B-lymphocytes

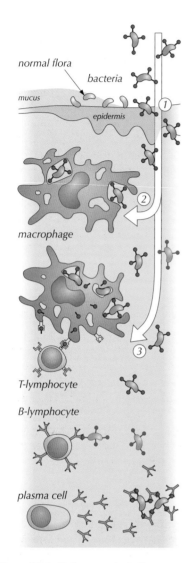

Figure 22.1 Defence against diseases. Mechanical and chemical barriers form the first-line defence (1). Phagocytosing cells form a second-line defence (2). The specific immune system forms the third-line defence (3).

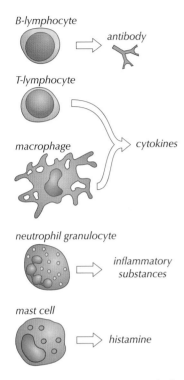

Figure 22.2 **The immune system.** Active cells in the immune defence system and the secretion of immunomodulating substances.

are especially active in bacterial infections and at destroying large foreign molecules such as proteins and toxins that are secreted from microorganisms. Drugs that subdue the activity of B-lymphocytes increase the risk of bacterial infections.

T-lymphocytes are stimulated by antigens that are presented to them by other cells in the immune system. This results in production of T-helper lymphocytes, T-suppressor lymphocytes and T-attack lymphocytes. These have somewhat different functions, but cooperate to remove antigens from the organism. The T-lymphocytes are active in fighting fungi, virus-infected cells or cells that are transformed to cancer cells, and cells in transplanted tissue that the body does not recognize as its own. Patients with deficient production of T-lymphocytes or those who use drugs that suppress the activity of the T-lymphocytes have an increased risk of infection with fungi and viruses. Additionally, cells that are starting to develop into cancer cells are less likely to be destroyed. T-lymphocytes are important for the cellular immune defence. Figure 22.2 shows the different cells that participate in the immune defence.

COOPERATION IN THE IMMUNE SYSTEM

Macrophages phagocytose antigens and break them down into smaller components. These components are presented on the surface of the macrophages, together with the macrophages' surface proteins (MHC protein II), in the form of an antigen–protein complex. When the cells of the body are infected with viruses or transformed for any other reason, they present antigens in addition to their own surface antigens (MHC protein I). T-helper lymphocytes bind to the complex of antigen/MHC protein II on the surface of macrophages and secrete cytokines. These agents activate T-attack lymphocytes to bind to the complex of antigen/MHC protein I on the surface of their own transformed cells. The binding of T-attack lymphocytes to transformed cells damages the cells so that they die, but can possibly also neutralize viruses in infected cells without killing the cell. See Figure 22.3.

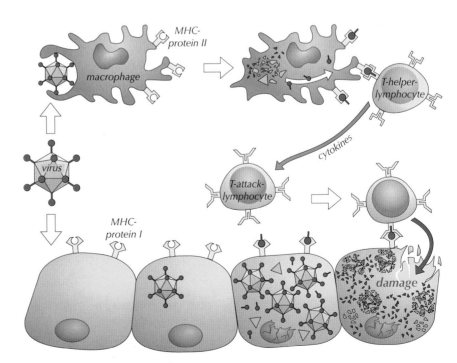

Figure 22.3 **Cooperation between phagocytosing cell and T-lymphocytes.** Refer to the text for a more detailed explanation.

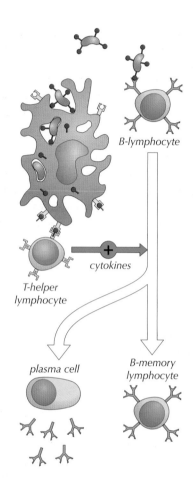

Figure 22.4 Cooperation between a phagocytosing cell and B- and T-lymphocytes. A B-lymphocyte presents an antigen to a macrophage. The macrophage then presents the antigen to a T-helper lymphocyte, which activates T-attack lymphocytes (see Figure 22.3) and stimulates B-lymphocytes to differentiate into plasma cells, resulting in the production of antibodies and the new production of B-memory lymphocytes.

Cytokines from T-lymphocytes are also important because they stimulate B-lymphocytes to produce plasma cells and memory B cells. With that, the production of antibodies increases. Antibodies from plasma cells bind again to antigens and increase the phagocytosing cells' ability for phagocytosis. See Figure 22.4.

Similarly, monocytes are important in optimizing the immune system. They exert their effect in the blood.

With the development of autoimmune diseases, changes occur in some 'self' cells, so that they are perceived as foreign. The immunological activity that occurs around these cells often results in tissue damage. After tissue transplantation, unknown antigens on the transplanted tissue will activate the immune system, which damages or rejects the tissue.

IMMUNOLOGICAL HYPERSENSITIVITY REACTIONS

Different properties of the different components in the immune system mean that immunological responses can present in different ways. In practice, it is possible to differentiate between four types of hypersensitivity reaction.

Type I reactions (anaphylactic reactions)

Type I reactions are the result of plasma cells forming excessive antibodies of the IgE type, which embed into the membrane of mast cells in tissues and basophilic granulocytes in blood. When antigens subsequently bind to these antibodies, the cells rupture and immediately release histamine and other active substances. See Figure 22.5. Antigens that bind IgE antibodies are called allergens. A hypersensitivity reaction between IgE antibodies and allergens is called an allergy. Cells that contain histamine are found in almost all tissues, but they occur in especially high concentrations in the mucous membrane of the airways, the gastrointestinal tract and the skin. Also, basophil granulocyte circulating in the blood may release histamine. Released histamine binds to specific histamine receptors (H_1 receptors).

H_1 receptors are found on smooth muscle and endothelial cells. Histamine binding to H_1 receptors in the airways results in bronchoconstriction and increased secretion of mucus, both of which compromise ventilation. Histamine binding to H_1 receptors on endothelial cells stimulates the release of nitric oxide (NO), which diffuses to smooth muscles in the vascular wall and causes vasodilation. At the same time, permeability through the endothelial cells increases. Vessel dilation leads to a fall in blood pressure. Increased permeability causes leakage of plasma and proteins from small blood vessels and local oedema. Histamine binding to H_1 receptors on smooth muscle in the intestine can cause cramps and diarrhoea. H_2 receptors are found in mucosa of the stomach. Histamine binding to these receptors causes increased secretion of hydrochloric acid. In the skin, histamine will stimulate sensory nerve ends and cause itching. With some insect bites, histamine is injected into the skin, which is the cause of swelling and itching.

Such reactions occur as soon as the antigen binds to the IgE antibodies. They are called immediate allergies, or anaphylactic reactions. Leukotrienes, which have a strong contractile effect on bronchial smooth muscle, can be released 4–6 h after the release of histamine. This is a typical late reaction that often follows an acute asthma attack.

Type I reactions can occur topically (locally) in the tissue or in the bloodstream, depending on how the antigen reaches the organism. With topical release of histamine, topical allergic reactions are seen, which result in runny eyes and nose, skin rashes or asthma. With the systemic release of histamine into the circulation, many blood vessels will be affected, causing vasodilation and leakage of plasma and

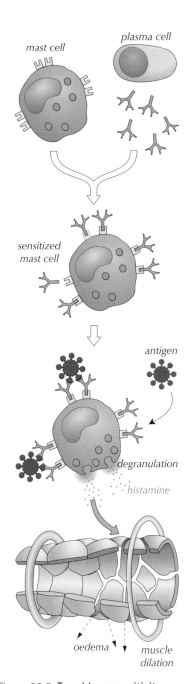

Figure 22.5 **Type I hypersensitivity.** Antigens bind to IgE antibodies embedded in mast cells. The binding results in degranulation and the release of histamine and other active substances, which particularly affect vascular and bronchial smooth muscle.

resulting in a fall in blood pressure and circulatory collapse – anaphylactic shock. Anaphylactic shock can also develop by topical release, if the histamine reaches the bloodstream in sufficient quantity before it is broken down.

Drug treatment of type I reactions aims to prevent the release of histamine or to prevent histamine binding to its receptors. Antihistamines (which prevent histamine binding to its receptors) are used in the prophylactic treatment against such reactions.

Type II reactions (cytotoxic type)

The basis for type II allergic reactions are IgG or IgM antibodies that bind to cellular receptors. Proteins in basal membranes and other cells can function as receptors for such antibodies. Parts of the immune system (the complement system) are activated and destroy the antibody binding cells – hence the term cytotoxic reactions. See Figure 22.6. Drugs that bind to proteins can change protein structures such that they are perceived as foreign. In drug-induced haemolysis of erythrocytes, it is thought that drugs bind to the surface of erythrocytes, which are thereafter damaged by the immune system and haemolysed. Myasthenia gravis is an autoimmune type II reaction where antibodies are formed against acetylcholine receptors in motor end-plates of skeletal muscle. Because these receptors are destroyed, the muscles lose the ability to respond to acetylcholine and become limp.

To reduce type II reactions, it is possible to suppress the antibody production from the plasma cells. Immunosuppressive drugs will prevent proliferation of plasma cells and reduce the production of antibodies.

Type III reactions (immunocomplex-mediated)

In this reaction, immunocomplexes are formed by antigens and antibodies, either in the circulation or locally in the tissue. The complexes can attach to different tissues, especially basal membranes in the kidneys or other tissues that filter the blood. By this filtering, the antigen–antibody complexes are trapped in the tissue, where they activate other parts of the immune system and induce damage. See Figure 22.7. Glomerulonephritis after streptococcal infection (poststreptococcal glomerulonephritis) is a type III reaction where immunocomplexes are precipitated in glomeruli. Immunocomplexes can also be responsible for infection reactions of unknown origin in the wall of small- and medium-sized arteries (polyarteritis).

Type III reactions can be suppressed with immunosuppressive drugs.

Type IV reactions (delayed cell-mediated reaction)

T-lymphocytes that bind antigens secrete cytokines and activate macrophages that aggregate in the area where the antigen is found. The reaction takes a few days to develop (i.e. it is delayed) and is called cell-mediated, since T-lymphocytes and

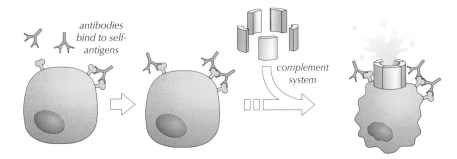

Figure 22.6 **Type II reaction.** Complement binds to antigens on a cell and haemolyses the cell. Also, T-attack lymphocytes can damage cells that have bound antibodies.

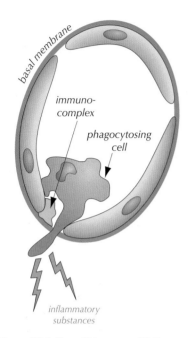

Figure 22.7 Type III hypersensitivity.
Immunocomplexes that are bound to basal membranes can trigger damage from both the complement system and phagocytosing cells.

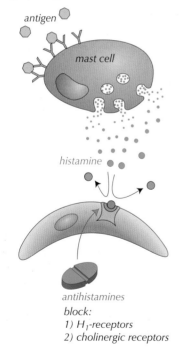

Figure 22.8 Antihistamines. By blocking histamine H₁ receptors, the effect of released histamine is reduced. They also block cholinergic muscarinic receptors and therefore possess some anticholinergic properties.

macrophages (not antibodies) are the central elements. Figure 22.3 shows a type IV reaction. The immune response towards the tuberculosis bacterium and a number of allergens that come into contact with the skin (contact allergy) involving T-lymphocytes are cell-mediated. Type IV reactions can be suppressed with immunosuppressive drugs.

Hypersensitivity reactions in tissue transplants

In reactions against foreign tissue transplants, several allergic mechanisms can be activated. A hyperacute reaction will occur if the recipient has circulating antibodies against the transplanted cells. The antibodies will attach to endothelial cells in the recipient's blood vessels and lead to thrombosis even while the transplant procedure is being undertaken. If this reaction occurs, the transplant must be discontinued immediately. An acute reaction that involves both antibody-mediated and cell-mediated allergy can develop during the first weeks after transplant. Antibody reactions damage mainly blood vessels, while cell-mediated mechanisms result in infiltration of lymphocytes and macrophages that damage the cells. A chronic reaction that involves both antibody and cellular mechanisms occurs gradually over months and years, and results in changes in blood vessels that cause constriction of the lumen and reduced perfusion, and thereby leads to cellular damage of the transplanted tissue.

To avoid these acute and chronic responses, the activity must be subdued with immunosuppressive drugs.

DRUGS USED TO TREAT IMMUNOLOGICAL DISORDERS

Drugs against unwanted immunological disorders can be divided into antiallergenics and immunosuppressives. Antiallergenics suppress type I reactions, where histamine release is an essential factor. Antihistamines and cromoglicate are drugs in this group. Glucocorticoids inhibit the release of histamine and other inflammatory substances, but also have an immunosuppressive effect, which consists of inhibiting the activation of immunological cells and suppressing cell proliferation.

ANTIALLERGENICS

Antihistamines (H₁ Antagonists)

Antihistamines are used in allergic rhinitis, allergic conjunctivitis and urticaria, where histamine is the most important mediator of the allergic response. They have little effect in asthma, since histamine is only one of many mediators in this disease. Antihistamines are also used to treat nausea and motion sickness and as sedatives.

Mechanism of action and effects. The antiallergenic effect results from blockade of histamine (H₁) receptors – the release of histamine is not inhibited. See Figure 22.8. The sedative effect and the effect against nausea and motion sickness are associated with an influence on the central nervous system.

Antihistamines are divided into first- and second-generation drugs. First-generation antihistamines are also referred to as sedating antihistamines while second-generation antihistamines are referred to as non-sedating. First-generation antihistamines pass easily across the blood–brain barrier. They have better sedative and antiemetic effects than second-generation antihistamines. First-generation antihistamines have the most pronounced adverse effects on the central nervous system. Because of their sedative effects, they should not be used by those about to drive or operate heavy machinery.

Antihistamines – first generation (sedating)
Alimemazine, Brompheniramine, Chlorphenamine, Clemastine, Cyproheptadine, Diphenhydramine, Doxylamine, Hydroxycine, Promethazine, Tripolidine

Antihistamines – second generation (non-sedating)
Acrivastine, Cetirizine, Desloratadine, Fexofenadine, Levocetirizine, Loratadine, Mizolastine, Terfenadine

Other antiallergics and antiinflammatory topical drugs
Antazoline Azelastine, Emedastine, Epinastine, Ketotifen, Levocabastine, Lodoxamide, Nedocromil, Olopatadine, Sodium cromoglicate

---

Table 22.1 Drugs used to treat allergic disorders

Histamine H_2-receptor antagonists are used exclusively in the treatment of ulcers to suppress the acid secretion from the stomach mucosa. They have no place in the treatment of allergy.

Adverse effects. Sedation, tinnitus, listlessness, confusion, poor coordination and tremors occur in varying degrees among the different antihistamines. A noticeable anticholinergic effect is associated with blockage of muscarinic receptors on the salivary glands and contributes to dryness of the mouth. Because of the reduced sedative effect of second-generation antihistamines, their use is preferred in the treatment of allergic disorders.

Interactions. Simultaneous use of drugs or intoxicants with subduing effects on the central nervous system will exacerbate the sedative effect of antihistamines.

Other antiallergics and antiinflammatory topical drugs

Cromoglicate, lodoxamide and nedocromil are used prophylactically against allergic rhinitis and allergic conjunctivitis. They are only used for topical application and have no effect if they are administered after an allergic response has been triggered.

The drugs probably inhibit immediate and delayed antigen-triggered release of histamine and other pro-inflammatory mediators from mast cells. They do not prevent histamine binding to its receptors. See Figure 22.9. Adverse effects are few. The use of cromoglicate in the treatment of asthma is discussed in Chapter 21, Drugs used to treat endocrinological disorders.

Drugs used as antiallergenics are listed in Table 22.1.

IMMUNOSUPPRESSIVE DRUGS

If it were possible, it would be advantageous to choose immunosuppressive agents that act selectively on B-lymphocytes and the production of antibodies or on the cellular immune system, depending on which reactions require suppression. This is only possible to a certain extent. There is general suppression of the immune system when immunosuppressive drugs are used, with increased risk of infection as the most important adverse effect.

Glucocorticoids, ciclosporin, tacrolimus, cytotoxics and anti-tumour necrosis factor-α are immunosuppressive drugs. Often, combinations of several of these drugs are used simultaneously.

Glucocorticoids

The immunomodulatory effects of glucocorticoids occur because the drugs inhibit signals that cause proliferation of both B- and T-lymphocytes, and this subdues immune responses. In addition, the release of fatty acids from cell membranes is

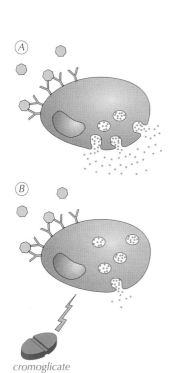

cromoglicate

Figure 22.9 **Cromoglicate** causes reduced degranulation of mast cells.

reduced because the activity of the enzyme phospholipase A_2 is reduced. As a result, the synthesis of several immunomodulating agents, e.g. prostaglandins and leukotrienes, is also reduced. Glucocorticoids have a general immunosuppressive effect and are often used together with other immunomodulating drugs. It is common to use glucocorticoids after organ transplants, when there is a risk of acute organ rejection, and after stem cell transplantation. Glucocorticoids are discussed in Chapter 21, Drugs used to treat endocrinological disorders.

Selective immunosuppressive drugs

Selective immunosuppressive drugs are drugs that mainly exert effects on B- and T-lymphocytes. Ciclosporin and tacrolimus (primary effect on T-lymphocytes), mycophenolate (effect on B- and T-lymphocytes) and immunosuppressive immune globulins belong to this group.

Ciclosporin, tacrolimus and sirolimus

Ciclosporin and tacrolimus exert a particular effect on T-lymphocytes. Sirolimus is a new immunosuppressant used to inhibit rejection after organ transplantation. The primary indication for the use of these drugs is to prevent rejection after organ and bone marrow transplantation. Ciclosporin is also used in serious rheumatoid arthritis, psoriasis and a number of other autoimmune disorders. The T-lymphocytes, in particular, are active in rejection reactions.

Mechanism of action and effects. Ciclosporin and tacrolimus inhibit the release of cytokines from T-helper lymphocytes, so that activation and proliferation of T-attack lymphocytes are reduced. See Figure 22.10. There is little effect on B-lymphocytes and antibody production. The drugs primarily provide cellular immune suppression, which is important after transplantation and occurs in autoimmune diseases such as rheumatoid arthritis and psoriasis.

Adverse effects and precautionary measures. Ciclosporin and tacrolimus have insignificant bone marrow suppressive effects. The chances of serious bacterial infections are few, as the activity of the B-lymphocytes and antibody production are intact. Because the T-lymphocytes are inhibited, there is an increased risk of infection with fungi and viruses. There may also be an increased risk of virus-induced cancer development with prolonged use, because the T-lymphocytes also neutralize virus-infected cells that can be transformed to cancer cells. In high concentrations, the drugs have a nephrotoxic effect and a tendency to cause hypertension. Early signs of infection and increases in blood pressure and changes in creatinine levels must be carefully monitored.

Immunosuppressive immune globulins

Immunosuppressive immunoglobulins are antibodies that bind to specific receptors on T-lymphocytes, so that the activity of the T-lymphocytes is inhibited and the cellular immune response is reduced. This drug group has been used in combination with glucocorticoids and ciclosporin after organ transplantation. However, they are also used in the treatment of serious forms of rheumatoid arthritis and Crohn's disease. Muromonab-CD3, basiliximab, daclizumab, infliximab and etanercept belong to this group.

Basiliximab and daclizumab

Both of these drugs are antibodies that bind to receptors for interleukin-2 on T-lymphocytes. This results in reduced cytokine production and thereby reduced

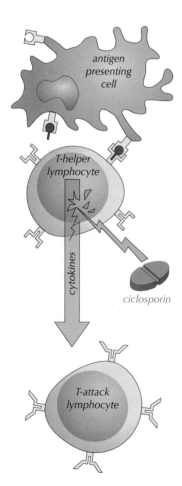

Figure 22.10 **Ciclosporin.** By inhibiting the release of cytokines from T-helper lymphocytes, the proliferation of T-attack lymphocytes is reduced, so cellular hypersensitivity is inhibited.

stimuli to proliferation of T-attack lymphocytes. In this way the cellular immune system is inhibited. Frequent adverse effects are constipation, urinary tract infections, pain, nausea, hypertension, upper respiratory tract infections, headaches and diarrhoea.

Infliximab and etanercept

These bind to and inhibit TNF-α, a cytokine that stimulates immunocompetent cells, especially T-lymphocytes. The result is a reduction in the number of inflammatory cells in inflamed tissue. Frequent adverse effects are nausea, diarrhoea, stomach pains, headaches, dyspepsia, rashes and respiratory tract infections. These drugs are also discussed in Chapter 15, Drugs used to treat inflammatory and autoimmune joint diseases.

Cytotoxics

Cytotoxics are used as immunosuppressive drugs when glucocorticoids alone do not provide sufficient effect or produce unacceptable adverse effects, or if the disease is of a particularly serious nature. The majority of cytotoxics inhibit cellular synthetic processes that are necessary for cell division. Therefore, they act best during the division phase of the cell cycle. Such drugs can be used to suppress the proliferation of immunomodulatory cells. Cytotoxics produce general and non-specific immune suppression which can be difficult to predict and varies from disease to disease. In addition, the drugs have an anti-inflammatory effect. The effect of these drugs can be evaluated based on measurements of C-reactive protein and sedimentation rate.

Azathioprine

Azathioprine is a cytotoxic that is only used as an immunosuppressive. The substance is metabolized to a metabolite that inhibits the synthesis of DNA, resulting in inhibition of cell division. Leucocyte proliferation is particularly inhibited. The metabolic processes influenced occur by the enzyme thiopurine methyltransferase (TMPT), which shows genetic variation. Individuals exhibiting low activity of the enzyme will have a greater effect at standard dosage of the drug. It can be useful to determine the activity of TPMT in order to establish whether a person should receive a reduced dosage.

Cyclophosphamide

Cyclophosphamide acts by creating cross-links between DNA strands, so that DNA does not function optimally for replication and transcription and, consequently, protein synthesis needed for proliferation of cells in the immune system is inhibited. Cyclophosphamide acts during both the division phase and resting phase of the cell cycle. Both B- and T-lymphocytes are affected.

Methotrexate

Methotrexate inhibits the enzyme dihydrofolate reductase, which is required for the conversion of folic acid to tetrahydrofolate, which in turn is needed for DNA synthesis and cell division. In low doses, methotrexate is used for refractory cases of rheumatoid arthritis, psoriasis and polymyositis.

Adverse effects

As cytotoxic drugs have toxic effects on cells in the division phase of the cell cycle, they can cause a number of serious adverse effects. Reduced immune defence increases the danger of infections from microorganisms that do not usually cause disease. Inhibition of bone marrow function may cause anaemia because of the

| Glucocorticoids |
| Methylprednisolone, Prednisolone |
| **Selective immunosuppressive drugs** |
| Ciclosporin, Sirolimus, Tacrolimus |
| **Immunosuppressive immunglobulins** |
| Basiliximab, Daclixumab, Etanercept, Infliximab |
| **Cytotoxics** |
| Azathioprine, Cyclophosphamide, Methotrexate, Mycophenolate mofetil |

Table 22.2 Drugs used as immunosuppressants

reduced production of erythrocytes, increased danger of haemorrhage due to reduced numbers of platelets, and increased risk of infection due to reduced production of leucocytes. Damage to mucous membranes, hair loss and reduced fertility are expressions of adverse effects on other proliferating cells. When used during pregnancy, cytotoxics can have teratogenic effects.

Mycophenolate
Mycophenolate inhibits the production of a nucleic acid base in B- and T-lymphocytes, while other cell types are little affected. The drug is used prophylactically against rejection after organ transplants, in combination with corticosteroids and ciclosporin. The most common adverse effects are diarrhoea, nausea, vomiting and leucopoenia.

Drugs used as immunosuppressants are listed in Table 22.2.

CANCER

Cancer is a generic term for malignant cell growth that results in death when untreated. Twenty per cent of the population die of cancer.

Cancer can develop in all organs and tissues. The cell growth can be localized as a solid tumour or it can spread, e.g. in bone marrow and blood/lymph (leukaemia and lymph cancer). The spread can occur by local infiltration or by remote spreading (metastases) to other organs. The malignant progress is caused by disturbance of the normal function of invaded tissue and by the effect of substances produced by cancer cells.

To understand the effect of drugs that are used in the treatment of cancer, it is necessary to know about growth by normal cell division and the pathophysiology of the development of cancer.

GROWTH BY NORMAL CELL DIVISION

Healthy cells that grow by cell division pass through a cell cycle consisting of several phases each time two daughter cells are created. Through each cell cycle, cellular structures must be replicated. The different phases in a cell cycle are of different duration. Stable cells (cells that do not divide) are in interphase. In this phase, necessary proteins and enzymes are produced. If a cell division starts, the regeneration of cellular structures starts in the last part of the interphase. The phase where the cell divides is called mitosis.

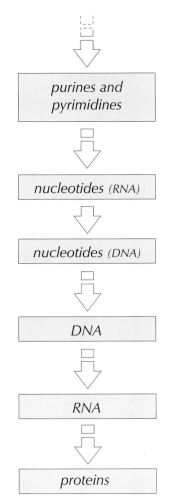

Figure 22.11 Synthesis steps in cell in resting phase.

Formation of RNA and DNA requires synthesis of bases (purines and pyrimidines) that are connected to the sugar and phosphate molecules. See Figure 22.11. Sugar, phosphate and bases form nucleotides (the basic units in DNA and RNA). During replication, existing DNA acts as a template for the production of new DNA. The nucleotides are 'converted' to RNA by the process of transcription. RNA, in turn, forms proteins by the process of translation. In order for the DNA chain to be read to make transcription and replication possible, the bonding between the base pairs in each strand of DNA must be broken. Before mitosis, DNA disperses to each of the cell's halves because spindle fibres (mitotic spindles) pull on the DNA. All of these processes can be affected by different drugs.

PATHOPHYSIOLOGY OF CANCER DEVELOPMENT

Growth and division of cells are subject to strict control. Cancer cells are characterized because they do not demonstrate normal control functions; they operate autonomously. Consequently, cancer cells repress and suppress growth, energy consumption, movements and special functions of normal cells.

It was previously thought that the most characteristic feature in the development of malignant growth was the uncontrolled and rapid cell growth. In fact, many cells die in a growing tumour and the cell division may take place at an even slower rate than in normal dividing tissue. In the beginning of the development of a tumour, a large proportion of the cells will be undergoing cell division. The tumour then has both a high growth fraction and high growth rate. Gradually, as the tumour grows, the number of cells that divide is reduced and the tumour has a low growth fraction and low growth rate. It is thought that it may take from 10 to 15 years from the time the first mutations occur until a clinical diagnosis of cancer can be made. This, of course, does not apply in children's cancer. At the point when the tumour is diagnosed, it usually has low growth fraction and low growth rate.

Cellular influences that cause change or damage to the genetic material (DNA) in a cell are called mutations. Such damage usually causes the cell to die. If the cell does not die and a mutation takes place in an area of the DNA molecule that helps to control the gene expression for growth-promoting or -inhibiting factors, this provides an opportunity for uncontrolled cell growth. If the new DNA structure can be transferred over to new daughter cells with the same properties, it can be the start of cancer development.

Proto-oncogenes are a group of normal genes that are important in growth regulation. Proto-oncogenes can be activated to oncogenes (carcinogenic genes) by infection with viruses, ultraviolet and radioactive radiation, or by the influence of chemical agents.

Tumour suppressor genes, also called anti-oncogenes, are another type of gene. It is thought that these genes prevent uncontrolled growth and cancer development. Damage to the suppressor genes opens up the possibility of the development of cancer.

It is possible that immunological active cells and the humoral immune defence system take care of a number of newly formed cancer cells. Empirical evidence supporting the theory of the importance of the immune defence system is that immune suppression that lasts several years, e.g. in patients who have received kidney transplants, results in increased incidences of cancer.

When a tumour grows, the need for space and blood supply increases. This problem is solved because the cells release substances that break down surrounding tissue and produce factors that increase infiltrating growth of the cancer cells and the growth of new blood vessels in the tumour. With that, the path is laid for remote metastases, through cells that reach the lymph and blood.

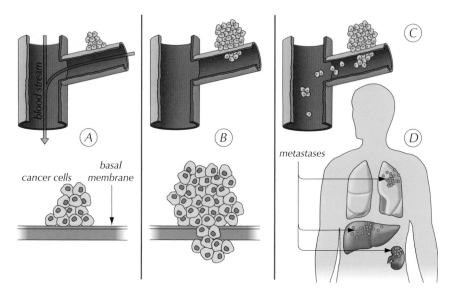

Figure 22.12 **Cancer cells spread** by infiltrating surrounding tissue or via the blood or lymphatic systems. By remote spreading, the cancer cells can grow up in incidental places in the body. (A) shows local growth. (B) shows spreading by infiltration. (C) shows spreading via the blood. (D) shows remote metastases.

Primary tumours and metastases

Primary tumours are cancer cells localized to the tissue from which the cells are originating. When cancer cells metastasize, the growth of the 'released' cells will establish growth of one or more new tumours. See Figure 22.12. Metastasized tissue will resemble the tissue of the primary tumours. If, with the help of different techniques, a tumour is discovered in the brain or in the liver that resembles tissue from the colon, the tumour represents metastases from the colon and cannot be a primary tumour.

To the extent that it is technically possible, it is common to remove primary tumours surgically. In many forms of cancer where metastases are discovered in the form of multiple tumours, surgical treatment is not generally applicable.

DRUGS USED TO TREAT CANCER

Drugs that are used to eradicate cancer cells are called cytotoxics or cytotoxins. Those that have been developed in the past 50 years have been directed mainly against suppressing cell growth. They have been designed to inhibit the function and synthesis of DNA, RNA and proteins. However, clinical experience shows that the majority of cytotoxics also cause damage to the cells, which causes them to start a programmed cell death – apoptosis. How this takes place is currently not fully understood.

The goal of cancer treatment is to remove the tumour masses completely and to cure the patient. See Figure 22.13. It is estimated that a tumour mass weighing 1 kg (not uncommon) has approximately 10^{12} cells, i.e. 1000 billion cells. If we remove all but 1 per cent of these, there still remains a tumour mass of 10 g (10 billion cells). If we further remove all the cells with the exception of 1 per cent, there still remains a tumour mass of 100 mg (100 million cells). These can continue to cause a relapse of the disease, known as recidivism. The cancer treatment therefore consists of surgical treatment, radiation treatment and chemotherapy where it is appropriate.

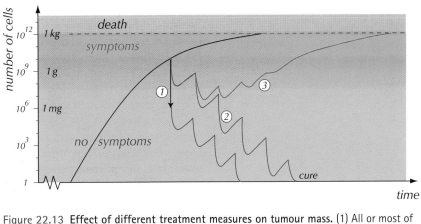

Figure 22.13 **Effect of different treatment measures on tumour mass.** (1) All or most of the tumour mass can be removed by surgery. (2) Use of adjuvant treatment with cytotoxics where all the tumour cells are removed. (3) Use of adjuvant treatment with cytotoxics where the tumour cells are not removed, but the growth rate is reduced and the time for death is postponed. The effect of cytotoxics on the cancer cells is dependent on the sensitivity of the cells.

With such combined treatment, the aim is to eradicate cells such that only approximately 100 tumour cells exist in the individual and with the hope that the immune system can remove the remaining cells. This is, however, a problem, since cytotoxic drugs suppress the effectiveness of the immune system. To reduce the number of cancer cells to about 100, repeated treatments are required. Because of the toxic effects on healthy (non-cancerous) cells, there must be pauses between the treatments, so that normal cells will not be irreversibly damaged.

If the goal is to cure the disease, then intensive treatment that usually consists of a combination of several cytotoxics is required. Such treatment regimes often have serious adverse effects.

If the cancer is such that it is incurable, the treatment goal will be extension of life or symptom-relieving effects (palliative treatment). In this situation, it is necessary to consider the patient's wishes, general condition and quality of life. The adverse effects of the treatment must not be greater than the effects of the disease.

When cytotoxics are administered together with other treatment (adjuvant treatment) such as surgery or radiation therapy, the purpose is to increase the possibility of preventing the spread of disease by surgery and to eradicate any remaining cancer cells in the area or any metastases of cancer cells. Adjuvant cytotoxic treatment has not found its final place in today's cancer treatment. It is an established part in some therapy regimes, but it is still being tested in others.

Cells are most vulnerable in the division phase of the cell cycle. With the use of cytotoxics, vulnerable links in the cell division process are attacked. Figure 22.14 shows possible points of attack for the most commonly used cytotoxics.

Antimetabolites

Antimetabolites are chemical compounds that resemble (are analogous to) molecules that the cell needs in order to mature and complete cell division. Because the antimetabolites are incorporated into cellular structures or inhibit essential enzymes, further cell maturation is inhibited. The antimetabolites are analogues to key molecules for the synthesis of purines and pyrimidines, DNA and RNA. Methotrexate is the best known in this group. Others are mercaptopurine and fluorouracil.

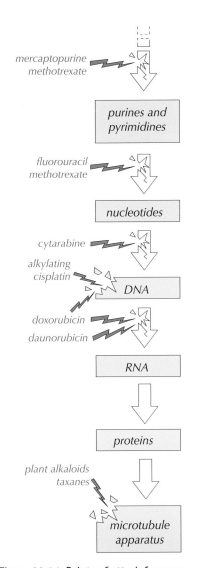

Figure 22.14 **Points of attack for some cytotoxics.** The majority of cytotoxics act by inhibiting the synthesis of necessary components in the cell.

Methotrexate is a folic acid analogue that inhibits the enzyme dihydrofolate reductase, which metabolizes folic acid to reduced folic acid. Reduced folic acid is needed in the synthesis of thymidylate, which is a building block in the synthesis of DNA. In this way, methotrexate inhibits DNA synthesis. Methotrexate reduces the ability for cell division in all tissues with a large turnover of cells.

High-dose methotrexate is a standard treatment in acute lymphatic leukaemia and in a number of other forms of cancer. In metastases to the central nervous system, methotrexate is injected intrathecally, i.e. into the cerebrospinal fluid. This treatment is necessary because methotrexate is poorly transported across the blood– brain barrier. Low-dose methotrexate is used in autoimmune diseases such as psoriasis and rheumatoid arthritis.

To avoid irreversible damage to the bone marrow during high-dose methotrexate therapy, leucovorin is administered. This is an active analogue of tetrahydrofolate, which saves the cells from the effect of methotrexate. Leucovorin is administered when methotrexate has had some time to act. Without administration of leucovorin, all patients who receive high-dose treatment with methotrexate would die of bone marrow depression. Leucovorin does not increase the elimination of methotrexate.

Mercaptopurine is a purine analogue that inhibits DNA synthesis after it is activated by metabolism. The drug is included as a standard treatment in acute lymphatic leukaemia. Azathioprine, which is used in immune suppression, is metabolized to mercaptopurine in the body.

Fluorouracil inhibits synthesis of thymidylate, and consequently DNA synthesis. The substance is a uracil (nucleic acid base) analogue and is used in the treatment of different forms of cancer in the intestinal tract.

Alkylating agents

Alkylating agents are compounds that bind covalently to DNA molecules by adding alkyl groups. This leads to a breakdown of DNA molecules and the formation of crossbridges between the two DNA strands, so that they cannot split in the normal way that is necessary in replication and transcription. See Figure 22.15.

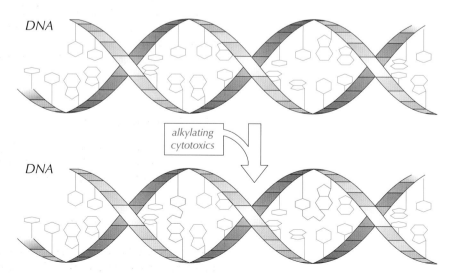

Figure 22.15 **Alkylating cytotoxics.** Formations of crossbridges between components in the DNA strands disturb the function of DNA.

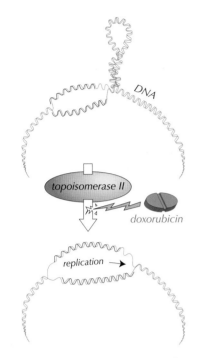

Figure 22.16 **Cytotoxic antibiotics.** By preventing the necessary splitting of DNA for replication or transcription, cytotoxic antibiotics inhibit regeneration of cellular structures.

Alkylating agents only slightly differentiate between cells in the resting phase and division phase of the cell cycle, but are most toxic for cells in the division phase. This group of drugs have nausea-provoking effects via actions on the central nervous system and pronounced toxic effects on the bone marrow.

Cyclophosphamide is an example of an alkylating substance. This drug must be metabolized to become active. Toxic metabolites are eliminated renally and can cause haemorrhagic cystitis. This effect can be limited by administering mesna, an antidote to the toxic metabolites.

Cytotoxic antibiotics

Some antibiotics exert effects on human cells by binding to DNA, so that replication and translation are inhibited. Doxorubicin belongs to this group. The cytotoxic effect of doxorubicin is caused by the inhibition of the enzyme topoisomerase-II, which cuts and pastes the DNA molecule during DNA replication and transcription. See Figure 22.16. Metabolism of cytotoxic antibiotics generates oxygen radicals, which are believed to be primarily responsible for the toxic effects on the heart.

Plant alkaloids – spindle toxins

Plant alkaloids are agents that inhibit mitosis because they bind to the microtubule apparatus (the spindles) in the cells. See Figure 22.17. Mitosis is inhibited so cell division stops. They are therefore also characterized as spindle toxins. Vinblastine and vincristine belong to this group.

Other cytotoxics

Cisplatin and carboplatin are complex compounds of platinum. DNA is damaged by the binding of these drugs, which is the basis for the cytotoxic effect. Asparaginase is an enzyme that breaks down the amino acid asparagine. A relatively selective effect is achieved because leukaemic lymphoblasts cannot themselves produce asparagine and are dependent on exogenous administration.

Tamoxifen and toremifene are anti-oestrogens that bind to oestrogen receptors and block the effect of endogenous oestrogen. They also have a weak oestrogen-like effect. The drugs are used in treatment of oestrogen-dependent breast cancer.

The anti-androgen bicalutamide is an example of a competitive blocker of androgen receptors and is used in the treatment of prostate cancer that is sensitive to testosterone.

In cancer therapy, the inhibitory effect of glucocorticoids on cell proliferation is utilized, especially in the treatment of lymphatic leukaemia.

RESISTANCE TO CYTOTOXICS

Cancer cells can be primarily resistant against cytotoxics or develop secondary resistance, i.e. become resistant after they have first responded to treatment. There are several mechanisms for such resistance.

ADVERSE EFFECTS OF CYTOTOXICS

The lack of selectivity between cancerous and non-cancerous cells is a fundamental problem in cytotoxic treatment. The intensity of adverse effects is a limiting factor in a number of treatment regimes. Different cytotoxic drugs have different adverse effect profiles.

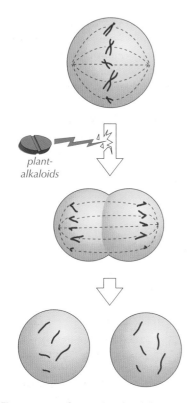

plant-alkaloids

Figure 22.17 Cytotoxics that inhibit spindle function. By preventing the chromosomes from being distributed to the two poles of the cell, these cytotoxics inhibit mitosis.

The adverse effects are primarily seen because the cytotoxics disturb normal cell function in organs and tissues with normal high cell division rate, such as bone marrow, the gastrointestinal tract and hair follicles. These adverse effects are dose-dependent and predictable. Adverse effects from the bone marrow first manifest themselves in the form of granulocytopenia, which can require prophylactic treatment with antibiotics to prevent the occurrence of infections and subsequent intense treatment if they do occur. There is also a reduction in the production of platelets – thrombocytopenia – which increases the danger of haemorrhage. Eventually anaemia occurs as a result of the reduction in the number of red blood corpuscles.

Nausea and vomiting are mainly triggered from influences in the central nervous system (i.e. the chemoreceptor trigger zone in the central nervous system). The group of cisplatin drugs has an especially potent ability to cause nausea. However, the use of modern antiemetics such as the serotonin antagonists and metoclopramide in high doses has come a long way to solving this problem.

Some drugs cause considerable hair loss (alopecia). This is usually reversible and the hair often has a better quality when it regrows after treatment has finished.

Large amounts of uric acid are produced as a result of the increased death of cells and subsequent breakdown of nucleic acids. The uric acid can be deposited in the form of uric acid crystals in joints and kidneys and cause gouty arthritis and kidney damage. Administration of the drug allopurinol inhibits the metabolism of nucleic acids to uric acid, such that these dangerous adverse effects can be avoided. Treatment of gouty arthritis is more thoroughly discussed in Chapter 15, Drugs used to treat inflammatory and autoimmune joint diseases.

Several cytotoxics are mutagenic and teratogenic. The mutagenic effect can trigger cancer. Follow-up studies show an increased frequency of cancer (secondary malignancies) in patients who have been treated for a cancer with cytotoxics and radiation. The teratogenic effect can cause fetal damage.

Antimetabolites
Capecitabine, Cladribine, Cytarabine, Fludarabine, Fluorouracil, Gemcitabine, Mercaptopurine, Methotrexate, Pemetrexed, Raltitrexed, Tegafur with Uracil, Tioguanine

Alkylating agents
Busulfan, Carmustine, Chlorambucil, Chlormethine, Cyclophosphamide, Estramustine, Ifosfamide, Lomustine, Melphalan, Thiotepa, Treosulfan

Cytotoxic antibiotics
Aclarubicin, Bleomycin, Dactinomycin, Daunorubicin, Doxorubicin, Epirubicin, Idarubicin, Mitomycin, Mitoxantrone

Plant alkaloids
Etoposide, Vinblastine, Vincristine, Vindesine, Vinorelbine

Other cytotoxics
Amsacrine, Bexarotene, Bortezomib, Carboplatin, Cetuximab, Cisplatin, Crisantaspase, Dacarbazine, Docetaxel, Hydroxycarbamide, Imatinib, Irinotecan, Pentostatin, Oxalplatin, Paclitaxel, Porfimer, Procarbazine, Tamoxifen, Temozolomide, Temoporfin, Topotecan, Trastuzumab, Tretinoin

Other drugs used to treat cancer
Crisantaspase (asparaginase), Bicalutamide and Flutamide (anti-androgens), Tamoxifen and Toremifene (anti-oestrogens)

Table 22.3 Drugs used to treat cancer (cytotoxics)

Treatment with cytotoxins can cause sterility in men and damage the eggs in the ovaries of women. Sperm can be frozen prior to treatment with such drugs. Menstrual disturbances and premature menopause are seen in women. A number of patients who have survived acute lymphatic leukaemia after intensive chemotherapy in childhood have nonetheless gone through a normal puberty and had healthy children.

In the same way as with other drugs, cytotoxics cause adverse effects in a number of organs. The heart is particularly affected by the doxorubicin drug group. The kidneys are affected by cisplatin and methotrexate, while the liver is affected by methotrexate.

Drugs used to treat cancer are listed in Table 22.3.

SUMMARY

- The immune system consists of chemical compounds and cells that differentiate between self and foreign structures called antigens. It prevents infections and removes diseased, damaged and dead cells.
- The non-specific immune system reacts to many different antigens.
- The specific immune system recognizes antigens that have previously activated the immune system by binding to specific receptors. B-lymphocytes are metabolized to plasma cells that secrete antibodies. Production of antibodies is especially important for preventing bacterial infections. T-lymphocytes have a direct cell toxic effect when they bind to antigens. The activity of T-lymphocytes is particularly important for fighting virus-infected cells, fungi and in rejection reactions after tissue transplants. The non-specific and specific immune systems enhance each other's effect by acting together.
- When the immune system is inappropriately activated, allergic reactions occur. Antigens that cause allergy are called allergens. Drugs can bind to proteins and thereby function as allergens.
- Type I reactions occur when the immune system is inappropriately activated. Allergic reactions occur when allergens bind to IgE antibodies on mast cells and basophilic granulocytes, which thereby degranulate and release histamine and other active substances. Type II reactions occur because antibodies bind to cellular structures and activate the complement system, which damages the cells. Type III reactions are mediated by complexes of antibodies and antigens that attach particularly to tissue that filters blood or are deposited in the wall of small- and medium-sized arteries. Type IV reactions are delayed immunological reactions that are mediated by T-lymphocytes and macrophages.
- Antihistamines are used against type I reactions and act by preventing histamine binding to histamine receptors. Adverse effects are sedation, listlessness, disturbances in coordination and anticholinergic effects. Cromoglicate stabilizes mast cells and reduces the release of histamine.
- Immunosuppressive drugs prevent proliferation of immunologically active cells. Glucocorticoids, ciclosporin and some cytotoxics belong to this group. Immunosuppressive drugs increase in the risk of infection. Glucocorticoids and cytotoxics have an inhibitory effect on the proliferation of cells of the immune system. Ciclosporin particularly inhibits the effects of T-lymphocytes and carries a particular increased risk of infections with virus and fungi.
- Cytotoxic drugs in cancer treatment are used curatively, palliatively or adjuvantly. Curative treatment is often a combination treatment with considerable adverse

effects. Different cytotoxics act by inhibiting the synthesis of necessary components in a cell, such that cell division is inhibited.

■ Cytotoxic drugs act primarily on cells in the division phase of the cell cycle. Because of small differences between cancer cells and healthy cells, the effect is relatively unselective, i.e. they also act on cells other than cancer cells. They therefore have many adverse effects. The adverse effects are particularly apparent in tissue that has a high cell turnover, e.g. bone marrow, hair follicles and mucous membranes in the intestinal system. Tissue toxicity that is not related to inhibition of cell division is also observed, e.g. nausea, liver and kidney damage and toxic effects on the urinary bladder and heart.

23 Drugs used to treat functional disorders of the bladder, prostatic hyperplasia and erectile dysfunction

The bladder functions as a reservoir for collecting urine and as a pump to expel the urine through the urethra. Whilst urine is collecting in the bladder no leakage should occur, and during micturition (expulsion) urine should flow freely and the bladder should empty completely. For the bladder to function optimally, a complex interaction between anatomy and neural regulation must take place.

There are different categories of functional bladder disorders. Incontinence may be caused by impaired closing of the neck of the bladder or dysfunction of the nervous regulation of the bladder. Obstruction of flow in older men is often caused by prostatic hyperplasia. The inability to achieve erection increases with age and leads to a reduction in sexual function for some men. Drug therapies constitute important treatment options for functional bladder disorders, prostatic hyperplasia and erectile dysfunction.

ANATOMY AND NERVOUS REGULATION OF THE BLADDER AND THE URETHRA

The bladder consists of an inner mucosal layer and a thick outer wall that is interwoven with smooth muscle. Sections of the muscle are arranged in such a way that they act as sphincters to control the flow of urine from the bladder (urethral sphincters). Bladder wall and sphincter tension is mediated by the autonomic nervous system. When the bladder is filling, sympathetic activity dominates,

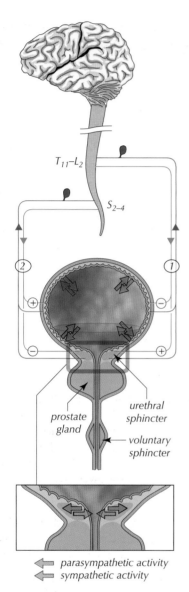

Figure 23.1 **Anatomy of the bladder and the urinary outlet.** (1) Sympathetic activity relaxes the bladder wall and contracts the internal sphincter such that the bladder can be filled without leaking. (2) Parasympathetic activity causes the bladder wall to contract and the internal sphincter to relax such that the bladder can be emptied.

ensuring that the tension in the internal urethral sphincter is high and preventing the passage of urine into the urethra. This effect is mediated by noradrenaline stimulating α_1-adrenoceptors causing the urethral sphincter to close more tightly. If the receptors are blocked, the internal urethral sphincter relaxes, allowing urine to pass into the urethra and be voided.

Filling the bladder leads to stretching of the bladder wall and distortion of baroreceptors within it. These baroreceptors are sensitive to stretching and, as a result, send signals from the bladder to both the micturition reflex centre in the sacral section of the spinal cord and the micturition control centre in the medulla oblongata. When the bladder reaches its normal maximum capacity, activity increases in the parasympathetic fibres that lead to it. Gradually, the parasympathetic signals will predominate over the sympathetic and lead to relaxation of the internal urethral sphincter and contraction of the bladder wall, resulting in urine flow. This happens because acetylcholine is released and acts at the cholinergic receptors. If the cholinergic receptors are stimulated, the bladder wall tolerates less tension (filling), and the bladder empties more frequently. If the cholinergic receptors are blocked, the bladder tolerates a greater volume before it empties spontaneously, and any tendency towards 'leakage' can be improved. Simply put, sympathetic activity ensures that the bladder remains closed, while parasympathetic activity initiates voiding. If the autonomic balance of the bladder is disturbed, functional bladder disorders arise. See Figure 23.1.

In addition to the autonomic emptying of the bladder, there is a degree of voluntary muscular control (somatic innervation), such that one can 'squeeze' and therefore avoid emptying of the bladder, or, alternatively, one can initiate emptying of the bladder. The muscle that controls the voluntary voiding of urine is the external urethral sphincter.

Muscles and ligaments in the pelvic floor should help to hold the bladder neck and the bladder itself in a favourable anatomical position so that it does not 'leak'. During pregnancy, the growing uterus presses against the muscles and ligaments of the pelvic floor, which then stretch. After childbirth, these structures can lose their natural tension and become weak, resulting in bladder leakage (incontinence). In some women, hormonal changes after menopause will lead to atrophy and reduced elasticity of the mucosa in the vagina and urethra. A weak pelvic floor together with postmenopausal altered mucosa can lead to leakage from the bladder, especially when the pressure in the abdominal cavity increases (coughing, sneezing, laughter, heavy lifting).

In men, the prostate gland gradually increases in size with age. Since the urethra passes through the prostate, the growth of the prostate gland gradually leads to constriction of the urethra's opening, leading to an obstruction of urinary flow when trying to empty the bladder. See Figure 23.1.

FUNCTIONAL DISORDERS OF THE BLADDER

Functional disorders of the bladder involve problems in the collection or voiding of urine. Such disturbances can be associated with disease or injury of the ligaments and muscles holding the bladder in the correct anatomical position, or damage to the nervous regulation of bladder function. Functional disorders can lead to incontinence or urine retention. Incontinence occurs when emptying of the bladder happens at inappropriate times, when a full bladder continuously 'runs over' without complete emptying, or when there is incompetence of the urethral sphincters. In urge incontinence, the person lacks control over active emptying. In stress incontinence, the bladder leaks because of poor urethral sphincter function.

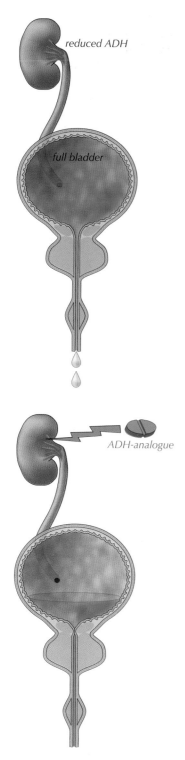

Figure 23.2 **Desmopressin** taken just before bedtime mimics the effect that naturally excreted antidiuretic hormone (ADH) has on the kidneys, and prevents the bladder from filling up during the night.

Urine retention is primarily caused by urinary outlet obstruction (prostatic hypertrophy or malignant hyperplasia), the anticholinergic effect of drugs, or when neurogenic control of the bladder is damaged.

ENURESIS

Enuresis is a condition characterized by repeated incontinence. The phenomenon occurs most frequently in children and is diagnosed after the age where one would expect a child to have bladder control. If such uncontrolled emptying of the bladder occurs when the child is awake, it is usually due to reduced bladder capacity or rhythmic contractions of the bladder wall over which the child has no control (increased parasympathetic activity). If the child does not achieve control, drugs reducing the parasympathetic activity (anticholinergics) may be tried (see 'Urge incontinence', below). Uncontrolled micturition while the child is sleeping (nocturnal enuresis) is usually associated with high nocturnal urine production. This is often because the child lacks the normal nocturnal increase in the secretion of antidiuretic hormone (ADH) from the pituitary gland, which reduces urine production. If this is the case, urine production will be so great that the bladder is filled early on in the night. If the child sleeps heavily, he or she will not be aware of the full bladder and will possibly wet the bed. Nocturnal enuresis can be treated with synthetic ADH.

DRUG TREATMENT OF NOCTURNAL ENURESIS

If, following examination, no other cause of nocturnal enuresis can be found other than a lack of nocturnal ADH increase, desmopressin is the drug of choice. Tricyclic antidepressants may be of some benefit because the anticholinergic effect contributes to relaxation of the detrusor muscle. They are now used less often because of adverse effects, and relapse often occurs after withdrawal. Tricyclic antidepressants are described in Chapter 13, Drugs used to treat psychiatric disorders.

Desmopressin
Desmopressin is a synthetically produced, ADH-like substance. By administering desmopressin as a nasal spray just before bedtime, nocturnal urine production will be reduced so that the bladder does not fill up and spontaneous micturition is avoided.

Mechanism of action and effects. Desmopressin binds to receptors in the distal tubules and collecting ducts of the kidneys and increases the permeability of the tubule to water such that water is reabsorbed from the tubular lumen into the blood. Because a large part of the tubule fluid created at night is reabsorbed into the blood, less urine is produced. The effect does not taper off with long-term treatment. In the majority of children, a treatment period of several weeks will usually lead to an improvement in the situation (increased production of nocturnal ADH) with a subsequent improvement in symptoms. See Figure 23.2. This treatment should be used in conjunction with fluid reduction in the early evening.

Adverse effects and precautionary measures. The use of large doses can result in an undesirable, drastic reduction in urine production leading to fluid retention.

ADH–analogue
Desmopressin

Table 23.1 Drug used to treat nocturnal enuresis

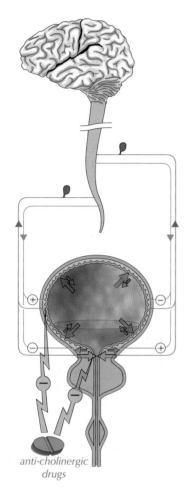

anti-cholinergic drugs

Figure 23.3 **Anticholinergic drugs** act by blocking muscarinic receptors, and thereby blocking the effects of acetylcholine on the bladder wall.

Some individuals also experience nasal congestion due to swelling of the nasal mucosa.

URGE INCONTINENCE

Urge incontinence is a strong, sudden and unstoppable need to micturate, resulting in the patient failing to reach the toilet in time. The urge to micturate is often accompanied by a strong involuntary contraction of the bladder wall that voluntary control, which acts against emptying of the bladder, is insufficient to restrain. These conditions are the result of increased parasympathetic activity within the bladder. Drug treatment is based on the reduction or complete blockade of parasympathetic activity.

DRUG TREATMENT OF URGE INCONTINENCE

As urge incontinence is associated with hyperactivity of the parasympathetic nerve supply (cholinergic stimulation of muscarinic receptors) and contractions of the detrusor muscle, anticholinergic drugs may be useful.

Anticholinergics
Oxybutynin and tolterodine are effective. Some newer antimuscarinic drugs are also licensed for urge incontinence. Trinsyclic antidepressants may be of some use but are not used so much now because of adverse effects.

Oxybutynin and tolterodine
Oxybutynin is an antimuscarinic drug with a direct relaxant effect inhibiting the detrusor overactivity. Also, tolterodine is used to treat urge incontinence because of its antimuscarinic effect.

Mechanism of action and effects. Both drugs block peripheral muscarinic receptors and prevent released acetylcholine from binding to the muscarinic receptors thereby initiating contraction of the bladder wall. By blocking muscarinic receptors (anticholinergic effect), a greater volume is tolerated before emptying of the bladder becomes necessary. In this way, longer intervals are achieved between voiding and a more controlled emptying of the bladder is achieved. See Figure 23.3.

Adverse effects and precautionary measures. Dryness of the mouth, constipation and dry eyes (reduced tear flow) are typical anticholinergic side-effects. These drugs should not be administered to individuals with glaucoma (increased pressure within the eye), since anticholinergics result in dilation of the pupils and can cause mechanical obstruction of the normal drainage of the aqueous humour within the eye. Caution should be exercised with the simultaneous use of other drugs with anticholinergic activity. In patients who have a history of urine retention (prostatic hyperplasia), anticholinergic drugs should be used very cautiously as they can exacerbate the problem.

Drugs used to treat urge incontinence are listed in Table 23.2.

Antimuscarinic drugs
Flavoxate, Oxybutynin, Propiverine, Solifenacin, Tolterodine, Trospium

Antidepressants
Amitriptyline, Imipramine

Table 23.2 Drugs used to treat urge incontinence

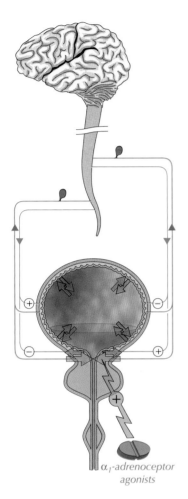

α₁–adrenoceptor
agonists

Figure 23.4 α_1–adrenoceptor agonists stimulate α_1–receptors in the internal sphincter, increasing tone and preventing leakage.

STRESS INCONTINENCE

Stress incontinence is associated with loss of urine without contraction of the detrusor muscle, and therefore insufficient closure of the internal urethral sphincter. This functional disorder occurs relatively frequently in women with pelvic floor weakness and reduced mucosal elasticity in the neck of the bladder and urethra after menopause. In some cases, stress incontinence occurs in men because of damage caused to the bladder neck as a result of prostatic hyperplasia surgery. In this context, 'stress' is related to an increase in abdominal pressure (coughing, sneezing, laughter, heavy lifting), which causes the pressure against the bladder to increase, squeezing out small amounts of urine without the patient feeling the need to micturate. Stress incontinence can be treated surgically by 'tightening up the bladder', thus improving the anatomical conditions for closing the neck of the bladder, or with drugs. Drug treatment of stress incontinence should be combined with pelvic floor exercises to strengthen muscles.

DRUG TREATMENT OF STRESS INCONTINENCE

Drug treatment of stress incontinence is aimed at increasing the sympathetic tone of the bladder, thus increasing the effectiveness of the internal urethral sphincter. To achieve this effect, α_1-adrenoceptor agonists (drugs which mimic the effect of noradrenaline), which stimulate α_1-adrenoceptors in the internal sphincter, are used to increase the closing pressure at the bladder outlet. Administration of oestrogens after menopause can improve the situation in some women by increasing the elasticity of the urogenital membranes. Drugs used for urge incontinence may also be of some use.

α_1-adrenoceptor agonists: phenylpropanolamine

α_1-adrenoceptor agonists stimulate α_1-adrenoceptors within the internal urethral sphincter. This results in increased sphincter tone and an increase in the closing pressure at the bladder outlet, possibly reducing the symptoms of stress incontinence. See Figure 23.4. It should be noted, however, that α_1-adrenoceptor agonists are primarily used to reduce mucosal oedema in the upper respiratory passages through vascular constriction, leading to reduced plasma leakage from the capillary bed. Unpleasant effects associated with the treatment of stress incontinence can therefore be dryness in the nose and mouth. Undesirable stimulation of α_1-adrenoceptors in the heart and other parts of the vascular system can result in a transient rise in blood pressure.

Oestrogens

After menopause, the mucosa in the urethra atrophies in common with the entire genital region. Topical or systemic administration of low-potency oestrogens can make the mucosa more elastic and reduce the likelihood of incontinence problems (and simultaneously reduce the risk of urinary tract infections). Oestrogens are thus an alternative in the treatment of stress incontinence. See Chapter 21, Drugs used to treat endocrinological disorders.

Drugs used to treat stress incontinence are listed in Table 23.3.

α_1–adrenoceptor agonist
Phenylpropanolamine
Antidepressants
Amitriptyline, Imipramine

Table 23.3 Drugs used to treat stress incontinence

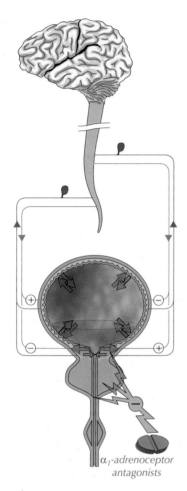

α₁-adrenoceptor antagonists

Figure 23.5 **α₁-adrenoceptor antagonists** block the effect of noradrenaline on α₁-adrenoceptors and cause the internal sphincter to relax. At the same time, the tension is reduced in the smooth muscle in the prostate gland and the proximal urethra, such that the passage of urine is easier.

NEUROGENIC BLADDER DISORDER

Injuries or diseases that affect neurogenic control of the bladder exhibit different symptoms depending upon which area of the nervous system the injury affects and whether or not the spinal parasympathetic and/or sympathetic reflex arc is damaged. Since innervation of the bladder is complex, neurogenic bladder disorders often require investigation by a specialist in urology. It is common to differentiate between supraspinal, spinal, sacral and peripherally related bladder disorders.

Supraspinal-related bladder disorder
In a supraspinal injury, the damage is found in the areas of the brain that regulate the voluntary emptying of the bladder. Cerebrovascular accidents (strokes) are a frequent cause. With this type of injury, there is no awareness of the bladder filling or emptying. Filling of the bladder continues until the tension in the bladder wall becomes so great that emptying is initiated spontaneously by increased parasympathetic activity. In reality, this leads to frequent and uncontrolled emptying of small urine volumes, with residual urine remaining in the bladder often urination.

Treatment of supraspinal bladder disorders consists primarily of intermittent or indwelling urethral catheterization. Drug treatment is based on inhibiting parasympathetic activity, so that the bladder can hold a larger volume and be emptied less frequently. A drug with anticholinergic effects may be appropriate. See 'Drug treatment of urge incontinence' above and Figure 23.3.

Spinal-related bladder disorder
If a spinal injury occurs above the level where sympathetic fibres leave the spinal cord (above S2), there may be an associated spinal-related bladder disorder. This type of injury involves both a loss of sensation and loss of control of bladder function. With this type of injury, frequent, uncontrolled emptying, with contraction of the bladder wall but without simultaneous coordinated opening of the internal sphincter, is seen. It is possible for the bladder to contract without simultaneous relaxation of the urethral sphincters, resulting in a significant increase in pressure within the bladder which can be transmitted up the ureters, leading to the development of hydronephrosis (swelling of the kidneys).

Treatment of spinal-related bladder disorders centres on urethral catheterization to drain the bladder, and, in some cases, the use of rhythmic tapping over the bladder can initiate emptying. This is thought to work because the tapping triggers activity in the parasympathetic fibres and thus contraction of the bladder. The use of α₁-adrenoceptor antagonists, which reduce sympathetic activity, can cause relaxation of the internal urethral sphincter and improve urinary outflow. Such treatment can improve the effectiveness of bladder emptying. See 'Drug treatment of prostatic hyperplasia', below, and Figure 23.5.

Sacral or peripherally related bladder disorder
Following sacral injury, it is possible for there to be either complete disruption of the autonomic nervous supply to the bladder or damage in a single branch only (parasympathetic or sympathetic). When efferent or afferent peripheral nerves are damaged, the spinal reflex is disrupted. If the spinal sympathetic reflex arc is preserved while the spinal parasympathetic reflex arc is damaged, the internal sphincter will remain competent, but contraction and emptying of the bladder cannot be initiated. These patients will suffer from incontinence when the bladder is full and will require urethral catheterization as part of their management. Spontaneous

emptying initiated by rhythmic tapping over the bladder is not possible since the spinal reflex is no longer present. If the spinal sympathetic reflex or both the sympathetic and the parasympathetic reflexes are damaged, the internal urethral sphincter will be incompetent with frequent leakage. Drug therapy is not helpful in the management of sacral or peripherally related bladder disorders.

PROSTATIC ENLARGEMENT

Enlargement of the prostate gland leads to a narrowing of the urethra. The growth is associated with stimulation of androgen receptors in the prostatic tissue. The increased tissue growth can be benign (hypertrophy – enlargement of cells) or malignant (hyperplasia – more cells). Gradually, as the growth increases, the urinary outlet obstruction worsens and patients will experience problems emptying their bladder. The outlet obstruction can also be associated with contraction of smooth muscles in the prostate tissue (via stimulation of α_1-adrenoceptor), which reduces the diameter of the urethra. Due to overdistension of the bladder, individuals experience an intense need to urinate. As a result of prostatic enlargement, there is difficulty/latency in commencing micturition (hesitancy), the urine stream is poor and the bladder does not empty completely, resulting in leakage immediately after micturition.

As there is residual urine volume, the bladder fills up again quickly; prostatic enlargement therefore results in the need for frequent micturition. Poor urine flow through the urethra also fails to dislodge bacteria found in the distal portion of the urethra and, combined with the residual urine volumes, leads to increased risk of urinary tract infections. The urinary outlet obstruction can be so severe that a sharp increase in pressure is seen in the bladder during micturition. This increased pressure can be transmitted up the ureters to the renal pelvis, often resulting in enlargement and damage to the renal pelvis (hydronephrosis) and widening of the ureters.

Surgical treatment of prostatic enlargement is common. Surgery is aimed at removing prostatic tissue to widen the opening through the prostate gland. A possible complication of this type of surgical procedure is inadvertent damage to the urethral sphincter leading to stress incontinence. In some cases, prostatic enlargement can be treated with drugs. In malignant prostatic enlargement, the malignant tissue is most often surgically removed.

DRUGS USED TO TREAT PROSTATIC ENLARGEMENT

Drug treatment of prostatic enlargement is aimed at reducing the contraction of smooth muscles in the internal urethral sphincter, the prostate gland and the proximal urethra, or slowing and reversing the growth of the prostate gland, leading to reduced urinary outlet obstruction.

α_1-adrenoceptor antagonists
The use of selective α_1-antagonists may be helpful in treating urinary outflow obstruction caused by prostatic enlargement.

Mechanism of action and effects. α_1-adrenoceptor antagonists block α_1-adrenoceptors in the neck of the bladder, proximal urethra and prostate tissue. This results in reduced tone of the internal urethral sphincter, the smooth muscles in the prostate and the proximal urethra, thus improving the passage of urine. Doxazosin, alfuzosin, and terazosin are α_1-adrenoceptor antagonists with such effects. The drugs are suited for use in mild-to-moderate obstructive urinary tract disorders and patients awaiting surgical treatment. See Figure 23.5.

α$_1$-adrenoceptor antagonist
Alfuzosin, Doxazosin, Indoramin, Prazosin, Tamsulosin, Terazosin

---

Table 23.4 Drugs used to treat urinary outflow obstruction due to prostatic enlargement

Adverse effects. The most common adverse effects are related to inhibition of sympathetic activity in organs other than the urinary tract. Because the drugs block α$_1$-adrenoceptors in arterioles and can cause vascular dilatation, hypotension can occur and result in dizziness, palpitations and, in rare cases, syncope. α$_1$-Adrenoceptors are also found in the central nervous system where stimulation contributes to increased wakefulness. Blockage can therefore result in lethargy. Dyspepsia and nausea may also occur.

Drugs used to treat urinary outflow obstruction due to prostatic enlargement are listed in Table 23.4.

ERECTILE DYSFUNCTION – IMPOTENCE

Erectile dysfunction is defined as the inability to achieve a satisfactory erection for the purposes of sexual intercourse. In order for an erection to occur, the blood supply to the penis and the neurogenic regulation of the blood flow within the penis must be intact.

PATHOPHYSIOLOGY OF ERECTILE DYSFUNCTION

When the penis is flaccid, vasoconstriction of the arterioles within the penis is present because of adrenergic stimulation (sympathetic activity) of α$_1$-adrenoceptors in the blood vessels. During sexual stimulation, the activity in parasympathetic efferent fibres increases and predominates over the adrenergic stimulation. This leads to the arterioles in the spongy bodies of the penis dilating and filling with blood. Dilatation is associated with the effects of nitric oxide (NO), which is synthesized in the endothelial cells of the blood vessels. Simultaneously, the arterioles dilate and are filled with blood; the veins are contracted, reducing the outflow of blood. In this way, the penis fills with blood and becomes erect. The parasympathetic fibres have their origins in the sacral region of the spine.

There are a number of possible causes of erectile dysfunction. Severe atherosclerotic narrowing of the pelvic arteries or the arteries in the penis can result in an inability to achieve erection due to inadequate blood flow. Disease or injury in the spinal cord and surgery in the pelvic region can damage the nerve supply and thereby prevent erection. A reduction in testosterone production also reduces the ability to achieve erection. There is also an important psychological component with anxiety about the ability to achieve erection often compounding the problem. Certain drugs (β-blockers, antidepressants) and excessive alcohol consumption can also reduce the ability to achieve erection. Before commencing drug treatment for erectile dysfunction, it is important to rule out any specific pathology.

DRUGS USED TO TREAT ERECTILE DYSFUNCTION

For drug treatment to be successful, the blood supply and the nervous regulation must be intact. The drugs that are most often used are inhibitors of phosphodiesterase, alprostadil (a prostaglandin) and apomorphine (a dopamine stimulant).

Phosphodiesterase inhibitors

Phosphodiesterase inhibitors (sildenafil) are the most frequently used drugs in the treatment of erectile dysfunction. They are administered orally and, with simultaneous sexual stimulation, an erection is possible about 1 h after taking the drug.

Mechanism of action and effects. The therapeutic effect of these drugs is achieved by the increased synthesis of nitric oxide (NO) in the arterioles within the spongy body, dilating the vessels and thus filling them with blood. The increase of NO requires an increase of cGMP (cyclic guanine monophosphate). There is usually only a moderate amount of cGMP in the vessel walls of the penis, since the compound is continuously broken down by the enzyme phosphodiesterase, found in conjunction with cGMP. Sildenafil, tadalafil and vardenafil inhibit phosphodiesterase and contribute to an increase in the amounts of NO. Phosphodiesterase is found in all tissues, but with small differences in structure (tissue-specific phosphodiesterase). These drugs are so specific in their effect that they primarily inhibit phosphodiesterase 5, which is predominantly found in the arterioles of the penis. Thus, a general vascular dilatation is avoided. If this were not the case, there would be dilatation throughout the body's blood vessels, which would result in a considerable drop in blood pressure with the use of these drugs. Maximum plasma concentration of the drugs is reached approximately 1 h after ingestion, and the concentration is maintained sufficiently to produce an erection that lasts 3–5 h.

Adverse effects and precautionary measures. The lowest effective dose should be used. With larger doses, there is a greater risk of systemic vascular dilatation. With higher plasma concentrations of the drug, other tissue-specific phosphodiesterases are affected, with the risk of systemic vascular dilation and a serious drop in blood pressure. The majority of adverse effects are associated with this mechanism. Some individuals experience dizziness, headache, flushing and nasal congestion. Altered colour vision, increased sensitivity to light and blurred vision are associated with the influence of phosphodiesterase in the retina. Simultaneous use of phosphodiesterase inhibitors and nitrates (e.g. nitroglycerine in ischaemic heart disease) can cause an increased vascular dilatation and a dangerous drop in blood pressure, reducing circulation to the vital organs and even causing cardiovascular collapse. Patients with a poor coronary circulation are particularly vulnerable. The combination of nitrates and sildenafil/vardenafil is therefore contraindicated.

Prostaglandin

Alprostadil is a prostaglandin (PGE_1) that is normally administered by injection into the spongy bodies in the penis. Intraurethral administration is also possible. Alprostadil is a possible alternative when the use of phosphodiesterase inhibitors is contraindicated.

Mechanism of action and effects. It is thought that alprostadil exerts its effect by inhibiting stimulation of α_1-adrenoceptors in the arterioles of the penis. This inhibition results in a relative dominance of parasympathetic tone and dilation and filling of the blood vessels in the spongy bodies of the penis. Alprostadil produces an erection even without sexual stimulation. Erection is usually achieved 5–15 min after injection.

Adverse effects and precautionary measures. Injection of alprostadil can result in pain at the injection site and haematoma formation. Too large a dose can cause priapism (prolonged, painful erection), and it should therefore be titrated such that the erection lasts about an hour. Repeated injections can cause the development of connective tissue, causing the penis to curve during erection. Use should therefore be limited to one injection per day, and no more than three injections per week.

Dopamine stimulant

Apomorphine is a morphine derivative that has dopamine-like effects. The effect in erectile dysfunction is somewhat weaker than that of phosphodiesterase inhibitors.

Mechanism of action and effects. Apomorphine stimulates dopamine receptors in the hypothalamus, which sends impulses to blood vessels in the penis. The effect is medicated via an increase in NO concentration in small vessels in a similar way to phosphodiesterase inhibitors. Apomorphine also requires sexual stimulation to produce an erection.

Adverse effects and precautionary measures. Adverse effects include nausea, dizziness and headache, which are related to the effect on dopamine receptors in the central nervous system. Drops in blood pressure are reported, especially in patients who experience postural hypotension. The preparation should not be used by patients who are taking nitrates (e.g. for ischaemic heart disease), since the combination can cause a pronounced drop in blood pressure. A number of antipsychotics act by blocking dopamine receptors and can reduce the effect of apomorphine.

Drugs used to treat erectile dysfunction are listed in Table 23.5.

Phosphodiesterase inhibitors
Sildenafil, Tadalafil, Vardenafil
Prostaglandin
Alprostadil
Dopamine stimulant
Apomorphine

Table 23.5 Drugs used to treat erectile dysfunction

SUMMARY

- The bladder's function is controlled by both autonomic and voluntary mechanisms. The sympathetic nervous system keeps the bladder shut while the parasympathetic nervous system controls bladder emptying.
- In uncontrolled nocturnal micturition in children, an evening dose of desmopressin may help, by reducing nocturnal urine production.
- In urge incontinence, the activity of the parasympathetic system increases quickly and initiates emptying of the bladder. Treatment with anticholinergic drugs that block muscarinic receptors in the bladder wall reduces the effect of increased parasympathetic activity.
- In stress incontinence, the internal urethral sphincter requires stimulation to ensure increased tone. Drugs that stimulate α_1-adrenoceptors are suitable. Low-potency oestrogens can be effective in women with stress incontinence.
- A specialist is necessary for the treatment of neurogenic bladder disorder, which requires correct diagnosis of disease/injury.

- Drug treatment in urinary outlet obstruction associated with prostatic hyperplasia aims to block α_1-adrenoceptors in the internal urethral sphincter, the prostate gland and the urethra, in order to reduce outlet obstruction.
- Erectile dysfunction can be treated with drugs.
- Phosphodiesterase inhibitors indirectly increase the amount of NO in small blood vessels in the penis and thereby contribute to vessel dilatation and increased filling of the spongy bodies of the penis with blood. These drugs should not be used in patients taking nitrates to manage ischaemic heart disease.
- Alprostadil, injected into the penis, leads to a local reduction of sympathetic activity and results in vessel dilatation with increased blood flow and therefore erection.
- Apomorphine acts via the central nervous system and causes local increase in the release of NO in the penis.

24 Drugs used to treat diseases of the skin

The skin is the body's largest organ. Its most important tasks are to function as a barrier against the surrounding environment and as an organ for temperature regulation, to receive and communicate different stimuli from the surroundings, and to synthesize vitamin D utilizing sunlight.

The most common skin diseases are eczemas, sebaceous gland diseases, infections and psoriasis. In many patients, these skin diseases are chronic. In some, they are periodically socially crippling and life-threatening. Parasites on the skin can be troublesome and, in some cases, can lead to secondary disease. It is these common diseases that are covered in this chapter.

Skin diseases are usually treated topically, but in some cases systemic therapy is required.

ANATOMY AND PHYSIOLOGY OF THE SKIN

In adult humans, the skin constitutes approximately 16 per cent of the body weight and covers approximately $1.8\,m^2$ of the body surface. It is usual to divide the skin

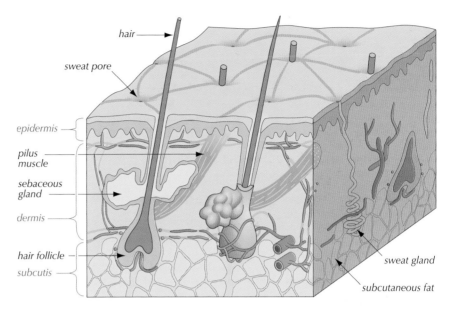

hair

sweat pore

epidermis

pilus muscle

sebaceous gland

dermis

hair follicle

subcutis

sweat gland

subcutaneous fat

Figure 24.1 **Structure of the skin.** The skin is divided into the epidermis, dermis and subcutis.

into three layers: epidermis, dermis and subcutis. See Figure 24.1. In the border between the epidermis and dermis, there is a constant division of new cells that move towards the outer surface. As they migrate, the skin cells increase their production of keratin and secrete a fatty glue-like substance which holds the cells tightly together. This helps to make the outer layer of skin hard and dense, which reduces water evaporation and the possibility of penetration and damage by chemical and biological substances. The epidermis contains melanocytes, cells that produce melanin. Melanin absorbs part of the energy in ultraviolet rays, thereby protecting against damage. The epidermis is thus an effective barrier against the external environment. Loss of this barrier function increases the risk of fluid loss, infections and radiation damage. Hair, nails and all skin except the mucous membranes contain keratin.

Hair and adjoining sebaceous glands are part of the epidermis, but penetrate deep into the dermis where there is a rich network of capillary vessels. The sweat glands start in the transition between the subcutaneous layer and the dermis, and form ducts that terminate on the skin surface. By varying the blood flow in the dermis and by the secretion of sweat, the skin functions as an important modulator of body temperature. Nerve fibres with different sensors that perceive different external stimuli are also found in the dermis. These are discussed in more detail in Chapter 11. The subcutaneous layer provides good heat insulation and is important for fat storage in the body.

The skin contains T-lymphocytes, mast cells and macrophages. These respond to harmful stimuli and release inflammatory substances. Allergic and toxic reactions are often expressed as skin changes.

The skin on the palm of the hand is firmer and thicker than on the back of the hand. The skin on the scalp is often densely filled with thick hair. Anatomical differences found in different skin areas are a result of a diversity of function associated with different body surfaces. These differences make different parts of the skin vulnerable to different diseases and can make it necessary to use specially adapted treatments depending on the location and extent of a skin disease.

DRUG FORMULATIONS FOR APPLICATION ON SKIN

Topical therapy of skin diseases makes it possible to administer drugs in smaller doses than would be necessary if using a systemic route. In this way, it is possible to achieve a topical effect with reduced adverse effects. For topically administered drugs to have an effect, the active substance must penetrate down into the epidermis and/or dermis. This is achieved by blending the active substance into different carrier media (vehicles) that provide contact and penetration into the skin. The purpose of the different preparations is to have drug formulations that are suitable for different types of skin and skin diseases. Different antimicrobial drugs can also be blended into topical forms that make the topical therapy of skin infections possible. These are used in bacterial, fungal and viral infections.

Liniments are liquid preparations with a water or alcohol base in which the active substance is dissolved. Liniments have a cooling effect and are well suited to the treatment of conditions with an inflammatory component.

Creams are emulsions where water constitutes the carrier substance. Since they have a water base, these creams will adhere to moist parts of the skin. They are therefore typically used in the acute phases of suppurating eczemas, but also on dry parts of the skin. Creams are absorbed relatively quickly into the skin and do not rub off onto clothing. They are cosmetically more acceptable than ointments and are often used on the hands and face. Creams are often used without an active substance. These creams can have moisture-retaining and softening effects on dry skin and, as such, prevent cracking and possible ingress of infection.

Ointments are emulsions with oil or fat as the carrier substance, but water can be blended in. The active substance can be dissolved in the oil or water, or added as particles. Ointments are particularly useful on dry parts of the skin in chronic eczemas. They have an occlusive and softening effect. Because of their fatty consistency, they are not suitable for moist skin surfaces. They rub off on clothing and can be cosmetically unacceptable.

Pastes are fats with powder blended in. This form is suitable if it is necessary to protect the skin against softening by aqueous solutions. It is also suitable for application on limited parts of the skin in psoriasis.

ECZEMA

Eczema is an inflammatory condition of the skin that is the result of toxic or allergic reactions from chemical substances, metals or biological allergens, such as solvents, detergents, cement, latex and rubber. In some individuals, eczema occurs without a demonstrable external cause. Atopic eczema is one such form, and is usually observed in children where there is history of allergic sensitivity within the family. Distribution is usually symmetrical, i.e. the right and left sides of the body are equally affected, and it is found in the creases of the elbows, knees, ankles and wrists, but also elsewhere.

CHARACTERISTIC SKIN CHANGES IN ECZEMA

In the acute phase, eczematous skin is often red and suppurating; in the chronic phase, it is dry and itchy. See Figure 24.2. Because of the intense itching experienced, scratching often results in damage to the skin, which becomes easily infected.

acute eczema

inflammatory cells
dilated vessels
vesicles

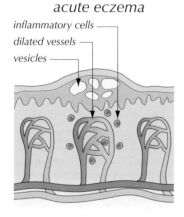

chronic eczema

inflammatory cells
elongated papilla
hyperkeratosis

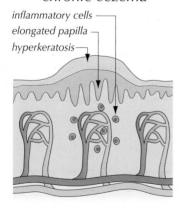

Figure 24.2 **Acute and chronic eczema.** In acute eczema, vesicles in the epidermis are seen. These can burst and cause moist skin surfaces. In chronic eczema, the vesicles are gone and the epidermis is thickened (hyperkeratosis).

If the skin changes have an *asymmetrical* distribution, this may be an indication that the skin changes are a result of an external cause e.g. latex allergy. A *symmetrical* distribution suggests a systemic reaction to a potential allergen/toxin such as a reaction to certain food types.

DRUGS USED TO TREAT ECZEMA

The choice of treatment depends on the severity of the condition. In cases where the eczema has a known cause, the trigger agent must be removed, if possible. Mild eczemas are treated with moisturizers and antipruritic drugs. Eczema of intertriginous areas (areas where skin lies against skin), such as the groin, under the arms and under the breasts in women, should be treated with creams or liniments. If the eczema is infected, it is important to treat the infection.

The most effective topical treatment is with glucocorticoids. In some cases, parenteral administration is chosen. The use of moisturizers can reduce the need for glucocorticoids. In some treatment-resistant cases, cytotoxic (methotrexate) or immunosuppressive (ciclosporin) drugs are used.

Glucocorticoids

Glucocorticoids for topical application on the skin are divided into four strengths that are used with increased severity of disease:

- mild (group I), e.g. hydrocortisone
- moderately potent (group II), e.g. flumethasone
- potent (group III), e.g. betamethasone
- very potent (group IV), e.g. clobetasol.

It is recommended the mildest preparation possible be used, and in cases where the eczema is difficult to treat, alternation between a potent and mild preparation is recommended. If two strengths of glucocorticoid preparation are to be used, then treatment should begin with the potent preparation and then be changed to the milder preparation or emollient alone when symptomatic improvement is noted. Gradual withdrawal is sometimes recommended in order to avoid a rebound appearance of symptoms.

Mechanism of action and effects. Topically applied glucocorticoids exert their most important therapeutic effects by reducing the formation of inflammatory substances in immunologically active cells. They have a good antipruritic effect, so that the skin is rested (constant scratching around eczematous parts of the skin serves to maintain the eczemas). Glucocorticoids are more thoroughly discussed in Chapter 22, Drugs used in allergy, for immune suppression and cancer treatment.

Pharmacokinetics. Only a small percentage of topically administered glucocorticoids are absorbed, although different parts of the body have different absorption rates. Thin skin with a good blood supply has the greatest rate of absorption. Once-daily application appears to be as effective as more frequent applications. The glucocorticoids diffuse down into the layers of skin; these layers then function as a depot, providing a long duration of action.

Adverse effects. Adverse effects depend on the duration of use and the potency of the formulation used. Any systemic effects also depend on the size of the skin area that is treated. The most important adverse effects are topical skin atrophy, delayed wound healing and increased risk of infection. These adverse effects are due to a reduction in the formation of new connective tissue and the inhibitory effect on immunomodulating cells within the skin. When used over longer periods of time,

Mild
Hydrocortisone

Moderately potent
Alclometasone dipropionate, Clobetasone butyrate, Fludroxycortide, Fluocinolone acetonide, Fluocortolone, Fluticasone propionate

Potent
Beclometasone dipropionate, Betametasone esters, Diflucortolone valerate, Hydrocortisone butyrate, Fluocinonide, Fluprednidene acetate, Mometasone furoate, Triamcinolone acetonide

Very potent
Clobetasol propionate, Halcionide

Table 24.1 Topical glucocorticoids (corticosteroids) according to potency

striae are observed, which are stripe-shaped scar formations and colour changes in the skin. These striae are caused by small rips in the corium that lead to haemorrhage, microembolism and scar formation. The damage occurs as a result of reduced connective tissue formation and loss of elasticity and strength, and is observed where strain on the corium is at its greatest.

There are a number of topical moisturizers – bath oils, fish oil ointments, zinc oxide preparations and allergen-free ointments and pastes – that do not contain glucocorticoids. Carbamide and propylene glycol in liniment are the most common additives. Both have moisture-retaining effect.

SEBACEOUS GLAND DISEASES

The most common sebaceous gland diseases are acne and rosacea. There is a significant inflammatory component to both these diseases.

ACNE

Acne is a chronic inflammation of the pilosebaceous units (sebaceous glands and a single hair follicle). Development progresses through several stages. Androgens (male sex hormones) stimulate the sebaceous glands to increase production of sebum. Acne is characterized by hyperkeratosis of the follicular epithelium, leading to horny impactions of the skin and clogging of the secretion duct. See Figure 24.3.

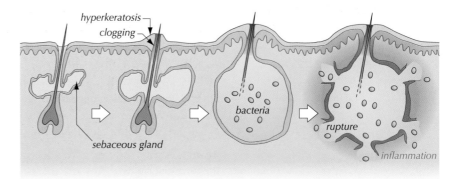

Figure 24.3 **Acne is created in the pilosebaceous unit.** Hyperkeratinization and clogging of the secretary duct result in a rupture of the gland and inflammation in the surrounding tissue.

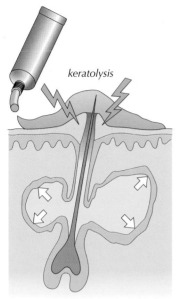

keratolysis

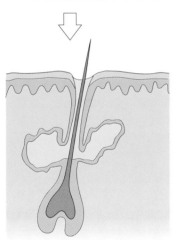

Figure 24.4 Keratolytic effect in acne.
The keratolytic effect removes the blockage of the sebaceous gland. Thus, the sebum can be secreted to the surface and the pressure in the gland decreases.

The sebaceous gland and the surrounding skin area are colonized by the bac-teria *Propionibacterium acnes*. The bacterial infection results in breakdown of the fat in the sebum and release of fatty acids and production of inflammatory substances. The gland can be damaged, so that inflammatory substances leak out to surrounding tissue. A typical presentation is the formation of comedones (black plugs with keratinaceous melanin at the outlet of the sebaceous glands), papules, pustules and cysts. In the most serious cases, cyst formation leads to pronounced scarring in the affected areas. The distribution of acne mirrors the skin areas that have the greatest numbers of sebaceous glands, and it is most commonly found on the face, neck and upper parts of the chest and back. Since androgynous stimulation is important, acne occurs most frequently during and after puberty.

DRUGS USED TO TREAT ACNE

Treatment has three key aims.

■ reduction of bacterial colonization
■ a keratolytic effect to enlarge the secretory ducts
■ suppression of inflammation.

Moderate forms of acne
The treatment strategy is to reduce colonization of bacteria and achieve a keratolytic effect. See Figure 24.4.

Azelaic acid
Azelaic acid is an organic acid that has an antibacterial effect on *Propionibacterium acnes* by inhibiting the synthesis of essential bacterial fatty acids. In addition, the production of horn cells is reduced through a keratolytic effect. These two effects can be enough to suppress acne development. The drug is usually applied twice daily and improvement is usually seen within 3–4 weeks. The treatment must often continue over several months. Adverse effects include skin irritation with reddening, stinging, flaking and itching, usually occurring immediately after application. When such problems arise, use is recommended once daily during the initial treatment period.

Benzoyl peroxide
Benzoyl peroxide is metabolized to benzoic acid in the skin. It has a keratolytic effect and reduces the number of *Propionibacterium acnes*. The substance is usually washed off after 1–2 h exposure during the initial treatment period. Thereafter, the treatment time is gradually increased up to 12 h before washing off.

Skin irritation with reddening, dryness and flaking is the most common adverse effect. Allergic contact eczema occurs in a small number of cases.

Clindamycin
Clindamycin is an antibiotic that is used for topical application in therapy-resistant acne. If benzoyl peroxide is used simultaneously, the risk of antibiotic resistance is reduced.

Serious forms of acne
Systemic therapy against acne consists of antibiotic therapy and use of retinoids. The treatment should last several months but is often poorly tolerated because of adverse effects.

Topical preparations for mild acne
Benzoyl peroxide, Azelaic acid

Topcial retinoides and related preparations
Adepalene, Isotretinoin, Tretinoin

Topical antibiotics
Erythromycin, Clindamycin, Tetracycline

Systemic antibiotics
Erythromycin, Tetracycline

Table 24.2 Drugs used to treat acne

Tetracycline and erythromycin

Tetracycline and erythromycin are used in serious forms of acne to treat the associated *Propionibacterium acnes* infection. The antibiotic course should last 4–6 months. The adverse effects are primarily diarrhoea and allergic reaction. Pregnant women should not use tetracycline, since it is known to affect the calcification of teeth in the fetus. Protracted use of antibiotics can also result in the emergence of bacterial resistance.

Isotretinoin

Isotretinoin belongs to the retinoid group, which resembles vitamin A. These drugs affect the growth and differentiation of epithelial cells and give a looser structure in keratinized skin. Keratinization is also inhibited, such that the hyperkeratosis in the secretion ducts of the sebaceous glands is reduced. In addition, activity in the sebaceous glands is also reduced. The mechanism of action is unknown. These drugs are administered systemically.

Systemic use of isotretinoin has many serious adverse effects. The preparation is strongly teratogenic. Fertile women should use reliable contraceptive measures 1 month before treatment, and for 2 years following the cessation of treatment. Many experience problems with dry skin that easily cracks. The retinoids also have a number of other adverse effects on the skin, mucous membranes, musculoskeletal system and central nervous system, and should always be used under the supervision of a consultant dermatologist.

ROSACEA

Rosacea is a disease with unknown aetiology. It is characterized by chronic inflammation and hyperplasia of sebaceous glands, pronounced erythema and formation of pustules. The veins in the skin are dilated and lymphoedema, particularly of the nose and cheeks, occurs in rare cases. In rosacea, there are no comedones such as are seen in acne. The disease has a later onset than is seen in acne and normally lasts for several years, but responds well to treatment.

Treatment consists of systemic antibiotic therapy, usually with tetracycline. Topical treatment with metronidazole ointment is an alternative.

Topical antibiotics
Metronidazole

Systemic antibiotics
Erythromycin, Tetracycline

Table 24.3 Drugs used to treat rosacea

PSORIASIS

Psoriasis is a chronic, inflammatory skin disease without accompanying infection. There is a considerable increase in the formation of new skin cells in demarcated areas, with thickening of the epidermis and increased keratin production in the cells. A thick and scaly layer of skin forms, with clear-cut boundaries against normal skin. There is an increase in neutrophil granulocytes, which may form microabscesses. In some cases, these can be so large that they form pustules. See Figure 24.5. All skin surfaces can be affected, including mucous membranes and nails, but the distribution is usually localized to the elbows and knees. In some cases, joints are attacked, which can result in significant disability. Different environmental factors appear to trigger outbreaks in predisposed individuals.

The treatment of psoriasis depends on its distribution and on how active the disease is. In cases where the joints are attacked, where there are large areas of skin affected and where there is formation of pustules in the palms of the hands and under the feet, treatment by a specialist is required.

Sun and saltwater baths have been shown to be beneficial, with many individuals demonstrating benefit from exposure to artificial ultraviolet rays (UVB rays).

DRUGS USED TO TREAT PSORIASIS

Topical treatment is used on small patches of keratinized skin. Since the disease is characterized by an increased, new formation of horny skin, drugs are used that dissolve keratin and reduce cell division. It is helpful to remove loose and scaly skin before ointment and creams are applied. See Figure 24.6.

Tar preparations

Tar preparations are used as topical treatment and probably act by inhibiting DNA synthesis. In hospitals, tar is often used together with UVB rays. The strong smell makes tar treatment unacceptable for many individuals.

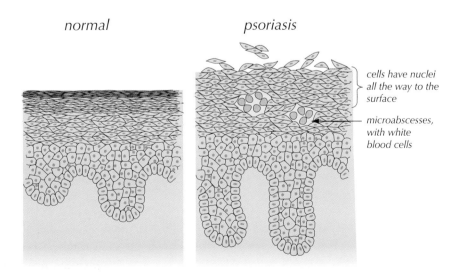

Figure 24.5 **Skin changes in psoriasis.** In psoriatic skin areas, the skin cells have nuclei all the way to the surface and the epidermis is thickened. In addition, microabscesses are seen.

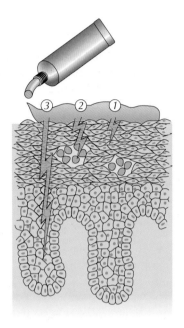

Figure 24.6 **Principles for treatment of psoriasis.** Drugs can have a keratolytic effect (1), suppress the release of inflammatory active substances (2), and suppress the formation of new cells (3).

Salicylic acid

Salicylic acid has a keratolytic effect and is used as a topical treatment on both the scalp and body skin. It is often blended with Vaseline and used prior to other topical treatment to improve penetration by reducing the thickness of the horn layer.

Dithranol

Dithranol is used as topical treatment. It is thought to act by inhibiting DNA synthesis and thereby the formation of new cells. Both hyperactive and normal skin cells are influenced. To avoid local irritation, contamination of healthy skin should be avoided. The preparation causes discoloration of the skin and clothing and for cosmetic reasons is unacceptable for many individuals. Otherwise, it has few adverse effects.

Calcipotriol

Calcipotriol is used as topical treatment. It is a vitamin D analogue that inhibits cell proliferation and increases differentiation and maturation of the skin cells. Skin changes can, in some cases, be normalized. The effect is potentiated if it is used with dithranol or topical glucocorticoids.

Since vitamin D increases the absorption of calcium from the intestines and its release from bone mass, hypercalcaemia can occur. However, the effect depends on the size of the area that is treated (the amount of calcipotriol that is used daily).

Tacalcitol

Tacalcitol is a vitamin D analogue that resembles calcipotriol.

Acitretin

Acitretin is a retinoid used in the systemic treatment of psoriasis that has proved resistant to topical treatment. It has similar effects and adverse effects to isotretinoin, which is used for treatment of serious acne.

Methotrexate and ciclosporin

Methotrexate and ciclosporin are used in therapy-resistant psoriasis. Methotrexate is a cytotoxic drug with anti-inflammatory and immunomodulating effects. Ciclosporin inhibits the proliferation of T-lymphocytes and reduces the formation of active inflammatory substances. Both are discussed in Chapter 22, Drugs used in allergy, for immune suppression and in cancer treatment.

Local treatment with glucocorticoids is often used together with other topical treatment (see p. 365 for a more detailed discussion of glucocorticoids).

Tar preparations and related preparations
Coal tar, Dithranol, Tazarotene

Salicylic acid
Salicylic acid

Vitamin D analogues
Calcipotriol, Tacalcitol

Retinoid for systemic use
Acitretin

Cytotoxic and immunosuppressive drugs
Methotrexate, Ciclosporin

Topical glucocorticoids
See Table 24.1

Table 24.4 Drugs used to treat psoriasis

INFECTIONS IN THE SKIN

Infections in the skin can occur as a result of bacteria, fungi and viruses. As micro-organisms not only colonize the surface of the skin but also penetrate down into it, systemic antibiotic treatment may be necessary in some cases. It is important that the specific antimicrobial susceptibilities are determined to ensure effective treatment and prevent the emergence of resistant organisms.

BACTERIAL SKIN INFECTIONS

The most important bacterial infections seen in the skin, except those associated with acne, are impetigo, folliculitis, furunculosis, carbuncles, exanthema, erysipelas and cellulitis. See Figure 24.7. Several of these infections involve the hair follicles. *Staphylococcus spp.* and *Streptococcus spp.* are the most frequently occurring bacteria. Staphylococcus infections often have a clear demarcation, while streptococcal infections demonstrate more diffuse spreading.

Topical treatment with neomycin or fucidin two to three times daily is often sufficient to treat the infection.

Impetigo is a superficial skin infection, often restricted to the face. The causative organisms are staphylococci or streptococci. The condition often requires systemic treatment with antibiotics.

Folliculitis is a bacterial infection of the hair follicles.

Furunculosis is further development of folliculitis with abscess formation.

Carbuncles are deep abscesses that involve many hair follicles. Staphylococcus organisms are usually the cause of these infections. Furuncles and carbuncles often require surgical drainage as well as systemic antibiotic therapy.

Ecthyma is a localized infection, usually caused by group A beta-hemolytic streptococci that occurs after small skin injuries. It is most frequently found on the extremities.

Erysipelas is caused by β-haemolytic streptococci (group A). The infection is most often restricted to the face. Phenoxymethylpenicillin is the primary choice of antibiotic; erythromycin can also be used. Both drugs are administered systemically.

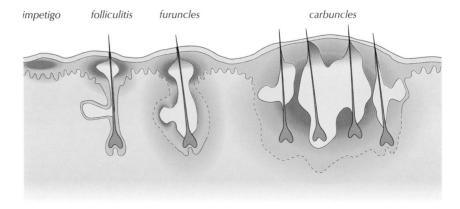

impetigo *folliculitis* *furuncles* *carbuncles*

Figure 24.7 **Bacterial skin infections.** Impetigo, folliculitis, furuncles and carbuncles.

Antibacterials for topical use
Fucidic acid, Mupirocin, Neomycin, Polymyxins
Antibacterials for systemic use
Flucloxacillin (see also Chapter 16, Antimicrobial drugs)

Table 24.5 Antibacterial drugs for skin infections

Cellulitis is an infection of the subcutaneous tissue, usually caused by streptococcal organisms. The condition differentiates itself from erysipelas with oedema, more intense redness and pain on touching.

Lyme disease is caused by the spirochaete *Borrelia burgdorferi*. The microbe is transmitted through bites of the arachnid tick. The infection is characterized by a ring-shaped, red rash that spreads concentrically from the bite site around 3–7 days after the injury. It is important to diagnose the infection correctly, as untreated Lyme disease can result in serious infection of the nervous system, joints and several other organs.

Antibacterial drugs are discussed in more detail in Chapter 16, Antimicrobial drugs.

FUNGAL SKIN INFECTIONS

Fungal infections are called mycoses. These can occur in horny skin, mucous membranes, hair and nails. Mould fungi thrive best in keratinized tissue, while the mucosa is usually infected by yeast fungi. Fungal infections in the skin are called tinea.

Tinea pedis (athlete's foot) is a fungal infection of the feet. It is characterized by flaking and cracking of the skin, particularly between the outer toes. Erythema, vesicles, pustule formation and white dry flaking in the soles of the feet are not uncommon.

Tinea mannum is a fungal infection localized to the palms of the hands. Mild erythema and keratotic process result in pronounced skin furrows (chalk lines) in the palm of the hand. The infection can be confused with eczema and psoriasis.

Tinea cruris (jock itch) is a fungal infection of the groin. Dry, scaly flaking with a sharp, distinct border against normal skin is typical.

Tinea corporis (ringworm) is a fungal infection of the upper part of the body. Ringworm often occurs in the form of topical, itchy, erythematous changes with pronounced border activity, with elements of different sizes.

Tinea capitis is a fungal infection of the hair and the scalp. One type of infection can present itself with scaly scalp skin and patchy hair loss without pronounced inflammation in the affected area. The other type causes severe inflammation, and a kerion (swollen mass) will appear on the scalp, often with secondary bacterial infection.

Tinea unguium is a nail fungus. Loose horn masses flake off under the nail, which lift it up and cause a thickened, yellowish and porous nail.

DRUGS USED TO TREAT FUNGAL INFECTIONS

Fungi have ergosterol in the cell membrane, while humans have cholesterol. Most fungicides act by inhibiting ergosterol synthesis or by damaging ergosterol in the

---

Topical treatment
Amorolfine, Clotrimaxole, Econazole, Miconazole, Nystatin, Terbinafine, Tioconazole

---

Table 24.6 Drugs used to treat fungal skin infections

fungal membrane. Superficial fungal infections in the skin can be treated with topical drugs. Exceptions to this are tinea capitis and tinea unguium, which often require systemic treatment.

Drugs for treatment of fungal infections are discussed in more detail in Chapter 16, Antimicrobial drugs.

VIRAL SKIN INFECTIONS

The most common viral skin infections are warts and herpes infections.

Warts
Warts can occur in both horny skin and mucosal epithelium on all body surfaces. The causative organism is the human papilloma virus (HPV). Common warts in children disappear in most cases within a few years. They do not require treatment if they are unproblematic. Plantar warts can cause pain and are best treated with liquid nitrogen (the cold damages infected cells such that the wart degenerates) or deep debridement. An alternative treatment can be tried with a blend of salicylic acid and podophyllin in acetone and collodium. This is brushed on the wart and then the area is covered with an occlusive dressing for 1 week.

Condyloma acuminata are genital warts caused by the same virus. They tend to resolve spontaneously within the course of months to years. Attempts can be made to remove them mechanically or by topical application with podophyllotoxin or imiquimod.

Podophyllotoxin
Podophyllotoxin is effective against warts by inhibiting cell division. Topical reactions such as pain and skin irritation can occur. By inadvertently applying to non-affected areas, skin necrosis can occur and systemic absorption of the drug can cause neurotoxic and cardiotoxic adverse effects. It is therefore not recommended for use on non-problematic common warts. This drug should also not be used by pregnant women.

Imiquimod
Imiquimod has no direct antiviral effect, but modifies the immune response by increasing the production of cytokines, which are important in the immune system's defence against viruses. Topical reactions occur, such as erythema, itching, peeling skin and vesicle formation, but usually disappear after about 2 weeks.

Herpes infections
Viral skin infections often cause sores in the form of blisters. The herpesvirus can be divided into different types. After the primary (first) outbreak, the virus lies dormant in the dorsal ganglia of sensory nerves. From here, it can be reactivated and travel to the skin area that is innervated by the infected nerve and cause new outbreaks. The outbreaks diminish after a number of days, but can be painful. It is important to commence treatment as early as possible, before virus replication causes clinical disease.

Preparations for warts
Imiquimod, Podophyllotoxin
Preparations for herpes infections
Aciclovir, Penciclovir, Idoxuridine, Valaciclovir

Table 24.7 Drugs used to treat viral skin infections

Herpes simplex type 1 usually infects mucous membranes and keratinized skin in and around the mouth and nose, but other parts of the skin can also be affected. Such infections can be treated with topical application of aciclovir or penciclovir creams. The treatment should start early in the clinical course of the disease.

Herpes simplex type 2 usually infects mucosal membranes on the genitals and causes herpes genitalis. Outbreaks can be treated with aciclovir or valaciclovir. With significant outbreaks and severe pain, systemic treatment may be necessary.

Herpes zoster (shingles) is caused by the varicella zoster virus. The infection occurs almost exclusively in individuals who have previously had chickenpox. Here, the virus lies dormant in sensory ganglia and is reactivated and moves along nerve fibres towards the skin. Distribution of the disease is usually found on the trunk and is dependent on the sensory ganglia infected. Post-herpetic neuralgia with persistent severe pain can occur after an outbreak. Herpes zoster infections can also attack the cornea of the eye.

Herpes zoster infections are treated both topically with aciclovir and systemically with aciclovir or valaciclovir.

Aciclovir and valaciclovir inhibit virus replication by inhibiting DNA synthesis of the virus. Valaciclovir is metabolized in the liver to aciclovir. Aciclovir is applied topically to the area several times daily. Topical treatment can cause transitory burning and prickling feelings in the area. Erythema, flaking and itching also occur.

Antiviral drugs are more thoroughly discussed in Chapter 16, Antimicrobial drugs.

PARASITES

Scabies and lice are parasites that are transmitted by contact with an infected person or infected clothing, bedclothes or towels. Itching is the most common presentation.

SCABIES

Scabies is caused by mites that burrow into the skin, where they lay eggs that first develop into larvae and then into mites. See Figure 24.8. Typical distribution is on the sides of fingers, wrists and ankles, but the parasites can also be found around the navel and genitals. Scabies are not found on the face or scalp. It is recommended that all family members of an infected person are treated to prevent reinfection. The itching can last several weeks after treatment, even if the mites are dead. Itching can be treated with a topical glucocorticoid.

Permethrin is used for individuals over 2 years of age. A 15 per cent solution of benzyl benzoate can be used for small children.

LICE

There are two varieties of lice: body/head lice and pubic lice (crab lice). See Figure 24.8. Both species live by sucking blood from the host and laying eggs that attach to hair.

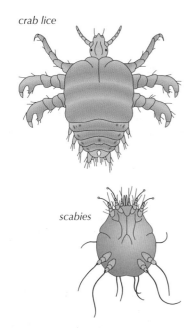

crab lice

scabies

Figure 24.8 **Crab lice and scabies.**

DRUGS USED TO TREAT PARASITES

Itching is a common problem when infected by these parasites, leading to scratching and contamination of skin wounds. Oral administration of antihistamine in the evening may relieve itching during the night. Antiparasitic drugs used to treat scabies or lice may all cause skin irritation.

Permethrin

Permethrin is an insecticide commonly used to treat scabies (and lice). Treatment should be applied to the whole body. Particular attention should be paid to the webs of the fingers and toes and under the ends of nails. Permethrin should be applied twice, one week apart. The drug is also effective in the treatment of lice.

Ivermectin

Ivermectin is an antiparasitic drug that acts by producing a paralysis of the parasite. It is taken orally in a single dose by patients where permethrin is not effective to treat scabies.

Carbaryl, malathion, permethrin and phenothrin

Carbaryl, malathion, permethrin and phenothrin are effective in treating lice. They are liquid or lotion formulations that should be applied for 12 hours. Treatment should be repeated after one week, to kill parasites that survive the first treatment in the egg phase.

Scabies
Permethrin, Ivermectin

Lice
Carbaryl, Malation, Permethrin, Phenothrin

Table 24.8 Drugs used to treat scabies and lice

SUMMARY

- The skin functions as a protective barrier against the environment, regulates body temperature, communicates stimuli from the surroundings, and synthesizes vitamin D after exposure to sunlight.
- In topical treatments, active substances are blended into carrier media that provide good contact with the skin area that is to be treated. In some cases, systemic therapy is necessary.
- The most common skin diseases are eczemas, sebaceous gland diseases, psoriasis, infections and parasites.
- Treatment for eczema is different in the acute and chronic phases. Glucocorticoids are the most effective drugs; they suppress inflammation, suppress the release of inflammatory substances and reduce the activity of immune cells. The glucocorticoids are divided into four strengths. Adverse effects are skin atrophy, increased tendency for infection and delayed wound healing.
- The most common sebaceous gland diseases are acne and rosacea. The treatment of acne is aimed at eradicating infection (*Propionibacterium acnes*) and achieving a keratolytic effect, such that sebum discharge is not blocked. Clindamycin is used topically. Tetracyclines and erythromycin are used in systemic antibiotic therapy.

Isotretinoin reduces hyperkeratosis in the secretion ducts and reduces activity in the sebaceous glands.

■ Rosacea is a chronic inflammatory disease, often complicated by secondary infection that leads to the formation of papules and pustules. The disease is treated with antibiotics.

■ Psoriasis is characterized by an increase in the formation of immature skin cells. The disease can also attack nails and joints. Accumulation of granulocytes can cause pustules to form. The treatment aims to reduce inflammation in affected parts of the skin and reduce the formation of new skin cells. Glucocorticoids are used for their anti-inflammatory effect. Tar preparations and dithranol probably inhibit DNA synthesis and thereby reduce formation of new skin cells. Calcipotriol inhibits cell proliferation and increases differentiation and maturation of skin cells.

■ Infections in the skin can be attributed to bacteria, fungi and viruses.

■ Most bacterial infections can be treated with topical antibiotic therapy, but systemic treatment may be necessary.

■ Most fungicides act by inhibiting ergosterol synthesis or by damaging ergosterol in the fungal membrane. Local treatment is often sufficient.

■ Viral infections in the skin can cause different kinds of warts. Different herpes infections also arise from viruses. Effective treatment requires early use. Wart viruses are treated with podophyllotoxin, which inhibits the division of virus-infected skin cells. Herpes infections are treated with idoxuridine aciclovir or valaciclovir, which inhibit virus replication.

■ Scabies and lice are dealt with by single-treatment preparations of insecticides. To prevent growth of hatched eggs, re-treatment may be necessary after approximately 1 week.

25 Drugs in anaesthesia

Anaesthesia literally means 'without feeling'. Drugs that induce anaesthesia are called anaesthetics. They are used primarily during surgical intervention, but they are also used in postoperative management of pain.

Anaesthesia can be achieved by blocking afferent pain impulses from certain areas of the body (local or regional anaesthesia) or by affecting the central nervous system so that the pain impulses are not perceived (general anaesthesia). See Figure 25.1.

Anaesthetics are divided into two main groups: local anaesthetics, which render parts of the body numb, and general anaesthetics, which render the patient unconscious, and without experience of pain. Not all anaesthetics have good analgesic effect so it may be necessary to administer analgesic drugs as well. If surgery requires relaxed muscles to ease the work of the surgeon, muscle relaxants can be used. These drugs also paralyse ventilatory muscles and the patient will require artificial ventilation.

As part of a typical anaesthetic regime, drugs are also used for premedication, to sedate the patient before surgery, to reduce pain, bradycardia and mucus secretion from the airways during the period of anaesthesia.

LOCAL AND REGIONAL ANAESTHESIA

Local anaesthesia includes surface anaesthesia, infiltration anaesthesia and blockade of peripheral nerves to small areas such as the fingers, ankles or intercostal dermatomes.

Regional anaesthesia includes blockade of nerves that supply large tissue areas. It can be an asymmetrical blockade of a nerve plexus to, for example, an arm, or a symmetrical blockade of spinal nerves (i.e. an epidural or spinal anaesthetic), which administers the same level of anaesthesia to the right and left sides. This results in nerve impulse traffic in the afferent fibres to the spinal cord being blocked.

Surface anaesthesia is used on mucous membranes (e.g. the surface of the eye, the airways, oesophagus and urethra) and sometimes the skin. For infiltration anaesthesia, the anaesthetic drug is administered to the tissue to be anaesthetized with the aid of a syringe.

In regional anaesthesia, the anaesthetic is injected into the tissue around a nerve or spinally or epidurally. In spinal anaesthesia, the drug is injected into the sub-arachnoid space, so that it mixes with the cerebrospinal fluid (CSF) and affects the spinal nerve roots. The way in which the anaesthetic is distributed in the spinal canal will determine whether the nerve roots of just a few or many spinal segments are affected. Drug mixtures are used that are denser than CSF. When given to patients who are lying down but tilted at an angle such that the head is above the level of the feet, the drug 'sinks' down in the spinal canal. This prevents the movement of the local anaesthetic 'up' the spinal cord. This ensures that the drug has no effect on the nerves that supply the muscles of ventilation. A hole is opened in the dura mater, so that some of the CSF can be lost from the spinal compartment. Loss of CSF can lead to headaches (spinal headaches). In epidural anaesthesia, the anaesthetic is administered outside the dura. This form of anaesthesia affects fewer spinal segments than spinal anaesthesia, depending on the dose, but is technically more difficult to carry out than spinal anaesthesia. See Figure 25.2.

Regional intravenous anaesthesia is a technique where the anaesthetic is injected intravenously into an area that has been exsanguinated (i.e. from which blood has been removed) and closed off with a tourniquet. The drug distributes itself in the blood vessels of the isolated region. The tourniquet prevents the drug from leaving the area. After a while, the drug diffuses out of the blood vessels and is distributed to the tissues of the isolated region.

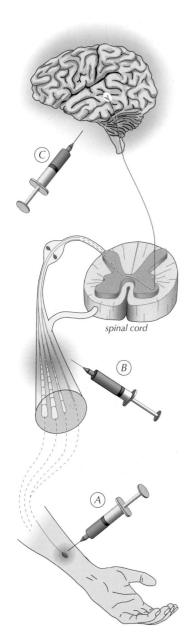

spinal cord

Figure 25.1 **Different forms of anaesthesia.** (A) infiltration anaesthesia; (B) conduction anaesthesia; (C) general anaesthesia.

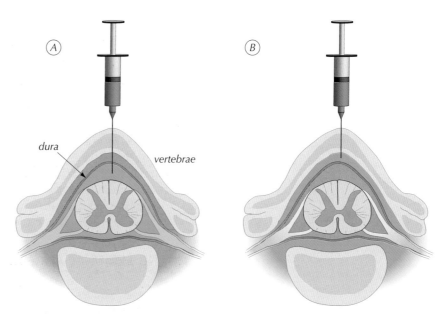

dura

vertebrae

Figure 25.2 **Spinal and epidural anaesthesia.**

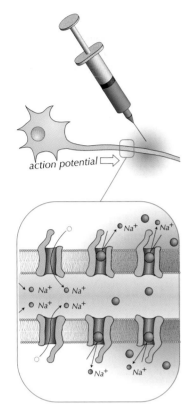

Local and regional anaesthesia is used in minor surgical interventions and when a greater risk is posed with the use of general anaesthetics, e.g. in elderly persons with heart or lung disease.

Patients who undergo major surgical interventions with the use of local anaesthetics should fast prior to the surgery. This is because complications may arise that make general anaesthesia and artificial ventilation necessary. The patient should not have stomach contents that can be aspirated and enter the airways.

LOCAL ANAESTHETICS

The most widely used local anaesthetics are lidocaine, bupivacaine and prilocaine. Different local anaesthetics differ from each other in terms of potency, duration of action, toxicity and their ability to penetrate mucous membranes.

Mechanism of action and effects. Local anaesthetics diffuse into neurons and block Na^+ channels so that Na^+ ions cannot flow across the neuronal membrane and transmission of action potentials is inhibited. See Figure 25.3. Blockade of Na^+ channels is reversible. When local anaesthetics diffuse out of the neuron, the ability to conduct action potentials is regained.

All neurons are sensitive to local anaesthetics, but generally neurons of a small diameter are more sensitive than larger diameter neurons, and unmyelinated neurons are more sensitive than those that are myelinated. This property can be exploited to create a differential block, which primarily affects nociceptive and autonomic neurons. Modalities such as movement and touch can be unaffected, but with increasing doses, these neurons are also affected. See Figure 25.4.

Local anaesthetics block action potentials most effectively in neurons that conduct action potentials at a high frequency. This means that they have their greatest effect when the action potential frequency increases. This explains the antiarrhythmic effect of lidocaine when used in the hyperexcitable state of ventricular fibrillation.

Figure 25.3 **Local anaesthetics** act by blocking sodium channels.

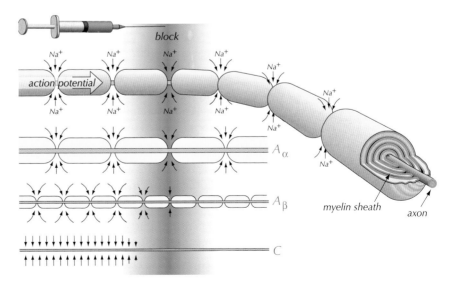

Figure 25.4 **A differential block** acts by blocking sodium channels, primarily in neurons with the smallest diameter.

Onset and duration of action are dependent on how close to a nerve the drug is deposited and how large a dose is used. The onset is shortest for procaine, and is increasingly longer for (in this order) mepivacaine, lidocaine, ropivacaine and bupivacaine. The duration of action is shortest for lidocaine, longer for prilocaine/mepivacaine and longest for ropivacaine/bupivacaine.

Pharmacokinetics. Local anaesthetics diffuse into mucous membranes and affect nociceptive neurons. Keratinized tissue, e.g. skin, acts as an effective barrier for the absorption of local anaesthetics. For minor surgical procedures on the skin, local anaesthetics may be administered in a cream (e.g. EMLA cream), which in turn is covered by a dressing that prevents fluid loss. The skin 'softens up' and the drug diffuses into the neurons.

The majority of local anaesthetics are weak bases that exist in an ionized form at physiological pH. In infiltration anaesthesia, they are distributed to nerves in an un-ionized, lipophilic form, but bind to the Na^+ channel in their ionized form. Local anaesthetics can also reach their target site in the ion channel via the ion channel itself in uncharged form. In local infection, the pH will often be low in the infected tissue, which results in an increased degree of ionization of local anaesthetics and thereby reduced diffusion into the nerves. This is a significant reason why local anaesthetics have a reduced effect in tooth root infection.

Drugs intended for local anaesthesia or infiltration anaesthesia are usually combined with a vasoconstrictor (e.g. adrenaline). This prolongs the duration of action in that the blood vessels in the anaesthetized area constrict, so that the blood flowing through the area does not rapidly remove, i.e. wash away, the anaesthetic that is deposited in the tissue.

Adverse effects. Absorption after administration of local anaesthetics in a tissue can lead to systemic adverse effects. The most sensitive organs are the central nervous system and the heart. Numbness of the tongue, malaise, tinnitus and slurred speech are signs of central nervous system toxicity. Cardiovascular toxicity manifests itself with myocardial depression and peripheral vasodilation with a drop in blood pressure. Anaphylactic reactions occur but are rare.

Lidocaine is the most commonly used substance when infiltration anaesthesia is needed in minor and brief surgical interventions. The onset is 1–2 min after it is deposited near the nerve. The duration of action is approximately 90 min when used as an infiltration and conduction anaesthetic. It is also used for conduction, spinal and epidural anaesthesia.

Bupivacaine is used extensively for local and regional anaesthesia. The onset is short and duration of action is considerably longer than for lidocaine (up to 8 h) when it is used in nerve blockage. It is also used for epidural and spinal anaesthesia when a long duration of action is required.

Mepivacaine is used for infiltration and conduction anaesthesia. The onset is short and its duration of action lies between that of lidocaine and bupivacaine. It is also used in dental anaesthesia.

Prilocaine is used for surface anaesthesia in the mouth and throat and as infiltration anaesthesia and conduction anaesthesia in dental treatment.

Articaine is used in dental treatment. It has a short onset and duration of action.

Ropivacaine is used for infiltration, conduction and epidural anaesthesia when a long duration of action is required.

Blockade of Na$^+$ channels
Bupivacaine, Lidocaine, Levobupivacaine, Prilocaine, Procaine, Ropivacaine, Tetracaine

Table 25.1　Drugs used for local anaesthesia

GENERAL ANAESTHESIA

Under general anaesthesia, patients are unconscious, pain-free and will not remember what happened while they were anaesthetized. It may also be necessary to paralyse skeletal muscles and to suppress coughing, vomiting, laryngeal spasms and mucus secretion. Increased mucus secretion is the result of physiological reflexes arising from the insertion of an endotracheal tube which is used in anaesthesia when the ventilatory muscles are paralysed.

General anaesthetics are administered via inhaled air or intravenously, and so are termed inhalation anaesthetics and intravenous anaesthetics. See Figure 25.5. Different anaesthetics cause different depths of anaesthesia, different degrees of pain relief, reflex suppression and muscular paralysis. The time it takes for effect depends on how rapidly the drug is distributed to the central nervous system.

THE ANAESTHESIA PERIOD

The anaesthesia period is divided into three phases: the induction, the maintenance phase and the recovery phase.

Induction is the period from the initial administration of an anaesthetic until the patient has reached a sufficient level of anaesthesia that the surgical procedure can start. This is a critical phase where the patient is unconscious, but easily aroused by external stimuli, especially sounds. The patient may exhibit restlessness, irregular breathing, unstable blood pressure and abundant eye movements with dilated pupils. In this stage, the blinking and vomiting reflexes are still functional. The environment around the patient should be quiet and no surgery should take place. The induction phase should be as short as possible. Duration of induction depends on how rapidly the anaesthetic is distributed to the central nervous system, which in turn is dependent on the anaesthetic used. Intravenous anaesthetics are primarily used during the induction phase.

The maintenance phase is the period where the surgical intervention takes place and is usually divided into light, medium and deep surgical anaesthesia. Administration of the anaesthetic is controlled, so that the anaesthesia has suitable 'depth'. This is checked, for example, by examining the eye reflexes. In surgical anaesthesia, the pupil has a normal opening, but the blink reflex cannot be triggered by touching the eyelashes. The length of the maintenance phase depends on the surgery that is being performed. If the anaesthesia is too deep, the patient goes into a paralytic stage with loss of respiratory and circulatory function.

The recovery phase lasts from the time the administration of the anaesthetic stops until the patient is awake. The duration depends on how rapidly the anaesthetic is redistributed from the central nervous system to the blood and is removed. How long the recovery phase lasts is, as with the induction, dependent on which anaesthetic is used. During the recovery, the patient passes through the same stages as during the induction, but in reverse order.

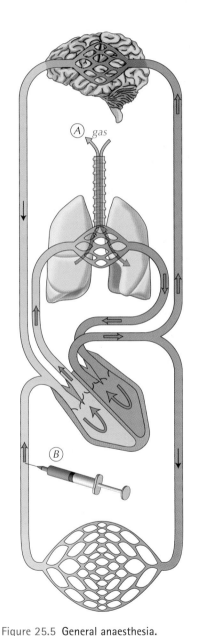

Figure 25.5 **General anaesthesia.**
(A) Inhalation anaesthetics diffuse from the alveolar compartment to the blood and are carried to the central nervous system.
(B) Intravenous anaesthetics are administered directly into the blood.

Mechanism of action of general anaesthetics

The precise mechanism of action of general anaesthetics is unclear, but several possibilities have been proposed. They may:

- alter the presynaptic release of neurotransmitter
- alter the removal of neurotransmitters from synapses
- alter the binding ratio of neurotransmitters to receptors
- alter postsynaptic events after the neurotransmitter has bound.

Whichever mechanism is operating, the final effect is a reduction or loss of consciousness, reduced response to sensory stimuli (especially pain) and reduced muscle tone.

INHALATION ANAESTHETICS

Inhalation anaesthetics are stored in liquid form, but administered to the patient in gas or vapour form in inhaled air. They are used primarily during the maintenance phase of the anaesthesia period, as the depth of the anaesthesia can be rapidly changed by varying the concentration in the inhaled air. Inhalation anaesthetics are the most widely used anaesthetic drugs in modern anaesthesia. Halogenated hydrocarbons (desflurane, isoflurane and sevoflurane) and nitrous oxide belong to this group. Previously used anaesthetic agents include ether (no longer used because of the danger of explosion), halothane (no longer used because of the risk of hepatocytic necrosis) and enflurane (replaced by similar substances with fewer adverse effects).

Desflurane, isoflurane and sevoflurane all provide total anaesthesia with unconsciousness, analgesia, reflex suppression and muscle relaxation. Achieving these effects, however, requires deep anaesthesia, with an increased risk of adverse effects. It is common to produce a lighter anaesthesia with these drugs and to administer separate analgesics and muscle relaxants. With the use of muscle relaxants, ventilation can be affected long after administration of the drug is stopped.

Pharmacokinetics of inhalation anaesthetics. Inhalation anaesthetics are mixed in the inhaled air and reach the alveoli. The less soluble the gas is in blood in relation to alveolar gas, the faster the blood is saturated. See Figure 25.6.

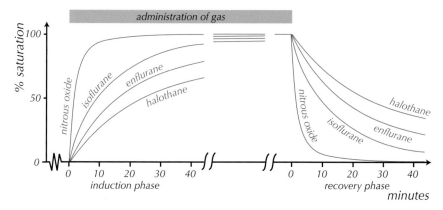

Figure 25.6 **Inhalation anaesthetics**. Saturation of inhaled gases in alveolar blood for some inhalation anaesthetics. Low solubility produces rapid saturation in the blood and rapid elimination when the anaesthetic is stopped. Nitrous oxide has the lowest solubility, while halothane has the highest solubility.

When the blood is saturated with anaesthetic gas, it diffuses to other tissue. The diffusion occurs most rapidly to tissue which has a rich blood supply. This is why high concentrations are rapidly achieved in the central nervous system. The higher the solubility of the gas in fat (the brain has considerable amounts of fatty tissue), the longer it takes for its removal from the central nervous system after anaesthesia is stopped. The depth of anaesthesia is regulated by varying how much anaesthetic is added to inhaled air. It is common to administer a combination of halogenated hydrocarbons and nitrous oxide in a mixture of air or oxygen.

Nitrous oxide has a very low solubility in blood and is the fastest acting of all inhalation anaesthetics. Since it also has low lipid solubility, it is rapidly redistributed back to the alveolar compartment when its administration is stopped and is thus rapidly removed with the exhaled air. Nitrous oxide is used in childbirth because of its rapid onset and termination of effect. Patients control the intake themselves. The effect of halogenated hydrocarbons has a slower onset than that of nitrous oxide.

By removing anaesthetic gas from the inhaled air, the gases are rapidly eliminated from tissues via the exhaled air.

Adverse effect profile of inhalation anaesthetics. Halogenated hydrocarbons cause a dose-dependent fall in arterial blood pressure, associated with peripheral vasodilation, while heart rate is increased. The drugs can cause malignant hyperthermia (see p. 388). Inhalation anaesthetics cause cerebral vasodilation leading to increased intracranial pressure.

Desflurane is not arrhythmogenic and does not lead to adverse redistribution of blood from poorly perfused areas to better perfused regions in the heart, but it does have an irritating effect on the respiratory passages.

Isoflurane is not arrhythmogenic but can lead to the adverse redistribution of blood from poorly perfused areas to better perfused regions in the heart. This is termed coronary steal syndrome, i.e. blood is 'stolen' from poorly perfused regions. Therefore there is an increased risk of myocardial infarction during the anaesthetic. A simultaneous fall in the blood pressure increases the risk even further.

Sevoflurane is not arrhythmogenic and does not lead to coronary steal syndrome. It does not cause irritation in the respiratory passages. Rapid distribution to the central nervous system makes it possible to induce anaesthesia with sevoflurane.

Nitrous oxide (N_2O) is a gas that produces rapid, light anaesthesia and rapid recovery. The gas does not have a respiratory depressant effect or a muscle-relaxing effect. A mild rise in blood pressure is associated with a sympathomimetic effect. Nitrous oxide has good analgesic properties but does not provide sufficient analgesia to be used as a general anaesthetic alone. It is therefore combined with other drugs in larger surgical interventions.

INTRAVENOUS ANAESTHETICS

All intravenous anaesthetics have a short duration of onset. There are differences in their ability to produce sleep, pain relief, reflex suppression and muscle relaxation. They are mainly used with other drugs for brief narcosis and induction of general anaesthesia. All the drugs are eliminated via the liver or kidneys, as they do not exist in gas form and cannot therefore be eliminated via pulmonary ventilation. Their elimination occurs slowly compared with inhalation anaesthetics.

Large doses therefore have a long-lasting effect even when the anaesthetic is stopped. Intravenous anaesthetics include barbiturates, propofol and ketamine.

Thiopental is a barbiturate with a good sleep-inducing effect, but without analgesic properties. It acts briefly and is distributed rapidly to the central nervous system. Recovery is swift because the drug is redistributed rapidly from the brain to the blood and other tissue. To maintain barbiturate anaesthesia, constant supplementary doses must be administered. The tissue depots will gradually become saturated and produce a long-lasting effect. The barbiturates are primarily used for short periods of anaesthesia and induction of longer periods of anaesthesia that are subsequently maintained with inhalation anaesthetics. Thiopental has anticonvulsive effects. In combination with analgesics, the amount of thiopental required to maintain anaesthesia is reduced. Thiopental produces a fall in blood pressure and transitory respiratory depression that can develop into respiratory failure, especially when administered by rapid injection. The substance is alkaline and toxic to tissues if it is administered extravasally or intra-arterially.

Propofol has a rapid onset of its sleep-inducing effect, and possesses properties similar to thiopental. It is used together with analgesics for sedation in local and regional anaesthesia and in some diagnostic procedures in patients over 3 years of age. It is quickly metabolized and produces little nausea. A fall in blood pressure and transitory respiratory depression are common during induction with this drug. Ventilation must be closely monitored.

Ketamine is an anaesthetic that produces light sleep where the patient appears to be awake, but distant – so-called dissociative anaesthesia. It has a pronounced analgesic effect, but does not produce muscle relaxation. The tendency for a fall in blood pressure and respiratory inhibition is small. In the recovery phase, there are hallucinations and unpleasant dreams. These can be reduced by administration of a benzodiazepine and by allowing the patient to wake in a quiet room with subdued lighting.

Neuroleptic anaesthesia

Neuroleptic anaesthesia requires a combination of several drugs that together produce full anaesthesia. A potent neuroleptic (usually droperidol) which makes the patient sleep, together with nitrous oxide, results in sedation of the patient, who is also given a strong-acting analgesic (usually fentanyl) and a muscle relaxant (usually pancuronium). This is an anaesthetic regime that was once much used in major surgery. It is used far less frequently today. When this form of anaesthesia is used now, droperidol is often replaced by a benzodiazepine.

Benzodiazepines are used as premedication, orally or rectally, for both children and adults. Strong-acting opioids are used with general anaesthetics to enhance their analgesic effect.

Drugs used in general anaesthesia are listed in Table 25.2.

Inhalation general anaesthetics
Desflurane, Enflurane, Isoflurane, Nitrous oxide, Sevoflurane

Intravenous general anaesthetics
Etomidate, Ketamine, Propofol, Thiopental

Opioid analgesics in general anaesthetics
Alfentanil, Fentanyl, Remifentanil

Table 25.2 Drugs used in general anaesthesia

PERIPHERAL-ACTING MUSCLE RELAXANTS

In thoracic, abdominal and major orthopaedic surgery, it is essential to relax muscles so that the surgeon can reach the operation site. In neurosurgery and surgery involving the inner ear or the eye, it is equally important to relax muscles to prevent the patient from moving or coughing during the surgery.

The drugs that are used to produce this relaxation interfere with the actions of acetylcholine between motor neurons and skeletal muscle. They are therefore called peripheral-acting muscle relaxants or neuromuscular blockers. See Figure 25.7.

Action potentials in motor neurons result in the release of acetylcholine. The binding of acetylcholine to its receptors in skeletal muscle cells triggers a depolarization and contraction. If many muscle cells are stimulated simultaneously, the entire muscle contracts and produces a coordinated movement. If the stimulation is uncoordinated, then small contractions (fasciculations) occur in different places in the same muscle. See Figure 25.8.

There are two main types of peripheral-acting muscle relaxants: non-depolarizing and depolarizing. Non-depolarizing muscle relaxants block the muscle without first causing depolarization, while depolarizing muscle relaxants first depolarize the muscle cells and thereafter block further impulse transmission. With the use of both of these drug groups, all ventilatory muscles are paralysed. Assisted ventilation is therefore necessary.

Depolarizing and non-depolarizing drugs block nicotine receptors in skeletal muscle but not in autonomic ganglia. Muscarinic receptors are not affected. The drugs therefore produce few effects in the sympathetic and parasympathetic nervous systems.

NON-DEPOLARIZING MUSCLE RELAXANTS

Non-depolarizing muscle relaxants prevent depolarization of the muscle in that the drugs compete with acetylcholine in binding to nicotinic receptors. The drugs themselves do not have stimulating properties and there is no muscle contraction. Different drugs have different onset and duration of action. Atracurium and cisatracurium are metabolized by enzymes in the synaptic cleft and the blood, while others are dependent on hepatic and renal elimination.

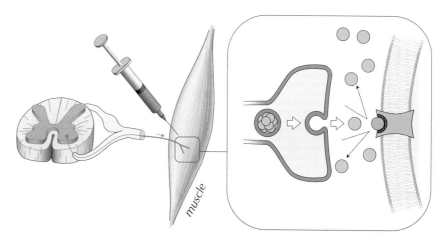

Figure 25.7 **Peripheral-acting muscle relaxants** affect receptors in the motor end-plate.

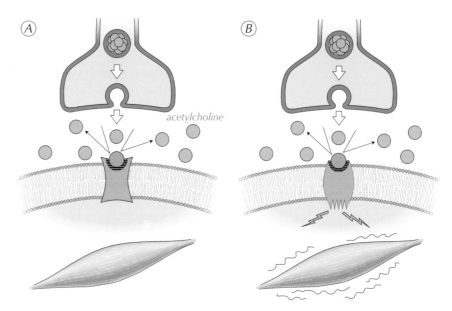

Figure 25.8 **Peripheral muscle relaxants.** (A) Non-depolarizing muscle relaxants relax muscles without causing depolarization. (B) Depolarizing muscle relaxants trigger a muscular depolarization before the muscles become relaxed.

DEPOLARIZING MUSCLE RELAXANTS

Depolarizing muscle relaxants bind strongly to nicotinic receptors on the muscle cells. The binding results in depolarization of the muscle cells. Continued depolarization of the membrane prevents repolarization and the repeated depolarizations that are necessary to stimulate the muscle cell to contract. With that, the muscle relaxes. Since the drug does not reach all the receptors simultaneously, different cells depolarize in a muscle at different times. Fasciculations are seen in skeletal muscle, but not coordinated muscle contractions.

Suxamethonium is the only drug in this group. It is not metabolized by acetylcholinesterase but rather by pseudocholinesterase, which is found in plasma and the liver. Suxamethonium remains in the synapse for a long time, and its effect lasts until the majority of it has been metabolized.

Depolarization and the temporary increase in muscle tone can cause temporary but undesired increases in pressure intracranially, intraocularly and intra-abdominally. Continued depolarization causes a leakage of potassium out of the muscle cells and contributes to hyperkalaemia. Suxamethonium can cause different arrhythmias, the risk of which is increased with concurrent hyperkalaemia.

Suxamethonium is the fastest acting muscle relaxant. It is particularly useful when there is an acute need for intubation. It is also suitable for use in Caesarean sections, as it does not cross the blood–placenta barrier and thus does not affect the fetus' respiration.

REVERSAL OF NEUROMUSCULAR BLOCKADE AND INHIBITION OF RESPIRATION

At the conclusion of a surgical intervention in which muscle relaxants are used or where there is a pronounced inhibition of ventilation by opiate analgesics, it is vital

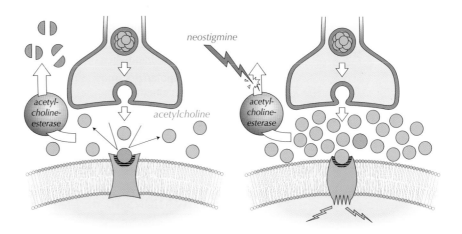

Figure 25.9 **Reversal of non-depolarizing muscle relaxants.** Neostigmine inhibits cholinesterase and contributes to an increase in the concentration of acetylcholine in the synapse.

for the patient to resume spontaneous ventilation. It is common to adapt the dosage so that the effects of these drugs are diminished at the end of the surgery. If inhibition of ventilation is pronounced at the conclusion of the period of anaesthesia, drugs may be used that reverse the paralysis of the ventilatory muscles.

Cholinesterase inhibitors

Muscle relaxation caused by non-depolarizing drugs can be reversed by increasing the concentration of acetylcholine in the synaptic cleft. This can be done by blocking its breakdown. This is achieved by using drugs which inhibit acetylcholinesterase, the enzyme which breaks down acetylcholine, i.e. cholinesterase inhibitors. See Figure 25.9.

Neostigmine is an example of a cholinesterase inhibitor. The elimination of neostigmine can occur more rapidly than the elimination of some non-depolarizing drugs, particularly if they are at high concentration at the end of the anaesthetic. It is important to observe if ventilatory depression returns. Neostigmine will also increase the concentration of acetylcholine at effector organs in the parasympathetic nervous system. This results in increased parasympathetic stimulation with increased mucus secretion and bradycardia. These effects can be avoided by administering a small dose of atropine or glycopyrronium, which inhibit the effect of acetylcholine at muscarinic receptors. The depolarizing drug suxamethonium cannot be reversed by increasing the levels of acetylcholine, as it has a long-lasting binding to the nicotinic receptors. Cholinesterase inhibitors cannot be used as an antidote. The effect of the drug disappears with diminishing concentration. It is important that the concentration of suxamethonium is not high at the end of the anaesthesia period. If the patient is still affected after the surgery is completed, artificial ventilation must be maintained until the effect stops. Opiates cause inhibition of ventilation by reducing the respiratory centre's sensitivity to elevated levels of carbon dioxide and reduced levels of oxygen in the blood. Naloxone is an opioid antagonist that reverses the effect of opioid analgesics.

Drugs acting at the neuromuscular junction used in anaesthesia are listed in Table 25.3.

Non–depolarizing muscle relaxants
Atracurium, Cistracurium, Gallamine, Mivacurium, Pancuronium, Rocuronium, Vercuronium

Depolarizing muscle relaxants
Suxemethonium

Cholinesterase inhibitors
Edrophonium, Neostigmine

Table 25.3 Drugs acting at the neuromuscular junction used in anaesthesia

OBSERVATIONS TO BE MADE DURING ANAESTHESIA

Circulatory collapse, ventilatory collapse and malignant hyperthermia are life-threatening adverse effects that can be caused by drugs used during anaesthesia. In addition, it is necessary to look out for insufficient analgesia, as the patient is unable to signal this if muscle relaxants are used. Postoperative nausea can be pronounced.

REDUCED CIRCULATION

Changes in blood pressure and peripheral circulation must be carefully monitored during the period of anaesthesia. All drugs that produce deep sleep reduce activity in the sympathetic nervous system and therefore the release of catecholamines. This results in peripheral vasodilation and bradycardia. Some anaesthetic drugs also have a direct vasodilating effect and can release histamine, which further enhances the vasodilatory effect. Several anaesthetics have cardiodepressive and arrhythmogenic effects. Insertion of a tracheal tube and the surgical intervention itself can also influence the circulation. Together these effects can cause serious circulatory disturbances. Patients with heart problems are particularly susceptible to complications. Epidural and spinal anaesthesia can cause a large fall in blood pressure, in that efferent impulses in sympathetic nerves are inhibited, resulting in vasodilation.

REDUCED VENTILATION

Ventilation rate and depth must be monitored from the time induction starts throughout the entire anaesthesia period. The possibility of a need for assisted ventilation is always present. Many of the drugs used in anaesthesia cause reduced ventilation. Rapid superficial ventilation produces a reduced tidal volume, resulting in an accumulation of carbon dioxide and a reduction in oxygen concentration. Opioids cause reduced ventilation. Muscle relaxants cause paralysis of the ventilatory muscles. Laryngeal spasms may cause contraction of the vocal cords and this may cause ventilatory failure. If the patient is not intubated, it is important to ensure that the tongue does not fall back and block the airways. Aspiration of stomach contents represents a risk in vomiting patients.

MALIGNANT HYPERTHERMIA

Malignant hyperthermia is an acute and life-threatening complication that can appear both during, and in the first 24 h after an anaesthetic. The risk increases with the simultaneous use of the depolarizing muscle relaxant suxamethonium. The cause of the rise in temperature is acute hypermetabolism in skeletal muscles and excessive heat development. Other accompanying symptoms are increased heart rate, cyanosis, rising blood pressure and muscle stiffness. If malignant hyperthermia is suspected, the anaesthetic must be stopped immediately and the patient hyperventilated with 100 per cent oxygen. Specific treatment consists of administering dantrolene, which has a muscle-relaxing effect by inhibiting the release of calcium from the sarcoplasmic reticulum in muscle cells.

SUMMARY

■ Local anaesthesia includes surface anaesthesia, infiltration anaesthesia and blockade of peripheral nerves to small tissue areas. Regional anaesthesia includes blockade of nerves which serve larger tissue areas, regional intravenous anaesthesia, spinal and epidural anaesthesia. In these forms of anaesthesia, local anaesthetics are used that act by blocking Na^+ channels so that afferent pain impulses are inhibited. Adding adrenaline to the local anaesthetic gives a longer duration of action because the blood flow through the tissue is reduced.

■ General anaesthesia should produce sleep, analgesia and suppression of adverse reflexes. Muscle relaxation is necessary for some surgical procedures. No single anaesthetic produces all these effects alone without some of the effects being undesirably potent.

■ The anaesthetic period is divided into three phases: induction phase, maintenance phase and the recovery phase.

■ General anaesthetics are divided into inhalation anaesthetics and intravenous anaesthetics. Both groups have unknown mechanisms of action. Inhalation anaesthetics are administered to the patient in gas or vapour form. The drugs diffuse to the central nervous system from the inhaled air via the blood. Drugs with low solubility in blood have a rapid onset. Inhalation anaesthetics are primarily used for maintenance anaesthesia.

■ Intravenous anaesthetics act more rapidly than inhalation anaesthetics. They are often used during the induction phase, followed by the use of inhalation anaesthetics in lengthy surgical procedures.

■ Some anaesthetics lack a good analgesic effect, so that the administration of separate analgesics may be needed.

■ Peripheral-acting muscle relaxants are divided into two groups: non-depolarizing and depolarizing muscle relaxants. The former compete with acetylcholine for nicotinic receptors at the motor end-plate in skeletal muscles, without causing muscular depolarization. The result is relaxed muscles. The effect can be reversed by increasing the concentration of acetylcholine in the synapse. Cholinesterase inhibitors have such an effect. Depolarizing muscle relaxants bind to receptors in the motor end-plate and block further neuromuscular impulse traffic after an initial depolarization. The effect of such drugs cannot be reversed with cholinesterase inhibitors, but gradually disappears after the drug is eliminated.

■ The most serious adverse effects under anaesthesia are circulatory collapse, ventilatory collapse and malignant hyperthermia.

SECTION IV: DRUG USE IN SPECIAL SITUATIONS

26 The use of drugs during pregnancy and the breastfeeding period

The growth and development of a fetus are dependent on substances that are supplied via umbilical cord blood. If the mother receives drugs, fetal development can be affected, because the physiological processes in the mother may be altered and because the drug is distributed to the fetus as well. The risk and nature of harm that may occur will vary with the type of drug, duration of use, and dose.

To decide whether a pregnant woman should be given a drug or not, three factors should be evaluated:

- the risk to the mother of not using the drug
- the risk to the child if the mother's illness is not treated
- the risk to the child if the mother uses the drug.

During pregnancy it is best to avoid the use of drugs if possible. If a pregnant woman needs treatment involving drugs, then drugs with well documented properties should be used and the smallest effective dose administered.

PHYSIOLOGICAL CHANGES IN THE MOTHER DURING PREGNANCY AND THE NEED FOR MODIFIED DOSING

The majority of physiological changes that happen in the mother favour fetal development. Some changes may affect the distribution and elimination of drugs. Since most drugs have an adequate safety margin, the dosage is seldom changed during pregnancy.

Reduction in the concentration of plasma proteins

Plasma protein concentration in the mother, especially albumin, falls during pregnancy. Drugs with a high level of binding to albumin will be bound to a lesser extent, so the total drug concentration (free plus bound) is less. However, the concentration of free (active) drug will be slightly altered. If the percentage of free drug were to increase considerably with the possibility of adverse effects in the mother and harm to the fetus, for drugs with a high degree of binding to plasma proteins it may be important to modify the dosage according to the concentration of free drug present.

Increased metabolic activity in the liver

Enzyme activity in the maternal liver can increase during the last stage of pregnancy. This can result in faster elimination of lipid-soluble drugs (altered by metabolism), and the dose needs to be increased to maintain therapeutic concentration (this is particularly true for antiepileptic drugs). In addition to the effect of simultaneously reduced albumin concentration, the need for good control is increased.

Increased renal blood flow and the percentage of water in the body

During pregnancy, the body weight increases because the percentage of extracellular water increases. At the same time, the renal blood flow and glomerular filtration increase to almost twice normal rates. Usually, during pregnancy, there is no need to adjust the dosage for drugs that are eliminated via the kidneys. An important exception, however, is the penicillin group. These drugs are eliminated quickly via the kidneys because of increased renal blood flow. The dose should be increased to maintain a drug concentration that provides sufficient bactericidal effect in cases of serious infection.

CAUSES OF FETAL HARM

Approximately 70 per cent of fetal harm has an unknown cause. It is estimated that environmental effects account for fewer than 5 per cent of all fetal effects. These consist of physical factors such as ionizing radiation, biological factors such as German measles, malaria, nutrition and lifestyle, and chemical factors such as drugs, chemicals, gases and intoxicating substances.

Drugs that cause developmental defects to a fetus are said to have a teratogenic effect. When drugs cause defects to the gene material, and the defect can be transmitted to new generations of cells, the drug is said to have a mutagenic effect.

In principle, there are two ways in which a fetus can be damaged when the mother is exposed to dangerous substances:

- Via an *indirect effect*, whereby the fetus is not affected directly by drugs or other harmful substances. Often the mother's circulation is altered in such a way that fetal nutrition and oxygenation are reduced. Damage is most pronounced in tissue that has a high metabolic rate and in tissue that is in the differentiation phase when the effect occurs.

■ Via a *direct effect*, where the harmful substance reaches the fetus's tissue and affects development.

Damage from both indirect and direct effects can occur throughout the entire pregnancy but is most pronounced during organogenesis (formation of organs).

CONDITIONS FOR FETAL INJURY

Fetal and maternal blood are separated by the placental barrier. This anatomical and physiological barrier, to a certain degree, selectively allows the passage of substances between the mother and the fetus, and reduces the possibility of damage. Drugs reach fetal blood primarily by passive diffusion across the placental barrier. The concentration of drugs in the mother's blood is therefore crucial for transport.

If the placental barrier slows the diffusion of a drug, then the longer the duration of the drug in the maternal circulation, the more likely it is that eventually some of the drug will enter the fetal circulation. Similarly, if a drug is used continuously over a long period of time, then there is enough time for it to be distributed to the fetus, with the potential to cause harm. Conversely, if a drug is metabolized or eliminated rapidly from maternal blood then any effect is minimized, as far less drug is likely to enter the fetal circulation.

The earliest cell divisions, after an egg cell and a sperm cell have fused, give rise to many identical cells. Gradually, the cells will develop into different organs and organ systems. During this phase, the cells differentiate and development continues by continuous new cell division and organ formation. The period of formation of the organs is called organogenesis (*genesis* = 'origin'). The cells differentiate at different points in time, and development and maturation of different organs occur at different times. See Figure 26.1.

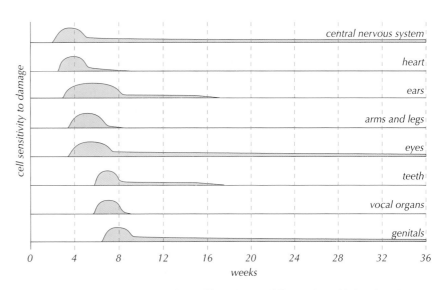

Figure 26.1 **Organ development.** Cells differentiate at different times. Notice that the central nervous system, the eyes and genitals have a long 'maturation period'. If damage occurs during this period, the chances of structural defects are greater. If the damage occurs during the maturation period, there is an increased chance of functional defects.

When the organs are formed, cell division will stop in some tissues. Further growth occurs by each cell growing and maturing, e.g. in muscle and fatty tissue. In other tissue, such as bone marrow, lymphatic tissue, cartilage, skin and mucous membranes, cell division will continue throughout the entire pregnancy and after birth.

SENSITIVITY OF CELLS TO DAMAGE

During the division phase, the cells can be affected to varying degrees depending on which stage they are at, and what affects them. For this reason, certain drugs will be more dangerous at certain times. For example, the extremities are formed between the 26th and 28th day after conception. Teratogenic effects during this time can result in structural deformities. Pregnant women who used thalidomide between the 23rd and 38th day after conception gave birth to children with defects in a high number of cases. Even a single tablet taken at a vulnerable point in time can cause a great risk of damage. Cells that form the extremities are thus very sensitive to thalidomide during the period of differentiation. The thalidomide disaster is described in Chapter 1, p. 4.

DEVELOPMENT OF NEW DRUGS

When evaluating whether the use of drugs represents a risk in pregnant women, it is important to ascertain which drug is involved, the dose and the time of use during pregnancy.

TYPES OF FETAL INJURY

The earlier in pregnancy a harmful effect occurs, the greater the potential for damage. Development is usually described in terms of the events of the first, second and third trimesters. However, this is only a rough guide that may not always be suitable when considering which periods demonstrate the greatest sensitivity to damage.

Fetal injuries can be divided into four types, which are described below.

Fetal death and miscarriage
Fetal death can occur at any time, but generally occurs early in pregnancy. Massive exposure to toxic agents immediately after conception, before the fertilized egg is implanted, usually results in a miscarriage. Similarly, harmful effects in the period from the second to third week after conception, when the cells are only slightly differentiated, often cause such fundamental damage that the fetus is aborted – an 'all or nothing' effect.

Structural injury
Active organ differentiation occurs in the third to 11th fetal week. Damage during this phase can lead to structural deformities, whereby the form and structure of the organs become abnormal. Typical examples of deformities are lack of closing of the membranes and vertebrae of the spinal cord (spina bifida), clubfoot and deformities of the urogenital tract.

Functional injury
Functional disturbances are said to occur when an organ or a body part is not functioning normally. During the eighth to 12th fetal week and beyond, the maturation of the differentiated structures dominates and the organs' functions are

developed. Fetal injuries during this period are often of a functional nature in consequence. Structural damage can also result in reduced function, such as deformed limbs or structural changes in the heart that produce pathology of the circulatory system.

The structural and physiological maturation of the central nervous system, kidneys and liver, and the development of a number of endocrine glands, continues for several months after birth. Functional disturbances are often discovered after birth.

Retardation of growth

Retardation of growth can occur throughout pregnancy, but is most common during the second and third trimesters and is often the result of poor nutrition associated with poor blood supply to the placenta. Body weight can be restored to within the appropriate range, but in some cases the concomitant intrauterine growth retardation or functional disturbances can affect the child for a long time, possibly even a lifetime. Retardation of growth can also give rise to functional injuries.

USE OF DRUGS DURING PREGNANCY

Untreated chronic illness and a number of acute illnesses in a pregnant woman can be a greater threat to fetal development than the adverse effects associated with any drug treatment. Where drug treatment is required, the lowest effective dose of a drug whose effects in pregnancy are well known should be used for preference. Chronic illnesses should be monitored by a specialist during pregnancy. This is particularly true for women with hypertension, kidney disease, diabetes mellitus and epilepsy. In addition, women with drug and/or alcohol problems should be encouraged to stop, or at the very least, reduce their use of intoxicating substances, as drug/alcohol abuse has harmful effects on the fetus.

The most commonly used drugs in pregnancy are analgesics, antiemetics, antibiotics and antiepileptics, as well as antihypertensive drugs towards the end of the pregnancy.

ANALGESIC AND ANTI-INFLAMMATORY DRUGS

Paracetamol is regarded as a relatively safe drug during pregnancy and should be the first choice of preparation when analgesics for light to moderate pain are required. Use of aspirin and other non-steroidal anti-inflammatory drugs (NSAIDs) towards the end of the pregnancy can cause intrauterine closing of the ductus arteriosus as a result of inhibiting prostaglandin synthesis, particularly prostaglandin E_1, which normally maintains the patency of this blood vessel. See Figure 26.2. As these drugs inhibit the aggregation of blood platelets, they have the potential to cause haemorrhage in a fetus that may have suffered mechanical trauma during parturition.

ANTIEMETIC DRUGS

Many pregnant women experience nausea during the first part of the pregnancy, but only a few will need drugs to counteract the problem. Where the problem persists and is accompanied by vomiting and weight loss, it may be necessary to take antiemetics. Antihistamines have long been used by pregnant women troubled by nausea. While there is no reason to suppose that antihistamines are harmful to the fetus, caution is recommended with the use of the newer antihistamines.

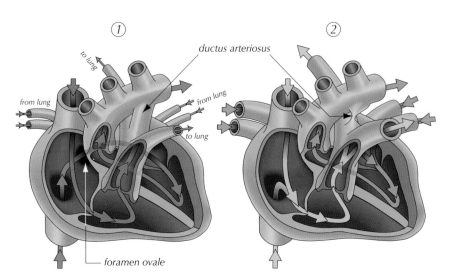

Figure 26.2 **The ductus arteriosus** is a fetal blood vessel between the aorta and the pulmonary artery. This vessel allows the blood to pass from the right ventricle to the aorta (1), which is necessary because the pulmonary vascular bed cannot receive the blood flow while the lungs are empty of air and compressed. If the ductus arteriosus is closed before the child is born, pulmonary hypertension will develop. The ductus arteriosus is normally closed immediately after birth (2) and the blood flow to the lungs increases. The use of non-steroidal anti-inflammatory drugs (NSAIDs) towards the end of the pregnancy can cause the ductus arteriosus to be closed prematurely.

ANTIMICROBIAL DRUGS

Infections occur just as frequently during pregnancy as at any other time, but the incidence of bacterial urinary tract infections and fungal infections may be increased. Penicillins, erythromycins and cephalosporins are regarded as safe antibiotics during pregnancy. Pivmecillinam and pivampicillin should not be used during pregnancy, as these drugs may result in the depletion of carnitine (a B vitamin) with the risk of fetal damage.

Sulphonamides aminoglycosides, tetracyclines and chloramphenicol should only be used if essential for treatment. Sulphonamides should not be administered during the last trimester of pregnancy, since sulphonamides compete with bilirubin for the binding to albumin in the fetal circulation and displace the bilirubin. Trimethoprim should be avoided during pregnancy as the drug inhibits the metabolism of folic acid in the fetus. Folic acid is necessary for growth and maturation of all cells, and its deficiency can lead to structural injuries, such as neural tube defects. Aminoglycosides can damage the fetus's VIIIth cranial nerve and cause hearing damage. Tetracyclines may accumulate in tooth enamel and cause brown discoloration of the child's teeth. The damage occurs if the drug is used after the mineralization process has started, around the 12th week. It is only the milk teeth that are damaged if the child is only exposed during pregnancy. Chloramphenicol (but not as eye drops that are used for short periods) can cause bone marrow damage in the fetus.

Sulphonamides in late pregnancy and the risk of 'nuclear icterus'
During the fetal life, two types of haemoglobin are found in the fetal circulation (fetal haemoglobin and adult haemoglobin). After the delivery, fetal haemoglobin is quickly broken down to form bilirubin, which is eliminated after conjugation to glucuronic acid. At the time of birth the liver is immature, with a reduced capacity

to conjugate bilirubin, giving rise to a high concentration of non-conjugated bilirubin. Most of the non-conjugated bilirubin is bound to albumin, but some will be free bilirubin. The free bilirubin is distributed to most tissues, including the skin, giving rise to neonatal jaundice.

If the delivery takes place before term, the liver is even more immature than it would be at term, and is less able to conjugate all the bilirubin formed. In this situation the concentration of free bilirubin will be even higher than in births at term, to the extent that there is a risk it will cross the blood–brain barrier and accumulate in the nuclei of the central nervous system (nuclear icterus) which becomes irreversibly damaged.

If the mother takes sulphonamides during late pregnancy and gives birth prematurely, the sulphonamides will be distributed to the fetal circulation and displace the non-conjugated bilirubin from albumin by competition. The use of sulphonamides in late pregnancy therefore represents an increased risk for nuclear icterus in the child.

ANTIEPILEPTIC DRUGS

Children of mothers with epilepsy are reported to have a higher frequency of deformities than children of healthy mothers. Many antiepileptics are teratogenic, even if the causal relation between the use of these drugs and the occurrence of fetal injuries is equivocal. However there is agreement that mothers with epilepsy should be treated during pregnancy, as frequent seizures present a greater risk to the child than drug treatment. When antiepileptics are used during pregnancy, monotherapy is advised, at as low a dose as possible, provided good control of seizure frequency is maintained. This is particularly important during the first trimester of pregnancy.

ANTIHYPERTENSIVE DRUGS

Use of antihypertensive agents during pregnancy can lead to reduced circulation in the placenta and, with that, poor growth and development. Hypotonia (floppy limbs) in the child after birth can be caused by antihypertensive treatment of the mother. Diuretics can result in electrolyte disturbances, and the haematocrit value can increase as a consequence of diuresis. The use of thiazide diuretics may result in neonatal thrombocytopenia. Use of angiotensin-converting enzyme (ACE) inhibitors during the last stage of pregnancy is associated with adverse effects on fetal renal function.

ENDOCRINE DRUGS

Little evidence exists concerning harmful effects to the fetus caused by the oral contraceptive pills that are used today. Use of sex hormones and anabolic steroids have been reported to cause genital deformities, especially in girls.

All pregnant women with diabetes should stop the use of oral antidiabetic agents and be maintained on insulin. Good glycaemic control is vital to reduce the risk of complications, deformities and fetal death. It is important the blood sugar is not elevated as this may lead to large overweight fetuses and increase the likelihood of complications during birth. Drugs such as carbimazole, which reduce the production of thyroid hormones in the mother, can lead to mild hypothyroidism and goitre in the fetus, but this usually subsides after birth.

Corticosteroids may cause slight growth retardation in the fetus. For serious illnesses requiring treatment with glucocorticoids, e.g. asthma, the benefits of treatment outweigh the risk of the illness to the fetus. Inhaled steroids in moderate doses can be used during pregnancy.

ANTICOAGULANT DRUGS

If there is a need for anticoagulant therapy in pregnant women, heparin should be used, although prolonged use should be avoided. Warfarin used during pregnancy can cause congenital malformations with the risk of fetal and neonatal haemorrhage, fetal death and miscarriage.

ANXIOLYTIC, NEUROLEPTIC AND ANTIDEPRESSANT DRUGS

Long-term use and large doses of benzodiazepines can affect the child at birth and cause withdrawal symptoms. Regular use should be avoided (unless needed for seizure control). Their use in late pregnancy may lead to neonatal hypothermia and respiratory depression.

Antipsychotics and antidepressants have been suspected of causing deformities, but no strong evidence exists for this. The use of lithium can cause deformities of the cardiovascular system in the fetus.

CYTOTOXIC AND IMMUNOSUPPRESSIVE DRUGS

Cytotoxic drugs act on cells in the division phase. Naturally this group has harmful effects on the fetus and should be avoided during pregnancy. Indeed, adequate contraception is advised for individuals undergoing therapy with cytotoxic drugs. Women who want to become pregnant after concluding treatment with cytotoxins are recommended to wait at least a year. Fertility is reduced after such treatment, probably because the eggs in the ovaries are affected.

Of the immunosuppressive drugs, azathioprine and ciclosporin a need not be discontinued in pregnant subjects as there is no evidence of teratogenicity; however, premature births and low birthweights have been reported with azathioprine.

USE OF DRUGS DURING BREASTFEEDING

Different drugs achieve different concentrations in the milk. Generally the concentration of drug in the mother's milk is somewhat lower than the concentration in the blood. Children who are nourished through breastfeeding alone can receive 0.5–2.0 per cent of the mother's daily dose. For the majority of drugs, this is such small dose that it is unlikely to injure the child and it is considered desirable that women should breastfeed their child even if they have to use drugs during the breastfeeding period. However, there are some drugs that should be avoided.

DRUGS AFFECTING MILK PRODUCTION AND MILK EJECTION

Oxytocin is a hormone produced in the hypothalamus that stimulates contraction of the myoepithelial cells that surround the ducts, the lactiferous ducts and alveoli, thereby increasing milk ejection. Obstruction of the lactiferous ducts during the breastfeeding period may lead to swollen, inflamed and painful breasts. Careful massage of the breast and the use of oxytocin may aid the ejection of milk in these situations.

High doses of oestrogen may inhibit the production of milk. The use of combined oral contraceptive pills may lead to reduced milk production. If contraception is required during the breastfeeding period, then progestogen-only contraceptives should be used. If the child is fully breastfed (and also fed during the night), the increased secretion of prolactin from the pituitary gland can inhibit ovulation during the first few months after delivery.

In some situations the mother may need to stop the breastfeeding, e.g. after delivery of a stillborn child or if she has to use drugs that will have a toxic effect on the child. Bromocriptine inhibits the secretion of prolactin (necessary for the production of milk) and may be used to terminate the lactation period.

CONCENTRATION OF DRUGS IN MILK

Most drugs have a lower concentration in mother's milk than in blood, but this varies from drug to drug. Some general guidelines apply:

- The higher the concentration of a drug in the mother's blood, the higher the concentration in the milk.
- Milk consists mostly of water, and so water-soluble drugs (those that are eliminated via the kidneys) will be distributed in the milk to a greater degree than lipid-soluble drugs.
- Drugs that bind extensively to plasma proteins (e.g. antiepileptics) will be distributed in the milk to a lesser extent, since proteins in the milk have less ability to bind drugs than proteins in the blood.
- Breast milk is slightly more acidic than blood. Alkaline drugs (e.g. tricyclic antidepressants and antipsychotics) are distributed to a greater extent into acidic tissue compartments than to alkaline tissue compartments, and can have a higher concentration in milk than in blood (the opposite is true for acidic drugs such as aspirin and penicillin).

DRUG EFFECTS ON THE CHILD

Neonates, in particular premature children, will eliminate drugs more slowly than older children and adults. For this reason, both the drug and its metabolites can accumulate during breastfeeding. In this way, a high concentration of a drug, sufficient to affect the child, may be achieved.

Adverse effects of drugs will usually be similar in both the child and the adult. However, it will be difficult to establish whether increased tiredness, listlessness, diarrhoea and/or failure to thrive are due to adverse effects of drugs rather than being caused by something else. It is important to consider whether the behaviour of a child can be ascribed to the effects of drugs that the mother has taken.

Antimicrobials

When antibacterial agents are used, there is a possibility that the intestinal flora of the child may be affected. There may also be allergic reactions. However, the majority of antibiotics tend to be found in low concentration in the mother's milk.

Sulphonamides should be avoided in newborns with jaundice, as they displace bilirubin from plasma proteins and increase the risk of jaundice. Tetracyclines should be avoided because of the danger of brown discoloration of the teeth. The risk is lower during the breastfeeding period than during pregnancy.

Antiepileptic drugs

Treatment of epileptic mothers during the breastfeeding period is usually advised, as during pregnancy. Use of antiepileptics can result in increased tiredness. This is particularly true for ethosuximide and phenobarbital, which are readily distributed to the mother's milk.

Anxiolytic, neuroleptic and antidepressant drugs

Breastfeeding is best avoided when there is extensive use of drugs of addiction which can result in dependence in the child, giving rise to tiredness, listlessness and reduced intake of nutrients.

Antipsychotics and antidepressants are eliminated in very small quantities in mother's milk. Use of low doses of these drugs by the mother can probably be tolerated by the child. However, some women eliminate antidepressants so slowly that even small doses can result in high plasma concentrations. Lithium is found in such high concentration in mother's milk that breastfeeding should be avoided. It is advisable to measure the concentration of such drugs in the blood of breastfeeding mothers in order to evaluate a possible reduction of the dose.

Analgesic drugs

If analgesics are necessary, paracetamol is recommended.

SUMMARY

- The general attitude towards drugs during pregnancy is to reduce or avoid their use.
- Drugs with a narrow therapeutic range and extensive binding to plasma proteins should be closely monitored during pregnancy.
- Fetal death may occur with toxic effects early in the pregnancy. Deformities occur mainly during organogenesis. Functional disturbances occur most readily during the fetal maturation stage. Growth retardation is most common during the two last trimesters of the pregnancy.
- Untreated chronic illness and a number of acute illnesses in a pregnant woman can be of greater threat to fetal development than the adverse effects risked by adequate drug treatment. If drug treatment is started, the lowest dose of a drug whose effects are clearly established should be used.
- NSAIDs, sulphonamides, trimethoprin and ACE-inhibitors should not be used during the last trimester.
- Aminoglycoids, tetracyclines and chloramphenicol should only be used during pregnancy if essential for treatment.
- If needed heparin should be used during pregnancy as an anticoagulant instead of warfarin. Insulin should be used instead of oral hypoglycaemic drugs.
- Lithium should be avoided during pregnancy.
- The majority of drugs are secreted in such small quantities in breast milk that mothers can still breastfeed their children even if they are taking drugs.
- If the mother uses drugs over a prolonged period of time and in large doses, the chance of adverse effects on children who are breastfed is increased.
- The higher the concentration of a drug in the mother's blood, the higher the concentration will be in breast milk.
- Drugs used by the mother can be accumulated in a child who is breastfed.
- Oxytocin increases the ejection reflex of milk by stimulating the myoepithelial cells around the milk ducts and alveoli. Bromocriptine reduces the production of milk by inhibiting the secretion of prolactin.
- Tetracyclines, sulphonamides and lithium should be avoided during the breastfeeding period.
- Key information on drugs that may or may not be used in pregnancy or breastfeeding are listed, respectively, in Appendices 4 and 5 of the *British National Formulary*.

27 Children and drugs

During the first year after birth, humans go through the greatest and fastest physiological changes of their entire life. When children are to be treated with drugs, it is necessary to consider the extent of the child's physiological development and the prevailing pharmacokinetic and pharmacodynamic conditions that apply. These considerations are important to ensure that the correct drug is chosen and its formulation, method of administration, dose and dosage schedule are appropriate. Because of the ethical issues involved in carrying out pharmacological studies on children, there is less knowledge in this area than there is for adults.

PHARMACOKINETICS IN CHILDREN

Premature and newborn babies have proportionally more water and less fat in their bodies than do older children. In addition, the organs and organ systems of the body need to mature and develop structurally and physiologically, particularly the liver and kidneys. The younger and more premature a child is, the greater the difference their organ function is from normal. Structural changes in tissues take place in step with the growth of the child and maturation of the organs. For instance, the concentration of plasma proteins increases, and the barrier properties of the skin change.

ABSORPTION

Gastric emptying is reduced in young and premature children until the age of about 6 months. Absorption of drugs from the intestine can be slightly delayed, but the significance of this is likely to be minimal.

The skin is thin in newborns and has a reduced barrier function compared with that of adults. More drugs are easily absorbed through the skin, especially, for example, in those areas with eczematous change. Consequently, caution is advised in the use of steroid preparations, and they are best avoided on large areas of skin and over a long period of time, if possible. However, it is not necessary to advise against treatment with mild steroids in small children with pronounced eczema. It is important to be careful when washing the skin with disinfectants that may be absorbed and cause damage.

Rectal administration is useful when vomiting prevents oral administration of a drug, and also for drugs that have a substantial degree of first-pass metabolism. For example, diazepam is particularly suited to rectal administration for the treatment of convulsions because of its fast absorption by this route.

DISTRIBUTION

Premature and newborn babies have a larger percentage of water in their body, which will result in an increased distribution volume for water-soluble drugs. See Figure 27.1. The dose of such drugs needs to be increased in order to ensure that appropriate concentrations are achieved in body fluids, but this should be considered against the ability of the kidneys to eliminate the drug. Administration of such drugs, particularly those with a narrow therapeutic range, requires specialized knowledge.

Concentration of plasma proteins
The concentration of plasma proteins is low immediately after birth. In very premature babies, the albumin concentration may only be half of that found in older children. With a reduced concentration of plasma proteins, the binding capacity of drugs is reduced. With less binding of a particular drug to plasma proteins, effectively there is an increase in the concentration of free drug. This is significant for drugs that display a high degree of binding (over 70 per cent protein binding), particularly those with a narrow therapeutic range. This is particularly important when certain antiepileptic drugs, e.g. carbamazepine, phenytoin and valproate, are used in young children.

Blood–brain barrier and pH
With an elevated body temperature, metabolism increases and the cells of the body produce more carbon dioxide than they do at normal body temperature. Small

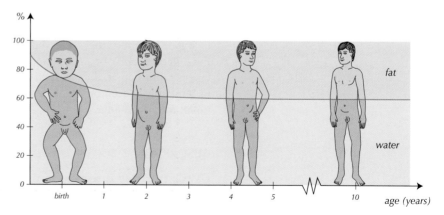

Figure 27.1 **Distribution of water and fat in the body.** In the early years of childhood, there is a greater percentage of water in the body than in later years. This results in an increased distribution volume for water-soluble drugs, and a reduced distribution volume for lipid-soluble drugs.

children can experience problems in removing this excess of carbon dioxide from the body. When carbon dioxide accumulates, acidosis occurs. With acidosis, the equilibrium of acidic drugs is shifted from the dissociated to the non-dissociated form. This results in an increase in the transport of acidic drugs across the blood–brain barrier.

If a person uses acetylsalicylic acid (aspirin) to lower the body temperature in this situation, more acetylsalicylic acid will pass from the blood to the central nervous system than with normal pH, i.e. the acidotic nature of the blood results in a greater proportion of non-dissociated acetylsalicylic acid, which crosses the blood–brain barrier more easily than the dissociated form. A high concentration of acetylsalicylic acid in the central nervous system acts on the respiratory centres of the brain stem and suppresses respiration. When respiration is lowered, the acidosis increases even more, which again drives more acetylsalicylic acid from the blood to the central nervous system. Paracetamol should be used when it is necessary to reduce the body temperature of small children with high temperature.

ELIMINATION

The ability of the kidneys to eliminate water-soluble drugs takes more time to reach maturity than it does for the liver to reach maturity in terms of its ability to metabolize lipid-soluble drugs.

With reduced elimination of drugs, there is an effective increase in their half-life. It takes a longer time before steady state is achieved using a standard dose. If a rapid effect is required there may be a need to use a loading dose. It takes a correspondingly longer time before a drug is eliminated from the body with reduced elimination.

Early renal and liver function
The ability of the kidneys to eliminate foreign substances develops quickly in childhood and reaches full maturity after about 6 months. See Figure 27.2. The enzymatic activity of the liver is poorly developed at birth but develops to full maturity at four weeks after birth. This is particularly apparent for the conjugation of bilirubin

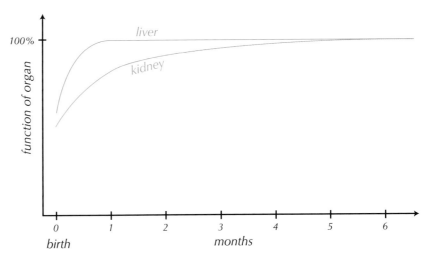

Figure 27.2 Organ function in children. Liver and renal functions develop gradually after birth. Immediately after birth, dosing of drugs must therefore be adapted to the function in the organ that eliminates the drug.

(which originates from the decomposition of fetal haemoglobin). Since the ability of the liver to conjugate bilirubin to glucuronic acid is lower in the newborn, the concentration of free bilirubin may increase and pass the blood–brain barrier where it causes irreversible brain damage.

A high concentration of bilirubin in the plasma can also displace drugs from albumin and contribute to increased concentration of free drug. Similarly, drugs can contribute to the displacement of bilirubin from albumin. For example, sulphonamides and phenytoin may compete with bilirubin for the binding sites on albumin. Clearly, such drugs must be used with caution in conditions such as neonatal jaundice (hyperbilirubinaemia).

Originally, drug doses for children were calculated according to the adult dose, and administered on a pro rata basis according to the child's weight. For example, if a drug was administered at 10 mg/kg, a 70 kg adult would receive 700 mg (10 mg × 70), whilst a child weighing 4 kg would receive 40 mg (10 mg × 4). In most cases, this resulted in a drug concentration that was too high. For example, if the antibiotic chloramphenicol is given to newborn babies on a pro rata adult dose, it exceeds the amount of chloramphenicol which can be conjugated with glucuronic acid in the liver. The result is a gradual increase in the concentration of chloramphenicol, and finally a toxic effect on the heart (grey baby syndrome).

Morphine is eliminated more slowly in newborn children than in older children and adults, because of their lack of ability to conjugate it. Therefore labour pains should not be treated with morphine but with another analgesic, as morphine crosses the placenta and enters the baby's circulation. Since it is eliminated slowly, its concentration can increase in the blood to the extent that it suppresses ventilation.

Dosing in the period immediately after birth

Dosing of drugs to premature and newborn babies should be lower (i.e. per kg body weight) than for older children. Drugs that are eliminated by biotransformation in the liver require gradually increasing doses (per kg of body weight) in the first 3–4 weeks, and then a more gradual increase up to the age of 6 months. Drugs that are eliminated through the kidneys require gradually increasing doses (per kg body weight) up to the age of 4–6 months, and then a more gradual increase up to the age of 6 months to 1 year. Because of different dose needs in different age groups, it is better to follow dosage regimen related to different age groups.

PHARMACODYNAMICS IN CHILDREN

Differences in pharmacodynamics between small children and adults are not well established. For some drugs, it is even possible to see an opposite effect to that which was anticipated. This is particularly true for drugs that act on the central nervous system. Diazepam, phenobarbital and other sedatives can cause hyperactivity, sleeplessness, irritability, anxiety and restlessness in children. Another example is seen by the fact that small children require larger doses of adrenaline and atropine (per kg body weight) than adults in order to achieve the desired effect.

The cause of altered effects in early childhood can be explained in part by modified receptor sensitivity and receptor density in different tissues at different ages.

DOSING IN NEWBORNS

When administering drugs to children, it is important to use precise measurement aids, such as measuring spoons, drop counters and finely graduated syringes, to

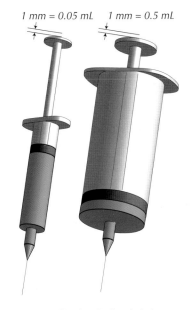

1 mm = 0.05 mL   1 mm = 0.5 mL

Figure 27.3 **Precise dosing.** It is important that the syringe is appropriate for the volume that is to be measured.

measure fluid drugs. See Figure 27.3. A large syringe would not be very suitable for drawing up exact small volumes. When it is necessary to withdraw a particular volume of a solution from a bottle or vial, the fluid will have a tendency to move up along the edges of the surfaces that limit it. This is why syringes with a large diameter are less accurate than graduated cylinders with a small diameter.

If the accuracy of a syringe is quoted as being ±0.5 mL, this means that a person normally draws up a volume that does not deviate by more than 0.5 mL from that volume which the person intends to draw up. Depending on how large a volume one draws up in such a syringe, the percentage error will vary.

For example, if a person draws up 19.5 mL in a syringe with an accuracy of ±0.5 mL when the person is planning to draw up 20 mL, the error will be:

$$\frac{0.5\,\text{mL}}{20.0\,\text{mL}} \times 100\% = 2.5\%$$

If a person draws up 9.5 mL instead of 10 mL, the error will be:

$$\frac{0.5\,\text{mL}}{10.0\,\text{mL}} \times 100\% = 5.0\%$$

If a person draws up 4.5 mL when the person wants to draw up 5 mL, the error will be large, i.e.:

$$\frac{0.5\,\text{mL}}{5.0\,\text{mL}} \times 100\% = 10.0\%$$

If a person uses a small syringe with an accuracy of 0.1 mL when the person wants to draw up 5 mL, the error will be small:

$$\frac{0.1\,\text{mL}}{5.0\,\text{mL}} \times 100\% = 2.0\%$$

From this it can be seen that the smaller the volume one wishes to draw up, the more precise the measurement must be if the error is to be acceptably small, i.e. a small volume requires a small syringe.

Generally, one should use syringes that are so small that one always draws up a volume that is greater than half the syringe's total volume. The greatest accuracy is achieved if a person uses the smallest syringe size that accommodates the entire desired volume in one draw.

ADVERSE EFFECTS IN CHILDREN

It can be difficult to distinguish certain adverse effects of drugs, e.g. changes in appetite, behaviour and sleep patterns, from the same non-drug-induced changes. It is important to observe children closely when they are administered drugs that may cause such effects. Because of pharmacokinetic differences seen in children compared with adults, the measurement of the plasma concentration of drugs, particularly those with a narrow therapeutic range, is useful.

POISONING IN CHILDREN

Poisoning in children occurs most frequently between the ages of 1 and 3 years. The most serious poisonings occur with acetylsalicylic acid (aspirin) preparations, iron tablets, sedatives and, in some cases, antiepileptics.

All drugs must be stored out of children's reach, and preferably locked away. This is also true for iron, vitamin and fluoride supplement tablets, which are often within children's reach, especially in the bathroom. Poisoning is discussed in more detail in Chapter 30, Poisoning.

SUMMARY

- Immediately after birth, the skin has poor barrier function. It is necessary to be careful with creams containing steroids and when washing the skin with disinfectants.
- Newborns have a larger percentage of water in their body than older children. Therefore, the volume of distribution for water-soluble and lipid-soluble drugs changes during the first year or so after birth.
- The concentration of plasma proteins is low in newborns, so the percentage of free (as opposed to protein-bound) drug will be high.
- Liver and kidney function is not fully developed in newborns. The dose of drugs with hepatic metabolism should be gradually increased during the first 3 weeks after birth. The dose of drugs with renal elimination should be increased gradually during the first 4–6 months after birth.
- The majority of drugs are administered in fluid form, and generally the volumes given are small. This means that the errors in the volume administered are amplified, i.e. a small error in the total volume administered may give rise to a large error in the intended drug concentration in plasma.

28 The elderly and drugs

With increasing age comes increased ill-health and reduced organ function. Increased ill-health leads to greater use of drugs. In conjunction with reduced organ function, this may contribute to a higher frequency of adverse effects and serious drug interactions in the elderly than in younger patients. The elderly may also have increased sensitivity to certain drugs' effects. It is important to observe the elderly closely, both after starting with new drugs and after cessation of medical treatment, to monitor whether the intended effects are achieved and whether troublesome or serious adverse effects or interactions have occurred.

It is important to remember that not all conditions can or should be treated with drugs. A good quality of care, a stimulating social environment and regular physical activity can be effective in preventing pain, preventing injuries from falling over, improving mental health and reducing constipation. These disorders are all too readily, and often unnecessarily, treated with drugs.

PHYSIOLOGICAL AND PATHOPHYSIOLOGICAL CHANGES AFFECTING DRUG RESPONSE IN THE ELDERLY

Changes in organ function can result in changes in the absorption, distribution and elimination of a number of drugs. In addition, physiological and pathophysiological changes can result in altered pharmacodynamics, thus affecting the sensitivity to some drugs.

ALTERED PHARMACOKINETICS

The most important age-related change that affects pharmacokinetics is reduced renal function, but altered distribution of water and fat in the body and reduced levels of plasma proteins can also result in changes in pharmacokinetic properties. Diseases that alter the distribution of blood flow in the intestine, kidneys and liver can affect absorption and elimination in different ways.

Absorption
Absorption is little affected with increasing age. However, there is the possibility of delayed gastric emptying and reduced intestinal motility. If blood supply to the

intestine is also decreased, absorption of some drugs is slowed, thus delaying the effect of drugs that are used occasionally, such as analgesics. Total absorption is not significantly affected by delayed gastric emptying or reduced motility in the intestine, so the effects of drugs taken on a regular basis will not as a rule be affected. Conditions that cause nausea may cause gastric retention and delayed absorption. Vomiting before the drug has passed out of the stomach reduces the availability of the drug. If parts of the stomach or small intestine have been removed, or if a malabsorption syndrome exists, drug absorption may be incomplete. Consequently, a smaller percentage of the dose enters the circulation, with a consequently reduced therapeutic effect.

Distribution
In the elderly, there is a reduction in the percentage of body water and increased percentage of body fat compared with young adults. A variation of 30 per cent from standard values is not uncommon. Thus, water-soluble drugs have a smaller volume of distribution, resulting in a shorter half-life and more rapid elimination. Conversely lipid-soluble drugs have a larger volume of distribution, which results in a longer half-life and less rapid elimination. However, in practice, these changes have little consequence for the dosage used. It is only in elderly patients with marked obesity or those who are very thin that it is appropriate to alter standard doses.

Concentration of plasma proteins
Plasma albumin concentration decreases with age, particularly in individuals with poor nutrition, liver disease or reduced renal function. The capacity of the plasma proteins to bind drugs is reduced, giving rise to a situation where the quantity of bound drug is much lower but the concentration of unbound drug is hardly affected (remember that it is only 'unbound' or 'free' drug that is available for pharmacological activity). The result is a lower total concentration of drug than would be seen with normal levels of albumin. It is important to bear this in mind when determining the plasma concentration of drug in the elderly, especially for drugs with high levels of binding to plasma proteins (e.g. antiepileptics, such as phenytoin, carbamazepine and valproate).

Elimination
As an individual ages, the body's organs have reduced function, which may be exacerbated by any existing disease. For example, acute hypovolaemic renal failure in association with urinary tract infection or pneumonia with high fever or acute cardiac failure are typical instances where renal elimination of drugs can be significantly reduced. If drug elimination is reduced, the half-life of that drug increases and its steady-state concentration will increase if the dose is not reduced. This is particularly important for drugs that are eliminated unchanged, such as lithium. Thus, when administering drugs to the elderly, the fact that reduced organ function can affect the elimination of drugs must be taken into consideration.

Renal elimination
Renal blood flow diminishes with increasing age. Glomerular filtration and tubular secretion are also reduced. The result is reduced elimination of water-soluble drugs and water-soluble metabolites of lipid-soluble drugs. See Figure 28.1. Kidney disease can exacerbate the situation. In addition, dehydration, cardiac failure, hypotension and arteriosclerotic disease in the kidneys will reduce renal blood flow and, in consequence, renal function. Renal function must be taken into consideration when administering drugs removed by renal elimination, especially

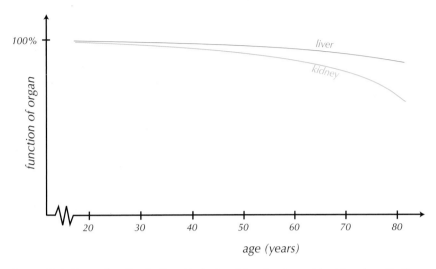

Figure 28.1 **Organ function in the elderly.** Renal function is considerably reduced in the elderly, while hepatic function is little altered. Dosing of drugs must be adapted to the failure in the organ that eliminates the drug.

drugs with a narrow therapeutic index, such as aminoglycosides, lithium, digoxin and oral hypoglycaemics.

Hepatic metabolism

Although liver size is decreased in the elderly, its metabolic ability is only slightly reduced with increasing age, which means that the elimination of drugs with hepatic metabolism is hardly affected. See Figure 28.1. Diazepam is an exception. It is metabolized to an active metabolite, desmethyldiazepam, which shows considerably reduced elimination and extended half-life in the elderly. This results in an accumulation of desmethyldiazepam with standard doses. For this reason, the elderly should use oxazepam when a sedative is required, as oxazepam is eliminated renally following conjugation. The ability to conjugate is reduced only slightly with increasing age. Diseases that affect the liver (hepatitis, obstruction of bile passages, cirrhosis) reduce the liver's ability to metabolize drugs to a much greater degree than the actual ageing process. However, simultaneous use of several drugs may increase the risk that enzymes that participate in hepatic drug metabolism will be affected (enzymatic inhibition or induction), such that the concentration of one or more drugs is altered.

ALTERED PHARMACODYNAMICS

Changes in drug concentration are not the only cause of altered drug response in the elderly. Increased sensitivity to drugs, a reduced ability to compensate when drugs affect physiological mechanisms, and polypharmacy, which causes drug interactions, also influence the response to drugs.

The nervous system

Some drugs used by the elderly affect central and autonomic nervous system functions more than when they are used by younger subjects. The ageing patient can demonstrate increased sensitivity to drugs with inhibitory effects on the central nervous system, which result in an increased tendency towards fatigue and confusion. Anxiolytic and sedative drugs, central-acting analgesics, the anti-Parkinson's disease drug, L-dopa, and many antidepressants, antipsychotics and antihistamines may cause such effects. These drugs may cause reduced neuromuscular control, resulting in unsteadiness and a risk of injury from falling. Antidepressants, antipsychotics and antihistamines cause marked anticholinergic effects in the elderly, particularly resulting in dryness of the mouth, delayed gastric emptying, reduced intestinal motility, constipation and urinary retention. Narcotic analgesic drugs also cause reduced intestinal motility and many elderly people experience constipation.

The cardiovascular system

The effectiveness of blood pressure-regulating mechanisms decreases with increasing age. This is especially pronounced for reflexes that are important in regulating rapid alterations in blood pressure, e.g. when shifting from a lying to a standing position. Elderly subjects who experience a rapid reduction in blood pressure and reduced blood flow to the brain and heart can exhibit symptoms of confusion, reduced attention span, fainting and, in the worst cases, stroke, angina pectoris and myocardial infarction.

A number of drugs can cause a fall in blood pressure as one of their adverse effects (e.g. antidepressants, antipsychotics and some analgesic drugs). In some instances, antihypertensive drugs may be too potent. The use of these drugs in the elderly demands care during the initiation of therapy. Patients should receive a low starting dose followed by careful increases in dose until the required effect has been achieved.

The intestinal tract

With increasing age, intestinal motility decreases, often resulting in constipation. Drugs that reduce intestinal motility (anticholinergic drugs) exacerbate the problem. The sensitivity of the mucous membrane of the stomach and duodenum to the effects of hydrochloric acid increases with age. There is an increased risk of gastric bleeding with the use of anti-inflammatory drugs (NSAIDs) in the elderly.

ADVERSE EFFECTS OF DRUG GROUPS FREQUENTLY USED IN THE ELDERLY

The elderly often have diseases of the cardiovascular system, of joints and muscles, depression, anxiety and sleep problems, and an increased risk of thrombosis.

Drugs for diseases in the cardiovascular system

Treatment of high blood pressure in the elderly has a beneficial effect in reducing the risk of strokes, myocardial infarction and heart failure. However, a rapid lowering of blood pressure can have a number of adverse effects. Poor cerebral blood flow, with confusion and agitation, can lead to symptoms of the onset of dementia. Orthostatic hypotension (rapid drop in blood pressure when rising from a lying or sitting to a standing position), which causes dizziness and increased risk of falling, can be exacerbated. Reduced circulation in the coronary arteries will exacerbate angina pectoris and may trigger myocardial infarction and heart failure. It is important to exercise caution when increasing doses in order to avoid such adverse effects.

Digitoxin and digoxin, used for treatment of cardiac failure and supraventricular rhythm disturbances, have a narrow therapeutic range. Overdose can cause rhythm disturbances, confusion, nausea, listlessness, dizziness and reduced appetite. Altered colour perception (yellow vision) is a typical symptom with a high plasma concentration of digitalis.

Diuretics can cause electrolyte disturbances (especially hypokalaemia), dehydration and hypotension. A low concentration of potassium and magnesium in the blood increases the heart's sensitivity to digitalis and increases the risk of arrhythmia. Thiazide diuretics can exacerbate diabetes by making the β cells in the pancreas less sensitive to low blood sugar, and can trigger gout by competition with uric acid for tubular secretion, leading to a reduced elimination of uric acid.

Non-steroidal anti-inflammatory drugs

Elderly people with joint problems and muscle pains frequently use NSAIDs. These drugs can cause ulceration and haemorrhage, as a result of irritation of the mucous membrane in stomach. The risk is increased considerably after a person reaches 65 years of age. If NSAIDs are needed then the mucous membrane may be protected by simultaneously giving misoprostol or a proton pump inhibitor such as omeprazole. NSAIDs reduce the synthesis of prostaglandins, which help to maintain renal blood flow, so long-term use can result in reduced renal blood flow and possibly lead to renal failure. To compensate for reduced renal blood flow, reabsorption of sodium and water in the kidneys is increased, which results in increased blood volume and hence increased blood pressure, which may exacerbate or trigger cardiac failure. If NSAIDs are taken with anticoagulants, the risk of haemorrhage is increased.

Anticoagulants

Complications from haemorrhage are common with the anticoagulant warfarin. For this reason, meticulous supervision is required for this type of treatment, particularly in elderly patients who do not demonstrate good compliance. Warfarin interacts with many different drugs, and can lead to death because of its serious adverse effects, which often occur as a result of drug interactions.

Antidepressant and antipsychotic drugs

Tricyclic antidepressants also have anticholinergic effects. This increases the risk of constipation, particularly in elderly patients with a low level of physical activity. Urinary retention can be pronounced in men with an enlarged prostate gland. Antidepressants of the selective serotonin reuptake inhibitors (SSRI) group of drugs have less anticholinergic effect than tricyclic antidepressants but can still cause headache, irritability, increased anxiety, sleep disturbances and tremors.

The increase in the use of antipsychotics in the elderly to reduce symptoms of senile dementia is not entirely appropriate as they may cause the development of irreversible tardive dyskinesias, with involuntary muscle twitches.

Sedative and anxiolytic drugs

Many elderly persons use sedatives and anxiolytic drugs. Drugs that suppress activity in the central nervous system can cause confusion and increase the risk of falling. Diazepam should be avoided because of its conversion to desmethyldiazepam, which has a long half-life in the elderly.

COMPLIANCE IN THE ELDERLY

Compliance refers to a patient's actual participation and cooperation following medical advice. Low compliance with regard to the use of drugs can help to explain why a particular therapy does not produce the anticipated result.

Motivation for treatment is the best guarantee that a particular therapy will be followed. Good motivation demands good information, particularly if the patient is uncomfortable with the treatment and it extends over a long period of time. The elderly patient should understand and be able to use the information that is given. Compliance is described in Chapter 2, Regulation and management of drug therapy and drug errors, p. 16.

SUMMARY

- Disease-related organ failure is the most important cause of changes that affect choice and dosing of drugs.
- Age-related reduction in renal function is the most important physiological change which affects choice and dosing of drugs.
- The elderly have a reduced ability to compensate when drugs affect physiological functions. Effects and adverse effects of drugs can be more pronounced in the elderly than in younger patients.
- Compliance may be poor among the elderly. The reason may be polypharmacy, complicated drug regimes, lack of understanding of the user instructions and poor information about therapy regimes from doctors and other health professionals.

29 Drugs of abuse

For as far back as there are records detailing human behaviour, we know that people have used intoxicating substances – psychoactive compounds that influence the central nervous system in such a way that the user's perception of reality and behaviour are altered.

Alcohol use has been found predominantly throughout Europe but there is evidence of many other intoxicating substances in use throughout the world. The cannabis plant was known to be cultivated in China in approximately 10 000 BC, and evidence of opium use in 2000 BC has been found in Crete. All the intoxicating substances used in historic cultures were derived from plants. Today, there are more than 4000 known plants that contain psychoactive substances.

The use of intoxicating substances was often related to social and religious rituals. Gradually, however, their use has become much more widespread, with individuals desiring the effects of intoxication. This is particularly true among young people in cultures where narcotics have become more readily available and many potent substances with both intoxicating effects and a likelihood for drug dependence are produced by simple chemical synthesis.

Among heavy users, a significant motive for the continued use of such substances is to prevent the emergence of unpleasant abstinence-related withdrawal symptoms and to 'escape' from difficult situations in life. Today, the production and sale of illicit narcotics are illegal. There are enormous social and personal costs associated with the chronic abuse of intoxicating substances. There is a clear connection between the use of intoxicating substances and disease as well as violent deaths such as accidents, murder and suicide.

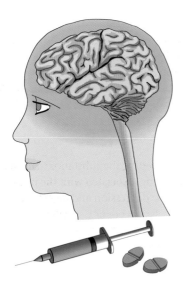

Figure 29.1 **Intoxication.** In order for a substance to have potential as an intoxicating substance, it must influence the signal transmission in parts of the central nervous system where processes for conscious experience take place.

DEFINITION OF CONCEPTS

The effects of intoxicating substances on the user are difficult to describe precisely, especially the subjective effects. There is considerable disagreement as to the definition of the concepts associated with intoxication. This becomes clearer if the concepts are described from a psychological, sociological, cultural or pharmacological point of view. In this text, an attempt is made to describe the concepts rather than provide strict definitions.

Intoxication

Intoxication is defined as the experience of altered mood and behaviour following the ingestion of chemical or biological substances. Intoxication is also associated with varying degrees of reduced concentration, learning ability and short-term memory. In the early phase of use, the intoxication often results in pleasurable experiences that contribute to a desire for continued use. Further use, however, can lead to increasing frequency of bad experiences associated with intoxication.

Intoxicating substances

These are chemical or biological substances that cause intoxication. Only substances that cause a noticeable alteration in behaviour can be regarded as having an intoxicating effect. In addition, the substances must have depressant or stimulating effects on the central nervous system that alter the psyche. See Figure 29.1.

The World Health Organization has a comprehensive description of the concept of a 'drug'. It is described as a chemical substance that alters biological functions but which is not necessary to maintain normal body functions. The substance is capable of being used both therapeutically and non-therapeutically. In addition, it produces different effects in the user by influencing or altering the frame of mind and the perception of reality or behaviour (psychoactive effect). Finally, there must be potential negative effects to health and/or social function, and the substance must be habit-forming.

Abuse

Abuse is the use of legal intoxicating substances that deviates from accepted social norms in a group, and all use of illegal substances, drugs and solvents for the purpose of achieving intoxication. In some environments and cultures, a particular use of intoxicating substances will be perceived as abuse, while it is accepted in other groups. In countries that do not prohibit the use of cannabis, moderate smoking of hashish will not be perceived as abuse. Acceptable use and abuse is thus a matter of attitude that changes with time in all cultures. Use of drugs with intoxication effects in non-therapeutic circumstances is regarded as an abuse of those substances.

In the case of narcotics, the distinction between use and abuse is coincident with medical and non-medical use. For alcohol, this distinction is less clear. The UK government has made an attempt to set safe drinking limits (14 units/week for women and 21 units/week for men) but this is related to health concerns rather than the prevention of abuse.

Dependence

Dependence on intoxicating substances is characterized by use that is not connected to medical indications and that is a result of the person's experience of the substance's effect. The user generally perceives the intoxicating substance as necessary for continued well-being. The use is often accompanied by 'negative' medical and social consequences.

Physical dependence

Physical dependence is a consequence of repeated administration of a substance that, on discontinuation, leads to unpleasant and potentially life-threatening abstinence reactions (withdrawal). Physical dependence is usually associated with the development of tolerance and is experienced as unpleasant and sometimes life-threatening physiological reactions when administration of the substance is reduced or stopped.

Mental dependence

Mental dependence is a conscious experience of needing the substance that causes intoxication in order to re-live the pleasurable feeling associated with the intoxication or to suppress unpleasant experiences, such as depression and dejection, after the effects of intoxication have stopped. Mental dependence usually manifests itself after the abuser experiences abstinence-related withdrawal symptoms. Users are generally reluctant to admit to physical and mental dependence.

Development of tolerance

The development of tolerance is a gradual process following repeated administration of a substance that leads to an increase in the dose of the substance required to achieve the same effect or to prevent undesired effects (abstinence-related withdrawal symptoms). Tolerance can be developed to the intoxicating effects of a substance without the person becoming tolerant to its physiological effects. With the use of cocaine, a person develops a tolerance for the intoxication experience, but not for the adverse effect (stimulation) on the heart. Tolerance of the intoxicating effect is also seen with the use of alcohol, but tolerance of the effects of alcohol on the respiratory centres is considerably lower. Tolerance development can lead the abuser to take larger and larger doses, with a life-threatening or fatal effect.

Abstinence reactions

These are mental and physical reactions to a reduction in the concentration of an intoxicating substance below a critical level. The reaction will, in all cases, be unpleasant and in some it will be life-threatening. Abstinence reactions can appear before all traces of the drug are excreted. They are strongest when stopping after large and frequent doses. The reactions can first manifest themselves as listlessness, anxiety, restlessness and insomnia, and thereafter an increasing feeling of illness with rapid pulse and respiration, an increase in blood pressure, increased saliva secretion, nausea, vomiting and diarrhoea. Pains and tingling in the muscles and joints are associated phenomena. Convulsions can occur.

Within every drug group, the abstinence-related withdrawal symptoms are most intense for substances that are eliminated quickly, but last longer for substances with slower elimination. See Figure 29.2.

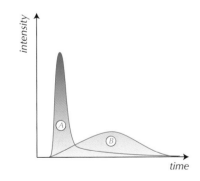

Figure 29.2 **Abstinence.** Substances with a short half-life (e.g. opiates) cause more intense but shorter abstinence periods than substances with a long half-life (e.g. benzodiazepines). Substance A has a short half-life, while B has a considerably longer half-life.

CLASSIFICATION OF INTOXICATING SUBSTANCES

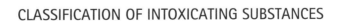

Intoxicating substances can be divided into those with depressive effects on the central nervous system, e.g. alcohol, cannabis, opiates and volatile solvents, and those with stimulating effects, e.g. cocaine, crack, ecstasy, amphetamines and methamphetamines. In addition to these substances, there are hallucinogenic substances, which are distinguished by their distortion of the normal perception of the environment and having a complex effect on the central nervous system.

Mechanism of action

In the central nervous system, different cells and areas connect with each other through a complex network of nerves. Impulses are generated when biochemical transmitters are released from nerve endings and influence receptors. An impulse that occurs in a nerve cell and spreads out via several branches can have both a stimulating effect on some nerve cells and an inhibitive effect on others.

All the intoxicating substances act by altering normal physiological processes in the central nervous system, primarily by altering the amount of signal transmitters that are available in the synapse or by altering the electrical potential across a membrane. The most important sites of action would appear to involve alteration of the signal transmitters dopamine, noradrenaline, serotonin and gamma-aminobutyric acid (GABA). Such an influence can occur because a nerve end increases the release of a signal transmitter, or because degradation or reabsorption of the signal transmitter is reduced. In all cases, the flow of ions across membranes is influenced in such a way that the signal transmission is disturbed. Different intoxicating substances produce different effects by influencing different receptors. With varying concentrations of the same intoxicating substance, the receptors will be influenced to different degrees, thereby producing different effects. When several intoxicating substances are taken simultaneously, the effects become unpredictable.

SUBSTANCES WITH A DEPRESSANT EFFECT ON THE CENTRAL NERVOUS SYSTEM

Substances that have a depressant effect on the central nervous system include alcohol, cannabis, opiates and volatile solvents. Almost all habit-forming drugs that are abused can also have a depressant effect.

ALCOHOLS

Among the intoxicating substances that suppress the central nervous system, ethanol dominates. Some chronic alcohol abusers also use isopropanol, found in windscreen washer fluid. Isopropanol ingestion results in a less pronounced intoxication than ethanol, but is more toxic because it is metabolized to acetone. Ingestion of methanol and ethylene glycol also occurs sporadically and accidentally. These compounds are very toxic and often require hospital treatment.

Ethanol

Ethanol is the intoxicating agent in all such substances.

Mechanism of action

Ethanol is known to cause changes in the structure of cells by increasing plasticity in cellular membranes. However, there is evidence to suggest that ethanol exercises the majority of its effect on the central nervous system by increasing the flow of chloride through ion channels connected to GABA receptors. This occurs because GABA binds more tightly to its receptor when ethanol is present and increases the flow of chloride ions into the cell. The cell thus has a lower resting potential and becomes more difficult to excite. See Figure 29.3. It is also thought probable that ethanol inhibits the influx of calcium into cells by preventing the opening of calcium channels. With low intracellular calcium levels, the release of transmitters is reduced.

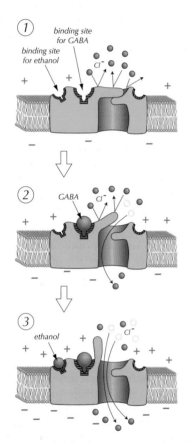

Figure 29.3 Mechanism of action of ethanol. Gamma-aminobutyric acid (GABA) is a signal substance in the central nervous system. When GABA binds to the GABA receptor, the chloride channel will partially open (2). Because ethanol binds to a receptor that is connected to the GABA receptor, the chloride channel opens wider (3). Increased concentrations of chloride ions on the inside of the membrane increase the electrical potential difference between the outside and the inside resulting in hyperpolarization. The nerve cell now needs a stronger stimulus to trigger depolarization. In this way, ethanol has a depressant effect.

Effects

The intoxication experienced with ethanol is due to effects on the central nervous system. With increasing concentrations, the user experiences altered mood, behaviour and emotions, reduced ability to concentrate and reduced motor and intellectual skills.

If someone maintains the blood alcohol concentration at approximately 0.1 per cent over several hours by ingesting the same amount of alcohol as he or she metabolizes, the effects of intoxication will diminish. To maintain the effects of intoxication a person has to ensure more alcohol is consumed than is metabolized. The level of cognitive impairment is often not recognized by alcohol users, leading to a potentially dangerous overestimation of their ability to perform skills and tasks.

The depressant effect increases with increasing ethanol concentration. In some people, the respiratory centre is affected with concentrations above 0.25 per cent, but some are able to tolerate concentrations exceeding 0.6 per cent. Chronic use of ethanol results in a certain amount of tolerance to both the physiological and intoxicating effects.

Use of ethanol during pregnancy will result in ethanol crossing the placenta and will result in similar ethanol concentrations in the fetus as in the mother. This can be detrimental during the first trimester, but fetal damage can also occur as the result of frequent ethanol ingestion during the latter stage of pregnancy. Fetal alcohol syndrome is a collection of symptoms associate with heavy ethanol ingestion during pregnancy which, amongst other things, includes irreversible brain damage.

NARCOTICS

The use of narcotics results in varying degrees of physical, mental and harmful social effects. The substances have different properties, but their use has a number of common characteristics. Anxiety, confusion and panic states increase with the length of use, and chronic users are frequently exposed to injuries, accidents and disease.

Cannabis

Cannabis is extracted from the cannabis plant. The psychoactive substance is tetrahydrocannabinol (THC). Different parts of the plant contain different quantities of THC. The highest concentrations are found in the resin and the flower shoots. Marijuana is obtained by drying and grinding up plant parts. Hashish is a further processing of marijuana. In cannabis oil, a further concentration of the active substance is found. Cannabis is usually ingested by smoking. Marijuana, hashish and cannabis oil are not water-soluble and it is therefore dangerous to inject these substances intravenously.

Mechanism of action

A receptor has been identified that has an affinity to THC and other cannabis analogues, and it is believed that this receptor is responsible for the effects we see with cannabis use.

Effects

Approximately 20 min after ingestion, the user will experience subjective feelings of euphoria, rapid heart rate, listlessness, fatigue/tiredness and altered perception of time. Some report that external stimuli such as light (colours) and sound are experienced more clearly with a heightened perception. Some describe the intoxication as similar to that experienced with the use of LSD, but less intense. Psychoses rarely occur and there is no increase in aggressiveness. Cognitive and motor functions are reduced during use. Ingestion of cannabis leads to a dilatation of the arteries in the conjunctiva and sclera, which can cause 'bloodshot' eyes. Cannabis use is now thought to be a risk factor for the development of mental illness.

Tolerance is known to develop quickly to the effects of euphoria.

Distribution

Tetrahydrocannabinol is largely distributed to tissues outside the bloodstream, especially fatty tissues. THC is metabolized in the liver. The half-life is approximately 20 h with single use, but increases with chronic use. Regular ingestion of cannabis can normally be traced in the urine for up to 3 weeks after use has stopped. With heavy use, it can be traced for an even longer period.

Dependence and social aspects

The risk of developing dependence to cannabis is regarded as small to moderate. However, the social settings in which the substance is used often result in the subsequent experimentation with and use of 'harder' drugs.

Opioids

Morphine and codeine are natural opiates that are extracted from the opium poppy. Pethidine and methadone are artificially produced opioid substances. Medicinal use of opioids is discussed in Chapter 14, Drugs with central and peripheral analgesic effect.

Mechanism of action

Opioids mediate their effects through different opioid receptors, mu (μ), delta (δ) and kappa (κ). Stimulation of the opioid receptors results in opening of potassium channels, which causes hyperpolarization and reduced excitability. See Figure 29.4. Opening of calcium channels is inhibited, which contributes to a reduction in the release of signal transmitters (see Figure 14.7). Stimulation of μ-receptors mediates pain relief, respiratory depression, euphoria and fatigue/tiredness, and contributes to the development of dependence. The δ-receptor is thought to mediate several effects associated with abuse. Stimulation of the κ-receptor results in analgesia at the spinal level, and possibly fatigue/tiredness and dysphoria.

The receptors are unevenly distributed throughout the central nervous system. Different opioids have different affinities to the different receptors.

Effects

Opioids have anaesthetic and analgesic effects that manifest themselves immediately after intravenous administration. They cause a feeling of well-being, sensory disturbances and an altered perception of reality. Estimation of time and distance is impaired and speech, movement and coordination are all affected. The most serious consequence of overdose is depression of the respiratory centres. Tolerance to the intoxicating effects of opioids occurs quickly, but not the toxic effect on respiration. It is believed that many deaths among opioid abusers are due to the user increasing the dose to achieve intoxication. There is also a great deal of variation in the 'purity' of the different preparations available, leading to many unintentional overdoses with unexpectedly pure products.

Distribution

Morphine is metabolized in the liver to the active metabolite morphine glucuronide. The glucuronide is eliminated through the kidneys. Codeine is metabolized partly to morphine, and the remainder to norcodeine. The metabolites are eliminated as

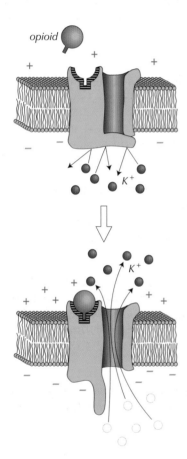

Figure 29.4 Mechanism of action of opioids. When opioids bind to their opiate receptors, potassium channels open increasing the flow of positive potassium ions flow out of the cell. A reduced intracellular potassium concentration increases the electrical difference between the outside and the inside leading to a hyperpolarized cell. A stronger stimulus is thus required to depolarize the nerve cell. In this way, opioids have a depressant effect on cell excitation. In addition, the opening of calcium channels is inhibited, thus reducing the release of signal substances into the synapse (not shown in the figure).

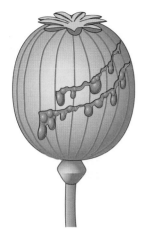

Figure 29.5 **Opium poppy.** By cutting the capsule, the plant juice seeps out.

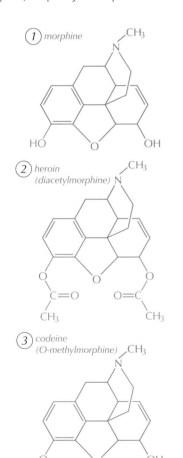

Figure 29.6 Morphine, heroin (diacylmorphine) and codeine (O-methylmorphine) are opiates. Differences in the molecular structure are indicated with red substitutes.

conjugates and inactive compounds. Ingestion of opiates can be traced in the urine 3–4 days after ingestion depending on the dose taken and length of use.

Dependence and social aspects
Opioids cause both early physical and mental dependence. The mental component is considerable, especially for heroin, making withdrawal from the drug difficult and often requiring structured withdrawal programmes. Since the abuse largely occurs via intravenous administration, many infectious diseases are transmitted by dirty syringes that are often shared by several people. Viral infections such as hepatitis B and C and human immunodeficiency virus (HIV) are the most serious.

Opium
Raw opium is a plant juice that is extracted from the seed capsule of the opium poppy. See Figure 29.5. Opium for smoking is obtained by grinding raw opium and dissolving it in water, filtering out the impurities. The most common form of ingestion is smoking, but it can also be eaten, drunk or injected. Opium contains morphine and codeine, which produce the intoxicating effect.

Morphine
Morphine is extracted from raw opium. The morphine base is added to an acid that renders it water-soluble and suitable for injection. See Figure 29.6. In the medical context, morphine is used as a potent analgesic in severe pain (see Chapter 14, Drugs with central and peripheral analgesic effect).

Heroin
Heroin is produced from morphine. Heroin is most often administered intravenously, but sniffing and smoking of heroin have gained increasing popularity as a route of ingestion. It is three times more potent than morphine, and it is believed to have a more significant habit-forming effect. Dependence develops quickly and abstinence symptoms can be seen after a short time. See Figure 29.6.

Codeine
Codeine is used mainly as a prescribed drug. It has analgesic and cough suppressive effects. Approximately 10 per cent of the ingested dose of codeine is metabolized to morphine.

Methadone
Methadone is a synthetic opioid compound that has many similarities to morphine. See Figure 29.7. However, it has a considerably longer half-life and is less sedating. Methadone has a greater biological availability than the other opioids, such that a significant portion of the orally ingested dose reaches the systemic circulation.

Dependence and social aspects
Methadone has a long half-life compared with other opioids, and therefore does not have the strong abstinence-related withdrawal symptoms of opioids. As methadone is suitable for oral administration, it is often used as an opiate substitute as part of a withdrawal programme. The individual is prescribed increasingly smaller doses of methadone in an attempt to gradually wean them from opiates. These withdrawal programmes have to be closely monitored. In order to be successful, the psychological and social aspects of dependence also need to be addressed.

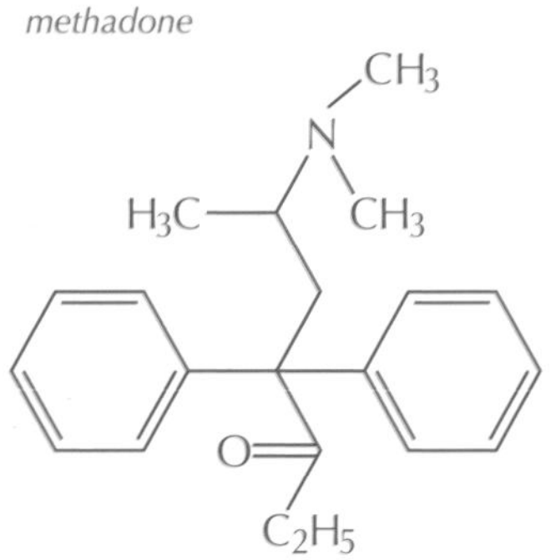

methadone

Figure 29.7 **Methadone** has a molecular structure that is different from that of morphine.

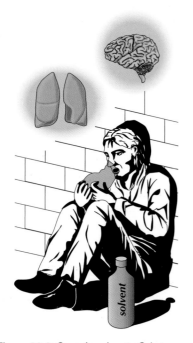

Figure 29.8 **Organic solvents.** Substances that are used for sniffing contain organic solvents that particularly damage the central nervous system and the lungs.

VOLATILE, ORGANIC SOLVENTS

Volatile, organic solvents that are inhaled or sniffed in sufficient quantities can result in intoxication. These substances are found in different products, such as thinners and cleaning agents for oily and fatty compounds. These include glue, gasoline, chloroform, trichloroethylene, ether, toluene, xylene and other substances that are relatively easy to obtain.

The substances are lipid-soluble and are distributed quickly to the central nervous system, where they exert their effect. Both the intoxication effect and abstinence-related withdrawal symptoms, which manifest themselves after long-term use, resemble those seen after alcohol use.

In addition to the depressant effects on the central nervous system, several of the substances can cause fatal heart rhythm disturbance, respiratory depression and pulmonary oedema. With long-term use damage is seen in the central nervous system, lungs, liver and kidneys. See Figure 29.8.

Solvent abuse is most commonly seen among young people.

HALLUCINOGENS

Hallucinogens are distinguished by their ability to distort perception of stimuli affecting thought, perception and mood. Mescaline and psilocybin are naturally occurring hallucinogens. LSD (lysergic acid diethylamide) and phencyclidine are synthetic compounds. See Figure 29.9.

Synthetic hallucinogens were used extensively after they came on the market, but consumption declined gradually as their harmful effects became known, especially LSD. There has, however, been a recent increase in their use.

The mechanisms of action of these substances are poorly understood, but it is believed that the effect is mediated by influencing serotonin receptors.

Effects

Lysergic acid diethylamide intoxication is often described as an intense revelation. The intoxication can last for several hours and can alternate from good experiences to anxiety, panic, acute depression and psychosis. Many users report 'out of body' experiences, delusions and suicidal thoughts. Users have committed murder and suicide under the influence of hallucinogens. A specific property of LSD is the experience of 'flashbacks'. This is where a user relives an experience they had during LSD use often many months or years later. These flashbacks can result in great distress.

SUBSTANCES WITH A STIMULATING EFFECT ON THE CENTRAL NERVOUS SYSTEM

Cocaine, crack, ecstasy, amphetamines and methamphetamines belong to this group.

Mechanism of action

Ingestion of substances that stimulate the central nervous system increase the amounts of noradrenaline, serotonin and dopamine in the synapses in the central nervous system. This is achieved by inhibiting reabsorption, or increasing the release, of these neurotransmitters. Noradrenaline is responsible for dilatation of the pupils, constriction of blood vessels, hypertension, rapid heart rate and increased respiration. Dopamine is responsible for the euphoric effect, anorexia, hyperactivity

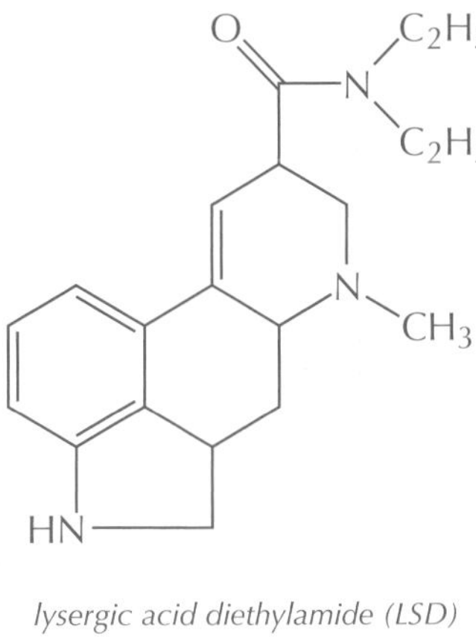

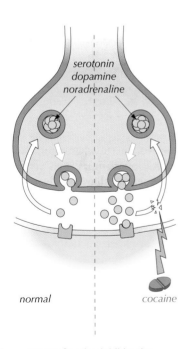

lysergic acid diethylamide (LSD)

Figure 29.9 LSD: lysergic acid diethylamide.

and increased libido. The stimulating effect on the central nervous system increases wakefulness and endurance as long as a moderate dose is used.

Cocaine and crack

Cocaine is a naturally existing, psychoactive substance that stimulates the central nervous system. It is extracted from the leaves of the coca plant. Crack is refined cocaine. Chewing coca leaves causes mild intoxication. Cocaine and crack can be administered intravenously, smoked, inhaled, eaten or drunk. Cocaine inhibits the reabsorption of neurotransmitters at the nerve terminal. See Figures 29.10 and 29.11.

Effects

Heavy ingestion of cocaine can cause psychosis, epileptic seizures, heart arrhythmias, elevated blood pressure and respiratory disturbances. The intoxication is short-lived; it lasts only minutes with intravenous use, and is even shorter with inhalation. The pleasurable feeling is intense and depression is considerable when use stops.

Crack has a more intense intoxicating effect than cocaine when inhaled, but is shorter lived than in cocaine use. The user often experiences severe rebound depression. Large doses have a local anaesthetic effect. The stimulating effects cause elevated blood pressure and increased strain on the heart.

Distribution

Cocaine is eliminated quickly from the body and can be traced for only 3–4 days after use has stopped.

Dependence and social aspects

Cocaine and crack are considered to have a potent habit-forming effect. The mental dependence is described as a loss of self-confidence and feelings of being lost without the drug. The desire to re-live the intoxication and the need to lift the depression result in a strong motive to continue use. Cocaine users do not seem to develop tolerance.

Amphetamine and methamphetamine (ICE)

Amphetamine is a synthetic, potent drug that stimulates the central nervous system. Methamphetamine (or 'ice' – the crystalline form) has many similarities with amphetamine. See Figure 29.12. Amphetamine can be administered intravenously, eaten, drunk or inhaled.

serotonin
dopamine
noradrenaline

normal   *cocaine*

Figure 29.10 **Cocaine** inhibits the reabsorption of noradrenaline, serotonin and dopamine. Thus, more signal substance is available in the synapse, enhancing signal transmission. Cocaine therefore has a stimulating effect.

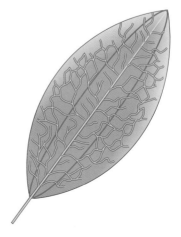

Figure 29.11 **Coca leaves** have a characteristic curved stripe on both sides of the midline.

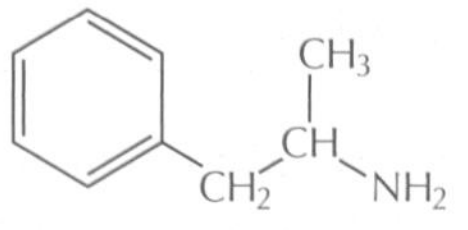

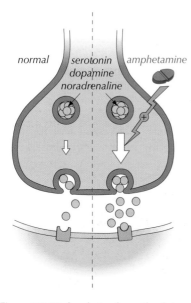

Figure 29.12 **Ecstasy, amphetamine and methamphetamine** have very similar molecular structures and have many similarities in effect. Changes to the amphetamine structure are indicated with red substitutes.

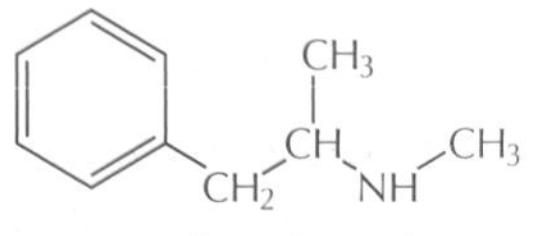

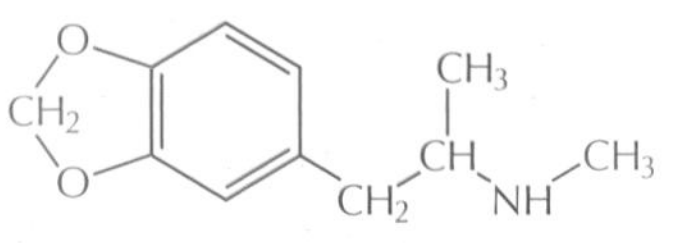

Figure 29.13 **Amphetamines** stimulate the release of noradrenaline, serotonin and dopamine. Thus, more signal substance is available in the synapse, which enhances the signal transmission. Amphetamines therefore have a stimulating effect.

Mechanism of action

Amphetamines increase the release of catecholamines (noradrenaline, serotonin and dopamine) into the synapse.

Effects

Amphetamines produce a euphoric effect with increased wakefulness, concentration, initiative and aggressiveness. The intoxication lasts considerably longer than with cocaine use. With increasing doses, toxic effects are much more pronounced. Paleness, flushing, palpitations, increased heart rate, elevated blood pressure and arrhythmias with varying degrees of atrioventricular block are all characteristic toxic effects.

Long-term use results in a reduction of catecholamine stores with resultant concentration difficulties, irritability, apathy, mental depression and fatigue. Schizophrenia-like amphetamine psychoses can occur.

Amphetamines and the amphetamine derivative methylphenidate are used to treat narcolepsy, a condition with uncontrolled, sudden sleep attacks.

Distribution

Amphetamines are eliminated quickly through the urine. The drug can usually be traced for only 1–2 days after use. The elimination rate increases with a low pH in the urine.

Dependence and social aspects

Amphetamine causes a lesser degree of dependence than is seen with cocaine and crack, but use is thought to lead to experimentation with other drugs. Methamphetamine is known to cause dependence quickly and some believe dependence can be present following a single exposure.

Ecstasy

Ecstasy is a slang term for methylenedioximethamphetamine (MDMA), a derivative of amphetamine. The molecular structure resembles that of amphetamine. See Figure 29.12.

Mechanism of action

The hallucinogenic effects seem to be associated with an increase in serotonin within the synapses, while the stimulating effects most probably stem from an increase in dopamine concentrations. Amphetamines increase the release of transmitter into the synapses. See Figure 29.13.

Effects

By using ecstasy, a person can sustain a high level of physical activity over a long period. Hallucinogenic experiences occur with increasing doses. In recent years, there have been reports from animal research of damage to the central nervous system, with the loss of serotonergic neurons after using ecstasy. Users can exhibit serious personality changes, possibly as the result of a loss of neurons, and possible irreversible damage.

Dependence and social aspects

The risk of developing dependence to ecstasy is considered high, as is the case for other substances that stimulate the central nervous system. The use of ecstasy has increased dramatically in recent years, particularly amongst young people. Many users mix several substances, both amphetamines and benzodiazepines, with ecstasy.

DRUGS THAT ARE POTENTIALLY INTOXICATING

Benzodiazepines, opioids, antiepileptics, antimigraines and centrally acting muscle relaxants have effects that are exerted via the central nervous system. They can cause intoxication and have the potential for abuse.

ANXIOLYTIC DRUGS/SEDATIVE DRUGS/HYPNOTIC DRUGS

There has been a decline in the use of benzodiazepines in recent years, but many people still take them. Some are introduced to them for the first time during a stay in hospital, often without the patient asking for drugs; for example: 'Take a tablet, and you'll surely sleep better tonight. You should be rested for the examination tomorrow.' Others take them for the first time when they are in a difficult life situation, e.g. anxiety problems, sleep disturbances, reactions to grief or stress problems associated with work. They thus learn to use chemical substances as a strategy for mastering problems that most people experience from time to time, and usually tackle without drugs. For some, this can be the start of a long-term use of habit-forming drugs. See Figure 29.14.

Mechanism of action
The benzodiazepines bind to receptors that are associated with GABA and increase the influx of negative chloride ions. This leads to an increase in the voltage between the inside and the outside of the cell. Thus, a stronger signal is required to excite the cell and transmit an impulse further. See Figure 29.15.

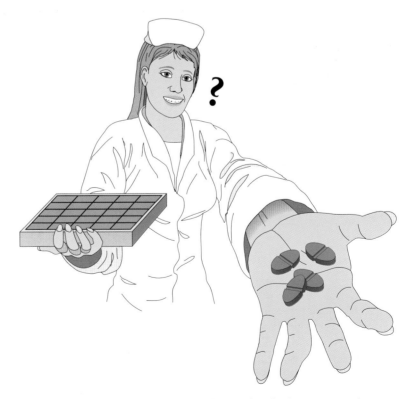

Figure 29.14 **Unfortunate practices.** Tranquillizers and analgesics are among the most abused drugs.

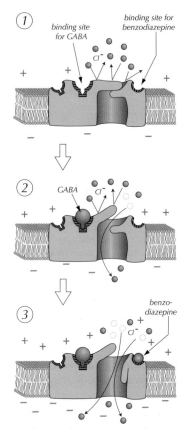

Figure 29.15 **Benzodiazepines** bind to a receptor that is associated with the gamma-aminobutyric acid (GABA) receptor, and thus the chloride channels open wider. An increased concentration of chloride ions on the inside of the membrane increases the potential difference between the outside and the inside, and requires a stronger stimulus for an impulse to occur. In this way, benzodiazepines produce a depressant effect on the cell, reducing excitation. The depressant effect is further enhanced with simultaneous use of ethanol (not shown in the figure).

Effects

Benzodiazepines act via benzodiazepine receptors in the central nervous system by enhancing the effect of the endogenous substance GABA. Drugs in this group have different degrees of anxiety-reducing, tranquillizing and soporific effects. They also have a muscle relaxant and antispasmodic effect.

Used together with alcohol or other drugs with a depressant effect on the central nervous system, a synergistic effect is seen which can depress respiration.

Distribution

These drugs are usually ingested orally. In cases of abuse, they can be dissolved and injected intravenously. This is a dangerous practice, both because of the chance of contamination and because undissolved particles can enter the blood. Benzodiazepines are lipid-soluble and are quickly distributed throughout the body's tissue, especially the central nervous system. They are metabolized in the liver to active metabolites that are eliminated in the urine.

The drug can be traced in the urine several weeks after use has stopped. The low-dose benzodiazepines can be difficult to trace in urine since they are used in small doses and thus produce low concentrations.

Dependence and social aspects

Abstinence-related withdrawal symptoms are most intense for substances that are eliminated quickly from the body. The most common withdrawal symptoms are sleep problems, anxiety, restlessness, concentration difficulties and myalgia (muscle pains). These withdrawal symptoms can last a long time.

Barbiturates

Barbiturates used as sedatives have largely been replaced by benzodiazepines because of the significant risks of dependence and abstinence problems with convulsions, delirium and cardiac arrest. The barbiturates bind to a receptor that is associated with the GABA receptor. The main clinical indications are for the treatment of epilepsy and in general anaesthesia.

ANALGESICS THAT ACT ON THE CENTRAL NERVOUS SYSTEM

Analgesics that act on the central nervous system exert their effect by influencing physiological processes within the central nervous system.

Opioids

Opioid substances are used clinically for the treatment of severe pain. In addition, these substances have anxiety-reducing, sedative and stress-relieving effects. They can result in intoxication when they are used in large doses, especially in situations without pain.

The opioids cause similar abstinence-related withdrawal symptoms as benzodiazepines, but are more intense and do not last as long. In addition, some people experience poor appetite, nausea, stomach pains and diarrhoea. Increased secretion from the eyes, nose and mouth are characteristic abstinence phenomena. Trembling and convulsions can also occur.

OTHER DRUGS WITH POTENTIAL FOR ABUSE

Drugs that belong to the groups listed below can cause varying degrees of fatigue/tiredness, confusion and partial hallucinations. They cause unexpected and strong effects, especially in combination with alcohol, and are potential intox-icating substances:

■ muscle relaxants, e.g. baclofen
■ anti-migraine drugs, e.g. ergotamine
■ antiepileptics, e.g. carbamazepine
■ centrally acting anticholinergics (anti-Parkinson's drugs), e.g. benzatropine.

SUMMARY

■ Intoxicating substances are chemically synthesized or naturally existing compounds that cause noticeable alteration in mood and behaviour.
■ Intoxicating substances cause different degrees of physical and mental dependence, tolerance development for the intoxicating experience and abstinence reactions when the concentration of the substance in the body drops below certain limits.
■ Abuse of intoxicating substances is the use of legal intoxicating substances that deviates from socially accepted norms and all use of prohibited intoxicating substances and chemical substances in such a way that they cause intoxication.
■ Ethanol causes reduced coordination of motor movements, reduced perception and ability to concentrate, reduced self-criticism and learning ability, and increased sleepiness/drowsiness.
■ Deaths resulting from acute alcohol poisoning are often associated with respiratory failure, but accidents and violent deaths occur more frequently under the influence of alcohol.
■ Chronic use of large amounts of ethanol leads to pronounced long-term effects that are most clearly seen in the form of damage to the liver, the central and peripheral nervous systems, endocrine functions and the immune system.
■ Cannabis is an illegal intoxicating substance that is used by many people. Few physical harmful effects have been proven in association with cannabis abuse. The social settings in which the substances are used often result in individuals 'experimenting' with other substances.
■ Opioids have a depressant effect on the central nervous system. The group includes many legal drugs, but also heroin. Large doses of heroin cause respiratory depression and bring about many deaths. Dependence develops quickly.
■ LSD is the most important compound in the group of hallucinogens. It causes unpredictable intoxication experiences and can lead to psychoses and a totally distorted perception of reality.
■ Volatile organic solvents cause intoxication when they are inhaled. The substances are lipid-soluble and particularly damage the central nervous system and lung tissue. Heavy users experience serious damage to the liver and bone marrow.
■ The most used central nervous system stimulating substances are amphetamines, but cocaine, crack and ecstasy belong to this group. The intoxication effect is a euphoric one with increased wakefulness and aggressiveness. Dependence is considerable after a period of use. The substances cause elevated blood pressure and can lead to life-threatening heart arrhythmias when they are taken in large doses.
■ The drugs that are abused most are benzodiazepines and opioids. Benzodiazepines produce anxiety-reducing, tranquillizing and soporific effects, while the opioids are mainly used as analgesics.
■ Use of illegal intoxicating substances contributes considerably to harmful social effects.

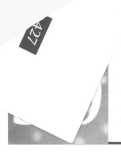

Poisoning

The majority of patients who die following poisoning do so as a result of respiratory failure, cardiac arrhythmias or cardiac arrest. Respiratory failure occurs because the toxin has a depressant effect on the respiration centres. This can be seen, for example, in overdoses with morphine, heroin, alcohol and many habit-forming drugs. In the unconscious patient, the tongue can fall backwards and result in airway obstruction.

Cardiac arrhythmias, cardiac arrest or hypotension occur as a result of direct effects on the heart and blood vessels. This applies, for example, to β-blockers, calcium channel blockers, tricyclic antidepressants, theophylline, antiepileptics, amphetamines and cocaine.

Large doses of some drugs can cause convulsions, e.g. tricyclic antidepressants, theophylline, antipsychotics and lithium. Insecticides and pesticides cause damage by disturbing nervous and neuromuscular signalling. Poisoning with some gases, e.g. carbon monoxide, disturbs the transport of oxygen in the blood.

Patients who survive the acute phase of poisoning can be left with serious organ damage, leading to a loss of function and possible fatal consequences.

The Poison Information Centre can provide information about the risks and treatment options following contact with toxic substances. Contact details can be found in the *British National Formulary* (www.bnf.org).

EPIDEMIOLOGY

A large number of poisonings in children occur by accident, most often in children under 4 years of age. More than 80 per cent of poisonings are due to careless storage of drugs and household chemicals.

In adults, the majority of acute poisonings are self-inflicted. The most common poisonings are mixed poisonings, i.e. they consist of more than one substance. They most frequently occur with alcohol, narcotic substances, antidepressants, paracetamol or salicylates. Approximately half of all adult patients with acute self-inflicted poisonings (ASPs) have drug and/or alcohol problems. Approximately 20 per cent of ASPs occur with true suicidal intent and these are far more frequent in cities/densely populated areas than in rural areas.

The mortality associated with ASPs in hospitals is approximately 1 per cent. For every patient who dies in hospital as a result of ASP, approximately 10 people will die before reaching hospital. Deaths due to overdoses with narcotic substances, especially heroin, are increasing.

DIAGNOSIS OF ACUTE POISONING

In cases involving the ingestion of toxic substances or an overdose of drugs, it is important to react quickly and implement measures such as gastric lavage, possibly preventing the toxins from being absorbed into the blood. It is therefore important to obtain information about possible poisonous substances as soon as possible.

OBTAINING INFORMATION

Patients who present with a self-inflicted poisoning may be suffering from mental health problems. In many cases, they will already have had contact with psychiatric services and been prescribed drugs. With drug overdoses, people often use drugs they have been prescribed. See Figure 30.1. It can be helpful to look for empty medicine packets or packaging from other products that may provide information about what has been ingested.

CASE HISTORY AND COURSE OF EVENTS

A case history and course of events can provide information on what an individual has been poisoned with, the time the poisoning occurred, and an indication of the degree of seriousness. If the patient is unconscious or unwilling to provide such information, friends, relatives and other key personnel should be contacted. If no

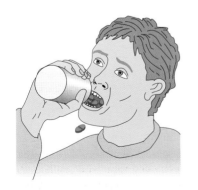

Figure 30.1 In drug overdoses people often take drugs they have been prescribed.

direct information is available with regard to the ingested substance, clinical examinations and laboratory tests are the only useful aids to diagnosis.

CLINICAL EXAMINATION AND TRANSPORT

The initial examination should concentrate on the patency of the airway, breathing and the circulation. Signs of needle marks indicating the possible injection of narcotic substances should be looked for. Unconscious patients should be managed and transported in a stable left lateral position to prevent airway occlusion and aspiration. Constant supervision is essential.

LABORATORY TESTS

Laboratory analyses are useful when managing the patient with acute poisoning. The most important fluids for analysis are blood and urine. On occasion, analysis of gastric content can also be useful.

Acid–base disturbances – pH and blood gases

pH is most often measured in arterial blood and demonstrates whether the patient has an acid–base disturbance. Determination of the blood gases will also distinguish whether the acid–base disturbance has a respiratory or metabolic cause. Respiratory acidosis is associated with reduced ventilation, which results in an accumulation of CO_2 with a virtually normal bicarbonate (HCO_3^-) value. With metabolic acidosis, HCO_3^- is low (used for buffering the acids) while CO_2 is normal.

Anion gap

The anion gap (AG) is the difference between positive and negative ions in the plasma. An increase in the anion gap is seen in metabolic acidosis.

$$AG = Na^+ + K^+ - Cl^- - HCO_3^- \text{ (normal approx. 16 mmol/L)}$$

An increase in the anion gap is associated with metabolic acidoses (the accumulation of organic acids: ketoacids in diabetic ketoacidosis, formic acid with methanol poisoning, and glycol acid with ethylene glycol poisoning). The increased anion gap is as a result of consumption of bicarbonate (HCO_3^-) to buffer the organic acids formed.

Osmolality gap

All particles that are dissolved in plasma contribute to its osmolality. The osmolality gap (OG) is the difference between measured osmolality (OM) and estimated osmolality (OB), i.e.:

$$OG = OM - OB \text{ (normal} < 10 \text{ mOsmol/kg H}_2O)$$

$$OB = \frac{1.86 \times Na^+ + glucose + urea}{0.93}$$

As shown above, sodium, glucose and urea influence estimated osmolality. In a 'healthy' person, alcohols are the only toxic substance that are ingested in such large molar quantities that they can result in an elevated osmolality gap.

In practice, metabolic acidosis with an elevated anion and osmolality gap is an indication of methanol or ethylene glycol poisoning (if diabetic ketoacidosis can be ruled out).

Concentration of drugs

In hospital laboratories the concentration of a wide array of drugs can be determined in blood to inform treatment. When using the result of such a measurement to inform a clinical decision, it is important to remember that the concentration of a drug or toxin in blood is dependent on the time elapsed after ingestion and the dose of drug or toxin taken.

Analysis of urine can reveal whether a compound is present or not, but is of little value when attempting to determine plasma concentrations.

ECG (electrocardiogram)

Some poisonings result in disturbances of the cardiac rhythm and bring about characteristic changes in the ECG. The ECG can therefore help to diagnose certain poisonings and evaluate whether or not specific treatments should be implemented. Tricyclic antidepressants are known to increase the width of the QRS complex.

TREATMENT OF ACUTE POISONING

Following acute poisoning, it is important to assess and support the airway, breathing and circulation and also to consider interventions related to the specific poison.

TREATMENT PRINCIPLES

Serious injuries and death following poisoning can often be avoided by early intervention. With acute poisoning, the same general rules apply as with all acute injuries. Poisons that depress respiratory and cardiovascular function will often require immediate life-saving interventions.

Organ support

The basic principles of acute illness management apply, e.g.:

- airway – the maintenance of a patent airway
- breathing – support with oxygen therapy and/or mechanical ventilation
- circulation – assessment and support of cardiovascular function.

Managing convulsions

- The benzodiazepine diazepam is the drug of choice.
- High concentrations of oxygen are administered if there is clinical evidence of hypoxia.
- Glucose is administered in the presence of hypoglycaemia.

Preventing further damage

- Gastric lavage or forced emesis should be attempted if the patient presents soon after ingestion. These procedures must always be closely supervised and the patient's airway protected to prevent gastric aspiration. Various emetics can be administered to induce vomiting.
- Antidotes should be administered if available.
- Activated charcoal is administered following gastric lavage/vomiting, if an oral antidote is not administered.

■ Clothes should be removed if they are contaminated by poisons that can be absorbed through the skin.

Treatment other than supportive measures will be dependent on whether the cause of the poisoning is known and if there is an effective treatment. In many cases, in the absence of a specific treatment, supportive therapies must be continued until the symptoms abate.

THERAPEUTIC ANTIDOTES

Antidotes are drugs used to counteract the effects of other substances.

Naloxone – counteracts the effects of opiates

Naloxone is an opiate antagonist (blocker) with a high affinity for opiate receptors. It is able to displace both pure and partial opiate agonists. The onset of action is approximately 1 min following intravenous injection. It is used to reverse the respiratory depression seen following opiate overdose. Clinical response to naloxone is also a useful diagnostic indicator of opiate use.

Neostigmine – inhibits decomposition of acetylcholine

Neostigmine is a reversible inhibitor of acetylcholinesterase, which breaks down acetylcholine. This enhances cholinergic effects within the body (bradycardia, micturition, increased gastrointestinal motility and increased mucous secretion in the respiratory passages). It is used in serious anticholinergic poisoning, e.g. atropine, antihistamines, tricyclic antidepressants and *Amanita* mushrooms (panther cap).

Neostigmine can result in potent cholinergic effects, resulting in increased bronchial mucus secretion, leading to lower airway obstruction. Atropine must therefore be immediately available to reverse potentially life-threatening adverse effects. Neostigmine must be administered cautiously to people with asthma, bradycardiac patients and patients with gastrointestinal obstruction.

Flumazenil – counteracts the effect of benzodiazepines

Flumazenil is a benzodiazepine antagonist that competitively inhibits the central nervous effects of substances that exert their effect via the benzodiazepine receptors at the GABA receptor complex (not effective in ethanol poisoning). The benzodiazepine effects are antagonized 30–60 s after an intravenous injection. The duration of action is 1–3 h. The effect of benzodiazepines can return when the effect of flumazenil disappears. Its use is indicated in severe benzodiazepine poisoning with life-threatening complications such as respiratory depression. As with naloxone a positive clinical response to flumazenil is an indicator of benzodiazepine use.

FORCED ELIMINATION

By removing toxins before they are absorbed, it is possible to limit damage. Activated charcoal will absorb the remains of toxins in the stomach and intestines. Dilution can limit local damage, especially following acid ingestion. Haemodialysis, haemoperfusion and peritoneal dialysis are methods used to remove some toxic substances from the blood. These methods are suitable for substances with a small volume of distribution; substances that are distributed to tissues outside the bloodstream are difficult to remove using these techniques.

Activated charcoal

Activated charcoal should be administered after gastric lavage. It must not be administered if an antidote is administered orally, e.g. when deferoxamine is used in iron poisoning, since charcoal will bind the antidote and reduce its effect. Activated charcoal is not absorbed into the blood. It must be administered in sufficient quantities, and the dose repeated after 4 h.

Activated charcoal does not absorb iron, lithium or potassium, and is of no use in alcohol poisoning. It is of no benefit when treating poisoning with acids.

Removal/dilution of toxic substances

Gastric lavage should be performed:

- if serious poisoning is suspected
- if administration of activated charcoal is considered inadequate
- if the period since ingestion is less than 1 h for fluid preparations and 2 h for solid preparations
- when drugs known to reduce gastric motility (anticholinergic drugs) are the source of poisoning.

Anticholinergic substances cause a delay in gastric emptying, which limits the toxin from reaching the intestine and being absorbed. Vomiting can be induced by administering emetics. Emetics have little effect if active charcoal has already been administered. Patients who have ingested caustic substances or petroleum products should not be encouraged to vomit as there is a high risk of aspiration and pulmonary damage and further damage to the oesophagus.

Following ingestion of caustic substances, the patient should be given water, milk or juice to drink in order to dilute the substance, but not so much that it induces vomiting.

With petroleum products, the patient should be given liquid paraffin or other fat-rich liquids (cream, heavy sour cream, cooking oil, etc.) to increase surface tension in the stomach and reduce the danger of vapour aspiration into the lungs. Aspiration of petroleum compounds destroys the surfactant layer in the alveoli and results in chemical pneumonitis, which is difficult to treat.

Haemodialysis

During haemodialysis, the concentrations of all solutes found in the blood and which can pass across the dialysis membrane are reduced. Dialysis also can help correct acid–base and electrolyte disturbances. Haemodialysis is useful in poisoning with alcohols, salicylic acid, theophylline, procainamide and lithium, all of which have a small volume of distribution. Large molecules, toxins with a large volume of distribution or high protein binding reduce the effectiveness of dialysis. The majority of toxins cannot be dialysed efficiently because of their large molecular weight. The principles of haemodialysis are shown in Figure 30.2.

Haemoperfusion

During haemoperfusion, the blood passes through a filter (charcoal or polystyrene) that absorbs certain toxins. The criteria for effective haemoperfusion is that the toxin must have an affinity for the filter material. The molecular size of the substance is less important than with haemodialysis (no membrane is passed). Haemoperfusion is suitable for substances with low plasma–protein binding and a small volume of distribution. Lipid-soluble substances are removed more efficiently than water-soluble substances. The principles of haemoperfusion are shown in Figure 30.3. Haemoperfusion is indicated in poisoning with barbiturates,

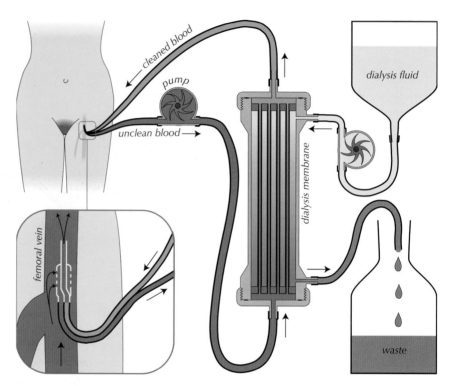

Figure 30.2 **Haemodialysis.** In the dialysis cell, the blood passes through a large number of capillaries made from permeable membrane surrounded by dialysis fluid. During haemodialysis, the blood is cleared by the passive diffusion of small molecular substances to the dialysis fluid.

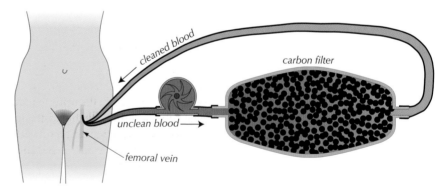

Figure 30.3 **Haemoperfusion.** With this technique, the blood is cleaned by a charcoal filter that absorbs toxins following direct contact with the blood.

meprobamate, theophylline, primidone, procainamide, phenytoin, ethosuximide, carbamazepine and sodium valproate.

Peritoneal dialysis

In principle, peritoneal dialysis removes the same substances as haemodialysis, but is less effective, especially with drug poisoning. The principles of peritoneal dialysis are shown in Figure 30.4.

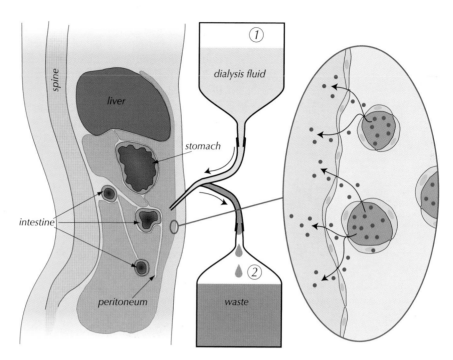

Figure 30.4 **Peritoneal dialysis.** The blood is cleared by infusing dialysis fluid into the peritoneal cavity (1). The peritoneal cavity and all abdominal organs are covered by peritoneum, rich in capillaries (red line). Toxic substances in the blood will diffuse from the capillaries of the peritoneum into the dialysis fluid. After the dialysis fluid has stayed in the peritoneal cavity for a set period of time, it is drained out, thus removing the toxins (2). The peritoneum and the capillary wall replace the permeable membranes used in haemodialysis.

FORCED ALKALINE AND ACID DIURESIS

Ionic substances pass across cell membranes less effectively than non-ionic substances. It can therefore be desirable to alter the pH of the urine, in order to ionize weak acids or bases in the urine to reduce the reabsorption of these toxins from the renal tube back into the bloodstream. By alkalinizing the urine, it is possible to increase the renal elimination of weak acids, e.g. salicylic acid and phenobarbital. By acidifying the urine, it is possible to increase the renal elimination of weak bases, e.g. amphetamines.

With forced diuresis, a large amount of fluid is infused intravenously to increase the glomular filtration and therefore urinary excretion of a toxin. Forced alkaline and acid diuresis must be used with caution and closely monitored in order to avoid electrolyte disturbances and fluid overload.

COMMON CAUSES OF POISONING

ALCOHOLS

The majority of alcohol poisonings occur with ethanol; however, poisoning with isopropanol is not uncommon. People may drink the deadly alcohols methanol

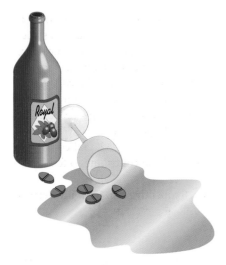

Figure 30.5 **Ethanol** is frequently used in self-inflicted poisoning, often in combination with drugs.

and ethylene glycol by mistake, most commonly by mixing them with ordinary alcoholic beverages. Ethanol is often used in combination with drugs in self-inflicted poisoning. See Figure 30.5.

The intoxicating experience from alcohol is caused by the substance's effect on the central nervous system. The person experiences altered mood, behaviour and emotions, reduced ability to concentrate and reduced motor and intellectual skills.

With alcohol ingestion resulting in serious poisoning, gastric lavage may be necessary to remove the remains of the ingested alcohol. Haemodialysis may be necessary in the cases of the most serious poisonings with isopropanol, methanol and ethylene glycol. See Figure 30.5.

Ethanol

Absorption

Some ethanol is absorbed from the stomach, but the majority is absorbed in the upper part of the small intestine. Absorption is dramatically increased if the stomach and intestine do not contain food. Fasting before ingestion of alcohol therefore results in a rapid increase in the blood alcohol concentration.

Distribution

Ethanol is distributed throughout the body's water phase. In men, approximately 70 per cent of the body mass is water, compared with 60 per cent in women. Therefore, for the same amount of alcohol in a man and a woman of equal weight, a higher blood alcohol level would be found in the woman than in the man.

Elimination

Approximately 90 per cent of alcohol consumed is metabolized in the liver by the enzyme alcohol-dehydrogenase to acetaldehyde, which is further metabolized to acetic acid by the enzyme acetaldehyde-dehydrogenase. The acetic acid is metabolized to water and carbon dioxide. See Figure 30.6.

In most people, acetaldehyde will be metabolized faster than ethanol, such that acetaldehyde does not accumulate. Disulfiram (sometimes used to promote abstinence in alcoholics) inhibits the metabolism of acetaldehyde. High concentrations of acetaldehyde result in tachycardia, hyperventilation, nausea and flushing. Many East Asians have a gene-associated lack of acetaldehyde-dehydrogenase, and therefore tolerate only small amounts of ethanol before they experience the adverse effects of acetaldehyde.

The liver's ability to metabolize ethanol is limited. With ingestion, a person quickly reaches a concentration that saturates the enzymes. There will thus be a fixed rate elimination of ethanol until the person has reached a low concentration.

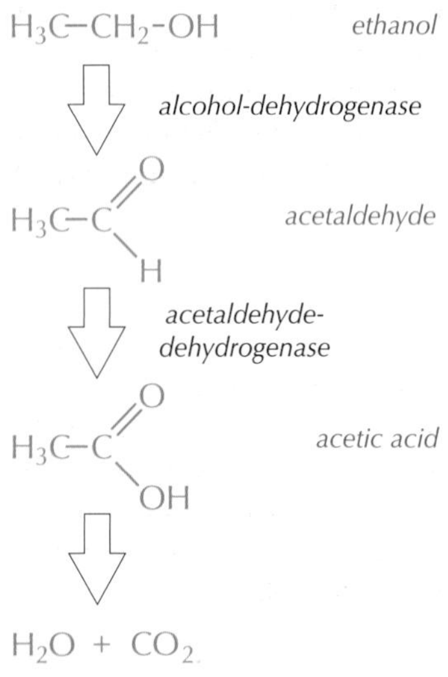

H_3C-CH_2-OH *ethanol*

⇩   *alcohol-dehydrogenase*

$H_3C-C\overset{O}{\underset{H}{\big\langle}}$ *acetaldehyde*

⇩   *acetaldehyde-dehydrogenase*

$H_3C-C\overset{O}{\underset{OH}{\big\langle}}$ *acetic acid*

⇩

$H_2O + CO_2$

Figure 30.6 **Metabolism/elimination of ethanol.** No toxic metabolites are formed.

Effects

The respiratory centres are affected in most people when the ethanol concentration is above 2.5 per cent blood alcohol concentration. With increasing concentrations, there is a noted reduction in the coordination of motor movements, speech is affected and increased drowsiness is seen. Some individuals will die with concentrations above 4.5 per cent, but some are able to tolerate concentrations exceeding 6 per cent.

Ethanol causes vasodilatation of the blood vessels in the skin. This leads to an increased feeling of warmth, but in fact there is increased heat loss from the skin. Ingestion of alcohol in cold conditions can therefore lead to hypothermia.

Alcohol stimulates an increase in the secretion of hydrochloric acid from the stomach wall, which irritates the mucosa and can lead to an increased risk of inflammation and haemorrhage. The secretion of antidiuretic hormone is decreased, thereby increasing urine production. Chronic use also results in structural changes in the liver. First fatty deposits are seen in the liver with eventual development of cirrhosis. These changes gradually result in a significant increase in the venous pressures within the portal vein system and a reduced circulation through the liver. This leads to the development of a collateral circulation. This leads to the formation of swollen tortuous veins inside the oesophagus (oesophageal varices) because of the increase in venous pressure. These varices can burst and lead to life-threatening haemorrhage. High chronic ethanol consumption also disturbs the synthesis of sex hormones and can contribute to feminization in men.

Central and peripheral nerve damage is also frequently seen. Both intellectual and physical skills are diminished with the chronic use of ethanol.

Treatment

Treatment of acute intoxication is only necessary if the poisoning is so severe that respiratory function is compromised. With high ethanol concentrations, it may be necessary to consider haemodialysis. Activated charcoal is of no use in the treatment of ethanol poisoning.

Isopropanol

Isopropanol is found in windscreen washer fluid, disinfectants and in antifreeze solutions.

Absorption

Approximately 80 per cent of the ingested quantity is absorbed within 30 min.

Distribution

This is as for ethanol.

Elimination

Twenty to fifty per cent is eliminated unchanged through the kidneys. The remainder is metabolized in the liver, with acetone as an intermediate product. Acetone is metabolized more slowly than isopropanol and results in an increase in acetone concentration while the concentration of isopropanol drops. The metabolism of isopropanol to acetone is catalysed by the enzyme alcohol-dehydrogenase. See Figure 30.7.

Effects

Isopropanol has a depressant effect on the central nervous system resembling that of ethanol. The effect manifests itself quickly because of rapid absorption, and is long-lasting since both isopropanol and acetone lead to intoxication. In addition, reduced motor coordination, palpitations, a fall in blood pressure associated with peripheral vasodilation, affected speech, reduced concentration and increased drowsiness are observed. Heavy ingestion can cause kidney and liver damage and haemolytic anaemia. Isopropanol is twice as toxic as ethanol.

Treatment

Gastric lavage is appropriate if the patient presents shortly after ingestion. Following significant ingestion with severe symptoms such as respiratory depression, hypotension and loss of consciousness, haemodialysis is appropriate.

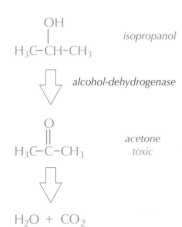

Figure 30.7 **Metabolism/elimination of isopropanol.** Acetone is toxic.

Methanol and ethylene glycol

Methanol is found in antifreeze solutions and in some solvent mixes. Ethylene glycol is used as an antifreeze solution.

Absorption

Absorption of methanol occurs rapidly. Absorption of ethylene glycol occurs slowly compared with the other alcohols.

Distribution

Both of the alcohols are distributed throughout the body's water phase, as with ethanol.

Elimination

Alcohol-dehydrogenase metabolizes methanol to formaldehyde, which is then metabolized to formic acid. Metabolism of formic acid occurs slowly, such that the concentration increases as the methanol is metabolized. The concentration of formic acid and the metabolic acidosis that develops are responsible for the organ damage seen in methanol ingestion. A fatal dose of methanol is approximately 1 g/kg body weight. See Figure 30.8.

Ethylene glycol is metabolized by alcohol-dehydrogenase, and after several intermediate products, oxalate is formed. The metabolites are harmful. See Figure 30.9.

Effects

Methanol has a depressant effect on the central nervous system but causes little intoxication and causes listlessness and nausea. The metabolites cause damage to the central nervous system, e.g. on the optic nerve, which results in a characteristic and permanent loss of vision. Hyperventilation is seen in response to the development of metabolic acidosis caused by acidic metabolites.

After ethylene glycol is metabolized to oxalate, it precipitates in the form of calcium oxalate in soft tissues like the kidneys, heart, pancreas and lungs, and damages these organs. Several of the intermediate products in the metabolism of ethylene glycol are acidic, causing metabolic acidosis. The precipitation of calcium oxalate leads to a reduction in serum calcium, which may trigger convulsions.

Treatment

Methanol, ethylene glycol and ethanol are metabolized by the same enzyme, alcohol-dehydrogenase. However, the enzyme has the greater affinity for ethanol. This means that ethanol will tax a considerable share of the enzyme activity if the alcohols are present simultaneously, and less methanol or ethylene glycol will metabolize per unit of time and therefore less harmful metabolites will be formed.

Vision disturbances, a methanol blood concentration above 0.6 per cent, severe metabolic acidosis and ingestion of more than 40 mL of concentrated methanol are indications for dialysis.

Hypocalcaemia due to ethylene glycol poisoning should not be treated before the onset of convulsions with administration of calcium because of the danger of increased precipitation of calcium oxalate. Severe poisoning with ethylene glycol is treated with haemodialysis, and/or by administration of ethanol. Fomepizole, an inhibitor of the enzyme alcohol-dehydrogenase, may also be used, resulting in the formation of less toxic metabolites per unit of time.

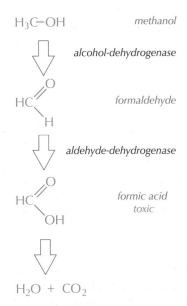

H_3C-OH *methanol*

alcohol-dehydrogenase

HC with $=O$ and H *formaldehyde*

aldehyde-dehydrogenase

HC with $=O$ and OH *formic acid toxic*

$H_2O + CO_2$

Figure 30.8 **Metabolism/elimination of methanol.** Formic acid is very toxic.

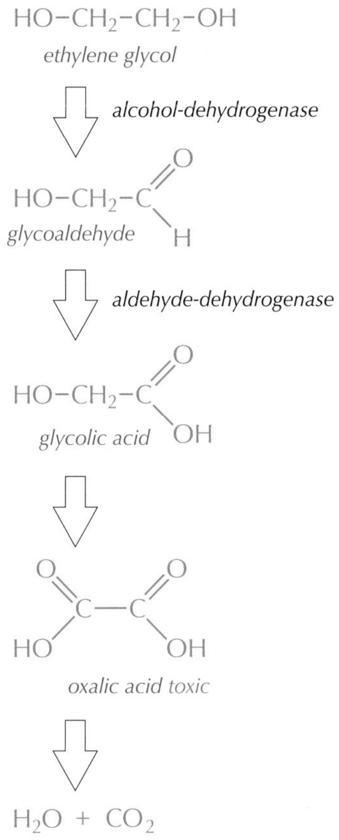

$$HO-CH_2-CH_2-OH$$

ethylene glycol

⬇ *alcohol-dehydrogenase*

$$HO-CH_2-C\!\!\begin{array}{c}O\\[-2pt]\diagdown\\[-2pt]H\end{array}$$

glycoaldehyde

⬇ *aldehyde-dehydrogenase*

$$HO-CH_2-C\!\!\begin{array}{c}O\\[-2pt]\diagdown\\[-2pt]OH\end{array}$$

glycolic acid

⬇

$$\begin{array}{c}O\qquad\quad O\\ \diagup\!\!C\!\!-\!\!C\diagup\\ HO\qquad\quad OH\end{array}$$

oxalic acid toxic

⬇

$$H_2O + CO_2$$

Figure 30.9 **Metabolism/elimination of ethylene glycol.** The metabolites formed, glycolate and oxalate, are very toxic. Glycolate leads to acute, serious acidosis. Oxalate reacts with calcium, forming calcium-oxalate crystals in the tissues, leading to organ damage and a low calcium level in the blood, which may trigger convulsions.

	Ethanol	Isopropanol	Methanol	Ethylene glycol
Acid metabolites	No	No	Yes	Yes
Acidosis	No	No	Yes	Yes
Increased anion gap	No	No	Yes	Yes
Increased osmolality gap	Yes	Yes	Yes	Yes
Toxic concentrations	2.5%	1.5%	0.6%	Metabolites are toxic
Other findings				Hypocalcaemia
Treatment	(Dialysis)	(Dialysis)	Ethanol, dialysis	Ethanol, dialysis

Table 30.1 Summary of alcohol poisonings

Summary of alcohol poisoning

Ingestion of alcohols in quantities that cause intoxication results in increased osmolality. In the early phase, an elevated osmolality gap is seen, while the anion gap is normal or only slightly elevated because the alcohol is not yet metabolized to its acidic metabolites. Gradually, the anion gap will increase, and the osmolality gap is reduced. This is because the acidic metabolites (the organic acids) are buffered by bicarbonate. Buffering of the acids results in a loss of bicarbonate. Since bicarbonate contributes to osmolality, this will also be reduced (see details earlier in the chapter). See Table 30.1.

In practice, metabolic acidosis with a simultaneously elevated anion and osmolality gap is a diagnostic indicator of methanol or ethylene glycol poisoning (if diabetic ketoacidosis can be ruled out). Treatment with bicarbonate and ethanol should be commenced and haemodialysis considered. Poisoning with acetylsalicylic acid may resemble intoxication with methanol or ethylene glycol in causing metabolic acidosis and an increased anion gap, but differs in not increasing the osmolality gap.

OPIOIDS

Poisonings with substances in this group are most often seen amongst elicit drug users. Heroin overdoses are the most frequent cause of life-threatening poisoning, but morphine, pethidine and codeine poisoning are also seen.

Poisoning by heroin occurs most commonly when the user unintentionally overdoses. Heroin is sold illegally in different purities and may be mixed with substances that can have harmful effects. Respiratory depression is the most serious adverse effect of opioid poisoning.

Treatment

Naloxone is an antidote for opiates that blocks opiate receptors. It is used to reverse respiratory depression and also as a diagnostic test in individuals who are suspected to have taken opiates. The opiates' duration of action is considerably longer than that of naloxone. Therefore it is possible for the adverse effects of the opiate to reoccur and further doses of naloxone may be required.

BENZODIAZEPINES

Benzodiazepines are often used in suicide attempts. If a benzodiazepine is taken on its own, the adverse effects are often not severe. However, if used in conjunction with alcohol and other drugs that depress the central nervous system, the combination can lead to the development of life-threatening complications, such as respiratory depression, hypotension and loss of consciousness.

Treatment

The antidote flumazenil which blocks the benzodiazepine receptor can be used both as a diagnostic test and as a therapeutic intervention in serious benzodiazepine poisoning.

ANTIPSYCHOTICS

Large doses of antipsychotics cause drowsiness and extrapyramidal side-effects, e.g. dystonia, rigidity and tremors of the entire body. Spasticity, restlessness and hyperreflexia can also occur, and general convulsions can be triggered.

Treatment

These preparations have anticholinergic effects that lead to a reduction in gastric emptying, such that the drug remains in the stomach many hours following ingestion. Gastric lavage can therefore be useful many hours following ingestion of the drug. The use of active charcoal is also recommended following lavage.

Drugs in this group typically have a large volume of distribution, which dramatically reduces the usefulness of interventions such as haemodialysis or haemoperfusion. Elimination occurs by metabolism in the liver.

Neostigmine can be used to counteract anticholinergic effects. With convulsions and severe rhythm disturbances, symptomatic treatment is required.

ANTIDEPRESSANTS

This group is dominated by the tricyclic antidepressants with regard to acute poisoning. They often result in life-threatening complications and large overdoses frequently result in death. The new selective serotonin reuptake inhibitors (SSRIs) are not as dangerous as tricyclic antidepressants in acute poisoning.

The main effects of tricyclic antidepressants are influenced by the monoaminergic processes in the brain with inhibited reabsorption of noradrenaline, serotonin and dopamine in the synapses.

Following overdose, the predominant effects are cardiac in origin. Pronounced rhythm disturbance can occur alongside myocardial depression. The ECG shows a characteristic increase in the width of the QRS complex. There is a good correlation seen between the increase in the width of the QRS complex and the seriousness of the overdose. Anticholinergic effects can also be pronounced. Metabolic acidosis may complicate severe poisoning.

Treatment

Gastric lavage can be performed even if it has been some time since ingestion. These preparations have an anticholinergic effect and reduce gastric motility and therefore emptying. Following lavage, the administration of active charcoal is known to be of benefit.

Drugs in this group have a large volume of distribution, which renders interventions such as haemodialysis or haemoperfusion of little use. Elimination occurs by metabolism in the liver.

There are no specific antidotes for this type of poisoning. Treatment is therefore supportive in nature, e.g. intravenous sodium bicarbonate to correct metabolic acidosis.

PARACETAMOL

Paracetamol has few adverse effects when used in therapeutic doses. In contrast, paracetamol overdose results in serious and, in some cases, fatal liver damage.

Paracetamol is conjugated in the liver to glucuronic acid and sulphate. With therapeutic doses, approximately 90 per cent will be removed this way. The remaining 10 per cent is metabolized to a toxic metabolite that can cause liver damage if it is not detoxified mainly by conjugation with glutathione, which is found in liver cells. In paracetamol overdose, the glutathione stores in the liver cells are depleted. The toxic metabolite then binds to macromolecules in the liver cells and causes damage. See Figure 30.10.

Serious paracetamol poisoning produces few symptoms in the first 2 days following ingestion. This can result in a failure to appreciate the severity of the poisoning. When the symptoms do appear, it may be too late to start treatment.

With serious poisoning, patients often report stomach pains after the second day (liver damage), and an increase in the level of liver enzymes is seen in the blood, indicating cellular damage. Because of damage to the liver cells and a reduction in the ability to conjugate bilirubin, the concentration of free bilirubin will gradually rise and lead to jaundice. Reduced synthesis of proteins needed for coagulation results in increased coagulation time and possible bleeding problems.

To determine the severity of the paracetamol poisoning, it is necessary to determine the concentration of paracetamol in the blood. If the measurement shows a concentration above a line drawn through the points 1330 and 465 μmol/L (200 and 70 mg/mL) on semilogarithmic paper, 4 and 10 h, respectively, after ingestion, this is an indication of serious poisoning. See Figure 30.11. If the time of ingestion is unknown, it is important to establish two known paracetamol concentration values at known points in time with at least a 3-h interval. A reduction in blood paracetamol concentration that demonstrates a half-life of more than 4 h indicates liver damage.

Chronic use of alcohol, phenytoin or the tuberculosis drug isoniazid increases the amount of the enzyme that metabolizes paracetamol to the toxic metabolite (enzyme induction). Overdoses by these individuals will result in liver damage at lower doses than is normally seen. Individuals who exhibit enzyme induction should therefore be treated with an antidote when there is a paracetamol concentration in the blood 30–50 per cent lower than indicated above.

In adults, it is estimated that as little as 10 g of paracetamol can be fatal.

Treatment of paracetamol poisoning

N-acetylcysteine is metabolized to glutathione in the liver and is an antidote for paracetamol poisoning. When there is a suspicion of the ingestion of a toxic dose, or with high plasma concentrations of paracetamol, N-acetylcysteine should be given intravenously or orally. If acetylcysteine is administered before the glutathione reserves are exhausted (within 10–12 h of ingestion), liver damage will usually not occur, but treatment is known to be effective even if the administration is delayed (within 24 h). If acetylcysteine is administered orally, activated charcoal must not be administered. In those who survive paracetamol poisoning, the liver damage is largely reversible.

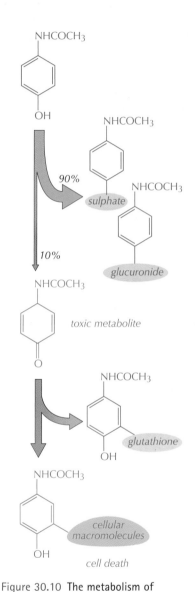

Figure 30.10 The metabolism of paracetamol. Approximately 90 per cent of a therapeutic dose of paracetamol is metabolized by binding to sulphates or glucuronides. About 10 per cent is metabolized to a toxic metabolite that is metabolized by conjugation to glutathione. If an overdose is taken, a greater percentage of the total dose will follow the toxic metabolic path. When all the glutathione is utilized, the toxic metabolite will react with intracellular components, giving rise to hepatocellular damage.

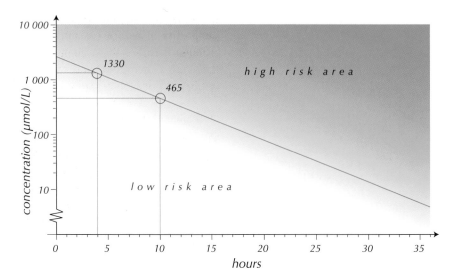

Figure 30.11 Paracetamol poisoning. Values above and to the right of the marked line indicate concentrations of paracetamol that will result in liver damage if the poisoning is not treated. The reference line has an angle of inclination corresponding to a half-life for paracetamol of 3.5 h. Elimination of paracetamol with a half-life exceeding 4 h is an indication of liver damage. Note that the axis showing concentration has a logarithmic scale.

LITHIUM

Lithium is used in manic-depressive disorders. Lithium has a narrow therapeutic range and, with chronic use, poisoning can occur. Such poisoning presents as neurological phenomena such as lethargy, confusion, tremors, dysarthria, ataxia, twitches and possible coma. Acute poisoning has few distinct symptoms in the early phase, as the distribution of lithium throughout the tissues is delayed.

Treatment
Gastric lavage can be utilized or forced emesis. Following gastric lavage, active charcoal is administered if there is a suspicion of mixed poisoning. In poisoning with lithium alone, active charcoal has little or no effect.

Haemodialysis will increase the elimination of lithium, but must often be performed several times because of the rebound effect from the tissue depots (slow passage across the membranes).

SALICYLIC ACID

Acetylsalicylic acid (ASA) overdose is frequently found in poisonings with suicidal intent among adults, and accidentally in children. Acute poisoning is often very serious. Because of an initially mild progression of symptoms, the seriousness of the overdose is often underestimated. The symptomatic progression of poisoning with ASA is usually divided into two phases.

Phase 1: respiratory alkalosis. Acetylsalicylic acid acts by directly stimulating the respiratory centres. This causes hyperventilation which will result in a lowering of pCO_2 in arterial blood. When the partial pressure of carbon dioxide (pCO_2) is sufficiently low, the equilibrium

$$CO_2 + H_2O \Leftrightarrow H_2CO_3 \Leftrightarrow H^+ + HCO_3^-$$

will move towards the left (H^+ is consumed, and respiratory alkalosis occurs). After some time, the kidneys will compensate for the respiratory alkalosis by excreting bicarbonate, sodium and potassium. With pronounced hypokalaemia, the kidneys attempt to conserve potassium, excreting hydrogen ions instead. This results in acidic urine despite an alkalosis in the blood (paradoxical aciduria).

Gradually, ASA is split into salicylic acid, and the initial respiratory alkalosis gradually moves towards acidosis (phase 2, metabolic acidosis).

Phase 2: metabolic acidosis. ASA inhibits oxidative phosphorylation in the cells where glucose is used as energy. This leads to the utilization of other metabolic pathways (which form acidic metabolites) for energy production, thus enhancing the acidosis. A 'problem' arises when the kidneys try to compensate for the acidosis. Hyperventilation is maintained by the metabolic acidosis by buffering with bicarbonate, since the majority of the bicarbonate has been secreted during the first phase by compensating for the respiratory alkalosis. The metabolic acidosis will result in continued hyperventilation, but if the acidosis is severe, it will gradually depress the respiratory system. The acidosis further increases the amount of undissociated ASA, which is then able to pass through the blood–brain barrier and depress respiration further, leading to a vicious circle.

More than 300 mg/kg results in serious poisoning. Concentrations higher than 5 mmol/L at 3–6 h after ingestion are serious, and higher than 7 mmol/L at 3–6 h after ingestion are life-threatening.

Presentation

The most common symptoms with ASA poisoning are nausea, vomiting, hyperventilation, reduced hearing and tinnitus. When the poisoning is sufficiently severe as to cause hyperventilation followed by respiratory depression, convulsions and coma may occur, and possibly cardiac arrest. ASA also increases the risk of haemorrhage.

Treatment

Gastric lavage or forced emesis should be carried out within 1–2 h following ingestion. Following gastric lavage, active charcoal is administered. Alkaline diuresis is useful when there is suspicion of serious poisoning. With an increase in the urine pH from 5 to 8, there is a considerable increase in the elimination of salicylic acid.

Since it is difficult to evaluate the seriousness of poisoning in the early phase, it is useful to measure the concentration of ASA in the blood. If the concentration is high, a further measurement may be taken 2 h later to determine if the concentration is increasing or falling. Salicylic acid has a low volume of distribution, and with concentrations over 7 mmol/L, haemodialysis is recommended. This is also true if blood sampling has been delayed following ingestion and plasma concentration is not falling.

Potassium supplementation is necessary for almost all patients developing metabolic acidosis because of potassium loss during acidosis. The potassium values must therefore be closely monitored. With ASA poisoning, the acidosis should be corrected quickly, since normalized pH will reduce the toxicity of the ASA (less ASA dissociated and less likely to cross the blood–brain barrier). Convulsions are treated with diazepam.

IRON

Poisoning with iron preparations is most common in children as a result of careless storage. Iron is caustic and can cause necrosis and perforation with haemorrhage in the intestinal tract and the subsequent development of shock. In addition, high concentrations of iron can have a direct toxic effect on the myocardium. High concentration of free iron inhibits the respiration chain within the mitochondria, leading to metabolic acidosis. A fatal dose is considered to be 50–300 mg Fe^{2+}/kg.

Serum iron concentrations greater than 90 mmol/L are considered to indicate severe poisoning. Leucocytosis, hyperglycaemia, diarrhoea, vomiting or remnants of tablets demonstrated on abdominal X-ray also indicate serious poisoning.

The progress of serious iron poisoning can be divided into four phases, as described below.

Phase 1 (0.5–1 h after ingestion). Early on, transitory symptoms such as nausea, listlessness, vomiting, diarrhoea and stomach pains may be seen. Metabolic acidosis, coma, convulsions and shock can occur in this phase and indicate serious poisoning. Vomiting and diarrhoea can be coloured black by the iron.

Phase 2 (6–12 h after ingestion). Many patients with serious poisoning have a symptom-free interval before the symptoms again increase, leading to phase 3.

Phase 3 (12–48 h after ingestion). Mild poisoning stops in phase 2. In cases with severe poisoning that result in the inhibition of respiration in the mitochondria and development of metabolic acidosis and intestinal haemorrhaging, there is a risk of shock, renal failure, liver necrosis and death 1–3 days after ingestion.

Phase 4 (2–6 weeks after ingestion). In those who survive a serious poisoning, scars and strictures (pyloric stenosis) may develop in the gastrointestinal tract, formed as a result of the caustic injuries.

Treatment
Gastric lavage and forced emesis can be used. Deferoxamine, an antidote for iron, is administered instead of active charcoal. Active charcoal should not be administered when an antidote is given orally. Deferoxamine binds with the remnants of the iron in the stomach and intestines. When there is a suspicion of gastrointestinal caustic injuries or with serum iron concentration higher than total iron binding capacity, deferoxamine is administered intravenously. The urine turns orange-red with this treatment. When the colour disappears, this is an indicator that no more free iron is binding to the deferoxamine and the treatment can be discontinued.

PETROLEUM PRODUCTS

This group includes benzene, diesel oil, white spirit, thinners, lighter fuels and lamp oils. These products contain mainly aliphatic hydrocarbons, but also some aromatic compounds. The aliphatic hydrocarbons are responsible for local effects in the lungs, while the aromatic hydrocarbons are responsible for systemic effects.

Aspiration of petroleum products destroys the surfactant layer in the pulmonary alveoli, resulting in collapse of pulmonary alveoli and the development of chemical pneumonitis. The seriousness of pulmonary complications observed is related to the amount of substance aspirated. In serious poisoning a persistent cough and tachypnoea is seen within 30 min of ingestion. Later, a change in the disease progression with tiredness, bronchospasms, cyanosis and coma may develop. Alveolitis is the most likely cause of the bronchospasm, alveolar oedema, exudation and haemorrhage that is seen.

The lipid solubility of the petroleum products and the resultant passage into the central nervous system explain the depressant effects on the CNS.

Treatment

Vomiting must not be induced and there must be no attempt at gastric lavage in these patients, because these procedures increase the danger of aspiration. Drinks with a high fat content (cream, heavy sour cream, cooking oil, etc.) increase the surface tension of the ingested substance and should be administered in moderate quantities to reduce the risk of aspiration.

Rapid deterioration can occur. Children with suspected poisoning should therefore be closely monitored in hospital. Respiratory problems are treated symptomatically with oxygen and and/or positive pressure ventilation with positive end-expiratory pressure, which keeps the alveoli dilated. The need for gastric lavage can be evaluated after intubation. There is uncertainty as to whether corticosteroids have a place in early treatment before signs of respiratory distress syndrome appear. Bronchospams are treated with nebulized adrenaline.

SUMMARY

- The majority of deaths by poisoning occur as a result of respiratory failure, arrhythmias or cardiac arrest.
- It is important to obtain information about the circumstances surrounding the poisoning, so that the correct treatment can be quickly implemented.
- Clinical and laboratory examination can provide important information about the poisoning's cause and degree of seriousness.
- With poisoning, it is important to maintain vital functions such as respiration and circulation. Likewise, it is important to stop convulsions and prevent further poisoning.
- Antidotes against some poisonings can be used both diagnostically and therapeutically.
- Forced elimination can be accomplished using several techniques. Gastric lavage or the use of emetics, activated charcoal, haemodialysis, haemoperfusion, peritoneal dialysis, and forced alkaline or acid diuresis are chosen based on which substances a person has been poisoned with.
- Of the alcohols, methanol and ethylene glycol result in the most serious poisonings, but ethanol and isopropanol are found far more frequently. Poisoning with methanol and ethylene glycol causes acidosis with an increased anion and osmolality gap.
- Opiates, benzodiazepines, neuroleptics and antidepressants are frequent causes of poisoning.
- Paracetamol, acetylsalicylic acid and iron tablets cause poisonings that first manifest themselves many hours after ingestion. It is important early on to determine the degree of poisoning by these substances, and to evaluate the necessity of treatment.

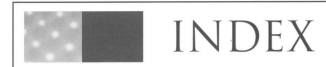

INDEX

Illustrations are well referred to from the text. Therefore, a page reference to significant material in an illustration has only been given in the absence of its mention in the associated text (on the same or adjacent pages) referring to the illustration.